Learning Disabilities: Assessment and Intervention

Learning Disabilities: Assessment and Intervention

Editor: Andy Parker

FOSTER ACADEMICS

www.fosteracademics.com

www.fosteracademics.com

FOSTER ACADEMICS

Cataloging-in-Publication Data

Learning disabilities : assessment and intervention / edited by Andy Parker.
p. cm.
Includes bibliographical references and index.
ISBN 978-1-63242-552-2
1. Learning disabilities. 2. Learning disabled. 3. Learning disabilities--Treatment.
I. Parker, Andy.
RJ506.L4 L43 2018
618.928 588 9--dc23

Foster Academics,
118-35 Queens Blvd., Suite 400,
Forest Hills, NY 11375, USA

ISBN 978-1-63242-552-2 (Hardback)

Printed and bound in China.

Contents

Preface

This book has been an outcome of determined endeavour from a group of educationists in the field. The primary objective was to involve a broad spectrum of professionals from diverse cultural background involved in the field for developing new researches. The book not only targets students but also scholars pursuing higher research for further enhancement of the theoretical and practical applications of the subject.

The disorders associated with difficulties in learning are referred to as learning disability. Dyslexia, dysgraphia, dyspraxia, dyscalculia are some common learning disorders. Heredity and genetics, problems during pregnancy and accidents are the primary causes for such disorders. This book is compiled in such a manner, that it will provide an in-depth knowledge about the assessment of learning disorders and intervention techniques associated with them. It is appropriate for students seeking detailed information in this area as well as for experts.

It was an honour to edit such a profound book and also a challenging task to compile and examine all the relevant data for accuracy and originality. I wish to acknowledge the efforts of the contributors for submitting such brilliant and diverse chapters in the field and for endlessly working for the completion of the book. Last, but not the least; I thank my family for being a constant source of support in all my research endeavours.

Editor

Evidence for the Late MMN as a Neurophysiological Endophenotype for Dyslexia

Nina Neuhoff[1], Jennifer Bruder[1], Jürgen Bartling[1], Andreas Warnke[2], Helmut Remschmidt[3], Bertram Müller-Myhsok[4], Gerd Schulte-Körne[1]*

1 Department of Child and Adolescent Psychiatry, Psychosomatics and Psychotherapy, University of Munich, Munich, Germany, **2** Department of Child and Adolescent Psychiatry and Psychotherapy, University of Würzburg, Würzburg, Germany, **3** Department of Child and Adolescent Psychiatry and Psychotherapy, University Hospital Gießen and Marburg, Marburg, Germany, **4** Statistical Genetics Max Planck Institute of Psychiatry, Munich, Germany

Abstract

Dyslexia affects 5–10% of school-aged children and is therefore one of the most common learning disorders. Research on auditory event related potentials (AERP), particularly the mismatch negativity (MMN) component, has revealed anomalies in individuals with dyslexia to speech stimuli. Furthermore, candidate genes for this disorder were found through molecular genetic studies. A current challenge for dyslexia research is to understand the interaction between molecular genetics and brain function, and to promote the identification of relevant endophenotypes for dyslexia. The present study examines MMN, a neurophysiological correlate of speech perception, and its potential as an endophenotype for dyslexia in three groups of children. The first group of children was clinically diagnosed with dyslexia, whereas the second group of children was comprised of their siblings who had average reading and spelling skills and were therefore "unaffected" despite having a genetic risk for dyslexia. The third group consisted of control children who were not related to the other groups and were also unaffected. In total, 225 children were included in the study. All children showed clear MMN activity to/da/−/ba/ contrasts that could be separated into three distinct MMN components. Whilst the first two MMN components did not differentiate the groups, the late MMN component (300–700 ms) revealed significant group differences. The mean area of the late MMN was attenuated in both the dyslexic children and their unaffected siblings in comparison to the control children. This finding is indicative of analogous alterations of neurophysiological processes in children with dyslexia and those with a genetic risk for dyslexia, without a manifestation of the disorder. The present results therefore further suggest that the late MMN might be a potential endophenotype for dyslexia.

Editor: Kevin Paterson, University of Leicester, United Kingdom

Funding: The study was suppoorted by the Deutsche Forschungsgemeinschaft (DFG). The funders had no role in study design, data collection and analysis, decision to publish, or preparation of the manuscript.

Competing Interests: The authors have declared that no competing interests exist.

* E-mail: Gerd.Schulte-Koerne@med.uni-muenchen.de

Introduction

Dyslexia is a specific disorder in learning to read and spell despite normal intelligence, adequate schooling, and no obvious sensory deficits [1]. With 5%–10% of school-aged children affected, dyslexia is one of the most common learning disorders [2,3].

Aside from reading and spelling deficits, a number of neurophysiological studies have revealed altered auditory event-related potentials (AERP) in both children and adults with dyslexia when passively discriminating between two phonemes, such as/ da/and/ba/(for review see [4,5,6]). The AERP component which is related to this type of speech processing is the mismatch negativity (MMN). MMN is a pre-attentive measure of the AERP and reflects both the obligatory response to successful discrimination between two acoustic stimuli presented in succession and short-term auditory memory capacity. The MMN is a negative curve which is obtained by subtracting the AERP to a frequently presented standard stimulus from the AERP of an infrequently presented deviant stimulus. This negativity is registered at the fronto-central and central scalp electrodes, peaking around 150–250 ms from change onset [6,7] and originates from sources in auditory and frontal cortices [6,8]. The MMN is an objective measurement of the speech discrimination ability, and is particularly well-suited for studies in children; because active attention to the speech stimuli is not required [6].

A late MMN component (also referred to as the late discriminatory negativity or LDN [9,10]) at a timeframe from 300–600 ms over fronto-central sites has also been described [10,11,12,13,14,15,16,17,18,19]. It is mainly elicited by complex auditory stimuli like syllables and words, however it also occurs for tones [20]. Hommet et al. (2009) investigated sink and source patterns of the late MMN in children and located generators primarily in centro-parietal areas of the right hemisphere. The authors did not find an involvement of the supratemporal auditory cortex. Overall, the characteristics of the late MMN suggest the involvement of other brain processes than those attributed to the early MMN. It is thought to be associated to higher cognitive processes, such as attention related processes [21], letter-speech sound integration [13] and long term memory [22].

Most studies on MMN and dyslexia have focused on the early MMN, and deficits to speech sounds have been generally reported (for review see [4,5]), although not always [18,23,24,25], or only in subgroups [26,27]. Bishop [5] states that studies on (early) MMN to speech sounds and dyslexia often suffer from low effect sizes, perhaps as a result from the employment of heterogeneous and small groups. Furthermore, the early MMN is often absent in a large percentage of healthy study participants and shows a very poor reliability on an individual level (ie. [28,29]. Altogether, the efficacy of early MMN in the study of language disorders has not been fully established and many questions remain to be answered. None-the-less, the literature on dyslexia, early MMN and speech sound processing suggests that a large number of individuals with dyslexia will show reduced early MMN amplitude. Studies have also reported reduced late MMN amplitudes in dyslexic individuals [17,18,30]; [14,18,31,32]; [12,33]. Because the functional significance of the late MMN is less well understood it is not yet clear what factors might underlie late MMN deficits.

Finally, dyslexia is also a disorder with a complex and heterogeneous genetic basis [34,35]. Four genes associated with dyslexia in particular are involved in the development of the cerebral neocortex, either in terms of axonal guidance (*ROBO1* [36]) or neuronal migration (*KIAA0319* [37], *DCDC2* [38], and *DYX1C1* [39]). Importantly, these genes are expressed in cortical brain regions that are part of the complex neuronal network for reading [40,41]. Among these are the temporo-parietal cortices, the occipito-temporal cortices, and the inferior frontal cortex [42]. All of these brain areas have been found to be differentially activated in subjects with dyslexia. Specifically, in the left temporo-parietal region reduced activity correlated with phonological processing (e.g. rhyme detection and segmentation) and word reading [43,44,45]. Increased activation of the left inferior frontal area was associated with articulation in dyslexic subjects and was attributed to compensatory activation [43,44]. Finally, abnormal activity reported in left-occipital temporal areas to word and pseudoword stimuli suggests a visual word processing deficit [41,46,47,48,49].

One major difficulty in dyslexia research is defining and characterizing dyslexia. This problem is inherently linked to the genetic heterogeneity of dyslexia [35] which contributes to the complex behavioural profiles observed. For example, many but not all dyslexic individuals present with speech processing deficits [5], phonological deficits or rapid naming deficits [50]. Further complicating the matter is that many, but not all, dyslexic individuals also show non-language related problems such as temporal processing deficits [51] or even arithmetic [52] and motor deficits [53]. These deficits or the lack of them seem to occur in no particular pattern, thus making it extremely difficult to acquire heterogeneous samples for investigation and indeed to describe and quantify dyslexia per se. Furthermore, the diagnosis of dyslexia is determined for study and clinical purposes based on behavioural criteria (i.e. low reading and/or spelling scores) in children. Adults are often classified retrospectively or according to non-standardized reading measures.

It is apparent that numerous genes will contribute in small ways to the manifestation of dyslexia, and the genetic profiles will differ from one group or individual to the next. Although candidate genes have been identified in dyslexia, and much has been understood about brain (dys)function in dyslexia it remains unclear how genetics impact brain function and how these areas are related to reading and spelling phenotypes.

The identification of endophenotypes has been proposed to bridge the gap between the genes involved in disorder pathophysiology and overt behavioural phenotypes (i.e. reading). Endophenotypes are intermediate phenotypes which are under strong genetic influence and present in the majority of individuals with a disorder. Because of their relevance for genetics, family members who are not affected by the disorder will show the endophenotype more frequently than control groups [44]. Endophenotypes can take on a number of forms, for example hormonal, anatomical or as investigated in the present study, electrophysiological. Endophenotypes more closely indicate "disorder" than overt phenotypes and are therefore substantially more straightforward to use for investigation purposes [54]. For example, using an endophenotype as inclusion criteria for a genetic study, as opposed to overt phenotypes, increases the likelihood of identifying genes related to the disorder. Understanding which genes are involved in a disorder has many consequences, including: implications for diagnostics; illumination of disorder heterogeneity; influencing the development of animal models to study disorder pathology; and the creation of early interventions for those individuals presenting with a particular endophenotype.

So far, endophenotypes have not been identified in dyslexia. However, two molecular genetic studies on dyslexia have investigated both early and late MMN elicited by speech stimuli as candidate endophenotypes for dyslexia. Both studies were able to detect a relationship of the late MMN to gene loci, but did not find any evidence for an influence of genetics on the early MMN [12,33] suggesting that late MMN might be under genetic influence. Roeske et al. (2011) were able to show how the late MMN was significantly associated to *SLC2A3*, a gene on chromosome 12 which had not yet been associated with dyslexia. The functionality of *SLC2A3* renders it a compelling candidate for developmental disorders, as it is the predominant facilitative glucose transporter in neurons during child development. In a subsequent study [12] the late MMN was associated to rare variants between the prominent dyslexia candidate genes *KIAA0319* and *DCDC2*, both located on chromosome 6. Together, these findings suggest that the late MMN component in dyslexia is influenced by genetics. Thus, the neurophysiological correlates of speech perception in dyslexia which are under genetic influence might be mainly related to later cognitive processes. Taken together, there are a number of convincing reasons to further explore MMN components as possible endophenotypes for dyslexia.

Present Study

We investigated both early and late MMN related to speech sound perception in dyslexic children and their unaffected siblings in order to further explore possible genetic influences on these components. To study these differences we employed the speech stimuli/ba/and/da/in a passive oddball paradigm. These same stimuli were used in earlier studies [17,18,23]. A small unrelated control group was included (see discussion for limitations).

Our primary goal was to determine if early and/or late MMN to speech sounds differed in dyslexic children and their unaffected siblings. Based on our previous findings [33,55] we did not expect to find any evidence to suggest that early MMN is influenced by the genetics underlying dyslexia. We expected to find a reduced late MMN in both the dyslexic and the unaffected sibling groups compared to the control group.

Methods

The children participating in this study were selected via a single proband sib-pair approach. The siblings were recruited from 2001–2004 at the Departments of Child and Adolescent Psychiatry and Psychotherapy at the Universities of Marburg and Würzburg in Germany, and was funded by DFG (Deutsche Forschungsgemeinschaft). Written informed consent was given by the parents for all participating children, and by the children themselves and the study was approved by the local ethic committees of the Universities of Marburg and Würzburg. All children were compensated with 10€ for taking part in the study. The families coming to the clinic were also refunded for transportation costs.

Children were selected for this study when at least two siblings were available and one sibling fulfilled the inclusion criterion of a discrepancy of ≥1 SD between the observed spelling score and that expected from the non-verbal IQ to be able to compare dyslexic children and there unaffected siblings [56]. Spelling was measured using an age-appropriate spelling-test (writing to dictation) [57], and an observed spelling score was calculated on the basis of a correlation of 0.4 between the proband's IQ (measured by using the Culture Fair Test) and spelling [58]. Because there were no standardized German reading tests for children at or above the 5th grade at the time of the study, a non-standardized reading test was performed with these children. This test requires children to read a list of 48 words as accurately and quickly as possible. The dependent variable was time needed to read words. All children included in the dyslexic group also fulfilled the criterion of a discrepancy of ≥1 SD between the observed reading performance and that expected from the non-verbal IQ. Although the probands with dyslexia in the current study had significantly poorer reading skills, they were recruited based on their below average spelling skills. Recruiting based on spelling disorder in German is often done because the German language represents a very transparent orthography. This transparency fosters reading skills, as phoneme-grapheme correspondences are very consistent [59]. Therefore, it is quite typical in German dyslexic populations to observe normal reading accuracy with potential fluency (speed) deficits [60,61,62,63]. Spelling on the other hand remains difficult in German and these deficits are more persistent in the dyslexic populations [63]. From the total sample of 390 probands [64,65] and their siblings, only affected probands and their matched unaffected siblings were chosen for the analysis. If any proband fulfilled the diagnostic criteria of ADHD the family was excluded from the study since their inclusion could have introduced further heterogeneity into the analysis. Additional exclusion criteria were a bilingual education, a non-verbal IQ<85, an uncorrected disorder of peripheral hearing or vision, and a psychiatric or neurological disorder influencing the development of reading and spelling ability [66].

The control group was recruited from a public school based on both a comparable school grade and age, and based on the same inclusion and exclusion criteria as mentioned above. In total a group of 225 children, aged 10–15 years, could be included in this present study (Table 1).

Table 1. Sample description, presenting the mean and standard deviation for sample number, age, spelling, reading, IQ, and handedness.

Sample	Dyslexic children	Siblings	Controls
N	105 (♂ 64, ♀ 41)	105 (♂ 26, ♀ 79)	15 (♂ 4, ♀ 11)
Age (years)	11.54 (1.65)	12.37 (2.11)	12.53 (0.33)
Spelling (T scores)	31.41 (5.63)	49.15 (6.85)	52.87 (5.07)
Reading (time, sec)	38.42 (10.33)	51.36 (10.22)	56.53 (12.08)
IQ	109.62 (11.84)	109.82 (12.85)	106.33 (7.5)
Handedness	91 right, 14 left	94 right, 11 left	15 right

In order to measure MMN a passive oddball paradigm was used which presented the consonant-vowel stimuli/da/and/ba/binaurally via headphones. The stimuli were synthetic speech stimuli synthesized with the Computerized Speech Research Environment (Computerized Speech Research Environment (CSRE) (1995) London: AVAAZ Innovations, Inc). The standard stimulus was/da/(85%) and the deviant stimulus was/ba/(15%). For both stimuli, stimulus duration was 240 ms. Stimuli were presented in a pseudorandom order with at least five standards between two deviants with a stimulus-onset asynchrony (SOA) of 980 ms [18,19,32]. The children were instructed to ignore the presented stimuli and their attention was directed towards a silent movie. Thirty-two electrodes (Fp1, Fp2, F7, F3, Fz, F4, F8, FT7, FC3, FCz, FT8, T3, C3, Cz, C4, T4, TP7, CP3, CP4, TP8, T5, P3, Pz, P4, T6, O1, Oz, O2 and four EOG-electrodes) were placed on the scalp, based on the expanded international 10/20-system, with reference to the left mastoid. The EEG was re-referenced offline to averaged mastoids, the ground electrode was positioned at Fpz. Eye movements were detected with electrodes placed above, below and next to the subject's eyes. The EEG was amplified with Neuroscan Amplifiers. EEG-recording was continuous and A/D converted at a sampling rate of 256 Hz. The recorded EEG was filtered with a 0.53–40 Hz band pass using Brainvision Analyzer. Eye artefacts were corrected by performing an independent component analysis (ICA), with manual identification and exclusion of the eye artefact components. Further artefacts were removed by excluding trials automatically with two gradients (allowed maximum of 50 µV per sample point; maximum allowed absolute difference 150 µV in 200 ms) and max-min criteria (maximum amplitude of +−100 µV). Signals were averaged into epochs of 1100 ms, including a pre-stimulus baseline of 100 ms.

The average accepted trials was 271 for deviant stimuli and 372 for standard stimuli. The lowest number of accepted trials for any proband was 47. Therefore, all children had an acceptable number of accepted trials and we did not exclude any children from the analysis. Difference waveforms (MMN curves) were calculated by subtracting the averaged standard from the averaged deviant AERP. Grand averages were generated over all subjects for each group separately. Based on the observed scalp topography of the MMN in the control group and on electrode choice in previous MMN studies, the following fronto-central electrodes were chosen for analysis: F3, F4, Fz, C3, C4, Cz, Fc3, Fc4, Fcz. This fronto-central region is also known to be of interest for auditory stimulus perception and processing [67] and these electrodes were also used for group comparisons between dyslexic probands and controls in former speech perception studies [18,19]. The grand average wave forms (figure 1) revealed three MMN components: labelled MMN1, MMN2, and late MMN. For the analysis of these components the grand averages were tested against zero using running t-tests in order to determine which time windows differed significantly from zero for each component. The following three time windows were determined: MMN1 (84–188 ms), MMN2 (188–300 ms) and late MMN (300–700 ms). Mean MMN peak amplitude and mean MMN peak latency for MMN1 and MMN2 were calculated using these time windows. Because late MMN revealed a broad amplitude with no obvious peak the value of the area under the curve (µV *ms) was taken.

We introduced a random factor variable into our statistical model to account for the dependency (familial relationship) between the probands with dyslexia and their unaffected siblings. Furthermore, due to the large differences in sample sizes we used a PQL method (penalized quasi likelihood) which is robust for small sample sizes. Age, IQ and sex were modelled as covariants. Independent sample t-tests were run over the groups "family" and

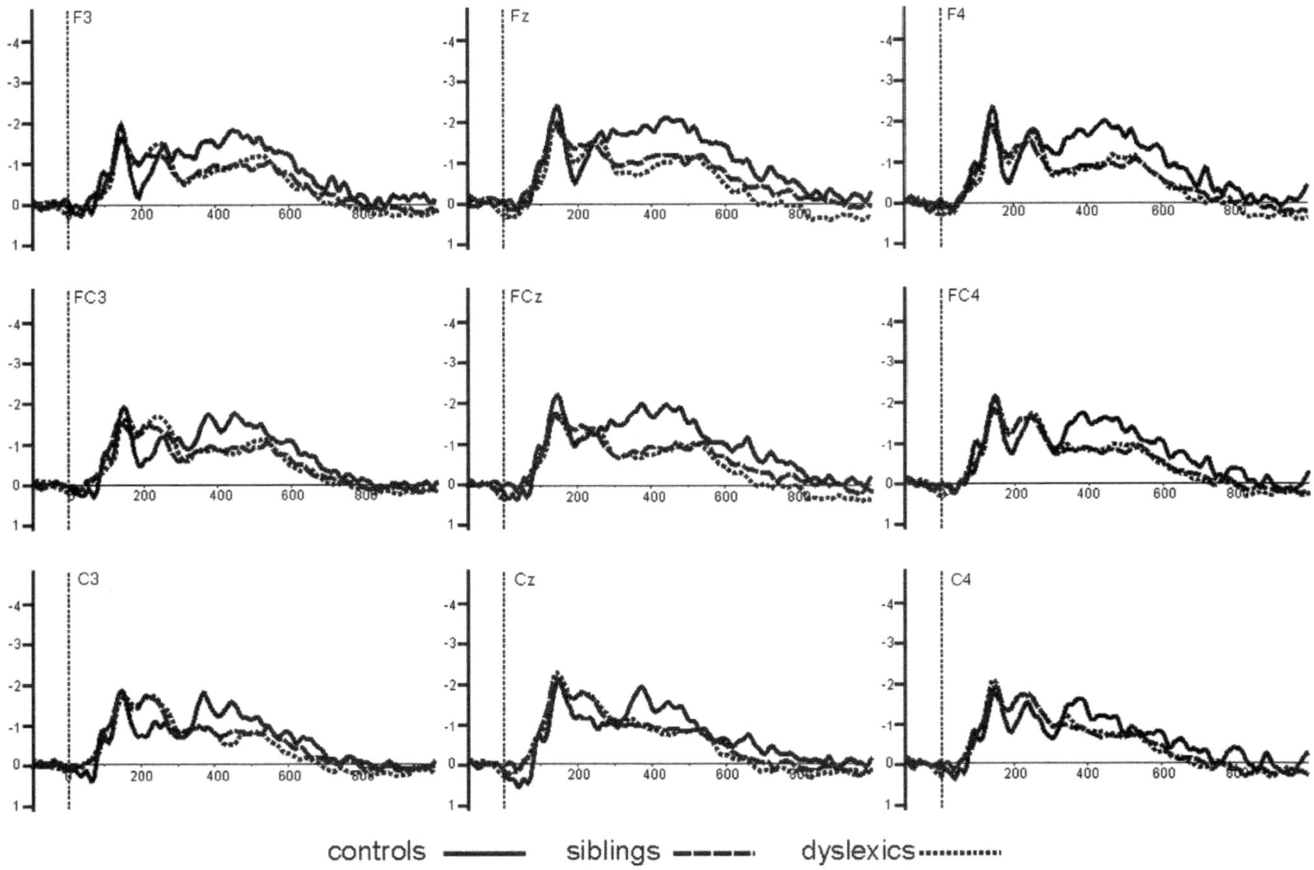

Figure 1. MMN1, MMN2, and late MMN for all 3 groups. MMN1, MMN2, and late MMN for dyslexic children (black line), unaffected siblings (dashed line), and unrelated controls (dotted line) at the nine fronto-central electrodes, giving the timeframes for the MMN1 (84–188 ms), MMN2 (188–300 ms), and late MMN (300–700 ms).

"control" for mean peak amplitude and mean peak latency for MMN1 and MMN2 and for mean area for the late MMN.

Results

MMN was generated for all three groups (dyslexic children, unaffected siblings, and unrelated controls) and revealed three distinct time windows (MMN1, MMN2, and late MMN) as can be seen in Fig. 1 and Table 2.

MMN1 and MMN2

Both MMN1 and MMN2 peaks were clearly visible in all three groups. We found no differences between groups for mean amplitude (MMN1: $p = .63$; MMN2: $p = .82$) or peak latency (MMN1: $p = .99$; MMN2: $p = .88$).

Late MMN

Control children revealed significantly greater late MMN than dyslexic and unaffected siblings ($t(117) = -2.38$, $p < .02$, d = −.64. Figure 2 depicts the scalp topography of the late MMN. In all three groups the greatest activity can be seen over the fronto-central electrode sites, however the activity is greater in the control group.

Table 2. Means and standard deviations of the MMN peak amplitudes, areas and latencies.

	Dyslexics Means (SD)	Siblings Means (SD)	Controls Means (SD)
MMN1, amplitude	−2.93 μV (1.65)	−2.84 μV (1.39)	−2.64 μV (1.25)
MMN2, amplitude	−2.75 μV (1.50)	−2.661 μV (1.38)	−2.48 μV (1.10)
late MMN (area under curve)	−260 μV*ms(412)	−350 μV*ms (376)	−480 μV*ms (276)
MMN1, latency	144.68 ms (19.92)	142.40 ms (21.18)	134.70 ms (24.14)
MMN2, latency	236.72 ms (28.01)	233.94 ms (28.06)	251.50 ms (26.56)

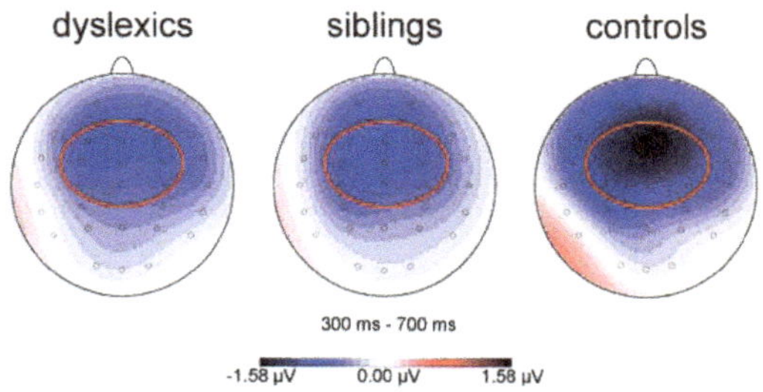

Figure 2. Topographic maps for the late MMN. Topographic maps for the time period 300–700 ms (late MMN) for dyslexic children, unaffected siblings, and unrelated controls, showing the ROI encircled in red.

Discussion

This present study was conducted to obtain further insight on the significance of early and late MMN elicited by differences in speech sounds as potential neurophysiological endophenotypes for dyslexia. For this purpose, children with a diagnosis of dyslexia, their unaffected siblings and unrelated control children were compared using a passive oddball paradigm with consonant-vowel stimuli.

We found three distinct MMN components of which the late MMN was reduced both in children with dyslexia and their unaffected siblings in comparison to control children. The early MMN components did not differentiate the groups. The first MMN component emerged in an atypical time window for MMN. Some studies on speech perception in dyslexia have reported group differences at similar early latencies (at 130 ms) [68], whereas others have not [18,69]. The second MMN component was typical of the early MMN latency. The amplitude of this component can be reduced in dyslexia, (for reviews see [4,6], but this has not always been found [18,28,29,70]. The present findings suggest that early MMN is not under genetic influence in dyslexia, which is supported by our previous research [33,55].

Late MMN: A Candidate Endophenotype for Dyslexia

Both the latency and scalp topography of the late MMN in the present study is consistent with reports in previous studies. These studies attributed the significance of the late MMN to higher cognitive processes, such as attention related processes [21], letter-speech sound integration [13] and to long term memory [22] as opposed to the detection of speech sound differences as associated to the MMN [6].

Previous studies have also found an attenuated late MMN to speech sounds in dyslexia [11,12,14,17,19,33,70]. However, this is the first report of attenuation of an ERP in relatives of dyslexic individuals, who therefore have a genetic risk for dyslexia, but have not developed reading and/or spelling disorders. The present findings complement recent molecular genetic research by our group [12,33] and further suggest that the late MMN might be a viable endophenotype for dyslexia research.

The identification of genes that contribute to a susceptibility to complex neuropsychiatric disorders is generally not successful when conventional genetic approaches are employed. Using endophenotypes (e.g. as study inclusion criteria) to investigate disorders with a complex genetic basis should aid molecular genetic studies because endophenotypes are more directly under genetic influence than the complex behaviours used to classify and diagnose psychiatric disorders (such as dyslexia, depression, schizophrenia and dementia). So far, research on the late MMN and dyslexia suggest that the area of late MMN to speech sounds might fulfil three criteria for endophenotype classification as suggested by Gottesman & Gould (2003): 1) the late MMN amplitude has been shown to be associated with dyslexia [11,14,17,18,19], 2) it has been associated with the genetics of dyslexia (for both known (*DCDC2* and *KIAA0319*) [12] and novel (*SLC2A3*) [33] candidate genes), and 3) as the present study demonstrates, it is also attenuated in individuals with a genetic risk for dyslexia, but who did not develop reading and spelling deficits.

Taken together, these findings suggest that the late MMN is influenced by the underlying genetics of dyslexia. Finding reduced late MMN in siblings with and without dyslexia opens the field for further investigations that might address protective environmental factors or compensatory mechanisms. Furthermore, future investigations of late MMN and dyslexia might reveal new insight for dyslexia interventions, since unaffected siblings master a normal reading and writing level even with reduced neurophysiological answers to speech sounds.

Despite these promising results, whether the late MMN can be classified as an endophenotype for dyslexia and if it can be concretely employed for future research still needs to be systematically examined. Although the late MMN seems to be a promising candidate for an endophenotype in dyslexia, replication of the present findings, as well as our previous findings [12,33] is essential and substantiation of the late MMN's heritability, occurrence throughout dyslexic families and presence after compensation or remediation remains to be established. In general, the identification of endophenotypes and the subsequent understanding of the genetics contributing to dyslexia have the potential to pave the way for improving diagnostics, treatment and understanding causality.

Limitations

We would like to address one major limitation of the potential study. Due to technical issues, we were unable to recruit a comparably sized control group. We have employed appropriate statistical tests robust for small and also unequal sample sizes. However, given the considerable individual variability of MMN these results are in need of replication.

Acknowledgments

The presented data are part of the dissertation from Nina Neuhoff at the Ludwig-Maximilians-University, Munich, Medical Faculty.

Author Contributions

Conceived and designed the experiments: NN GSK J. Bartling AW HR. Performed the experiments: NN J. Bartling GSK. Analyzed the data: NN J. Bruder GSK BMM. Wrote the paper: NN J. Bruder J. Bartling GSK.

References

1. Dilling H, Mombour W, Schmidt MH, Schulte-Markwort E (1994) Internationale Klassifikation psychischer Störungen - ICD-10 Kapitel V (F)/ Forschungskriterien. Weltgesundheitsorganisation. Bern: Verlag Hans Huber.
2. Shaywitz SE, Shaywitz BA, Fletcher JM, Escobar MD (1990) Prevalence of reading disability in boys and girls. Results of the Connecticut Longitudinal Study. The Journal of the American Medical Association 264: 998–1002.
3. Katusic SK, Colligan RC, Barbaresi WJ, Schaid DJ, Jacobsen SJ (2001) Incidence of reading disability in a population-based birth cohort, 1976–1982, Rochester, Minn. Mayo Clin Proc 76: 1081–1092.
4. Schulte-Korne G, Bruder J (2010) Clinical neurophysiology of visual and auditory processing in dyslexia: a review. Clin Neurophysiol 121: 1794–1809.

5. Bishop DV (2007) Using mismatch negativity to study central auditory processing in developmental language and literacy impairments: where are we, and where should we be going? Psychological bulletin 133: 651–672.
6. Naatanen R, Paavilainen P, Rinne T, Alho K (2007) The mismatch negativity (MMN) in basic research of central auditory processing: A review. Clinical Neurophysiology.
7. Tiitinen H, May P, Reinikainen K, Naatanen R (1994) Attentive novelty detection in humans is governed by pre-attentive sensory memory. Nature 372: 90–92.
8. Naatanen R (1992) Attention and Brain Function. Hillsdale: Lawrence Erlbaum.
9. Ceponiene R, Lepisto T, Soininen M, Aronen E, Alku P, et al. (2004) Event-related potentials associated with sound discrimination versus novelty detection in children. Psychophysiology 41: 130–141.
10. Ceponiene R, Yaguchi K, Shestakova A, Alku P, Suominen K, et al. (2002) Sound complexity and 'speechness' effects on pre-attentive auditory discrimination in children. Int J Psychophysiol 43: 199–211.
11. Alonso-Bua B, Diaz F, Ferraces MJ (2006) The contribution of AERPs (MMN and LDN) to studying temporal vs. linguistic processing deficits in children with reading difficulties. International Journal of Psychophysiology 59: 159–167.
12. Czamara D, Bruder J, Becker J, Bartling J, Hoffmann P, et al. (2011) Association of a rare variant with mismatch negativity in a region between KIAA0319 and DCDC2 in dyslexia. Behav Genet 41: 110–119.
13. Froyen DJ, Bonte ML, van Atteveldt N, Blomert L (2009) The long road to automation: neurocognitive development of letter-speech sound processing. J Cogn Neurosci 21: 567–580.
14. Hommet C, Vidal J, Roux S, Blanc R, Barthez MA, et al. (2009) Topography of syllable change-detection electrophysiological indices in children and adults with reading disabilities. Neuropsychologia 47: 761–770.
15. Korpilahti P, Lang HA (1994) Auditory ERP components and mismatch negativity in dysphasic children. Electroencephalogr Clin Neurophysiol 91: 256–264.
16. Maurer U, Bucher K, Brem S, Benz R, Kranz F, et al. (2009) Neurophysiology in Preschool Improves Behavioral Prediction of Reading Ability Throughout Primary School. Biological Psychiatry.
17. Maurer U, Bucher K, Brem S, Brandeis D (2003) Altered responses to tone and phoneme mismatch in kindergartners at familial dyslexia risk. Neuroreport 14: 2245–2250.
18. Schulte-Korne G, Deimel W, Bartling J, Remschmidt H (1998) Auditory processing and dyslexia: evidence for a specific speech processing deficit. Neuroreport 9: 337–340.
19. Schulte-Korne G, Deimel W, Bartling J, Remschmidt H (2001) Speech perception deficit in dyslexic adults as measured by mismatch negativity (MMN). International Journal of Psychophysiology 40: 77–87.
20. Ceponiene R, Cheour M, Naatanen R (1998) Interstimulus interval and auditory event-related potentials in children: evidence for multiple generators. Electroencephalogr Clin Neurophysiol 108: 345–354.
21. Shestakova A, Huotilainen M, Ceponiene R, Cheour M (2003) Event-related potentials associated with second language learning in children. Clin Neurophysiol 114: 1507–1512.
22. Zachau S, Rinker T, Korner B, Kohls G, Maas V, et al. (2005) Extracting rules: early and late mismatch negativity to tone patterns. Neuroreport 16: 2015–2019.
23. Heim S, Eulitz C, Kaufmann J, Fuchter I, Pantev C, et al. (2000) Atypical organisation of the auditory cortex in dyslexia as revealed by MEG. Neuropsychologia 38: 1749–1759.
24. Paul I, Bott C, Heim S, Wienbruch C, Elbert TR (2006) Phonological but not auditory discrimination is impaired in dyslexia. The European Journal of Neuroscience 24: 2945–2953.
25. Shafer VL, Morr ML, Datta H, Kurtzberg D, Schwartz RG (2005) Neurophysiological indexes of speech processing deficits in children with specific language impairment. J Cogn Neurosci 17: 1168–1180.
26. Banai K, Nicol T, Zecker SG, Kraus N (2005) Brainstem timing: implications for cortical processing and literacy. J Neurosci 25: 9850–9857.
27. Lachmann T, Berti S, Kujala T, Schroger E (2005) Diagnostic subgroups of developmental dyslexia have different deficits in neural processing of tones and phonemes. International Journal of Psychophysiology 56: 105–120.
28. Dalebout SD, Fox LG (2001) Reliability of the mismatch negativity in the responses of individual listeners. J Am Acad Audiol 12: 245–253.
29. Picton TW, Alain C, Otten L, Ritter W, Achim A (2000) Mismatch negativity: different water in the same river. Audiol Neurootol 5: 111–139.
30. Stoodley CJ, Hill PR, Stein JF, Bishop DV (2006) Auditory event-related potentials differ in dyslexics even when auditory psychophysical performance is normal. Brain Research 1121: 190–199.
31. Schulte-Korne G, Deimel W, Bartling J, Remschmidt H (1999) Pre-attentive processing of auditory patterns in dyslexic human subjects. Neurosci Lett 276: 41–44.
32. Schulte-Korne G, Deimel W, Bartling J, Remschmidt H (1999) The role of phonological awareness, speech perception, and auditory temporal processing for dyslexia. Eur Child Adolesc Psychiatry 8 Suppl 3: 28–34.
33. Roeske D, Ludwig KU, Neuhoff N, Becker J, Bartling J, et al. (2011) First genome-wide association scan on neurophysiological endophenotypes points to trans-regulation effects on SLC2A3 in dyslexic children. Molecular Psychiatry.
34. Paracchini S, Scerri T, Monaco AP (2007) The Genetic Lexicon of Dyslexia. Annual Review of Genomics and Human Genetics.
35. Scerri TS, Schulte-Korne G (2010) Genetics of developmental dyslexia. Eur Child Adolesc Psychiatry 19: 179–197.
36. Hannula-Jouppi K, Kaminen-Ahola N, Taipale M, Eklund R, Nopola-Hemmi J, et al. (2005) The axon guidance receptor gene ROBO1 is a candidate gene for developmental dyslexia. PLoS Genet 1: e50.
37. Cope N, Harold D, Hill G, Moskvina V, Stevenson J, et al. (2005) Strong evidence that KIAA0319 on chromosome 6p is a susceptibility gene for developmental dyslexia. Am J Hum Genet 76: 581–591.
38. Meng H, Smith SD, Hager K, Held M, Liu J, et al. (2005) DCDC2 is associated with reading disability and modulates neuronal development in the brain. Proc Natl Acad Sci U S A 102: 17053–17058.
39. Taipale M, Kaminen N, Nopola-Hemmi J, Haltia T, Myllyluoma B, et al. (2003) A candidate gene for developmental dyslexia encodes a nuclear tetratricopeptide repeat domain protein dynamically regulated in brain. Proc Natl Acad Sci U S A 100: 11553–11558.
40. Shaywitz SE, Shaywitz BA (2008) Paying attention to reading: the neurobiology of reading and dyslexia. Dev Psychopathol 20: 1329–1349.
41. McCandliss BD, Noble KG (2003) The development of reading impairment: a cognitive neuroscience model. Ment Retard Dev Disabil Res Rev 9: 196–204.
42. Richlan F, Kronbichler M, Wimmer H (2011) Meta-analyzing brain dysfunctions in dyslexic children and adults. NeuroImage 56: 1735–1742.
43. Brunswick N, McCrory E, Price CJ, Frith CD, Frith U (1999) Explicit and implicit processing of words and pseudowords by adult developmental dyslexics: A search for Wernicke's Wortschatz? Brain 122 (Pt 10): 1901–1917.
44. Pugh KR, Mencl WE, Jenner AR, Katz L, Frost SJ, et al. (2000) Functional neuroimaging studies of reading and reading disability (developmental dyslexia). Mental retardation and developmental disabilities research reviews 6: 207–213.
45. Rumsey JM, Horwitz B, Donohue BC, Nace K, Maisog JM, et al. (1997) Phonological and orthographic components of word recognition. A PET-rCBF study. Brain 120 (Pt 5): 739–759.
46. Shaywitz BA, Shaywitz SE, Pugh KR, Mencl WE, Fulbright RK, et al. (2002) Disruption of posterior brain systems for reading in children with developmental dyslexia. Biol Psychiatry 52: 101–110.
47. McCrory EJ, Mechelli A, Frith U, Price CJ (2005) More than words: a common neural basis for reading and naming deficits in developmental dyslexia? Brain 128: 261–267.
48. Salmelin R, Service E, Kiesila P, Uutela K, Salonen O (1996) Impaired visual word processing in dyslexia revealed with magnetoencephalography. Ann Neurol 40: 157–162.
49. Cohen L, Dehaene S (2004) Specialization within the ventral stream: the case for the visual word form area. NeuroImage 22: 466–476.
50. Wolf M, Bowers PG (2000) Naming-speed processes and developmental reading disabilities: an introduction to the special issue on the double-deficit hypothesis. J Learn Disabil 33: 322–324.
51. Tallal P, Miller S, Fitch RH (1993) Neurobiological basis of speech: a case for the preeminence of temporal processing. Ann N Y Acad Sci 682: 27–47.
52. Simmons FR, Singleton C (2008) Do weak phonological representations impact on arithmetic development? A review of research into arithmetic and dyslexia. Dyslexia 14: 77–94.
53. Nicolson RI, Fawcett AJ (2005) Developmental dyslexia, learning and the cerebellum. J Neural Transm Suppl. pp 19–36.
54. Gottesman, II, Gould TD (2003) The endophenotype concept in psychiatry: etymology and strategic intentions. The American Journal of Psychiatry 160: 636–645.
55. Ludwig KU, Roeske D, Schumacher J, Schulte-Korne G, Konig IR, et al. (2008) Investigation of interaction between DCDC2 and KIAA0319 in a large German dyslexia sample. Journal of Neural Transmission 115: 1587–1589.
56. Weiß RH, Osterland J (1997) Grundintelligenztest Skala 1 (CFT 1). Göttingen: Hogrefe.
57. Brähler E, Holling V, Leutner D, Petermann F (2002) Brickenkamp Handbuch psychologisccher und pädagogischer Tests. Göttingen: Hogrefe.
58. Schulte-Körne G, Deimel W, Remschmidt H (2001) Diagnosis of reading and spelling disorder. Zeitschrift für Kinder- und Jugendpsychiatrie und Psychotherapie 29: 113–116.
59. Ziegler JC, Goswami U (2006) Becoming literate in different languages: similar problems, different solutions. Dev Sci 9: 429–436.
60. Wimmer H (1993) Characteristics of developmental dyslexia in a regular writing system. Applied Psycholinguistics 14: 1–33.
61. Wimmer H (1996) The early manifestation of developmental dyslexia: Evidence from German children. Reading and Writing: An Interdisciplinary Journal 8: 171–188.
62. Landerl K, Wimmer H, Frith U (1997) The impact of orthographic consistency on dyslexia: a German-English comparison. Cognition 63: 315–334.
63. Landerl K, Wimmer H (2008) Developmental of word reading fluency and spelling in a consitent orthography: An 8-year follow up. Journal of Educational Psychology 100: 150–161.
64. Schumacher J, Anthoni H, Dahdouh F, Konig IR, Hillmer AM, et al. (2006) Strong genetic evidence of DCDC2 as a susceptibility gene for dyslexia. American Journal of Human Genetics 78: 52–62.
65. Schulte-Korne G, Ziegler A, Deimel W, Schumacher J, Plume E, et al. (2007) Interrelationship and familiality of dyslexia related quantitative measures. Annals of Human Genetics 71: 160–175.

66. Unnewehr S, Schneider S, Margraf J (1998) Kinder-DIPS: diagnostisches Interview bei psychischen Störungen von Kindern und Jugendlichen. Berlin: Springer.
67. Giard MH, Perrin F, Pernier J, Bouchet P (1990) Brain generators implicated in the processing of auditory stimulus deviance: a topographic event-related potential study. Psychophysiology 27: 627–640.
68. Meng X, Sai X, Wang C, Wang J, Sha S, et al. (2005) Auditory and speech processing and reading development in Chinese school children: behavioural and ERP evidence. Dyslexia 11: 292–310.
69. Sebastian C, Yasin I (2008) Speech versus tone processing in compensated dyslexia: discrimination and lateralization with a dichotic mismatch negativity (MMN) paradigm. Int J Psychophysiol 70: 115–126.
70. Schulte-Korne G, Deimel W, Bartling J, Remschmidt H (1998) Role of auditory temporal processing for reading and spelling disability. Perceptual and Motor Skills 86: 1043–1047.

2

Do Students with Dyslexia Have a Different Personality Profile as Measured with the Big Five?

Wim Tops[1]*, Ellen Verguts[2], Maaike Callens[1], Marc Brysbaert[1]

1 Department of Experimental Psychology, Ghent University, Ghent, Belgium, **2** vzw Kinsbergen Oriëntatiecentrum, Antwerp, Belgium

Abstract

Background: Few studies are available about the personality profile of higher education students with dyslexia and to which extent this could be any different from their non-dyslexic peers.

Aims and Sample(s): To obtain empirical evidence, we compared the personality profile of a group of 100 Dutch-speaking students with dyslexia with that of a control group of 100 students without learning disabilities.

Methods: The NEO-PI-R based on the Big Five in personality research was used.

Results and Conclusions: Our study showed no differences in the personality between both groups. This agrees with a recent meta-analysis of English findings (Swanson & Hsieh, 2009), suggesting that students with dyslexia do not perceive themselves differently than their non-dyslexic peers. Practical implications and directions for future research are considered.

Editor: Kevin Paterson, University of Leicester, United Kingdom

Funding: This study was made possible by an Odysseus Grant awarded by the Government of Flanders to Marc Brysbaert. The funders had no role in study design, data collection and analysis, decision to publish, or preparation of the manuscript.

Competing Interests: The authors have declared that no competing interests exist.

* E-mail: wimtops@gmail.com

Introduction

Although reading and writing are mastered well by most persons, they can be a source of frustration for people with dyslexia. This is particularly true during the school years, when good reading and writing skills are important for academic achievement and career building [1]. All beginning readers experience difficulties but for most of them automatization builds up rapidly and after a while they can read effortlessly. This is not true for a group that keeps on having difficulties into adult life, despite normal intelligence, adequate instruction, and often intensive remedial teaching. These persons are confronted with extra challenges compared to their non-dyslexic peers.

Although reading and writing are the core deficits in adults with dyslexia [2–3], various authors have suggested that other cognitive skills may be affected as well. Adults with dyslexia have been reported to experience (working) memory problems [4], attentional deficits [5], reduced processing speed [2], problems with fast word finding and arithmetic [6–7], and less elaborated vocabulary skills [8]. Dyslexia has also been associated with less sophisticated study strategies and metacognitive skills [9–10], higher anxiety, lower self-esteem, problems with coping, and deficient academic achievement and motivation throughout the life-span [11–13].

To our knowledge, little is known about the consequences of this adversity on the personality development of students with dyslexia. The only empirical study we could find was Waldo, McIntosh, and Koller [14]. These authors examined the MMPI-derived personality profiles of 165 adults with learning disabilities. Three groups were distinguished on the basis of a comparison of verbal and performance IQ [15]. People with a verbal IQ significantly below their performance IQ were assumed to have a verbal learning disorder; people with the reverse pattern were classified as having a non-verbal learning disorder. These two groups were compared to a control group with similar scores on verbal and performance IQ. No overall differences between the groups were observed, but the two groups with learning disabilities scored higher on some MMPI scales than the control group. The study of Waldo et al. [14] was included in the meta-analysis of Swanson and Hsieh [3], who concluded that there was only a small effect size of d = .28 between the personalities of adults with and without dyslexia.

The MMPI-test is typically used for clinical populations. Therefore, it would be interesting to know whether larger differences can be found on personality tests meant for non-clinical research. The most widely used tests in personality research measure personality traits. A personality trait is a hypothetic attribute that influences a person's behavior, thoughts and feelings across situations. According to the trait approach, differences in personality can be described with a limited set of dimensions. A trait usually is a continuum between two opposed characteristics (e.g., happy versus sad). The approach was introduced in the second half of the twentieth century, when authors like Cattell and Eysenck used factor analysis to examine the pattern of correlations between personality characteristics. Cattell [16] concluded that 16 bipolar traits were needed for a detailed description of one's personality, whereas Eysenck argued that three traits were enough (e.g., [17]). Gradually agreement emerged that five traits represented the optimal number. These five traits became known as the Big Five [18].

Table 1. General Information About the Student Groups With and Without Dyslexia.

		students without dyslexia N M (*SD*)		students with dyslexia N M (*SD*)		Effect size Cohen's *d*
Gender	Male	46		46		
	Female	54		54		
Studies	University	66		66		
	College for higher education	34		34		
Age		19.40	*(1.00)*	19.11	*(0.70)*	NA
Fluid IQ		106.80	*(10.80)*	105.40	*(11.00)*	−0.13
Word reading		100.40	*(10.60)*	77.00	*(14.20)*	−1.97
Pseudoword reading		59.70	*(13.10)*	40.90	*(10.50)*	−1.59
Word spelling		24.60	*(2.80)*	17.50	*(4.00)*	−2.05

Note. TIQ = Total IQ score (KAIT; Dekker, Dekker, & Mulder, 2004); Word reading = Dutch word reading, number of words read correctly in 1 minute time (EMT; Brus & Voeten, 1991); Pseudoword reading = number of pseudowords read correctly in 1 minute time (de Klepel; van den Bos et al., 1999); word spelling = number of words spelled correctly in a word dictation task (GL& De Pessemier & andries, 2009). Effect sizes calculated according to Cohen's *d* (positive d-values represent better performance of the controls and negative values better performance of the students with dyslexia).

The first dimension of the Big Five is *extraversion*. Extraverted people have more attention for and are more oriented towards aspects outside themselves. They are more sociable, more active, and more cheerful. They like excitement and action. They are also strongly focused on their direct environment. In contrast, introverted people are more distant and prefer to be alone. They have a focus on their inside, on their emotions, feelings, and thoughts. The second aspect within the Big Five is *neuroticism*. On the one end of the continuum, there is emotional lability. This is associated with generalized fear and negative feelings such as anger, frustration and shame. On the other end, there are people with high emotional stability who can better dismiss these negative feelings. The third dimension is *openness* to experiences, intellectual or cultural challenges. Open minded people are more (intellectually or culturally) curious and have a rich imagination. They like variation and are able to make independent judgments. There is a positive correlation between this factor and intelligence and educational level. People who lack openness show more conventional behavior and are more conservative. Fourth, *agreeableness* is a measure for interpersonal behavior and orientation to other people's experiences, interests and goals. One gets a high score for agreeableness, if one is cooperative, friendly and helpful. People with low scores tend to be more egocentric and antagonistic. The final dimension of the Big Five is *conscientiousness*. This refers to an individual's conscience as a directive and control mechanism for one's behavior. Expediency, self discipline and thoughtfulness are important facets of this category. Traditionally the Big Five are measured with a personality questionnaire. Two of the most frequently used are the NEO-PI-R [18] and the Five-Factor Personality Inventory [19].

We compared the answers of students with and without dyslexia on a Big Five questionnaire, to see whether the two groups perceive their own personality differently. Each group consisted of 100 participants, so that we could obtain stable estimates of the effect sizes.

Methods

This study was approved by the ethical comity of Ghent University, meaning that the researchers followed the ethical protocol of the university. All students gave written informed consent and were informed that they could stop at any time if they felt they were treated incorrectly.

Participants

Two hundred first-year undergraduate students of higher education participated in the study, both non-academic students and university students. One group consisted of 100 students diagnosed with dyslexia, the other was a control group of 100 students with no known neurological or functional deficiencies. All had normal or corrected-to normal vision and were native speakers of Dutch. They all attended higher education in Ghent, one of the major cities of Flanders (the Dutch-speaking northern half of Belgium). Students were paid for their participation.

The students with dyslexia have been thoroughly assessed [2,20] and meet the three criteria for dyslexia as outlined by the SDN [21]. The SDN uses a descriptive definition of dyslexia. In their guidelines dyslexia is defined as an impairment characterized by a persistent problem in learning to read and/or write words or in the automatization of reading and writing. First, the level of reading and/or writing of the students with dyslexia was significantly lower than what could be expected on the basis of their educational level and age. All students with dyslexia had (sub) clinical scores (<pc 10) on a word reading test (*EMT* [One Minute Test] [22]) and/or, pseudo word reading test (*De Klepel* [23]) and/or word spelling test (GL&SCHR [24]). Secondly, most students had low scores despite taking some form of remedial teaching, which meant they met the criterion "resistance to instruction" [25]. Finally, the SDN definition requires ensuring that the reading and writing impairment cannot be attributed to external and/or individual factors such as socio-economic status, cultural background or intelligence, which was the case for the group we examined.

A group of 100 control students was recruited matched on age, gender and field of study, using the social networks of the students, student coaches and electronic learning platforms. None of the members of the control group had known neurological or functional disorders.

There was no difference between the two groups in socio-economical level based on the educational level of the mother [$\chi^2(3) = 4.855$, $p = .183$] and father [$\chi^2(3) = 2.634$, $p = .452$]. Educational levels were: lower secondary education, higher secondary education, postsecondary education either at university or non-university college. Both groups had slightly above average fluid intelligence and did not differ from each other. Table 1 shows the main characteristics of the groups (see [2] for more details).

Table 2. Results for NEO-PI-R for Both Student Groups Expressed as Effect Sizes (Cohen's d).

	Students with dyslexia		Students without dyslexia			
	M	(SD)	M	(SD)	d	
Neuroticism	**147.180**	*(19.77)*	**150.76**	*(19.44)*	**−0.26**	
Anxiety	25.77	*(5.09)*	26.30	*(4.89)*	−0.15	
Angry hostility	21.86	*(4.67)*	22.76	*(4.10)*	−0.30	
Depression	25.08	*(5.14)*	26.17	*(5.43)*	−0.29	
Self consciousness	24.82	*(4.68)*	24.96	*(4.59)*	−0.04	
Impulsiveness	28.07	*(4.34)*	28.87	*(3.69)*	−0.28	
Vulnerability	21.66	*(4.33)*	21.68	*(4.20)*	−0.01	
Extraversion	**165.23**	*(18.66)*	**167.88**	*(19.81)*	**0.20**	
Warmth	29.49	*(4.36)*	29.54	*(4.29)*	0.02	
Gregariousness	28.18	*(5.039)*	28.81	*(4.66)*	0.18	
Assertiveness	24.04	*(4.368)*	23.79	*(5.25)*	−0.07	
Activity	26.03	*(3.84)*	25.80	*(4.21)*	−0.08	
Excitement seeking	27.70	*(4.10)*	29.20	*(4.12,*	0.52	*
Positive emotion	29.79	*(4.33)*	30.50	*(4.611*	0.22	
Openness	**167.85**	*(16.64)*	**168.97**	*(17.45)*	**0.10**	
Fantasy	29.58	*(5.26)*	29.60	*(4.57)*	0.01	
Aesthetics	27.30	*(7.21)*	27.61	*(5.44)*	0.07	
Feelings	29.140	*(4.50)*	30.06	*(4.00)*	0.31	
Actions	23.81	*(3.92)*	24.33	*(4.74)*	0.17	
Ideas	27.29	*(5.01)*	27.34	*(5.448)*	0.02	
Values	29.76	*(3.38)*	29.90	*(3.90)*	0.06	
Agreeableness	**165.69**	*(19.55)*	**165.44**	*(14.74)*	**−0.02**	
Trust	28.47	*(4.65)*	27.65	*(4.43)*	−0.26	
Straightforwardness	27.05	*(5.27)*	27.24	*(4.65)*	0.05	
Altruism	29.86	*(3.47)*	30.33	*(3.24)*	0.20	
Compliance	23.49	*(4.38)*	22.93	*(4.02)*	−0.19	
Modesty	27.99	*(4.59)*	27.80	*(3.98)*	−0.06	
Tender mindedness	28.72	*(4.00)*	29.47	*(3.53)*	0.28	
Conscientiousness	**152.35**	*(20.29)*	**150.36**	*(20.52)*	**−0.14**	
Competence	26.62	*(3.16)*	26.29	*(3.92)*	−0.13	
Order	23.22	*(5.02)*	23.19	*(5.09)*	−0.01	
Dutifulness	28.14	*(3.89)*	28.24	*(4.35)*	0.03	
Achievement striving	27.35	*(4.07)*	26.57	*(4.77)*	−0.25	
Self discipline	24.19	*(4.81)*	23.39	*(4.58)*	−0.23	
Deliberation	22.97	*(5.41)*	22.79	*(5.22)*	−0.05	

Note. * p<.05.

Test

We administered a computerized Dutch version of the NEO-PI-R [18,26]. This is a self-report questionnaire comprising 30 facet scales (based on 240 items) that can be reduced to the five dimensions of the Five Factor Model. Administration took 40 to 50 minutes on average. Because half of the participants had reading problems, no time constraints were imposed.

Procedure

The personality test was part of a larger protocol about dyslexia in higher education [2]. The complete test battery involved additional tests such as an intelligence test, reading and spelling tests, and a structured interview about the functioning and the well-being of the student. It was administered in two sessions of about three hours each. The protocol was divided into two counterbalanced parts. The order of tests in part one and two was fixed and chosen to avoid succession of similar tests. The two parts were counterbalanced (i.e., half of each group started with part one, the other half with part two).

For the personality test, students were seated in front of a computer screen in a well-lit and quiet room. The test administrator was present, but could not see the computer screen, nor the answers the students gave. If necessary, students could ask to have a question read aloud or explained to them. The latter usually involved the explanation of an unfamiliar word, for which the test administrator

Table 3. Results for NEO-PI-R for the Male Students Expressed as Effect Sizes (Cohen's d).

	Men with dyslexia		Men without dyslexia		
	M	(SD)	M	(SD)	d
Neuroticism	**141.45**	*−20.93*	**144.10**	*−19.72*	**−0.09**
Anxiety	23.98	−5.31	24.27	−4.79	0.04
Angry hostility	22.00	−5.10	22.59	−4.25	0.09
Depression	23.55	−4.99	24.88	−5.64	0.18
Self consciousness	23.83	−4.55	23.61	−4.58	−0.04
Impulsiveness	28.00	−3.76	28.59	−3.72	0.11
Vulnerability	20.05	−4.33	20.17	−4.24	0.02
Extraversion	**163.48**	*−20.28*	**164.02**	*−22.73*	**0.02**
Warmth	27.76	−4.62	27.73	−4.12	−0.01
Gregariousness	27.36	−5.65	27.66	−5.07	0.04
Assertiveness	24.79	−4.01	23.54	−5.36	−0.19
Activity	26.38	−4.29	25.57	−4.65	−0.13
Excitement seeking	28.17	−4.12	29.88	−4.30	0.29
Positive emotion	29.02	−4.62	29.66	−4.95	0.09
Openness	**166.14**	*−15.49*	**164.78**	*−15.78*	**−0.06**
Fantasy	30.38	−4.79	29.61	−4.06	−0.12
Aesthetics	26.62	−5.36	25.46	−5.53	−0.15
Feelings	27.76	−4.33	28.56	−3.90	0.14
Actions	23.41	−4.23	23.83	−4.76	0.07
Ideas	28.62	−4.71	28.29	−5.90	−0.04
Values	29.35	−3.48	28.79	−3.72	−0.11
Agreeableness	**156.57**	*−19.62*	**159.95**	*−14.85*	**0.14**
Trust	27.60	−5.31	26.83	−5.03	−0.11
Straightforwardness	24.57	−5.21	25.95	−4.65	0.20
Altruism	28.41	−3.47	29.17	−3.06	0.17
Compliance	22.79	−4.16	23.02	−3.66	0.04
Modesty	26.10	−4.96	26.78	−4.26	0.11
Tender mindedness	27.12	−4.26	28.39	−3.23	0.24
Conscientiousness	**148.71**	*−19.10*	**148.78**	*−21.08*	**0.00**
Competence	26.83	−3.01	26.92	−4.25	0.02
Order	21.64	−4.64	22.83	−4.18	0.19
Dutifulness	27.50	−4.20	27.41	−4.58	−0.01
Achievement striving	26.81	−4.16	25.78	−4.73	−0.16
Self discipline	23.19	−4.61	22.83	−5.11	−0.05
Deliberation	22.93	−5.31	23.00	−5.53	0.01

gave a synonym or a meaningful context. Students could also ask for breaks if necessary. If more than 40 answers (on a total of 240) were left open, the participant's results were excluded for further analysis. This was the case for one student from the dyslexia group. Other missing answers were replaced by the mean, neutral score. This was done in less than 0.01% of the questions for both groups.

Results

For many practical purposes, statistical significance is secondary to effect size, because statistical significance depends on the sizes of the groups tested as much as on the difference between the groups. Therefore, all results are additionally given as effect sizes derived from parametric t- tests (conclusions were not different when we used a non-parametric Mann-Whitney U-test). These are calculated as follows:

$$d = \frac{Mean_{dyslexic} - Mean_{control}}{\sqrt{\frac{SD^2_{dyslexic} + SD^2_{control}}{2}}}$$

Values of t are not given, as these can easily be calculated from the d-scores:

$$t = \frac{d * \sqrt{N_{dyslexic} + N_{control}}}{2} = \frac{d * \sqrt{100 + 100}}{2}$$

$$= 7.07 * \mathrm{d}\ (\mathrm{df} = 198).$$

The sign of the d-values was adapted so that positive d-values always represented better performance of the controls and negative values better performance of the students with dyslexia. Because we had two groups of 100 participants, the 95% confidence intervals of the obtained d-scores are ±.4, (calculated with ESCI-CI delta [27]). Effect sizes smaller than d = .4 do not exceed the normal variability observed within the population much and are often considered not to be of practical relevance.

As can be seen in Table 2, there was only one effect size above.4: Students with dyslexia reported that they were less sensation seeking than the controls. All other differences were smaller than.3. The largest effect size was observed for neuroticism (d = .26) in the advantage of the students with dyslexia (meaning that they reported lower levels of neuroticism) but without practical relevance.

Because gender is known to have impact on personality scores [28], we also ran separate analyses for the male and female participants. As can be seen in Tables 3 and 4, the lack of a difference in personality profile between students with dyslexia and controls was true for both genders.

Discussion

Students with dyslexia in higher education above all are confronted with serious reading and spelling impairments [3,5]. This was also true for the group we tested [2,20]. Reading and writing skills were the most impaired, resulting in effect sizes around d = 2.0. As for other cognitive skills, such as verbal and visual memory, problem solving and abstract reasoning, students with dyslexia differed much less from their non-dyslexic peers. All these factors resulted in small to moderate effect sizes [2].

Within the dyslexia literature there is, however, a debate about whether dyslexia is an isolated reading and/or writing deficit or a broader deficit affecting multiple cognitive, metacognitive, and socio-emotional domains, which may affect the personality. For instance, Mason and Mason [29] argued that students with learning disabilities frequently experience low self-esteem, which has negative consequences for their emotional state and well-being. The authors even claimed that because of the adversity people with dyslexia are confronted with the social dimensions of life can be bigger challenges for them than for their peers without reading and writing deficits. Unfortunately, this debate is not based on a rich set of empirical data. The few studies that exist were summarized by Swanson and Hsieh [3] as part of a wide-

Table 4. Results for NEO-PI-R for the Female Students Expressed as Effect Sizes (Cohen's d).

	Women with dyslexia		Women without dyslexia		
	M	(SD)	M	(SD)	d
Neuroticism	**151.33**	***−17.94***	**155.39**	***−17.99***	**−0.16**
Anxiety	27.07	*−4.54*	27.71	*−4.48*	−0.10
Angry hostility	21.76	*−4.37*	22.91	*−4.03*	−0.19
Depression	26.19	*−5.00*	27.12	*−5.10*	−0.13
Self consciousness	25.53	*−4.69*	25.89	*−4.40*	−0.06
Impulsiveness	28.12	*−4.84*	29.07	*−3.68*	−0.16
Vulnerability	22.83	*−3.97*	22.73	*−3.87*	0.02
Extraversion	**166.50**	***−17.46***	**170.56**	***−17.21***	**0.17**
Warmth	30.75	*−3.72*	30.80	*−3.97*	0.01
Gregariousness	28.78	*−4.50*	29.60	*−4.22*	0.13
Assertiveness	23.50	*−4.57*	23.97	*−5.21*	0.07
Activity	25.78	*−3.49*	25.97	*−3.90*	0.04
Excitement seeking	27.36	*−4.09*	28.73	*−3.97*	0.24
Positive emotion	30.35	*−4.06*	31.09	*−4.30*	0.13
Openness	**169.09**	***−17.46***	**171.88**	***−18.08***	**0.11**
Fantasy	29.01	*−5.54*	29.59	*−4.93*	0.08
Aesthetics	29.47	*−5.21*	29.10	*−4.89*	−0.05
Feelings	30.14	*−4.39*	31.10	*−3.76*	0.17
Actions	24.10	*−3.69*	24.68	*−4.73*	0.10
Ideas	26.33	*−5.03*	26.69	*−5.05*	0.05
Values	30.06	*−3.31*	30.68	*−3.86*	0.12
Agreeableness	**172.29**	***−16.77***	**169.25**	***−13.52***	**−0.14**
Trust	29.10	*−4.04*	28.22	*−3.90*	−0.16
Straightforwardness	28.85	*−4.57*	28.14	*−4.47*	−0.11
Altruism	30.91	*−3.08*	31.14	*−3.14*	0.05
Compliance	24.00	*−4.50*	22.86	*−4.27*	−0.18
Modesty	29.36	*−3.77*	28.51	*−3.65*	−0.16
Tender mindedness	29.88	*−3.40*	30.22	*−3.65*	0.07
Conscientiousness	**154.98**	***−20.88***	**151.46**	***−20.23***	**−0.12**
Competence	26.47	*−3.28*	25.86	*−3.65*	−0.12
Order	24.36	*−5.01*	23.44	*−5.66*	−0.12
Dutifulness	28.60	*−3.61*	28.81	*−4.12*	0.04
Achievement striving	27.75	*−3.99*	27.12	*−4.76*	−0.10
Self discipline	24.91	*−4.85*	23.78	*−4.89*	−0.17
Deliberation	23.00	*−5.54*	22.64	*−5.04*	−0.05

range meta-analysis. They reported only a small difference in personality between participants with and without dyslexia, but the data were mainly based on studies with the MMPI, a test mostly used for clinical populations. We addressed the shortage of data by examining the answers of two large groups on a widely used Big Five personality questionnaire.

Like the previous studies, summarized in Swanson and Hsieh [3], we too failed to find big differences between students with and without dyslexia (Tables 2, 3, 4). Furthermore, the small differences we found were often in favor of the students with dyslexia, who had better scores on neuroticism, agreeableness, and conscientiousness. Only for extraversion and openness did they score slightly lower (Table 2). The fact that this pattern was not exactly the same for males and females (Tables 3 and 4) testifies to the small sizes of the differences.

The similarity of the personality profiles of students with and without dyslexia goes against the claims made by some authors about the consequences of dyslexia (see above). The fact that the extra challenges students with dyslexia are faced with do not affect their scores on personality tests, is more in line with the view of personality as a stable construct over time and across circumstances [30], rather than with a view of personality as moldable and influenced by specific experiences [31].

Two comments should be made about our findings, however. The first is that our data are based on self-reports. So, a more valid summary of our findings might be that students in higher education do not perceive their own personality differently than control students. Theoretically, it is possible that students with dyslexia differ from those without, but do not notice it themselves. This possibility is made less plausible, however, by the observation of Swanson and Hsieh [3] that students with dyslexia are perceived similarly by third parties as controls. If anything, according to the meta-analysis third parties have a slightly more positive relationship with dyslexic students than with controls, a finding in agreement with our data.

The second comment to be made about our findings is that they pertain to a group of students with dyslexia, who despite all adversity have been reasonably successful. After all, they have managed to get into higher education. It is possible that the more negative personality consequences of dyslexia prevent other people from reaching this potential. This is a limitation that should be kept in mind when interpreting our findings. On the other hand, there are two factors mitigating this interpretation. The first is that in Belgium all students are allowed to enter higher education when they successfully completed secondary education. This is different from the Anglo-Saxon system in which institutes of higher education are allowed to impose extra entrance requirements such as SAT-scores or A-levels. Because of the lack of entrance requirements, the first year of higher education in Belgium is considered as a selection year, with only half of the students expected to complete the study they started. So, the students we tested were not sure of successful completion of their study (which by itself can be considered a potential source of stress). The second mitigating factor is that two thirds of the students we tested did not go to university but to a college of higher education providing a so-called professional bachelor directly applied to specific professions. Given that a university degree by many is considered as the ideal to strive for, not all of our students may have perceived themselves as fully successful.

All in all, we believe that our empirical data (together with those of Swanson and Hsieh [3]) give a quite realistic picture of the personality of students who come to higher education with an assessment (or suspicion) of dyslexia. These students seem to have more resilience to deal with the extra challenges they are confronted with than the doom scenarios sometimes portrayed. At the same time, we agree that our findings are limited to those students who start studying in higher education. Only a prospective, longitudinal study can inform us about the implications of dyslexia (and other learning difficulties) on personality for the full range of abilities.

Acknowledgments

The authors thank Valérie Van Hees and Charlotte De Lange from Cursief for their help in the study and the recruitment of participants. They also thank Joke Lauwers for her assistance in testing the participants.

Author Contributions

Conceived and designed the experiments: WT MC MB. Performed the experiments: WT MC JL. Analyzed the data: WT MC. Wrote the paper: WT EV MC MB.

References

1. Gerber PJ (2009) Impact of learning disabilities on adults. In JM Taymans (Ed.). Learning to achieve: A review of the research literature on serving adults with learning disabilities.Washington, DC:National Institute for Literacy, 231–252.
2. Callens M, Tops W, Brysbaert M (2012) Cognitive profile of students who enter higher education with an indication of dyslexia. Plos One 7: e38081.
3. Swanson HL, Hsieh CJ (2009) Reading Disabilities in Adults: A Selective Meta-Analysis of the Literature. Review of educational Research 79: 1362–1390.
4. Szmalec A, Loncke M, Page MPA, Duyck W (2011) Order or Disorder? Impaired Hebb Learning in Dyslexia. Journal of Experimental Psychology, Learning, Memory and Cognition 37: 1270–1279.
5. Hatcher J, Snowling MJ, Griffiths YM (2002) Cognitive assessment of dyslexic students in higher education. British Journal of Educational Psychology 72: 119–133.
6. De Smedt B, Boets B (2010) Phonological processing and arithmetic fact retrieval: evidence from developmental dyslexia. Neuropsychologia 48: 3973–3981.
7. Göbel SM, Snowling MJ (2010) Number-processing skills in adults with dyslexia. Quarterly Journal of Experimental Psychology 63: 1361–1373.
8. Rose LT, Rouhani P (2012) Influence of verbal memory depends on vocabulary: Oral reading fluency in adolescents with dyslexia. Mind, Brain, and Education 6: 1–9.
9. Borkowski JG & Thorpe PK (1994) Self-regulation and motivation: a life-span Perspective on underachievement. In DH Schunk & BJ. Zimmerman (Eds.). Self-regulation of learning and performance.\Hillsdale, NJ:Lawrence Erlbaum Associates, 45–73.
10. Sideridis GD, Morgan PL, Botsas G, Padeliadu S, Fuchs D (2006) Predicting LD on the basis of motivation, metacognition, and psychopathology: An ROC analysis. Journal of Learning Disabilities 39: 215–229.
11. Alexander-Passe N (2006) How dyslexic teenagers cope: an investigation of self-esteem, coping, and depression. Dyslexia 12: 256–275.
12. Carroll JM, Iles JE (2006) An assessment of anxiety levels in dyslexic students in higher education. British Journal of Educational Psychology 76: 651–662. http://wrap.warwick.ac.uk/385/1/WRAP_Carroll_anxietyJMC_140305.pdf
13. Trainin G, Swanson HL (2005) Cognition, metacognition, and achievement of college students with learning disabilities. Learning Disability Quarterly 28: 261–272.
14. Waldo SL, McIntosh DE, Koller JR (1999) Personality profiles of adults with verbal and nonverbal learning disabilities. Journal of Psycho-educational Assessment 17: 196–206.
15. Rourke BP (1989) Nonverbal learning disabilities: The syndrome and the model. New York, United States of America:Guilford Press.
16. Cattell RB (1946) The description and measurement of personality. New York:World Book.
17. Eysenck HJ (1991) Dimensions of personality - 16, 5 or 3 – Criteria for a taxonomic paradigm. Personality and Individual Differences 12: 773–790.
18. Costa PT, McCrae RR (1992) NEO PI-R: Professional Manual: Revised NEO PI-R and NEO-FFI. Florida, United States: Psychological Assessment Resources, Inc.
19. Hendriks AAJ, Hofstee KBW,de Raad B (1999) The Five-Factor Personality Inventory (FFPI). Personality and Individual Differences 27: 307–325.
20. Tops W, Callens M, Lammertyn J, Van Hees V, Brysbaert M (2012) Identifying students with dyslexia in higher education. Annals of Dyslexia 62: 186–203.
21. Stichting Dyslexie Nederland (2008) Diagnose en Behandeling dyslexie. Brochure van de Stichting Dyslexie Nederland (SDN). Geheel herziene versie. [Diagnosis and treatment of the Foundation Dyslexia Netherlands. Revision]. Bilthoven, The Netherlands:Stichting Dyslexie Nederland.
22. Brus B, Voeten M (1991) Eén-minuut-test vorm A en B, schoolvorderingstest voor de technische leesvaardigheid bestemd voor groep 4 tot en met 8 van het basisonderwijs. Verantwoording en handleiding [One Minute Test, Manual]. Lisse, The Netherlands:Swets & Zeitlinger.
23. van den Bos K, Spelberg H, Scheepsma A, de Vries J (1999) De klepel vorm A en B, een test voor leesvaardigheid van pseudowoorden. Verantwoording, handleiding, diagnostiek en behandeling [Test for pseudoword reading. Manual]. Lisse, The Netherlands:Swets & Zeitlinger.
24. De Pessemier P, Andries C (2009) Test voor Gevorderd Lezen en Schrijven [Test for advanced reading and writing].Antwerpen, Belgium:Garant Uitgeverij.
25. Vaughn S, Fuchs LS (2003) Redefining learning disabilities as inadequate response to instruction: The promise and potential problems. Learning Disabilities Research & Practice 18: 137–146.
26. Hoekstra HA, Ormel J, de Fruyt F (1996) Handleiding NEO persoonlijkheids-vragenlijsten NEO-PI-R en NEO-FFI [NEO-PI-R and NEO-FFI personality questionnaires. Manual]. Lisse, The Netherlands:Swets Test Services.
27. Cumming G, Finch S (2001) A primer on the understanding, use and calculation of confidence intervals based on central and noncentral distributions. Educational and Psychological Measurement 61: 530–572.
28. Feingold A (1994) Gender differences in personality: a meta-analysis. Psychological bulletin 116: 429–456.
29. Mason A, Mason M (2005) Understanding College Students with Learning Disabilities. Pediatric Clinics of North America 52: 61–70.
30. McCrae RR, Costa PT, Ostendorf F, Angleitner A, Hrebickova M, et al. (2000) Nature over nurture: Temperament, personality, and life span development. Journal of Personality and Social Psychology 78: 173–186.
31. Roberts BW, Wood D, Smith JL (2005) Evaluating Five Factor Theory and social investment perspectives on personality trait development. Journal of Research in Personality 39: 166–184.

Differences in Learning Volitional (Manual) and Non-Volitional (Posture) Aspects of a Complex Motor Skill in Young Adult Dyslexic and Skilled Readers

Itamar Sela[1]*, Avi Karni[1,2]

1 The Edmond J. Safra Brain Research Center for the Study of Learning Disabilities, University of Haifa, Haifa, Israel, 2 The Segol Department of Neurobiology & Ethology, and the Department of Human Biology, Faculty of Natural Sciences, University of Haifa, Haifa, Israel

Abstract

The 'Cerebellar Deficit Theory' of developmental dyslexia proposes that a subtle developmental cerebellar dysfunction leads to deficits in attaining 'automatic' procedures and therefore manifests as subtle motor impairments (e.g., balance control, motor skill learning) in addition to the reading and phonological difficulties. A more recent version of the theory suggests a core deficit in motor skill acquisition. This study was undertaken to compare the time-course and the nature of practice-related changes in volitional (manual) and non-volitional (posture) motor performance in dyslexic and typical readers while learning a new movement sequence. Seventeen dyslexic and 26 skilled young adult readers underwent a three-session training program in which they practiced a novel sequence of manual movements while standing in a quiet stance position. Both groups exhibited robust and well-retained gains in speed, with no loss of accuracy, on the volitional, manual, aspects of the task, with a time-course characteristic of procedural learning. However, the dyslexic readers exhibited a pervasive slowness in the initiation of volitional performance. In addition, while typical readers showed clear and well-retained task-related adaptation of the balance and posture control system, the dyslexic readers had significantly larger sway and variance of sway throughout the three sessions and were less efficient in adapting the posture control system to support the acquisition of the novel movement sequence. These results support the notion of a non-language-related deficit in developmental dyslexia, one related to the recruitment of motor systems for effective task performance rather than to a general motor learning disability.

Editor: Natasha M. Maurits, University Medical Center Groningen UMCG, Netherlands

Funding: This research was funded by the Edmond J. Safra Philanthropic Foundation.The funders had no role in study design, data collection and analysis, decision to publish, or preparation of the manuscript.

Competing Interests: The authors have declared that no competing interests exist.

* E-mail: isela01@campus.haifa.ac.il

Introduction

In a series of studies and theoretical papers during the last two decades, Nicolson and Fawcett developed the 'Cerebellar Deficit' theory to explain evidence for non-verbal, sensory-motor, impairments among dyslexic readers [1–5]. The theory is an attempt to elaborate on why developmental reading impairment is often accompanied by non-linguistic symptoms; although whether such deficits are a consistent feature of developmental dyslexia has been contested [6–10]. The proposal is that the phonological deficits in developmental dyslexia arise from developmental deficits that are not specific to language and that in order to understand developmental dyslexia it is important to identify and consider the neurological substrates of these non-language-related, presumably more basic, deficits. Two specific impairments were suggested: posture and balance deficits ascribed to an unspecified cerebellar dysfunction [1,11] and deficits in "automaticity" or skill (procedural) learning [12]. However, these deficits have not been verified in several studies[6,7,13] and it is not clear whether dyslexic reader individuals suffer from deficits in their posture control system or in their ability to acquire a novel (volitional motor) skill. Here, we tested whether dyslexic readers would show a deficit in the acquisition of a new volitional skill (a manual movement sequence) while maintaining a stable upright posture.

Almost every task (action) related movement of the human body can be conceptualized as consisting of primary (volitional or otherwise) movements, in parallel to posture and equilibrium movements, with the latter providing an effective base for the execution of the primary movements [14,15]. The acquisition of experience and skill can result in quantitative as well as qualitative changes in task related, primary motor movements [16–18]. Postural responses as well can be altered by repeated experience [19]. For example, in adult participants exposed to repeated perturbations, responses become gradually reduced in magnitude and fewer or different muscles were recruited to maintain posture and balance [20–22]. It is not clear, however, whether and to what degree the posture and balance control mechanisms in adults can undergo experience-dependent changes when a novel volitional skill is acquired and retained in long-term procedural memory. There are, nevertheless, some indications that posture maintenance movements can be acquired and retained in a time course similar to that of volitional procedural knowledge [23].

The time-course of volitional motor and non-motor skill acquisition has been intensively studied in recent years, and can be conceptualized as a series of distinct phases wherein quantitative but also qualitative changes occur in both performance and the brain representation of the practiced task [16,17,24–30]. The initial phases of skill learning occur within-session ('on-line'), starting with a 'fast learning' phase in which performance rapidly improves with repeated iterations of the task, but the rate of improvement slows down and subsequently, a plateau phase, in which no additional gains occur despite continued practice is attained [16,17,27,31]. Studies have shown that these within-session gains can be followed by an 'off-line', between-sessions, latent phase wherein the gains in performance become resistant to interference and additional performance gains, in both speed and accuracy, may evolve. These later, delayed gains in performance, require time, and often sleep, to be established and expressed [17,27,29] reflecting procedural memory consolidation processes [16,17,24,27,28,30]. The completion of each phase is essential for a successful initiation of the next phase and for an effective learning process [25,31].

The purpose of the current study was to test whether young adult dyslexic readers would show a deficit in procedural learning or a dysfunction of the posture and balance control system, or both, when compared to skilled reading peers. To this end, a variant of the hand-writing sequence task developed by Sosnik et al [18,32] in which both quantitative and qualitative changes in motor performance were described, was designed. In the new task, the Touch Sequence Task (TST) the required movements were performed while standing on a force plate and required the rapid and accurate generation of 3-D hand trajectories. An additional aspect of the TST was that each task-iteration was cued, i.e., was not self initiated, thus affording a measure of pre-motor processing speed. Pre-motor processing time includes aspects such as visual perception [33,34], decision making [35], the initiation of a movement [31,36–39] as well as the recruitment of motor systems for task performance, engaging a complex feed-forward process and sensorimotor loops [18,32]. Because participants performed the task while standing on a force plate, several measures of balance and posture maintenance were available for study. The ability to maintain balance and posture can be measured by computing the displacement of the body's center of pressure (COP) on a given surface, in the anterior-posterior and medio-lateral directions. The COP is not a stationary point. Rather, it moves at all times even while standing quietly [40,41]. The COP location is maintained by: *i.* the ankles which control the posterior/anterior axis of the COP movement through forward or backward corrective motion; and *ii.* movements of the waist that control the medio/lateral axis of the COP movement. Thus, the TST affords the assessment of the training related changes in the execution of the primary, task related, hand movements, the dynamics of balance and posture maintenance, as well as a measure of the experience related changes in readiness and pre-motor processing. Our working hypothesis was that both reading level groups, dyslexic and typical, would demonstrate an ability to acquire the novel sequence of touch movements and show consolidation phase gains as well as effective retention. However, we were expecting, given a recent study on the learning of a finger movement sequence in young female adults with ADD [42] and the data summarized by Nicholson and colleagues on adult dyslexic readers [5], that the memory consolidation phase (expression of between-sessions gains) may be atypical, slower, in the dyslexic readers. We also hypothesized that given that both reading level groups, typical readers as well as the dyslexics, were healthy high-performing young adult university students, both groups would show effective postural adaptation to the task demands on each training-test session, with, perhaps, a slight advantage for the typical readers [1–5]. Because the execution of the TST required movements in the medio-lateral axis, stronger adaptation effects were expected in this direction (COPx). Some slowing in reaction time (reflecting pre-motor processing) and in overall task performance was also expected, given previous reports on reduced 'speed of processing' in healthy young adult dyslexics [43].

Materials and Methods

Participants

Seventeen dyslexic readers (age 28.5±5.1 years, 10 females and 7 males, 14 right handed) and 26 skilled readers (age 24.5±3.4 years, 14 females and 12 male, 22 right handed) were paid to take part in a three-session training program in which a touch sequence task was performed while standing in a quiet stance position. All participants were university students or graduates. Handedness was assessed using the Oldfield questionnaire [44]. The skilled readers were recruited by notices posted on bulletin boards on the university campus. The dyslexic readers were recruited from a large pool of participants through the Student Support Service of the University of Haifa, which assists students with learning disabilities. They were diagnosed as dyslexic during childhood and classified as impaired readers by the Student Support Service using normative reading skills test in Hebrew [45]. The participants in the dyslexic readers' group were only subjects that received a score of −1.5 S.D and below in the MATAL Reading Test (measuring decoding accuracy and fluency in words and pseudowords, reading a text read orally, reading time, and reading comprehension) and who were eligible to receive learning accommodations according the Israeli Higher Education Center for testing and evaluation criteria. No significant between-group differences were found on nonverbal IQ percentile scores, as measured by the Raven Matrices Test [46] and by verbal ability, measured by Similarities [47] (Table 1). All participants were screened with the DSM-IV questionnaire [48] to assess co-morbidity with Attention Deficit/Hyperactivity Disorder (ADHD) (Table 1). Because co-morbidity with ADHD was suggested as a factor in the expression of balance and procedural learning deficits [8,49,50] participants with clinically relevant symptoms of ADHD were excluded. Participants reported good health with no history of neurological, medical or musculoskeletal disorders that may affect motor performance, and no chronic use of medications. Informed consent approved by the University of Haifa Ethics Committee was obtained prior to each participant's participation in the study.

Background and reading measurements

General ability. Performance ability was measured by the Raven Matrices Test [46], in which the participants were introduced to visual matrices with one part of the matrix missing, and had to choose, from four options, the one that matched the missing part, based on missing patterns and orientation. Verbal ability was measured by Similarities subtest WAIS 2003 [47].

Reading Measurements

1. Decoding- one list of 168 words and one list of 96 pseudowords [51] were given to the participants. The Participants were asked to read each list in a minute and the number of correct items read in each of the lists was documented.
2. Fluency: Oral reading task [51]. In this task, the participants were asked to read a text (276 words) and the reading time was measured.

Table 1. Performance of dyslexic and skilled readers on the IQ tests, the DSM-IV, OMT, background, and reading measurements.

Test (measure)	*Dyslexic readers*	*Skilled readers*	*T*	*p*
Raven	64.94 (15.59)	65.12 (12.81)	−.14	=.314
Similarities (SD)	11.56 (2.26)	11.94 (2.49)	−.898	=.371
DSM (attention)	3.65 (2.6)	1.5 (2.2)	2.87	<.01
DSM (hyperactivity)	1.06 (1.3)	.38 (.7)	1.9	=.07
DSM (impulsivity)	1.24 (1.3)	.46 (.8)	2.2	<.05
OMT (words correct)	65.65 (31.2)	112.65 (20.4)	−5.98	<.001
OMT (words Incorrect)	2.31 (2.2)	1.81 (2.3)	.7	=.485
OMT (pseudo-words Correct)	36.71 (11.6)	62.68 (13.6)	−6.43	<.001
OMT (pseudo-words Incorrect)	10.06 (7.8)	5 (4.3)	2.37	<.05
Fluency (reading time) (s)	285.49(22.1)	175.53(11.5)	5.99	<.001
Comprehension	20.20(3.15)	21.01(1.15)	1.03	=.09
Phonological accuracy %	80.5(6.04)	96.11(2.91)	4.98	<.001
Phonological time (s)	294.5(85.9)	166.7(35.02)	6.11	<.001
Orthographic correct %	88.21(8.0)	98.4 (4.1)	5.78	<.001
RAS time (s)	32.64 (5.61)	27.25 (5.41)	4.36	<.001
RAN (s)	35.31 (8.41)	26.42 (3.21)	5.68	<.001
Digit Span (forward and backward computed Standard score)	10.45 (7.18)	12.91(3.24)	4.59	<.001

3. Comprehension: Silent reading comprehension test [52] containing 319 words and 24 multiple choice questions.

Word Recognition

1. Phonological Processing [51] contained 1. Phonemic Deletion (total score: 25) and b. Segmentation Test (total score: 16). The accuracy (the number of correct answers) and the total response time were measured for the two tests and combined in one score.
2. Orthographic Processing: Parsing Test [53] containing 46 rows of words. Each line contained four words printed without spaces between them. The participants had to identify the words in each row by drawing a line to specify where the spaces should be. Performance accuracy was measured.

Cognitive abilities

1. RAS Naming [54].
2. RAN Naming letters [54].
3. Short term memory and capacity- digit span backward and forward subtests standard score WAIS-III [47].

Experimental Measures

Apparatus. The training-test setup included a touch-sensitive (19″ ELO Touchsystems) screen and an AMTI AccuSway balance and posture sway measurement forceplate (Advanced Mechanical Technology, Inc., Watertown, MA). The touch screen, which was used to display the touch sequence targets and to collect touch times, was positioned in front of the forceplate at a distance of approximately 50 cm from the participant's shoulder at a height of approximately 170 cm (Figure 1). The distance to the touch screen was set for each individual separately to ensure slight flexion of the elbow during performance of the task. The touch sequence presentation and response recordings as well as the forceplate output recording were controlled by a desktop computer using an in-house application and the AMTI data collection software. Matlab software (Version 2008a, The MathWorks, Natick, MA) was used to prepare data for statistical analysis with SPSS (Version 15, SPSS Inc., Chicago IL).

The Touch Sequence Task (TST). Participants were trained to perform a sequence of touch movements on the touch-sensitive screen using the index finger of the dominant hand with minimal body movements. The touch targets were four black circles (diameter 45 mm) that appeared on the screen in the same four locations (Figure 2a) throughout the three sessions of training. The

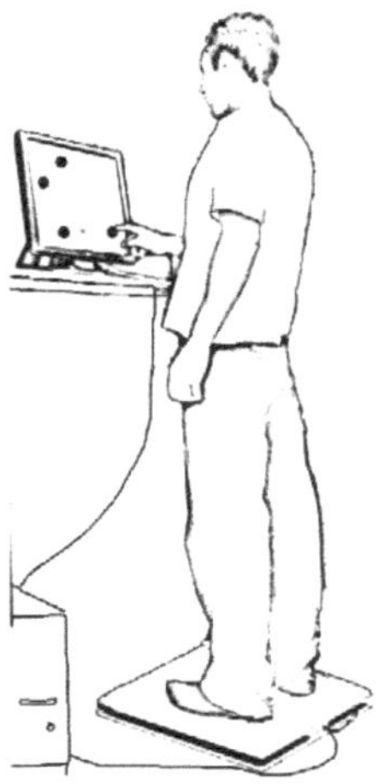

Figure 1. The experiment setup. The participant was instructed to stand on the forceplate in a quiet stance position, in front of the touch screen. The forceplate's output data was streamed into the same desktop PC that presented and controlled the touch sequence task.

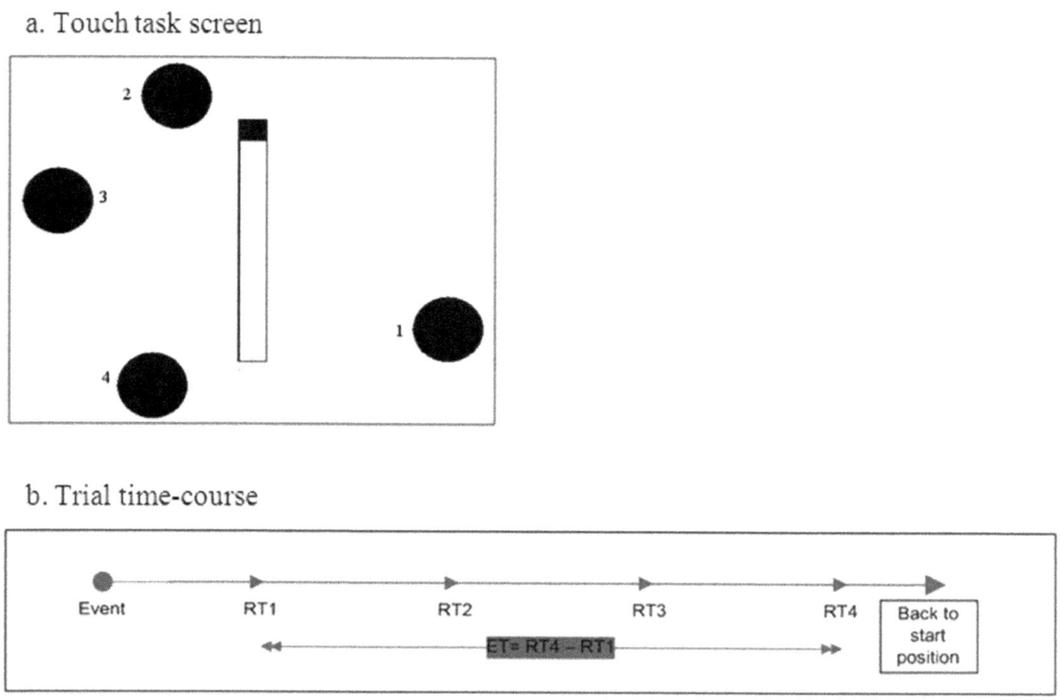

Figure 2. Task screen and time-course of a single trial. a) The relative positions of the four targets (black circles) (the numbering is for illustration purposes only and was not included in the actual display). As the targets changed color from black to yellow, the participant was instructed to turn them back to black by touching them, as fast as possible, following a predefined order (1→2→3→4), and to return to the starting point and wait for the next trial to begin. b) The time-course of a given trial was divided into two continuous time periods: RT1 (Reaction Time for target 1)- the time between the 'start' cue (the targets' color change) and the touching of the first target. ET (Execution Time) - the time between touching the first target and touching the fourth target.

touch targets were arranged in a left-right flipped manner for left-handed individuals.

The participants were instructed to stand in a quiet stance position with the index finger of their dominant hand located near, but not touching, the first target (the lower right target for right-handed participants and the lower left for left-handed individuals), and to wait for the cue to begin the trial. The start cue was a simultaneous change of all four target circles from black to yellow. The participants were instructed to touch the targets, as quickly and as accurately as possible, in the given sequence (Figure 2a). The targets were to be touched only in the predefined order in a counter-clockwise direction (clockwise for left-handed individuals). A switch in color from yellow back to black signaled a correct touch (on target and in the right order). Participants were instructed to return to the starting position with the index finger just above, but not touching, the first target circle after completing each touch sequence and wait for the next trial to start. There was a set interval of three seconds between the beginning of each trial and the following trial.

A successful trial was defined as one in which the participant did not miss any of the 4 targets in the specified sequence. Visual indications of current trial performance and the individual's performance relative to his or her best performance were provided in the form of a small time indicator that went on when the touch sequence was initiated and was stopped when the final target was touched. A small arrow indicated the best time achieved within the current block.

Procedure. Each participant took part in three identical sessions: initial training (first session), 24 hours later (second session), and one week after the initial training session (third session). Task instructions were provided at the beginning of each session and participants were allowed to touch the screen in multiple random sequences to familiarize themselves with its activation. Feedback for an effective touch was provided by the movement of the mouse cursor to the touched location. The training-testing blocks were initiated only when the participant and the experimenter were both satisfied with the participant's ability to consistently produce effective touch movements. Each training-testing block consisted of a 5-second interval of quiet stance followed by 20 touch sequence trials (60 seconds) and a final 5-second interval of quiet stance. Ten blocks were performed in each session.

TST performance analysis. Accuracy and speed were calculated for each block. The measure for accuracy was the percentage of trials within the block in which at least one target circle was missed (the error rate, ER). The measure for speed of performance was the average time for completing the sequence in each block of trials. Unsuccessful trials and successful trials that immediately followed unsuccessful ones were excluded from the analysis. This 'double exclusion criteria' allowed for the included trials to be more unified.

The time for completing the sequence in each trial was divided into two sub-periods, intervals, which were analyzed separately (Figure 2b). The first sub-period was the time from the trial start cue (the targets' color change) to the time when the first target was touched (RT1). This interval was considered to reflect task initiation, including visual perception and the decision to respond to the 'go' cue, as well as the time for preparation and execution of the first touch movement. The second interval included the touch times and movement times starting with the first target touch and ending with the fourth target touch (sequence execution time, ET).

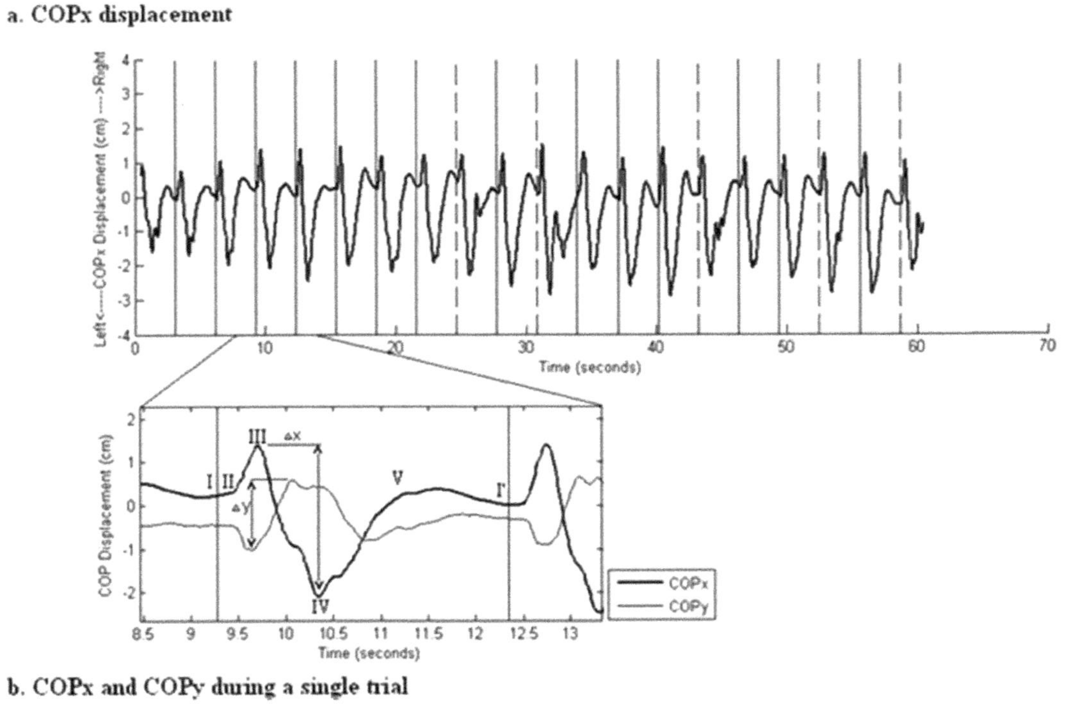

Figure 3. COP displacement during a block and a single trial. a) Representative results of COPx displacement during a block. Vertical solid lines represent the 'start' event of a successful trial. Vertical dashed lines represent the 'start' event of an unsuccessful trial. b) Detailed examination of the COPx (medio-lateral) and COPy (anterior-posterior) sway movements displacements during a trial (positive values are right and backward displacement of the COPx and COPy, respectively): (I) the 'start' cue, (II) as the hand moves toward the first target the COP starts to travel to the right and toward the screen, (III) as the hand starts to move toward target 2 the COP stops traveling to the right and forward and begins its shift backward and left, (IV) as the hand touches targets 2 and 3 and moves toward target 4, the COP stops traveling backward and left and turns again to forward and right, (V) the trial ends as the hand returns to its original location and the body posture is stabilized; (I') the beginning of the next trial. Δx and Δy are the absolute difference between the extreme values in each of the COP axes within a given trial; SDΔx and SDΔy are the standard deviations of all successful trials Δx and Δy within a block, respectively.

ET was calculated by subtracting the touch time of target 1 from the touch time of target 4 (ET = RT4-RT1).

Non-volitional task performance COP Analysis. The maximal amplitude of the movement of the center of pressure (COP) in the x (Δx) and y (Δy) directions (medio-lateral and anterior-posterior sway movements, respectively) within each trial, as well as the trial by trial block variance (standard deviations) of the maximal amplitude of the movement of the COP in both directions (SDΔx, SDΔy) were computed as measures of posture maintenance. Representative results of COPx and COPy displacements during a block of touch-sequence task iterations are shown in Figure 3. The COP is the point location of the vertical ground reaction force vector, representing a weighted average of the pressure vectors on the contact surface [40,55]. Block by block and session by session changes in these parameters were considered as measures of experience-dependent changes in posture control. It was hypothesized that as the main axis that is used in the current study's task is the medio-lateral axis, stronger learning effects will be found in the COPx as compared to the COPy.

Results

Background and reading measurements

T-test analyses revealed significant differences between the two reading groups on decoding reading fluency word identification and cognitive measures. The dyslexics read significantly fewer words and pseudowords in a minute and were slower in text reading than the controls. They also obtained lower scores in the phonological and orthographic tests as well as in the RAS and RAN naming tests. However no significant differences were found between the two groups in general ability (Raven and Similarity Tests) attention (DSM) and in reading comprehension test (Table 1).

Experimental measurements

Training on the given set of hand movements led to significant within- and between-session improvements in both the volitional touch-sequence task performance (Figure 4) and the non-volitional, posture control measures (Figure 5), but these measures were differentially affected by training. The training led to significant gains in performance by both reading-level groups. Nevertheless, the dyslexic readers showed smaller learning effects than the skilled readers and in some parameters failed to show significant experience-dependent changes.

The results of the analyses of variance (ANOVAs) for the TST performance measures (ER, RT1, ET) and the postural movements' parameters (Δx, Δy, SDΔx, SDΔy) are summarized in Tables 2 and 3, respectively. Each parameter was analyzed separately with the two reading-level groups as the between-subject factor and with the three sessions and the 10 blocks comprising each session as within-subject factors. In addition, to test for within-session gains the first and final 4 blocks of the sessions were compared. To test for between-session gains, the final 4 blocks of a session were compared to the initial blocks of the

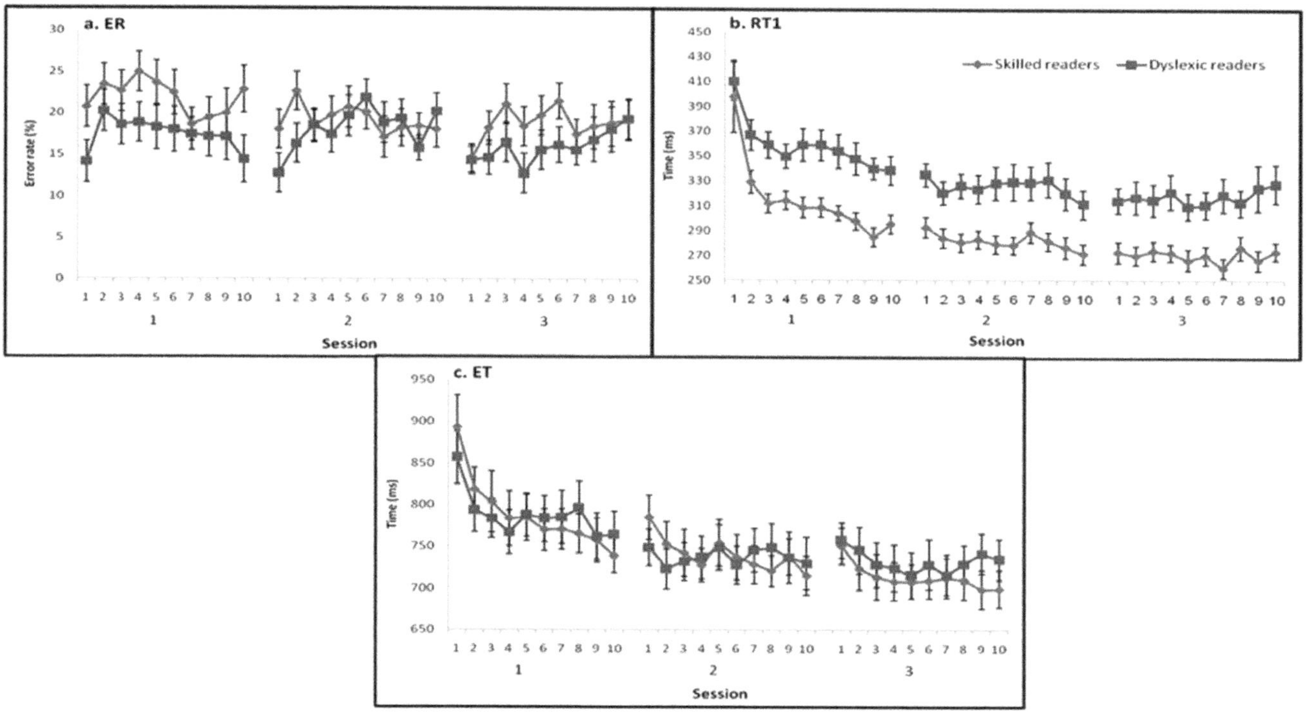

Figure 4. The group mean value of the volitional manual task parameters for dyslexic and skilled readers throughout the training program. a. ER. b. RT1, and c. ET. Error bars indicate group standard error.

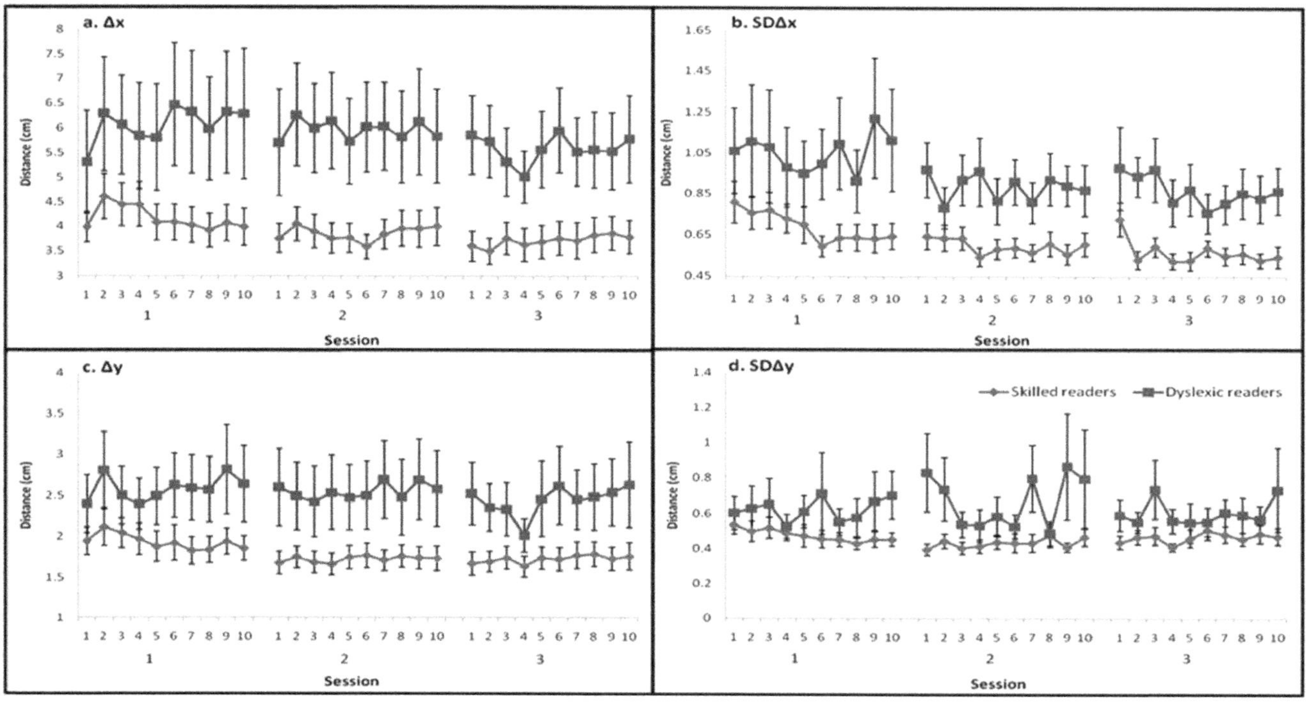

Figure 5. The posture control parameters throughout the training program in the dyslexic and skilled readers. a. Δx – block mean value of the maximal amplitude of the movement of the COP in the medio-lateral direction within a given trial; b. SDΔx – block standard deviation of the individual trials' Δx. c. Δy – block mean value of the maximal amplitude of the movement of the COP in the anterior-posterior direction within a given trial; d. SDΔy – block standard deviation of the trials' Δy. Error bars indicate group standard error.

Table 2. ANOVA results for the volitional manual movement parameters for a) skilled and b) dyslexic readers.

Group	*Comparison*	*ER*	*RT1*	*ET*
a) Skilled readers	Sessions effect	$F_{(2, 50)}=4.99$**	$F_{(2, 50)}=41.16$***	$F_{(2, 50)}=26.55$***
	Blocks effect	$F_{(2, 50)}=2.39$*	$F_{(9, 225)}=11.18$***	$F_{(9, 225)}=15.41$***
	Sessions and blocks interaction	$F_{(2, 50)}=.64$ (NS)	$F_{(18, 450)}=6.54$***	$F_{(18, 450)}=2.63$***
	1st session within-session gains	$F_{(1, 25)}=2.18$ (NS)	$F_{(1, 25)}=24.64$***	$F_{(1, 25)}=15.92$***
	2nd session within-session gains	$F_{(1, 25)}=2.34$ (NS)	$F_{(1, 25)}=1.03$ (NS)	$F_{(1, 25)}=15.61$**
	3rd session within-session gains	$F_{(1, 25)}=.16$ (NS)	$F_{(1, 25)}=.55$ (NS)	$F_{(1, 25)}=4.23$*
	2nd to 1st between-session gains	$F_{(1, 25)}=12.32$**	$F_{(1, 25)}=38.06$***	$F_{(1, 25)}=23.69$***
	3rd to 2nd between-session gains	$F_{(1, 25)}=.00$ (NS)	$F_{(1, 25)}=13.40$***	$F_{(1, 25)}=10.95$**
	2nd session delayed gains	$F_{(1, 25)}=.96$ (NS)	$F_{(1, 25)}=8.59$**	$F_{(1, 25)}=.50$ (NS)
	3rd session delayed gains	$F_{(1, 25)}=.12$ (NS)	$F_{(1, 25)}=7.39$**	$F_{(1, 25)}=.02$ (NS)
b) Dyslexic readers	Sessions effect	$F_{(1.37, 23.33)}=.57$ (NS)	$F_{(1.27, 20.34)}=20.69$***	$F_{(2, 32)}=5.99$**
	Blocks effect	$F_{(9, 153)}=1.51$ (NS)	$F_{(3.73, 59.70)}=2.87$**	$F_{(3.01, 48.15)}=3.44$*
	Sessions and blocks interaction	$F_{(18, 306)}=1.12$ (NS)	$F_{(6.25, 100.07)}=4.60$***	$F_{(18, 288)}=2.38$**
	1st session within session gains	$F_{(1, 16)}=.781$ (NS)	$F_{(1, 16)}=11.84$**	$F_{(1, 16)}=2.01$(NS)
	2nd session within session gains	$F_{(1, 16)}=2.96$ (NS)	$F_{(1, 16)}=.29$ (NS)	$F_{(1, 16)}=.43$ (NS)
	3rd session within session gains	$F_{(1, 16)}=2.80$ (NS)	$F_{(1, 16)}=.37$ (NS)	$F_{(1, 16)}=.58$ (NS)
	2nd to 1st between sessions gains	$F_{(1, 16)}=.26$ (NS)	$F_{(1, 16)}=24.26$***	$F_{(1, 16)}=1.24$***
	3rd to 2nd between sessions gains	$F_{(1, 16)}=1.77$ (NS)	$F_{(1, 16)}=3.65$ (NS)	$F_{(1, 16)}=.12$ (NS)
	2nd session delayed gains	$F_{(1, 16)}=.14$ (NS)	$F_{(1, 16)}=17.99$***	$F_{(1, 16)}=15.20$***
	3rd session delayed gains	$F_{(1, 16)}=7.70$*	$F_{(1, 16)}=1.03$ (NS)	$F_{(1, 16)}=.63$ (NS)

The session and block effects, interaction between sessions and blocks, as well as the within-session, between-session, and delayed gains effects, were analyzed using separate ANOVAs on ER, RT1, ET.
*p<.05,
**p<.01,
***p<.001; NS– not significant.

subsequent session. Thus, time-point (2) and blocks (4) were within-session factors. Whenever sphericity was not supported, the Greenhouse-Geisser method was used to correct the degrees of freedom and determine the significance of results.

Manual (TST) performance

ER. The skilled readers showed an overall significant main effect for both sessions and blocks (Table 2a), indicating a significant improvement in the accuracy of task performance throughout the three sessions (Figure 4a). There was no significant interaction between sessions and blocks, indicating a similar rate of improvement across blocks within the three sessions. No significant gains in accuracy were found within any of the three sessions ($\Delta\% = -2.75$; -1.77; .38, for the first, second and third sessions, respectively) although there was a significant difference decrease in the average ER across the three sessions (ER = 21.9%; 19.2%; 18.79%, for the first, second and third sessions, respectively).

The dyslexic readers group showed no significant main effects for either sessions or blocks (Table 2b), indicating no significant reduction in the number of error trials during training (Figure 4a). There were no significant gains either within the sessions or between the sessions, although significant delayed gains occurred between the end of the second session and the beginning of the third.

There was no significant group effect when the dyslexic readers were compared to the skilled readers ($F_{(1, 41)} = 1.08$, $p = .18$, Figure 4a), and no significant group by sessions or group by blocks interactions ($F_{(2, 82)} = 1.46$, $p = .18$; $F_{(9, 369)} = .98$, $p = .66$, respectively). The dyslexic readers committed fewer errors during the first session compared to the skilled readers (17.4% vs. 21.9%) but the difference was not significant ($F_{(1, 41)} = 2.74$, $p = .10$). The between groups gap in error rates decreased to less than 2% at the second and third sessions.

RT1. The skilled readers showed a significant main effect for both sessions and blocks (Table 2a), with increasingly shorter RT1 intervals across the sessions and within the sessions across blocks (Figure 4b). However, there was a significant interaction of sessions and blocks, reflecting the fast improvement within the first session (a mean difference of 43 ms between the initial four and final four blocks of the session) but no significant within-session improvements in sessions 2 and 3 (a mean difference of 5.6 ms and 3 ms, respectively). There was significant fast learning during the initial blocks of the first session indicating a novelty effect [17], but by the end of the first session performance was almost at asymptote. There was a significant difference in RT1 between sessions, and significant gains in performance that evolved between-sessions (i.e., significant delayed gains) (Figure 4b). Thus, RT1 was significantly reduced at 24 hours after the termination of the first training session. Also, there was a small but significant improvement across the week-long interval between sessions 2 and 3.

The dyslexic readers showed significant training effects for both sessions and blocks (Table 2b) as well, with a significant improvement in speed throughout the training program (Figure 4b). There was also a significant sessions by blocks interaction, with significant within-session gains only in the first session. There were clear between-sessions gains: mean RT1 values of 358 ms, 325 ms and 317 ms in the first, second, and

Table 3. ANOVA results for the posture maintenance parameters for a) the skilled readers and b) the dyslexic readers.

	Comparison	*Δx*	*SDΔx*	*Δy*	**SDΔy**
a) Skilled readers	Sessions effect	$F_{(2, 50)} = 2.25$ (NS)	$F_{(1.52, 38.11)} = 5.70$**	$F_{(1.46, 36.69)} = 3.11$*	$F_{(1.55, 38.76)} = 1.76$ (NS)
	Blocks effect	$F_{(9, 225)} = .82$ (NS)	$F_{(5.53, 7.29)} = 3.80$***	$F_{(3.86, 96.62)} = .62$ (NS)	$F_{(5.01, 125.37)} = .20$ (NS)
	Sessions and blocks interaction	$F_{(18, 450)} = 2.02$ (NS)	$F_{(8.85, 221.32)} = 1.18$ (NS)	$F_{(4.58, 114)} = 1.19$ (NS)	$F_{(7.27, 181.88)} = 1.01$ (NS)
	1st session within-session gains	$F_{(1, 25)} = 2.33$ (NS)	$F_{(1, 25)} = 8.88$**	$F_{(1, 25)} = 2.42$ (NS)	$F_{(1, 25)} = 4.45$*
	2nd session within-session gains	$F_{(1, 25)} = .18$ (NS)	$F_{(1, 25)} = 1.08$ (NS)	$F_{(1, 25)} = .28$ (NS)	$F_{(1, 25)} = 1.49$(NS)
	3rd session within-session gains	$F_{(1, 25)} = 1.23$ (NS)	$F_{(1, 25)} = 2.20$ (NS)	$F_{(1, 25)} = 1.79$ (NS)	$F_{(1, 25)} = 1.36$ (NS)
	2nd to 1st between-session gains	$F_{(1, 25)} = 1.88$ (NS)	$F_{(1, 25)} = 6.35$**	$F_{(1, 25)} = 4.02$*	$F_{(1, 25)} = 3.95$ (NS)
	3rd to 2nd between-session gains	$F_{(1, 25)} = 1.12$ (NS)	$F_{(1, 25)} = 1.12$ (NS)	$F_{(1, 25)} = .00$ (NS)	$F_{(1, 25)} = 2.78$ (NS)
	2nd session delayed gains	$F_{(1, 25)} = .42$ (NS)	$F_{(1, 25)} = .34$ (NS)	$F_{(1, 25)} = 3.57$ (NS)	$F_{(1, 25)} = 2.12$ (NS)
	3rd session delayed gains	$F_{(1, 25)} = 2.63$ (NS)	$F_{(1, 25)} = .06$ (NS)	$F_{(1, 25)} = .45$ (NS)	$F_{(1, 25)} = .00$ (NS)
b) Dyslexic readers	Sessions effect	$F_{(1.24, 19.82)} = .24$ (NS)	$F_{(1.20, 19.30)} = 1.45$ (NS)	$F_{(1.41, 22.63)} = .17$ (NS)	$F_{(1.27, 20.47)} = .67$ (NS)
	Blocks effect	$F_{(2.07, 33.19)} = .74$ (NS)	$F_{(2.96, 47.44)} = .81$(NS)	$F_{(2.47, 39.4)} = 1.18$ (NS)	$F_{(1.59, 25.44)} = 1.25$ (NS)
	Sessions and blocks interaction	$F_{(18, 288)} = .98$ (NS)	$F_{(18, 288)} = .80$ (NS)	$F_{(18, 288)} = .10$ (NS)	$F_{(18, 288)} = 1.26$ (NS)
	1st session within-session gains	$F_{(1, 16)} = .77$ (NS)	$F_{(1, 16)} = .15$ (NS)	$F_{(1, 16)} = .35$ (NS)	$F_{(1, 16)} = .18$ (NS)
	2nd session within-session gains	$F_{(1, 16)} = .06$ (NS)	$F_{(1, 16)} = .42$ (NS)	$F_{(1, 16)} = .92$ (NS)	$F_{(1, 16)} = 1.00$ (NS)
	3rd session within-session gains	$F_{(1, 16)} = .18$ (NS)	$F_{(1, 16)} = 1.56$ (NS)	$F_{(1,16)} = 1.89$ (NS)	$F_{(1, 16)} = .23$ (NS)
	2nd to 1st between-sessions gains	$F_{(1, 16)} = .08$ (NS)	$F_{(1, 16)} = 1.96$ (NS)	$F_{(1, 16)} = .02$ (NS)	$F_{(1, 16)} = .98$ (NS)
	3rd to 2nd between-sessions gains	$F_{(1, 16)} = .34$ (NS)	$F_{(1, 16)} = .01$ (NS)	$F_{(1, 16)} = .48$ (NS)	$F_{(1, 16)} = .74$ (NS)
	2nd session delayed gains	$F_{(1, 16)} = .66$ (NS)	$F_{(1, 16)} = 3.11$ (NS)	$F_{(1, 16)} = .51$ (NS)	$F_{(1, 16)} = .67$ (NS)
	3rd session delayed gains	$F_{(1, 16)} = .46$ (NS)	$F_{(1, 16)} = .52$ (NS)	$F_{(1, 16)} = 1.62$ (NS)	$F_{(1, 16)} = .96$(NS)

The session and block effects, interaction between sessions and blocks, as well as the within-session, between-session, and delayed gains effects were analyzed using separate ANOVAs on Δx, SDΔx, Δy, and SDΔy.
*p<.05,
**p<.01,
***p<.001; NS– not significant.

third sessions, respectively, with significant delayed gains after the first, but not the second, session.

A comparison of the RT1 of dyslexic readers and skilled readers yielded a significant group effect ($F_{(1, 41)} = 14.19$, $p = .001$). Nevertheless, both groups showed effective gains in RT1 (Figure 4b) and there was no significant group by sessions interaction ($F_{(2, 82)} = .20$, $p = .82$), and no group by blocks interaction ($F_{(9, 378)} = 1.27$, $p = .38$). Although both groups started at a nearly equal level of performance (approximately 400 ms in the first block of the first session) (Figure 4b), a significant time-gap (40–50 ms) developed by the second block of the first session in favor of the skilled readers. This time gap was maintained throughout the training program; thus, RT1 by the end of the third session was 273 ms in the skilled readers and 327 ms in the dyslexic readers.

ET. Similar to RT1, the skilled readers significantly improved the sequence ET throughout training with a significant main effect of both sessions and blocks (Figure 4c). A significant interaction effect was found between sessions and blocks: ET significantly diminished throughout and within all three sessions, but at a different rate across sessions. Significant between-session effects were also found (Table 2a).

The dyslexic readers group also exhibited significant sessions and blocks effects (Table 2b), with a significant reduction in ET throughout the training period, and a sessions and blocks interaction. There was a significant improvement between the first and second sessions; however, there were no significant within-sessions gains in any of the three sessions. There were significant delayed gains only after the end of the first session.

There was no significant group effect when the two groups of readers were compared ($F_{(1, 41)} = .00$, $p = .99$) and no significant group by sessions ($F_{(2, 82)} = .59$, $p = .59$) or group by blocks ($F_{(3.76, 154.32)} = 2.31$, $p = .06$) interaction. Both groups demonstrated a robust, significant reduction in ET throughout the training program (Figure 4c).

Posture control

There were significant changes in posture, reflected in the COP measures, as participants executed the touch sequence task. As can be seen in Figure 3b, participants spent the between-trial intervals (on average about 2 seconds) in a quiet stance position and the COP remained relatively stable. When a trial was initiated, the COP shifted from its original location toward the first target to the right (COPx). Then, as the performing hand moved to targets 2 and 3, the COP was shifted to the left. Finally, to facilitate the touching of the fourth target and the return to the starting position, the COP shifted to the right (with a small overshoot). In the orthogonal axis (COPy, Figure 3b), the initial shift of the COP was oriented forward, toward the touch screen. As the trial progressed and the hand moved toward the second, third, and fourth targets, the COP shifted backward with an overshoot; it was re-stabilized in close proximity to the starting location, while participants were waiting for the next trial to start (Figure 3b).

The working hypothesis was that the establishment of a posture control routine would be manifested by decreasing values for SDΔx and SDΔy rather than for Δx or Δy [56]. Also, because movement in the medio-lateral axis reflected more closely the required volitional movement sequence, changes in this axis (Δx and SDΔx) were expected to be more task specific than in the orthogonal antero-posterior axis (Δy and SDΔy).

Δx and SDΔx. The skilled readers (Table 3a) showed no significant changes in Δx (Figure 5a) as a function of training, either within or between the training sessions. There was, however, a robust decrease in variance (SDΔx) across the three sessions (comparing the initial 4 blocks of the first session to the final 4 blocks of the third session) in 22 of the 26 skilled readers, with each individual experiencing, on average, 45% less variance in Δx across the task iterations within the test block. Altogether, SDΔx significantly decreased across blocks within the training sessions (Table 3a), as well as between the first and second sessions (Figure 5b). The average value of SDΔx tended to increase at the beginning of the third session, but this trend was reversed in the second block, with a significant decrease in the mean value of SDΔx in the following 9 blocks ($t_{(25)} = 2.98$, $p<.01$).

Δy and SDΔy. The skilled readers also showed a significant decrease in the value of Δy across sessions (Table 3a, Figure 5c). There was a significant decrease in Δy between the first and second sessions but not between the second and third sessions. Similarly, except for a rapid decrease in SDΔy within the first session (Figure 5d), there was no indication of an experience-dependent change in terms of COP movements in the y direction.

In contrast to the robust learning effects in the manual aspect of the touch sequence task, and the training effects in the skilled readers' posture-related parameters, the dyslexic readers showed no training effects in any of the 4 parameters that reflected the posture control system (Table 3b). There were significant group effects for parameters Δx (Figure 5a), SDΔx (Figure 5b), and Δy (Figure 5c) ($F_{(1,\ 41)} = 7.15$, $p = .01$, $F_{(1,\ 41)} = 7.93$, $p<.01$, $F_{(1,\ 41)} = 5.33$, $p<.05$, respectively), but not for SDΔy (Figure 5d) ($F_{(1,\ 42)} = 3.65$, $p = .06$). There were no significant group-by-sessions interactions in any of the posture control system parameters ($F_{(1.28,\ 52.65)} = .05$, $p = .95$; $F_{(1.26,\ 51.67)} = .37$, $p = .59$; $F_{(1.43,\ 58.84)} = .29$, $p = .67$; $F_{(1.67,\ 68.75)} = 1.92$, $p = .16$, for Δx, SDΔx, Δy, and SDΔy, respectively).

The relationships between attention, motor learning and dyslexia

Pearson correlation analyses were applied to test for a possible relationship between the TST performance measures (the values of ER, RT1, ET) and the SDΔx in each of the three training sessions, and the DSM Attention and ADHD scores (as assessed in the screening phase). Among the skilled readers, significant correlations were found between ET in each of the three sessions and the Attention score ($r = .529$, $p<.01$; $r = .618$, $p = .01$; $r = .669$, $p<.001$; for the first, second, and third sessions, respectively). No significant correlations were found between the skilled readers' posture control and the DSM variables. No significant correlations were found between any of the above variables among the dyslexic readers.

Discussion

Altogether, the skilled readers' results support the notion that the balance control system is recruited to support the acquisition of a new volitional motor movement sequence. Moreover, the current results suggest that although the dyslexic readers were as effective as skilled readers in their abilities to acquire and robustly retain the trained movement sequence, they were impaired in the recruitment and integration of some aspects of the task compared to skilled readers. The current results therefore, support the notion of a non-language-related deficit in developmental dyslexia [57], one related to the recruitment of motor systems for effective task performance. Nevertheless, the results do not support a strong notion [3] of a general procedural (motor) learning disability as a core deficit in developmental dyslexia.

Learning the volitional aspects of the task

The skilled readers showed robust improvement in the performance of the explicitly trained volitional manual task. The time-course of learning as indicated by the three performance measures (RT1, ET, and ER), reflected distinctive phases; phases that were suggested as characteristic of procedural skill acquisition, specifically motor sequence learning [16,17,31]. However, the current results suggest that different aspects of the task may require a different amount of practice to be mastered. Fast within-session gains were noted in the first training session on all three parameters; however, within-session gains in ET occurred also during the second and even the third sessions. Clear delayed, 'off-line' gains [17,30,58] were apparent only for RT1. These differences suggest that different aspects of the task may require different amounts of experience (practice) to be mastered. That is, different amounts of practice may be needed to attain sufficient experience, to continue to a subsequent stage in the learning process, for different task aspects [25,31]. Previous studies have shown that a minimum of task iterations is needed in order to successfully shift between a given phase in the learning process to the next; for example, the triggering of delayed gains may require the attainment of asymptotic performance (plateau phase) within the session [17,25,31,59]. The delayed gains in RT1, expressed in sessions 2 and 3, can be accounted for by the plateau phase attained at the end of the first and second sessions, respectively. On the other hand, the length of each training session was apparently insufficient for triggering robust delayed gains for ET. ET continued to improve throughout each of the consecutive training sessions (a significant within-session learning effect was noted in all three sessions), and in terms of this parameter, task performance failed to reach any level of saturation in any of the three sessions. Thus, it may be that the fast learning phase was not successfully completed in any of the training sessions so the next phase in the learning process could not be initiated [17,25,31,59].

This conjecture suggests that different task parameters reflect different aspects and perhaps sub-systems engaged in the performance of the task. Thus, RT1 may encompass processes such as visual perception [33,34], decision making [35], and motor planning, as well as the initiation of the motor movement sequence [31,36–39]. ET may reflect different processes involved in the appropriate choice, ordering, and timing of the sequence of the different pointing movements that constitute the task, as well as processes such as hand-eye coordination needed to maintain accuracy [18,32]. Nevertheless, the same parameter may reflect different sub-systems and sub-routines at different levels of experience (stages of practice), a notion proposed to explain behavioral and brain imaging data indicating that the performance of a given task may be sub-served by different neural representations at different levels of experience [16,17,60,61]. In later stages of practice, for example, the movement routine employed for task performance may change through processes such as chunking or co-articulation [18,60,62], which presumably may be differentially reflected in changes in RT1 and ET [37]. From this perspective, a number of sub-systems (i.e., neural representations) may have been subject to experience-driven modification across the three training sessions, and the improvement of different performance measures was expressed at different rates (Table 2a).

The current results clearly show that the dyslexic readers were very effective in learning the volitional (manual) aspects of the movement sequence, in retaining the gains between sessions (intervals of a day and a week) and even in improving upon their performance in subsequent sessions. There were robust gains and no significant group differences in the speed of sequence execution (ET). The dyslexic readers were able to execute the sequence of movements as quickly as the skilled readers and showed significant and robust improvement in movement speed as a function of experience and time. This suggests that there was no deficit in their ability to execute and to learn from experience a given sequence of volitional motor movements. These gains in speed were not at the expense of accuracy in both reading-level groups. Indeed, the dyslexics tended to be more accurate in their performance. Thus, in both reading-level groups the gains in speed cannot be explained as reflecting a speed-accuracy tradeoff [16,17,63].

RT1 was the only measure in which a significant group difference was found. Nevertheless, both groups showed effective gains in RT1 (Figure 4b) and there were no significant group differences in the rate of improvement. The significant difference between the groups, expressed in RT1, reflected the opening of a time-gap (40–50 ms) early on in the first session in favor of the skilled readers. This time-gap in RT1 was maintained throughout the experiment. The finding that the dyslexic readers' improvements in RT1 paralleled those of the skilled readers (Figure 4b), suggests that the ability of the dyslexic readers to improve on the initiation of the sequence, as a function of accumulating experience, did not differ from that of the skilled readers. The time-gap in RT1 may relate to the general motor (in reading and non-reading related tasks) slowness of response that has been noted in developmental dyslexia [11,43] perhaps reflecting a deficit in executive functions in dyslexic readers [64]. One cannot rule out, however, that the dyslexics' slowness in RT1 may reflect a deficit in non-motor processing, for example in perceiving the visual task initiation cue [65].

A recently proposed model [66,67] suggests that there are two distinct cortex-subcortex-cortex loops involved in procedural, motor task, learning: the cortex-striatum-cortex loop is involved in learning to perform task-related movement sequences, and the cortex-cerebellum-cortex loop is involved when basic sensorimotor routines need to be adapted to changing task conditions and task environments (motor adaptation) [67,68]. Given this model, the current study's data on ET suggest that the basal ganglia loop is largely intact (in function) in adult dyslexic readers. The latest version of the Nicolson and Fawcett hypothesis [3], which directly refers to the Doyon model of skill learning, suggested that dyslexic readers suffer from a cerebellar dysfunction but not from a deficit in the functioning of the basal ganglia. Our results are compatible with this notion. They are not compatible, however, with Nicholson and Fawcett's findings that suggested that manual motor skill learning is deficient in developmental dyslexia [11]. There is an ongoing debate whether the dyslexic reader suffers from an impaired, general domain, procedural learning deficit. Several studies found evidence for a motor deficit among dyslexic readers [69–71] while others found no between-group differences [72,73]. Some authors have suggested that the inconsistent results in studies on sequence learning in dyslexia may be due to factors such as differences in participants' age, the heterogeneity of the subject groups, and comorbidity with other learning disabilities such as ADHD [8,49,50]. Participants with clinically relevant symptoms of ADHD were excluded from our study in order to reduce the dyslexic readers' in-group variability. Our results indicate, based on the similarity between the reading-level groups in both RT1 and ET, no evidence for a general domain, procedural learning deficit among the group of dyslexic readers.

In a recent study [5], dyslexic readers were compared to skilled readers in their ability to learn a movement sequence in the Finger Opposition Sequence (FOS) learning task. The study's protocol included a training session and a test 24 hours later. Overall, the dyslexic readers were slower and less accurate. Moreover, on the second day of the study a subgroup of dyslexic readers showed a reduction in accuracy [5] rather than the expected improvement [17]. The authors [5] proposed that some dyslexic readers may express insufficient memory consolidation for the novel motor sequence. A more recent study [42] suggests somewhat similar results in young adults with ADHD who have never received pharmacological treatment trained in the same (FOS learning) task. Evidence for an effective procedural memory consolidation phase was found, although the time-course of expression of delayed gains was longer and atypical [42]. The current results are in line with the notion that memory consolidation processes in individuals with developmental dyslexia may be atypical in some aspects, or more difficult to mobilize, but the potential for effective procedural memory consolidation seems to be preserved.

One should also note, when comparing the different studies, important differences in the nature of the training experience. For example, in the current study, a clear indication of the accuracy of the performance was provided using a visual feedback cue following each successful performance step during training, while in the FOS protocol no feedback was provided.

The relationships between attention, motor learning and dyslexia

In the current study, the presence of symptoms of ADHD was an exclusion criteria. Nevertheless, a significant correlation was found between ET in each of the three sessions and the DSM-Attention score for the group of skilled readers. Such correlation between attention resources and motor control has been described [74]. However, there was no correlation between ET or any other measure of TST performance and the DSM-Attention score in the dyslexic readers group. This is in line with previous studies suggesting that motor control and attention do not significantly correlate in dyslexic readers. The absence of significant correlation in the current study cannot be accounted for by differences in accuracy of performances (ET means), which were comparable for both reading level groups across all three sessions (Figure 4). Young adult high performing dyslexic readers may be able to reduce the dependence of motor control on general attention resources by way of compensation.

Learning in the posture control system

The current results indicate a significant difference in the manner and extent to which posture control mechanisms can be recruited to support the performance of a manual task in young adults with developmental dyslexia compared to skilled (typical) readers. All participants in the current study were instructed to maintain a quiet stance position while performing the volitional touch sequence task. The COP measurements, however, show that there were significant changes in posture control, but only in the skilled readers. Thus, in skilled readers, significant changes occurred in measures of posture control – a decrease in postural sway and in sway variance – both effects compatible with the establishment of a task specific posture control routine. A decrease in the variance of performance parameters as a function of training can indicate the establishment of a stable routine and automaticity [31,56,75–77].

A major role of the posture control system is to support volitional action [78] by maintaining body position and dynamically modulating muscle activities and joint stiffness [79]. A recent study [80] suggests that posture maintenance movements can be combined with volitional task aspects into a unitary movement representation. The current results extend those of Berret et al. [80] in which the postural changes were necessary for task performance, by demonstrating that postural changes that were not entailed by the volitional task could evolve in parallel to the volitional skill and be well maintained across a week long interval. The results of the dyslexic readers may be taken as an indication that volitional skill acquisition can nevertheless proceed, in adults, without specific, measurable, experience-driven modifications in posture maintenance.

Practice effects were more robustly reflected in the decreasing value of the variance of displacement than in the value of displacement itself. Some postural adjustments occurred only early on in training. The variance in the maximal COPx displacement diminished within the first session and between the first and second sessions (Figure 5b). Also, as the bending forward towards the screen was found to be unnecessary, this movement was quickly reduced to a minimum (Figure 5c). Importantly, these adjustments were retained both from the first to the second session and over the week-long interval between the second and third sessions. Thus, the current data support the notion that the posture and balance control system can retain the acquired task-related settings in the form of long-term memory [16].

The dyslexic readers displayed little or no learning effects in their posture control system (Table 3b, Figure 5). This apparent deficit is in line with the notions proposed by Nicolson, Fawcett and colleagues of a (cerebellar) balance control deficit in dyslexia [2,12,81,82]. In a more recent version of their model [3], Nicolson & Fawcett proposed a developmental deficit in a putative cortex-cerebellum-cortex loop [3,67,83], an impairment that may prevent dyslexic individuals from developing effective procedural memory, and suggested that motor sequence learning tasks be included in the diagnostic battery for developmental disabilities. The current results suggest that young adult dyslexic readers are not impaired in their ability to acquire and effectively retain experience-dependent procedural knowledge, specifically, the volitional aspects of a task related movement sequence; adult dyslexic readers are capable of learning as robustly as skilled reading peers. The current results do suggest, however, that dyslexic readers are encumbered by a pervasive slowness in the initiation of volitional performance and may be less efficient in adapting the posture control system to support the acquisition of novel movement sequences. These results support the notion of a non-language-related deficit in developmental dyslexia, one related to the recruitment of motor systems for effective task performance, but do not support the notion of a general motor skill learning impairment or a general automatization deficit.

Author Contributions

Conceived and designed the experiments: IS AK. Performed the experiments: IS AK. Analyzed the data: IS AK. Contributed reagents/materials/analysis tools: IS AK. Wrote the paper: IS AK.

References

1. Fawcett A, Nicolson RI (2008) Dyslexia and the cerebellum. In: Reid G, Fawcett A, Manis F, Siegel L, editors. The SAGE Handbook of Dyslexia. London: SAGE Publication Ltd. pp. 11–29.
2. Nicolson RI, Fawcett A (2005) Developmental dyslexia, learning and the cerebellum. Journal of Neural Transmission. Supplementum (69): 19–36.
3. Nicolson RI, Fawcett A (2007) Procedural learning difficulties: Reuniting the developmental disorders? Trends in Neurosciences 30(4): 135–141.
4. Nicolson RI, Fawcett A (2008) Learning, cognition and dyslexia. In: Reid G, Fawcett A, Manis F, Siegel L, editors. The SAGE Handbook of Dyslexia. London: SAGE Publication Ltd. pp. 11–29.
5. Nicolson RI, Fawcett A, Brookes R, Needle J (2010) Procedural learning and dyslexia. Dyslexia 16(3): 194–212.
6. Bishop DVM (2002) Cerebellar abnormalities in developmental dyslexia: Cause, correlate or consequence? Cortex 38(4): 491–498.
7. Ivry R, Justus T (2001) A neural instantiation of the motor theory of speech perception. Trends in Neurosciences 24(9): 513–515.
8. Raberger T, Wimmer H (2003) On the automaticity/cerebellar deficit hypothesis of dyslexia: Balancing and continuous rapid naming in dyslexic and ADHD children. Neuropsychologia 41(11): 1493–1497.
9. White S, Milne E, Rosen S, Hansen P, Swettenham J, et al. (2006) The role of sensorimotor impairments in dyslexia: A multiple case study of dyslexic children. Developmental Science 9(3): 237–269.
10. Wimmer H, Mayringer H, Landerl K (1998) Poor reading: A deficit in skill-automatization or a phonological deficit? Scientific Studies of Reading 2(4): 321–340.
11. Nicolson RI, Fawcett A, Berry EL, Jenkins H, Dean P, et al. (1999) Association of abnormal cerebellar activation with motor learning difficulties in dyslexic adults. The Lancet 353(9165): 1662–1667.
12. Nicolson RI, Fawcett A (1990) Automaticity: A new framework for dyslexia research? Cognition 35(2): 159–182.
13. Zeffiro T, Eden G (2001) The cerebellum and dyslexia: Perpetrator or innocent bystander? Trends in Neurosciences 24(9): 512–513.
14. Lacquaniti F (1992) Automatic control of limb movement and posture. Curr Opin Neurobiol 2(6): 807–814.
15. Pollock AS, Durward BR, Rowe PJ, Paul JP (2000) What is balance? Clin Rehabil 14(4): 402–406.
16. Karni A, Meyer G, Rey-Hipolito C, Jezzard P, Adams MM, et al. (1998) The acquisition of skilled motor performance: Fast and slow experience-driven changes in primary motor cortex. Proc Natl Acad Sci U S A 95(3): 861–868.
17. Korman M, Raz N, Flash T, Karni A (2003) Multiple shifts in the representation of a motor sequence during the acquisition of skilled performance. Proc Natl Acad Sci U S A 100(21): 12492–12497.
18. Sosnik R, Hauptmann B, Karni A, Flash T (2004) When practice leads to co-articulation: The evolution of geometrically defined movement primitives. Exp Brain Res 156(4): 422–438.
19. Galgon AK, Shewokis PA, Tucker CA (2010) Changes in standing postural control during acquisition of a sequential reaching task. Gait Posture 31(2): 265–271.
20. Chong RK, Jones CL, Horak FB (1999) Postural set for balance control is normal in alzheimer's but not in parkinson's disease. J Gerontol A Biol Sci Med Sci 54(3): 129–135.
21. Horak FB, Nashner LM (1986) Central programming of postural movements: Adaptation to altered support-surface configurations. J Neurophysiol 55(6): 1369–1381.
22. Horak FB, Diener HC, Nashner LM (1989) Influence of central set on human postural responses. J Neurophysiol 62(4): 841–853.
23. Elion O, Bahat Y, Sela I, Siev-Ner I, Weiss P, et al. (2008) Postural adjustments as an acquired motor skill: Delayed gains and robust retention after a single training session within a virtual environment. Virtual Rehabilitation, 2008 : 50–53.
24. Fischer S, Hallschmid M, Elsner AL, Born J (2002) Sleep forms memory for finger skills. Proc Natl Acad Sci U S A 99(18): 11987–11991.

25. Hauptmann B, Karni A (2002) From primed to learn: The saturation of repetition priming and the induction of long-term memory. Brain Res Cogn Brain Res 13(3): 313–322.
26. Karni A (1995) When practice makes perfect. Lancet 345(8946): 395.
27. Karni A, Sagi D (1993) The time course of learning a visual skill. Nature 365(6443): 250–252.
28. Maquet P, Laureys S, Perrin F, Ruby P, Melchior G, et al. (2003) Festina lente: Evidences for fast and slow learning processes and a role for sleep in human motor skill learning. Learning Memory 10(4): 237–239.
29. Roth D, Kishon-Rabin L, Hildesheimer M, Karni A (2005) A latent consolidation phase in auditory identification learning: Time in the awake state is sufficient. Learning Memory 12(2): 159–164.
30. Walker M, Brakefield T, Morgan A, Hobson JA, Stickgold R (2002) Practice with sleep makes perfect: Sleep-dependent motor skill learning. Neuron 35(1): 205–211.
31. Adi-Japha E, Karni A, Parnes A, Loewenschuss I, Vakil E (2008) A shift in task routines during the learning of a motor skill: Group-averaged data may mask critical phases in the individuals' acquisition of skilled performance. J Exp Psychol Learn Mem Cogn 34(6): 1544–1551.
32. Sosnik R, Flash T, Hauptmann B, Karni A (2007) The acquisition and implementation of the smoothness maximization motion strategy is dependent on spatial accuracy demands. Exp Brain Res 176(2): 311–331.
33. Gilbert C, Li W, Piech V (2009) Perceptual learning and adult cortical plasticity. The Journal of Physiology 587(12): 2743–2751.
34. Li W, Piech V, Gilbert C (2004) Perceptual learning and top-down influences in primary visual cortex. Nature Neuroscience 7(6): 651–657.
35. Song J, Nakayama K (2009) Hidden cognitive states revealed in choice reaching tasks. Trends in Cognitive Sciences 13(8): 360–366.
36. Rosenblum S, Parush S, Weiss PL (2003) The in air phenomenon: Temporal and spatial correlates of the handwriting process. Percept Mot Skills 96(3 Pt 1): 933–954.
37. Verwey WB (1993) Effects of extended practice in a one-finger keypressing task. Acta Psychologica 84: 179–197.
38. Cisek P (2007) Cortical mechanisms of action selection: The affordance competition hypothesis. Philosophical Transactions - Royal Society. Biological Sciences 362: 1585–1599.
39. Warren W (2006) The dynamics of perception and action. Psychological Review 113(2): 358–389.
40. Winter DA (1995) Human balance and posture control during standing and walking. Gait and Posture 3: 193–214.
41. Winter DA, Prince F, Frank JS, Powell C, Zabjek KF (1996) Unified theory regarding A/P and M/L balance in quiet stance. J Neurophysiol 75(6): 2334–2343.
42. Adi-Japha E, Fox O, Karni A (2011) Atypical acquisition and atypical expression of memory consolidation gains in a motor skill in young female adults with ADHD. Res Dev Disabil 32(3): 1011–1020.
43. Breznitz Z, Misra M (2003) Speed of processing of the visual-orthographic and auditory-phonological systems in adult dyslexics: The contribution of "asynchrony" to word recognition deficits. Brain and Language 85(3): 486–502.
44. Oldfield RC (1971) The assessment and analysis of handedness: The edinburgh inventory. Neuropsychologia 9(1): 97–113.
45. MATAL (2007) Diagnostic battery for the assessment of learning functions. Jerusalem, Israel: The Council for Higher Education and the Center for Psychometric Tests.
46. Raven JC (1960) Guide to the standard progressive matrices. London: H. K. Lewis.
47. Wechsler D (1997) Wechsler adult intelligence scale. New York: The Psychological Corporation.
48. American Psychiatric Association (1994) Diagnostic and statistical manual of mental disorders.
49. Ramus F (2003) Developmental dyslexia: Specific phonological deficit or general sensorimotor dysfunction? Current Opinion in Neurobiology 13(2): 212–218.
50. Wimmer H, Mayringer H, Raberger T (1999) Reading and dual-task balancing: Evidence against the automatization deficit explanation of developmental dyslexia. Journal of Learning Disabilities 32(5): 473–478.
51. Shany M, Lachman D, Shalem Z, Bahat A, Zeiger T (2006) "Aleph-taph" A test for the diagnosis of reading and writing disabilities, based on national israeli norms. Tel Aviv, Israel: Yesod.
52. The Center of Psychometric Tests (1994) Oral and silent comprehension test. government council on higher education.
53. Breznitz Z (2006) Fluency in reading : Synchronization of brain processes. Mahwah: Lawrence Erlbaum Associates.
54. Denckla MB, Rudel RG (1976) Rapid 'automatized' naming (R.A.N.): Dyslexia differentiated from other learning disabilities. Neuropsychologia 14(4): 471–479.
55. Winter DA, Patla AE, Frank JS (1990) Assessment of balance control in humans. Med Prog Technol 16(1–2): 31–51.
56. Cohen RG, Sternad D (2009) Variability in motor learning: Relocating, channeling and reducing noise. Experimental Brain Research 193(1): 69–83.
57. Savage R (2004) Motor skills, automaticity and developmental dyslexia: A review of the research literature. Reading and Writing 17(3): 301–324.
58. Robertson EM (2009) From creation to consolidation: A novel framework for memory processing. PLoS Biol 7(1): e1000019.
59. Hauptmann B, Reinhart E, Brandt SA, Karni A (2005) The predictive value of the leveling off of within session performance for procedural memory consolidation. Brain Res Cogn Brain Res 24(2): 181–189.
60. Hikosaka O, Nakahara H, Rand MK, Sakai K, Lu X, et al. (1999) Parallel neural networks for learning sequential procedures. Trends Neurosci 22(10): 464–471.
61. Bock O, Schneider S (2001) Acquisition of a sensorimotor skill in younger and older adults. Acta Physiologica Et Pharmacologica Bulgarica 26(1–2): 761–767.
62. Engel KC, Flanders M, Soechting JF (1997) Anticipatory and sequential motor control in piano playing. Exp Brain Res 113(2): 189–199.
63. Stelmach G (1996) Motor learning: Toward understanding acquired representation. In: Bloedel J, Ebner T, Wise SP, editors. The acquisition of motor behavior in vertebrates. Cambridge, MA: The MIT Press. pp. 391–408.
64. Reiter A, Tucha O, Lange K (2005) Executive functions in children with dyslexia. Dyslexia 11(2): 116–131.
65. Stein J (2001) The magnocellular theory of developmental dyslexia. Dyslexia 7(1): 12–36.
66. Doyon J, Song A, Karni A, Lalonde F, Adams M, et al. (2002) Experience-dependent changes in cerebellar contributions to motor sequence learning. Proceedings of the National Academy of Sciences of the United States of America 99(2): 1017–1022.
67. Doyon J, Penhune V, Ungerleider L (2003) Distinct contribution of the cortico-striatal and cortico-cerebellar systems to motor skill learning. Neuropsychologia 41(3): 252–262.
68. Doyon J, Ungerleider L (2002) Functional anatomy of motor skill learning. In: Squire LR, Schacter DL, editors. Neuropsychology of Memory. New york, NY: The Guilford Press.
69. Menghini D, Hagberg G, Caltagirone C, Petrosini L, Vicari S (2006) Implicit learning deficits in dyslexic adults: An fMRI study. NeuroImage 33(4): 1218–1226.
70. Menghini D, Hagberg G, Petrosini L, Bozzali M, Macaluso E, et al. (2008) Structural correlates of implicit learning deficits in subjects with developmental dyslexia. Annals of the New York Academy of Sciences 1145: 212–221.
71. Vicari S, Finzi A, Menghini D, Marotta L, Baldi S, et al. (2005) Do children with developmental dyslexia have an implicit learning deficit? Journal of Neurology, Neurosurgery and Psychiatry 76(10): 1392–1397.
72. Kelly S, Griffiths S, Frith U (2002) Evidence for implicit sequence learning in dyslexia. Dyslexia 8(1): 43–52.
73. Waber DP, Marcus DJ, Forbes PW, Bellinger DC, Weiler MD, et al. (2003) Motor sequence learning and reading ability: Is poor reading associated with sequencing deficits? Journal of Experimental Child Psychology 84(4): 338–354.
74. Wulf G, McNevin N (2010) The automaticity of complex motor skill learning as a function of attentional focus. The Quarterly Journal of Experimental Psychology Section A 54(4): 1143–1154.
75. Chein JM, Schneider W (2005) Neuroimaging studies of practice-related change: FMRI and meta-analytic evidence of a domain-general control network for learning. Cognitive Brain Research 25(3): 607–623.
76. Logan G (1988) Toward an instance theory of automatization. Psychological Review 95(4): 492–527.
77. Harris CM, Wolpert DM (1998) Signal-dependent noise determines motor planning. Nature 394(6695): 780–784.
78. Massion J, Woollacott MH (1996) Posture and equilibrium. In: Bornstein AM, Brandt T, Woollacott MH, editors. Clinical Disorders of Balance, Posture and Gait. USA: Oxford University Press, Inc, New York. pp. 10–18.
79. Vernazza-Martin S, Martin N, Le Pellec-Muller A, Tricon V, Massion J (2006) Kinematic synergy adaptation to an unstable support surface and equilibrium maintenance during forward trunk movement. Experimental Brain Research 173(1): 62–78.
80. Berret B, Bonnetblanc F, Papaxanthis C, Pozzo T (2009) Modular control of pointing beyond arm's length. The Journal of Neuroscience 29(1): 191–205.
81. Fawcett A, Nicolson RI (1992) Automatisation deficits in balance for dyslexic children. Perceptual and Motor Skills 75(2): 507–529.
82. Stoodley C, Fawcett A, Nicolson RI, Stein J (2005) Impaired balancing ability in dyslexic children. Experimental Brain Research 167(3): 370–380.
83. Nicolson RI, Fawcett AJ (2011) Dyslexia, dysgraphia, procedural learning and the cerebellum. Cortex 47(1): 117–127.

The Dyslexia Candidate Locus on 2p12 Is Associated with General Cognitive Ability and White Matter Structure

Thomas S. Scerri[1¤], Fahimeh Darki[2], Dianne F. Newbury[1], Andrew J. O. Whitehouse[3], Myriam Peyrard-Janvid[4], Hans Matsson[4], Qi W. Ang[5], Craig E. Pennell[5], Susan Ring[6], John Stein[7], Andrew P. Morris[1], Anthony P. Monaco[1], Juha Kere[4,8,9], Joel B. Talcott[10], Torkel Klingberg[2], Silvia Paracchini[1,11]*

1 Wellcome Trust Centre for Human Genetics, University of Oxford, Oxford, United Kingdom, **2** Department of Neuroscience, Karolinska Institutet, Stockholm, Sweden, **3** Telethon Institute for Child Health Research, Centre for Child Health Research, University of Western Australia, West Perth, Australia, **4** Department of Biosciences and Nutrition at Novum, Karolinska Institutet, Stockholm, Sweden, **5** School of Women's and Infants' Health, University of Western Australia, Crawley, Australia, **6** School of Social and Community Medicine, University of Bristol, Bristol, United Kingdom, **7** Department of Physiology, University of Oxford, Oxford, United Kingdom, **8** Molecular Medicine Research Programme, University of Helsinki, and Folkhälsan Institute of Genetics, Helsinki, Finland, **9** Science for Life Laboratory, Karolinska Institutet, Stockholm, Sweden, **10** Aston Brain Centre, School of Life and Health Sciences, Aston University, Birmingham, United Kingdom, **11** School of Medicine, University of St Andrews, St Andrews, United Kingdom

Abstract

Independent studies have shown that candidate genes for dyslexia and specific language impairment (SLI) impact upon reading/language-specific traits in the general population. To further explore the effect of disorder-associated genes on cognitive functions, we investigated whether they play a role in broader cognitive traits. We tested a panel of dyslexia and SLI genetic risk factors for association with two measures of general cognitive abilities, or IQ, (verbal and non-verbal) in the Avon Longitudinal Study of Parents and Children (ALSPAC) cohort (N>5,000). Only the *MRPL19/C2ORF3* locus showed statistically significant association (minimum $P = 0.00009$) which was further supported by independent replications following analysis in four other cohorts. In addition, a fifth independent sample showed association between the *MRPL19/C2ORF3* locus and white matter structure in the posterior part of the corpus callosum and cingulum, connecting large parts of the cortex in the parietal, occipital and temporal lobes. These findings suggest that this locus, originally identified as being associated with dyslexia, is likely to harbour genetic variants associated with general cognitive abilities by influencing white matter structure in localised neuronal regions.

Editor: Jean-Claude Baron, University of Cambridge, United Kingdom

Funding: This work was funded by the UK Medical Research Council (G0800523/86473 to SP) and was supported by a Wellcome Trust core grant (075491/Z/04, 090532/Z/09/Z). The UK Medical Research Council (74882) the Wellcome Trust (076467) and the University of Bristol provided core support for ALSPAC. The RAINE study is supported by the National Health and Medical Research Council (NHMRC) the University of Western Australia (UWA), the UWA Faculty of Medicine, Dentistry and Health Sciences, the Raine Medical Research Foundation, Curtin University, the Telethon Institute for Child Health Research, and the Women and Infants Research Foundation. The imaging study was supported by Knut and Alice Wallenberg Foundation, The Swedish Research Council and a Swedish Royal Bank Tercentennial Foundation grant in the program "Learning and Memory in Children and Young Adults" (KAW 2005.0179, 2010.0105, K2010-61X-21441-01-3 and PDOKJ028/2006:12 to TK and JK). All laboratory work and the collection of Guy's and Manchester's families of the SLIC collection were funded by The Wellcome Trust. The collection of families from Cambridge (CLASP) was funded by The Wellcome Trust, British Telecom, The Isaac Newton Trust, a National Health Service (NHS) Anglia & Oxford Regional R&D Strategic Investment Award, and an NHS Eastern Region R&D Training Fellowship Award. The funders had no role in study design, data collection and analysis, decision to publish, or preparation of the manuscript.

Competing Interests: The authors have declared that no competing interests exist.

* E-mail: sp58@st-andrews.ac.uk

¤ Current address: The Walter and Eliza Hall Institute for Medical Research, Melbourne, Australia

Introduction

Dyslexia (or reading disability, RD) and specific language impairment (SLI) are common neurodevelopmental disorders, reflecting specific deficits in the acquisition of literacy skills and oral language, respectively [1]. For both disorders, a diagnosis is achieved by excluding known causes of the deficits, such as co-occurring sensory or neurological impairment or lack of educational opportunity. RD and SLI are complex traits resulting from the interaction of multiple factors of both genetic and environmental origin, yet the biological underpinnings and cascading cognitive deficits remain poorly understood. Several genes have been proposed as susceptibility candidates for both RD and SLI. The RD candidates include the *ROBO1*, *KIAA0319*, *DCDC2* and *DYX1C1* genes and the *MRPL19/C2ORF3* locus [2]. The SLI candidates include the *CMIP*, *ATP2C2* and *CNTNAP2* genes [3]. It has been shown that most of the dyslexia risk genes (*KIAA0319*, *DCDC2*, *DYX1C1* and *ROBO1*) are involved in cortical development and specifically in neuronal migration [4]. An important unanswered research question is how genes involved in such a general process as cortical development contribute to the risk for specific neurodevelopmental disorders. Several studies have addressed this research question by investigating whether candidate genes implicated in a specific disorder show pleiotropic effects, which could, for example, help explain the high comorbidity observed between SLI, RD and ADHD [5,6,7]. To date only modest associations have been reported for shared genetic factors across these separate conditions [8,9,10]. Recently

Table 1. Details of phenotypic measures.

	ALSPAC	SLI families	Dyslexia families	Dyslexia cases	Raine
VIQ (mean± SD)	WISC (109.1±16.3)	WISC (100.1±15.4)	BAS/WAIS (60.8±8)	BAS/WAIS (56.9±8)	PPVT (104.9±11.5)
PIQ (mean ± SD)	WISC (101.3±16.7)	WISC (95.4±16.7)	BAS (55±9)	BAS (55.5±7.4)	RCPM (61.8±25.8)
Age at test in years	8	6–16	6–25	8–18	10
Male:female (ratio)	2,946:2,959 (1.00)	319:186 (1.70)	384:254 (1.51)	196:87 (2.25)	708:683 (1.03)
VIQ:READ correlation	0.57	0.62	0.40	0.44	0.40
PIQ:READ correlation	0.35	0.37	0.32	0.41	0.20

VIQ (verbal IQ); PIQ (performance (non-verbal) IQ); SD (standard deviation); WISC (Wechsler Intelligence Scale for Children); BAS (British Abilities Scales); WAIS (Wechsler Adult Intelligence Scale); PPVT (Peabody Picture Vocabulary Test); RCPM (Raven's Coloured Progressive Matrices).

we conducted an association study in the Avon Longitudinal Study of Parents and Children (ALSPAC) cohort to explore potential genetic overlaps between SLI and RD [11]. We analysed a panel of single nucleotide polymorphisms (SNPs), previously reported to be associated with either RD or SLI, and tested them for association with literacy and language related phenotypes. We reported highly specific effects for *DCDC2*, *KIAA0319* and *CMIP* with measures of single-word reading and spelling [11]. These data suggested genetic effects on specific and independent aspects of cognitive function rather than on multiple or more generalised phenotypes.

A direct genetic effect of the impact on broader cognitive abilities for RD and SLI candidate genes has never been tested. General cognitive ability, assessed with standardised intelligence tests, is a highly heritable trait [12,13], yet very few genes have been identified that impact upon these trait [14]. Most of the reported candidate genes have lacked adequate sample size and replications [15]. A recent genome-wide association study (GWAS) supports the strong heritability of cognitive abilities, but with effects that are spread across a large number of genetic factors and therefore not easily detectable in isolation [16]. In the present study, we used a candidate gene approach to investigate a precise question, namely whether genetic risk factors for RD and SLI have a broader impact on general cognitive function. This hypothesis is supported by the consistent observation of significant correlation between reading abilities and general cognition. We analysed RD and SLI candidate genes for association with general cognitive ability in the ALSPAC cohort and detected a statistically significant association at the chromosome 2p12 dyslexia-associated locus. The effect size was small but reproducible in independent samples. Given previous associations between white matter structure and both language-related phenotypes [17] and IQ [18], we looked for any correlations between genotypes at the *MRPL19/C2ORF3* locus and white matter structure. We found associations in the posterior corpus callosum and cingulum, connecting large sections of the parietal, occipital and temporal cortices. The widespread connectivity of this white matter region is consistent with a more general effect on both language and intellectual function.

Results

We analysed 19 SNPs for association with verbal IQ (VIQ) and non-verbal IQ (performance IQ; PIQ) in the ALSPAC child cohort (**Table 1**) across the *MRPL19/C2ORF3*, *KIAA0319*, *DCDC2*, *ATP2C2* and *CMIP* genes (**Table 2**). These markers were selected for previously reported associations with reading- and language-related phenotypes [11]. We detected significant associations (p-values$<$0.001) with VIQ and the SNPs rs714939 (*MRPL12/C2ORF3* locus) and rs6935076 (*KIAA0319*). The rs714939 SNP was also the only marker that showed a trend for association with PIQ ($P = 0.006$). A marker in *CMIP*, rs6564903, also showed a trend of association for VIQ ($P = 0.004$). Our previous study [11] showed that *KIAA0319* and *CMIP* are associated with a measure of single word reading (READ) [19] in a subset of the ALSPAC sample. Given the high correlation between VIQ and READ ($r = 0.571$; Table 1) [11], it is plausible that the association we observed here was driven by reading ability. Therefore, we included READ as covariate when analysing the association with VIQ (**Table 2**). This analysis showed that the associations with rs6935076 (*KIAA0319*) and rs6564903 (*CMIP*) became attenuated, whereas rs714939 remained significantly associated with VIQ. Therefore, while the association with the *KIAA0319* and *CMIP* markers may have been driven by the correlation with reading, the associations at the 2p12 locus appeared to be specific to IQ.

Another SNP at the *MRPL19/C2ORF3* locus, rs917235, also showed a trend of association with VIQ (**Table 2**). For both rs917235 and rs714939, the G alleles are associated with lower performance. These were the same alleles associated with dyslexia in the original report [20]. The most robust association in this previous study was reported for two haplotypes, in different populations, that overlapped for rs917235 and rs714939; specifically, the "GG" haplotype formed by these two markers increased susceptibility to dyslexia. Accordingly, we also tested the rs917235/rs714939 haplotypes for association with VIQ (**Table 3**) in the ALSPAC cohort. The "GG" haplotype gave the strongest association with lower VIQ scores ($P = 0.00009$). When READ was used as a covariate, the association became weaker but remained significant ($P = 0.00024$). Furthermore, the "AA" haplotype showed significant association with higher VIQ scores and with an effect size of similar magnitude.

To replicate these results, we tested the *MRPL19/C2ORF3* markers for association with VIQ and PIQ in four independent samples (**Table 4**). We consistently found a trend of association across the four collections, where either of the two originally associated markers had the G allele associated with lower performance. Associations were particularly evident in the SLI families (rs714939; $P = 0.009$; PIQ) and in the unrelated cases with dyslexia (rs917235; $P = 0.0004$; VIQ). The same SNPs did not show association with single word reading measures in previous studies using the same samples [9,11,21] excluding the possibility that these associations are driven by the high correlation between VIQ and reading ability. We also re-analysed all of the samples for association with reading using IQ as covariate, but again none of the samples including the ALSPAC cohort showed any associa-

Table 2. Single-SNP analyses in the ALSPAC cohort.

			Verbal IQ			Performance IQ			Verbal IQ with READ as a covariate		
Chr	**Gene (locus)**	**SNP**	**N**	**Beta**	**P**	**N**	**Beta**	**P**	**N**	**Beta**	**P**
2	*MRPL19/C2ORF3*	rs1000585	5565	−0.038	0.06859	5560	0.005	0.8475	5159	−0.037	0.03911
2	*MRPL19/C2ORF3*	rs917235	5796	−0.043	0.03136	5789	−0.01	0.6773	5330	−0.044	0.0102
2	*MRPL19/C2ORF3*	rs714939	5555	0.069	**0.00099**	5550	0.068	0.00631	5149	0.061	**0.00066**
6	*DCDC2*	rs793862	5636	−0.034	0.148	5627	−0.018	0.5077	5182	−0.017	0.3908
6	*DCDC2*	rs807701	5837	−0.009	0.6705	5831	0.02	0.4176	5369	−0.003	0.8591
6	*DCDC2*	rs807724	5671	−0.026	0.2885	5664	−0.024	0.4166	5210	−0.013	0.5418
6	*DCDC2*	rs1087266	5850	−0.006	0.7773	5843	0.003	0.8914	5380	−0.001	0.9315
6	*KIAA0319*	rs761100	5825	−0.046	0.02341	5816	0.004	0.8837	5362	−0.045	0.00871
6	*KIAA0319*	rs6935076	5468	0.083	**0.00011**	5463	0.026	0.3026	5C71	0.048	0.00862
6	*KIAA0319*	rs2038137	5569	−0.052	0.01319	5564	−0.015	0.5587	5161	−0.045	0.01142
6	*KIAA0319*	rs9461045	5641	−0.044	0.09869	5634	−0.013	0.6763	5190	0.002	0.9172
6	*KIAA0319*	rs2143340	5554	−0.053	0.06262	5549	−0.011	0.7384	5148	0.001	0.9517
16	*CMIP*	rs12927866	5570	−0.053	0.01085	5565	−0.017	0.4918	5163	−0.038	0.02997
16	*CMIP*	rs6564903	5750	−0.058	0.00385	5743	−0.024	0.3224	5289	−0.036	0.03382
16	*CMIP*	rs4265801	5565	0.028	0.1667	5560	0.013	0.5895	5159	0.02	0.2499
16	*CMIP*	rs16955705	5563	−0.035	0.0867	5558	0.001	0.9578	5158	−0.022	0.2104
16	*ATP2C2*	rs16973771	5503	0	0.985	5499	0.016	0.5133	5100	0	0.995
16	*ATP2C2*	rs2875891	5569	−0.007	0.728	5564	0.014	0.593	5161	−0.005	0.7846
16	*ATP2C2*	rs8045507	5560	−0.009	0.6748	5555	0.018	0.4787	5153	−0.003	0.8716

p-values<0.001 are emboldened.
BETA are relative to the minor allele.

tions (data not shown). The unrelated cases with dyslexia was the only sample that showed stronger association with VIQ, while the other samples showed associations mainly with PIQ. The dyslexia families and Raine samples only showed a modest trend of association, but it was in the same allelic direction (rs917235; $P = 0.064$ and rs714939; $P = 0.059$, respectively). Haplotype analysis in all replication sets revealed a similar trend, with the "GG" haplotype associated with lower performance, but did not show associations stronger than single SNP analyses (data not shown).

We assessed the effect of genetic variants at the *MRPL19/C2ORF3* locus on white matter structure in the Swedish cohort. Among seven genotyped markers, only rs917235 showed significant association with variation in white matter volume ($P_{corrected} = 1.27 \times 10^{-3}$ at cluster level with the threshold of $P<0.01$). Specifically, the G allele, already shown to be associated with lower IQ, was associated with lower white matter volume. This white matter cluster was located bilaterally and confined mainly to the posterior part of the corpus callosum and the cingulum (**Figure 1A**).

The significant cluster in the posterior corpus callosum (**Figure 1A**) was then used as a seed region for fiber tracking (see **Figure 1B** for tracking in one individual) performed in 30 randomly selected subjects. The pathways from each subject were then overlaid on a common template to identify the most consistent localization of pathways (**Figure 1C**). Next, we identified the parts of cortex that were closest to the end-points of the white matter tracts. This analysis showed that the pathways

Table 3. Summary results for rs917235/rs714939 haplotype associations with VIQ in the ALSPAC cohort.

	N = 5428	Haplotype N = 5428		Haplotype analysis with READ as a covariate N = 5030	
HAPLOTYPE	**%**	**BETA**	**P**	**BETA**	**P**
GG	0.317	−0.093	**0.00009**	−0.074	**0.00024**
AG	0.299	0.004	0.857	−0.005	0.821
AA	0.236	0.063	0.0175	0.072	**0.00116**
GA	0.148	0.076	0.0231	0.038	0.176

p-values statistically significant are in bold.

Table 4. P-values from single-SNP analyses for VIQ and PIQ in replication samples.

	ALSPAC			SLI families			Dyslexic families			Dyslexic cases			Raine		
SNP	N	VIQ	PIQ	N	VIQ	PIQ	N	VIQ	PIQ	N	VIQ	PIQ	N	VIQ	PIQ
rs1000585	5565	0.069	0.848	411 sib	0.393	0.272	604 sib	0.796	0.397	279	0.011	0.745	NT		
rs917235	5795	0.031	0.677	418 sib	0.574	0.304	599 sib	0.416	0.064	282	**0.0004**	0.464	1094	0.335	0.955
rs714939	5555	**0.001**	0.006	413 sib	0.034	0.009	592 sib	0.928	0.567	277	0.639	0.079	1080	0.846	0.059

p-values statistically significant are in bold.
RA = Risk alleles are given only for results showing trend of association ($p<0.1$); NT = not tested.
Risk allele was G for all SNPs in all samples.

passing through the region connected the right postcentral gyrus, superior parietal lobule, precuneous, lateral occipital cortex and fusiform gyrus to analogous areas in the left hemisphere (**Figure 1D**).

Discussion

We evaluated the effect of candidate genes for RD and SLI on measures of general cognitive ability in the ALSPAC cohort. The *MRPL19/C2ORF3* locus showed a statistically significant association with general cognitive abilities (VIQ and PIQ). *KIAA0319* and *CMIP* variants also showed associations, but these genes have previously been found associated with reading ability in the ALSPAC sample [11], hence the associations detected here could be an artefact due to the correlation between VIQ and measures of single word-reading. Indeed, the associations between the *KIAA0319* and *CMIP* markers and VIQ were attenuated when a reading measure was used as a covariate. Conversely, *MRPL19/ C2ORF3* markers did not show any association with single-word reading in the ALSPAC cohort [11]. Furthermore, this association remained significant when reading ability was used as a covariate and is supported by a consistent trend of association with IQ in four independent samples. The association would not stand a genome-wide correction for significance level, but this would be consistent with a recent GWAS that predicts multiple and small-size factors contributing to IQ [16]. Our candidate gene approach

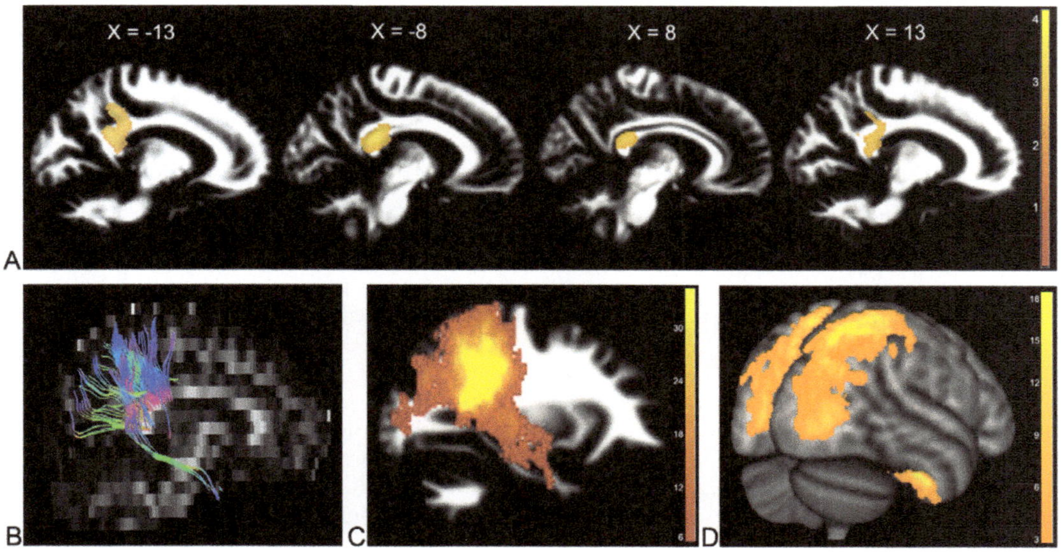

Figure 1. Imaging results. (A) Main association of rs917235 with white matter volume. Sagittal view of the significant cluster associated with rs917235 at the MNI coordinates of X = −13, −8, 8, and 13 mm relative to the midline. The background image is the average of all individuals' white matter segmented images. The colour-bar shows the z-scores of the statistical analysis. (B–D) Structural connectivity. (B) A sample of fiber tracking from one individual passing through the region associated with rs917235. Different colours show the direction of pathways (red for left-right, blue for superior-inferior, and green for anterior-posterior). (C) Overlay of tract tracing from 30 randomly selected individuals. The colour-bar is a count for the number of subjects; yellow shows the most probable pathways. (D) Cortical end-points of the white matter pathways showing that the fibers connect right postcentral gyrus, superior parietal lobule, precuneous, occipital cortex and temporal fusiform gyrus to the analogous left regions.

was based on the selection of previously reported disorder-associated genotypes, suggesting a more generalised effect across multiple cognitive traits. Our interpretation is that the chromosome 2 locus has an effect on cognition by influencing neurodevelopment. The effect on specific endophenotypes will depend on ascertainment criteria, methodology for phenotypic assessment and differences in genetic background. All these elements will have a significant role in the outcome of association analyses when sample sizes are relatively small.

To date, only a few common genetic variants have been associated with measures of verbal and nonverbal reasoning. These include variants in the *CHRM2*, *COMT* and *BDNF* genes [14]. GWASs, which have recently had an enormous success in identifying genetic variants contributing to complex traits, had little success in mapping variants associated with cognitive abilities, with no indication of major genetic contributing loci [16,22,23]. The generally accepted model proposes that cognitive abilities are influenced by many genes of small effect [24] and are therefore difficult to map in the relatively small-sized samples currently available. Gene group-base analysis might be more effective by testing biological functions determined by multiple genes [25].

Both rs714939 and rs917235 are within an intergenic region between the *FAM176A* and *MRPL19*/*C2ORF3* loci. The original study associating this locus with dyslexia showed an effect on gene expression of the co-regulated genes *MRPL19* and *C2ORF3*, and differential expression across a set of brain regions [20]. These genes are transcribed in a head-to-head orientation on chromosome 2p12. Visualisation of *MRPL19* and *C2ORF3* in the Allen Brain Atlas (a resource of human gene expression data derived from 3 post-mortem males aged 24 to 57 years old at time of death; http://www.brain-map.org/), show that these two genes are most highly expressed in white matter of the corpus callosum and the cingulum when compared to all other regions. This is in contrast to *KIAA0319*, *CMIP* and *ATP2C2* which show very low expression in white matter, and *FAM176A* which shows moderate expression. There is no direct evidence that these two SNPs are the causative variants and it is likely that together they tag the effect of a nearby functional factor. The *FAM176A* gene, also expressed in fetal brain, cannot be ruled out as being influenced by these two SNPs. Interestingly, rs714939 is located in a region of high H3K4Me1 marks (ENCODE ChIP-Seq data, GRCh37/hg19 assembly visualised in the UCSC Genome Browser (http://genome.ucsc.edu/cgi-bin/hgGateway)). H3K4Me1 is a monomethylation of lysin 4 of the H3 histone protein and this modification is often found near regulatory elements. This region of high H3K4Me1 spans 9–10 kb and could be involved in the cis-regulation of any of the three neighbouring genes.

The imaging results provide a neural correlate to the genetic polymorphism. Our interpretation is that the genetic variants contribute to structural variation in a relatively large area of white matter which affects both reasoning and reading. It should be pointed out, however, that this is an association study that does not provide any direction of causality. It cannot be excluded that genes affect behavior, which in turn affect the white matter. Our neuroimaging analysis revealed a significant association between rs917235 and white matter volume of the posterior part of the corpus callosum and cingulum. The G allele, associated with lower IQ in the behavioural analysis, was specifically associated with lower white matter volume in this region. Previous studies have reported correlations between white matter structure and measures of IQ [26,27,28,29], supporting the idea that neural connectivity of the brain is an endophenotype underpinning general intellectual ability [18]. Tract tracing of fibers passing through the correlated white matter region showed that they establish long-range connections with large regions of the parietal and occipital cortices, and a smaller region within temporo-occipital cortex. Intra- and superior parietal have been associated with performance on reasoning tasks [30] and the inferior parietal cortex is important for language-related functions [31]. The thickness of the splenium of the corpus callosum, which connects large parts of the occipital, parietal and temporal lobes, has been previously associated with intelligence [32]. Based on parieto-frontal integration theory of intelligence (P-FIT) [30], the lateral cortex and fusiform gyrus from the temporal lobe are involved in cognitive ability since they participate in visual perception, recognition and imagination. The superior parietal, supramarginal and angular gyri are involved in structural symbolism and abstraction. These regions are also important for language-related functions. The posterior part of the corpus callosum has been previously reported as a white matter region with structural differences between normal and dyslexic readers. [33,34,35,36]. It has been also shown that the posterior part of the corpus callosum is bigger in children with dyslexia rather than in typically developing children [37] The widespread connectivity of the white matter region associated with rs917235 is thus consistent with the previous neuroimaging associations to both language and general cognitive abilities. However, substantially more cortical regions and associated brain functions are likely to underlie general cognitive abilities. The integration of genetics with structural and functional imaging approaches holds potential for further elucidating the effects of genes on the normal and atypical development of cognitive function. With a similar approach we showed that three dyslexia susceptibility genes *DYX1C1*, *DCDC2* and *KIAA0319* are associated with white matter volume in distinct but overlapping regions of the left temporo-parietal hemisphere, and that the white matter volume in these regions also correlated with reading ability [38]. A recent study found association between candidate genes for language and reading impairment (*FOXP2* and *KIAA0319*, respectively) and regionally specific brain activations assessed with fMRI [39]. Another study reported two independent SNP associations, both on chromosome 12, with brain volume measures as well as suggestive evidence of an effect on cognitive abilities [40]. Most recently, a study has found a genome-wide significant association between a SNP (rs2298948) within *C2ORF3* (called *GCFC2* in that study) and hippocampal volume [41]. The hippocampus plays an important role in learning and spatial memory, and this is correlated with hippocampus volume.

The association of cognitive abilities with a genetic locus, originally identified as a candidate for dyslexia susceptibility, is independent from a clinical diagnosis of dyslexia and SLI. The association was statistically significant in the ALSPAC sample, which represents the general population, and we did not observe any associations with reading-related measures in either ALSPAC or the other replication samples, including the ones selected for dyslexia or SLI. It is possible that the original association with developmental dyslexia at the *MRPL19*/*C2ORF3* locus [20] was due to a sampling effect and the high correlation between the verbal component of cognitive abilities and reading. Alternatively, the same genetic variants may have different phenotypic effects when combined with alternative genetic or environmental factors and would become apparent in separate sample subgroups. Multivariate genetic analysis have consistently suggested a correlation of about 0.6 between general cognitive ability and learning [42] but there is less agreement in estimating the effects across the range of the entire phenotypic distribution [43]. This would imply that some factors may have specific effects only at the extremes of the phenotype where disorder diagnosis would apply.

In summary, we report an association of measures of general cognitive abilities with the chromosome 2p12 locus implicated in dyslexia. We show, for the first time, that the same genetic locus is associated with white matter volume in the posterior corpus callosum. Furthermore, fibers throughout this region connected cortical regions involved in both language and general cognitive abilities. Follow-up studies might identify the functional genetic variant(s) and the gene(s) implicated. Such findings will contribute to our understanding of the biological pathways underlying normal and atypical cognition and the possible shared factor(s) mediating general cognitive functions and highly prevalent developmental disorders such as dyslexia.

Materials and Methods

Ethics Statement

Informed written consent was obtained from the parents, with the option for them or their children to withdraw at any time. Ethical approval for the ALSPAC cohort was obtained from the ALSPAC Law and Ethics Committee and the Local Research Ethics Committees. Ethical approval for the SLIC cohort was granted by local ethics committees. Ethical approval for the Oxford/Reading and Aston studies was acquired from the Oxfordshire Psychiatric Research Ethics Committee (OPREC O01.02). For the Raine Study, participant recruitment and all follow-ups of the study families were approved by the Human Ethics Committee at King Edward Memorial Hospital and/or Princess Margaret Hospital for Children in Perth. For the Swedish sample, the study was approved by the Ethics Board of the Karolinska University Hospital (Stockholm).

Initial Sample

The ALSPAC cohort consists of over 14,000 children from the southwest of England that had expected dates of delivery between 1st April 1991 and 31st December 1992 [44]. From age 7 years, all children were annually assessed for a wide range of physical, behavioural, and neuropsychological traits, including reading and language-related measures. DNA is available for approximately 11,000 children. For this study, individuals with a non-white ancestry were excluded and after filtering for missing genotypic or phenotypic data we conducted the analysis in a sample of 5905 children. Cognitive ability was assessed using the Wechsler Intelligence Scales for Children (WISC-III) [45] for both verbal and performance IQ (VIQ and PIQ, respectively; **Table 1**). The VIQ scale included the subtests for Information, Similarities, Arithmetic, Vocabulary, Comprehension and Digit span. The PIQ scale included the subtests for Picture completion, Coding, Picture arrangement, Block design and Object assembly.

Replication Samples

The SLI Consortium (SLIC) cohort has been described in detail previously [46,47,48]. This family-based sample includes approximately 400 individuals from 181 families. The samples were assessed at one of five separate centres across the UK: The Newcomen Centre at Guy's Hospital, London, the Cambridge Language and Speech Project (CLASP [49]), the Child Life and Health Department at the University of Edinburgh [50], the Department of Child Health at the University of Aberdeen and the Manchester Language Study [51,52]. Cognitive ability of all children in the SLIC sample was assessed using the WISC-III [45] applying the same VIQ and PIQ subtests listed for ALSPAC. In the SLIC sample, the PIQ score (cut-off at PIQ>80) was used to exclude children whose language problems were accompanied by deficits in non-verbal skills.

The dyslexia-based sample has been described previously [53,54]. It includes 684 siblings from 288 unrelated nuclear families and 282 unrelated cases with dyslexia, recruited through the Dyslexia Research Centre clinics in Oxford and Reading, and the Aston Dyslexia and Development Assessment Centre in Birmingham. VIQ and PIQ were obtained from the BAS similarities and BAS matrices subtests respectively [55]. The similarities sub-scale of the Wechsler Adult Intelligence Scales (WAIS), a measure analogous to the BAS similarities test, was used when age was >17.5 years [45].

The Western Australian Pregnancy Cohort (Raine) study is a longitudinal investigation of 2900 pregnant women and their offspring recruited between 1989 and 1991 [56]. From the original cohort, 2868 children have been followed over two decades. The Raine sample is representative of the larger Australian population (88% Caucasian); only those children with both biological parents of white European origin were included in the current analyses. Verbal and non-verbal ability was assessed at 10 years of age using the Peabody Picture Vocabulary Test–Revised (PPVT-R) [57] and the Raven's Coloured Progressive Matrices (RCPM) [58], respectively. The PPVT-R provides a measure of receptive vocabulary, requiring children to select which of four pictures corresponds to an aurally presented word. Raw scores are converted to a Verbal IQ, standardized for age 2 years and above (based around a mean of 100 and a SD of 15). RCPM is a 36 item multiple choice test that presents a matrix-like arrangement of figural symbols and requires the child to select the missing symbols from a set of six alternatives. Raw scores are converted to percentiles, which provide an indication of performance relative to other children of a similar age. This assessment is standardized for children between 4.9 and 12.0 years of age.

The Swedish sample used for neuroimaging consists of 76 Swedish speaking children and young adults (age range 6 to 25 years) randomly selected from the "Brainchild" study, a longitudinal study of typical development [59,60]. The participants were from the population register in the town of Nynäshamn, Sweden, and showed no evidence of neurological or psychological disorders. DNA was available for all subjects.

Genotyping and statistical analysis

We analysed 19 SNPs across the *MRPL19/C2ORF3*, *KIAA0319*, *DCDC2*, *ATP2C2* and *CMIP* loci that were recently genotyped in the ALSPAC child cohort [11]. The sample size in the present study is larger because we did not apply an IQ filter as described in the previous analysis. SNPs were genotyped using either Sequenom iPLEX assays according to the manufacturer's instructions or the KBiosciences service using their in-house technology (http://www.kbioscience.co.uk/). The genotyping in the samples selected for dyslexia and SLI was conducted with Sequenom iPLEX assays as part of previous studies [9].

For the Raine study, DNA samples were genotyped on an Illumina 660 Quad Array [61].

For the Swedish sample, seven SNPs (rs3088180, rs4853169, rs917235, rs6732511, rs714939, rs17689640 and rs17689863) located at the *MRPL19/C2ORF3* locus were genotyped using the Sequenom iPLEX system as previously described [59].

Quantitative analyses were performed within PLINK (1.07) [62] using additive tests of association. We included two additional phenotypes (VIQ and PIQ) to the multiple testing correction applied in our previous study of the ALSPAC sample [11] which corrected for the analysis of 11 clusters of SNPs showing significant linkage disequilibrium (LD; $r^2>0.6$) and 2 phenotypes. Therefore we corrected here the significance level of $P=0.05$ for 44 independent tests (11 SNP clusters analysed for four phenotypes) resulting in P = 0.001. The ALSPAC cohort has been tested previously for other SNPs and phenotypes, therefore these tests should be considered in calculating a significant threshold p-value, or the genome-significant threshold of 5×10^{-8} should be applied. However, this would be too conservative for the scope of this study which analyses previously reported genetic markers and tests a specific hypothesis rather than conducting an explorative exercise. Family-based cohorts were analysed using QTDT [63].

Image analysis

For the Swedish sample, three-dimensional structural T1-weighted imaging with magnetization-prepared rapid gradient echo sequence (TR = 2300 ms, TE = 2.92 ms, 256×256 mm, 176 sagittal slices and 1 mm^3 voxel size) with the field of view of 256×256 mm, 256 slices, and 1 mm^3 voxel size was carried out on all the participants and repeated two years later for 69 subjects. White matter segmentation, followed by an alignment technique, was performed on the structural data using the Diffeomorphic Anatomical Registration using Exponentiated Lie algebra (DARTEL) toolbox in SPM (www.fil.ion.ucl.ac.uk/spm/software/spm5). Images were then spatially smoothed with an 8 mm Gaussian kernel. The DARTEL outputs are white matter segmented images which reflect the signal intensity modulated by volume transformations applied to individual images to register them into the MNI template.

Diffusion tensor imaging (DTI) was also acquired using a field of view 230×230 mm, matrix size 128×128 mm, 19 slices with 6.5 mm thickness b-max 1000 s/mm^2 in 20 directions. Eddy current and head motion were corrected using affine registration to a reference volume using FSL (www.fmrib.ox.ac.uk/fsl/). The diffusion tensors were then computed for each voxel and the DTI and fractional anisotropy (FA) data were then constructed.

The seven SNPs were entered separately as a main factor in a flexible factorial design second-level SPM analysis. This included both the individual images with and without repeated measures, to assess the variation of white matter with respect to the genetic markers and was corrected for the effect of age, sex, handedness and total white matter volume. Age X gene and gender X gene interaction effects were also included in the model. As a part of this exploratory analysis, the significance level was corrected at the cluster level using non-stationary cluster extent correction [64] for multiple comparisons resulting from searching the entire white matter volume as well as for the seven SNPs (Bonferroni correction, $P_{corrected} < 0.0014$ for comparison of searching the entire brain with a threshold of $P < 0.01$, as implemented in the SPM software).

The region showing the significant effect was saved as a binary region of interest (ROI). This ROI was then transformed to each individual's DTI space, to be used as a seed ROI for white matter fiber tracking. Deterministic fiber tracking was applied on 30 randomly selected subjects by starting tractography from the ROI following the principal eigenvector direction using 1 mm steps, considering thresholds of 0.15 for FA values and 30 for angular degree using ExploreDTI v4.7.3. (www.exploredti.com). Computed tracts from all individuals were then averaged across all 30 participants to derive a probabilistic map of the white matter pathways passing through the overlapping areas.

Acknowledgments

We are grateful to all the families and sample donors who took part in this study. We are grateful to Dorothy Bishop for her guidance in handling cognitive phenotypes and useful discussion. SP is a Royal Society University Research Fellow. DFN is an MRC Career Development Fellow and a Junior Research Fellow of St John's College, Oxford. AW is a NHMRC Career Development Fellow. This publication is the work of the authors and SP will serve as guarantor for the contents of this paper.

Author Contributions

Conceived and designed the experiments: CEP SR JS A.P. Monaco JK JBT TK SP. Performed the experiments: TSS FD DN AJOW MP HM SP. Analyzed the data: TSS FD DN AJOW MP HM QWA A.P. Morris JBT SP. Wrote the paper: TSS FD DN AJOW MP HM JK JBT SP.

References

1. Pennington BF, Bishop DV (2009) Relations among speech, language, and reading disorders. Annu Rev Psychol 60: 283–306.
2. Scerri TS, Schulte-Korne G (2010) Genetics of developmental dyslexia. Eur Child Adolesc Psychiatry 19: 179–197.
3. Newbury DF, Monaco AP (2010) Genetic advances in the study of speech and language disorders. Neuron 68: 309–320.
4. Galaburda AM, LoTurco J, Ramus F, Fitch RH, Rosen GD (2006) From genes to behavior in developmental dyslexia. Nat Neurosci 9: 1213–1217.
5. Snowling M, Bishop DV, Stothard SE (2000) Is preschool language impairment a risk factor for dyslexia in adolescence? J Child Psychol Psychiatry 41: 587–600.
6. McArthur GM, Hogben JH, Edwards VT, Heath SM, Mengler ED (2000) On the "specifics" of specific reading disability and specific language impairment. J Child Psychol Psychiatry 41: 869–874.
7. Pennington BF (2006) From single to multiple deficit models of developmental disorders. Cognition 101: 385–413.
8. Rice ML, Smith SD, Gayan J (2009) Convergent genetic linkage and associations to language, speech and reading measures in families of probands with Specific Language Impairment. J Neurodev Disord 1: 264–282.
9. Newbury DF, Paracchini S, Scerri TS, Winchester L, Addis L, et al. (2011) Investigation of dyslexia and SLI risk variants in reading and language-impaired subjects. Behav Genet 41: 90–104.
10. Bates TC, Luciano M, Medland SE, Montgomery GW, Wright MJ, et al. (2011) Genetic Variance in a Component of the Language Acquisition Device: ROBO1 Polymorphisms Associated with Phonological Buffer Deficits. Behav Genet 41: 50–57.
11. Scerri TS, Morris AP, Buckingham LL, Newbury DF, Miller LL, et al. (2011) DCDC2, KIAA0319 and CMIP are associated with reading-related traits. Biol Psychiatry 70: 237–245.
12. Bouchard TJ, Jr., McGue M (1981) Familial studies of intelligence: a review. Science 212: 1055–1059.
13. Plomin R, Spinath FM (2002) Genetics and general cognitive ability (g). Trends Cogn Sci 6: 169–176.
14. Deary IJ, Johnson W, Houlihan LM (2009) Genetic foundations of human intelligence. Hum Genet 126: 215–232.
15. Chabris CF, Hebert BM, Benjamin DJ, Beauchamp JP, Cesarini D, et al. (2012) Most reported genetic associations with general intelligence are probably false positives. Psychological Science In press.
16. Davies G, Tenesa A, Payton A, Yang J, Harris SE, et al. (2011) Genome-wide association studies establish that human intelligence is highly heritable and polygenic. Mol Psychiatry 16: 996–1005.
17. Klingberg T, Hedehus M, Temple E, Salz T, Gabrieli JD, et al. (2000) Microstructure of temporo-parietal white matter as a basis for reading ability: evidence from diffusion tensor magnetic resonance imaging. Neuron 25: 493–500.
18. Deary IJ, Penke L, Johnson W (2010) The neuroscience of human intelligence differences. Nat Rev Neurosci 11: 201–211.
19. Rust J, Golombok S, Trickey G (1993) WORD: Wechsler Objective Reading Dimensional Manual. Sidcup, UK: Psychological Corporation.
20. Anthoni H, Zucchelli M, Matsson H, Muller-Myhsok B, Fransson I, et al. (2007) A locus on 2p12 containing the co-regulated MRPL19 and C2ORF3 genes is associated to dyslexia. Hum Mol Genet 16: 667–677.
21. Paracchini S, Ang QW, Stanley FJ, Monaco AP, Pennell CE, et al. (2010) Analysis of dyslexia candidate genes in the Raine cohort representing the general Australian population. Genes Brain Behav 10: 158–165.
22. Davis OS, Butcher LM, Docherty SJ, Meaburn EL, Curtis CJ, et al. (2010) A three-stage genome-wide association study of general cognitive ability: hunting the small effects. Behav Genet 40: 759–767.
23. Pan Y, Wang KS, Aragam N (2011) NTM and NR3C2 polymorphisms influencing intelligence: family-based association studies. Prog Neuropsychopharmacol Biol Psychiatry 35: 154–160.
24. Plomin R (1999) Genetics and general cognitive ability. Nature 402: C25–29.
25. Ruano D, Abecasis GR, Glaser B, Lips ES, Cornelisse LN, et al. (2010) Functional gene group analysis reveals a role of synaptic heterotrimeric G proteins in cognitive ability. Am J Hum Genet 86: 113–125.

26. Deary IJ, Bastin ME, Pattie A, Clayden JD, Whalley LJ, et al. (2006) White matter integrity and cognition in childhood and old age. Neurology 66: 505–512.
27. Schmithorst VJ, Wilke M, Dardzinski BJ, Holland SK (2005) Cognitive functions correlate with white matter architecture in a normal pediatric population: a diffusion tensor MRI study. Hum Brain Mapp 26: 139–147.
28. Chiang MC, Barysheva M, Shattuck DW, Lee AD, Madsen SK, et al. (2009) Genetics of brain fiber architecture and intellectual performance. J Neurosci 29: 2212–2224.
29. Fjell AM, Westlye LT, Amlien IK, Walhovd KB (2011) Reduced white matter integrity is related to cognitive instability. J Neurosci 31: 18060–18072.
30. Jung RE, Haier RJ (2007) The Parieto-Frontal Integration Theory (P-FIT) of intelligence: converging neuroimaging evidence. Behav Brain Sci 30: 135–154; discussion 154–187.
31. Richlan F, Kronbichler M, Wimmer H (2011) Meta-analyzing brain dysfunctions in dyslexic children and adults. Neuroimage 56: 1735–1742.
32. Luders E, Thompson PM, Narr KL, Zamanyan A, Chou YY, et al. (2011) The link between callosal thickness and intelligence in healthy children and adolescents. Neuroimage 54: 1823–1830.
33. Vandermosten M, Boets B, Poelmans H, Sunaert S, Wouters J, et al. (2012) A tractography study in dyslexia: neuroanatomic correlates of orthographic, phonological and speech processing. Brain 135: 935–948.
34. Frye RE, Hasan K, Xue L, Strickland D, Malmberg B, et al. (2008) Splenium microstructure is related to two dimensions of reading skill. Neuroreport 19: 1627–1631.
35. Dougherty RF, Ben-Shachar M, Deutsch GK, Hernandez A, Fox GR, et al. (2007) Temporal-callosal pathway diffusivity predicts phonological skills in children. Proc Natl Acad Sci U S A 104: 8556–8561.
36. Odegard TN, Farris EA, Ring J, McColl R, Black J (2009) Brain connectivity in non-reading impaired children and children diagnosed with developmental dyslexia. Neuropsychologia 47: 1972–1977.
37. Hasan KM, Molfese DL, Walimuni IS, Stuebing KK, Papanicolaou AC, et al. (2012) Diffusion tensor quantification and cognitive correlates of the macrostructure and microstructure of the corpus callosum in typically developing and dyslexic children. NMR Biomed.
38. Darki F, Peyrard-Janvid M, Matsson H, Kere J, Klingberg T (2012) Three Dyslexia Susceptibility Genes, DYX1C1, DCDC2, and KIAA0319, Affect Temporo-Parietal White Matter Structure. Biol Psychiatry.
39. Pinel P, Fauchereau F, Moreno A, Barbot A, Lathrop M, et al. (2012) Genetic Variants of FOXP2 and KIAA0319/TTRAP/THEM2 Locus Are Associated with Altered Brain Activation in Distinct Language-Related Regions. J Neurosci 32: 817–825.
40. Stein JL, Medland SE, Vasquez AA, Hibar DP, Senstad RE, et al. (2012) Identification of common variants associated with human hippocampal and intracranial volumes. Nat Genet.
41. Melville SA, Buros J, Parrado AR, Vardarajan B, Logue MW, et al. (2012) Multiple loci influencing hippocampal degeneration identified by genome scan. Ann Neurol 72: 65–75.
42. Plomin R, Kovas Y (2005) Generalist genes and learning disabilities. Psychol Bull 131: 592–617.
43. Haworth CM, Dale PS, Plomin R (2009) Generalist genes and high cognitive abilities. Behav Genet 39: 437–445.
44. Golding J, Pembrey M, Jones R (2001) ALSPAC–the Avon Longitudinal Study of Parents and Children. I. Study methodology. Paediatr Perinat Epidemiol 15: 74–87.
45. Wechsler D, Golombok S, Rust J (1992) WISC-IIIUK: Wechsler Intelligence Scale for Children. Sidcup, UK: The Psycological Corporation.
46. SLIC (2002) A genomewide scan identifies two novel loci involved in specific language impairment. Am J Hum Genet 70: 384–398.
47. SLIC (2004) Highly significant linkage to the SLI1 locus in an expanded sample of individuals affected by specific language impairment. Am J Hum Genet 74: 1225–1238.
48. Falcaro M, Pickles A, Newbury DF, Addis L, Banfield E, et al. (2008) Genetic and phenotypic effects of phonological short-term memory and grammatical morphology in specific language impairment. Genes Brain Behav 7: 393–402.
49. Burden V, Stott CM, Forge J, Goodyer I (1996) The Cambridge Language and Speech Project (CLASP). I. Detection of language difficulties at 36 to 39 months. Dev Med Child Neurol 38: 613–631.
50. Clark A, O'Hare A, Watson J, Cohen W, Cowie H, et al. (2007) Severe receptive language disorder in childhood–familial aspects and long-term outcomes: results from a Scottish study. Arch Dis Child 92: 614–619.
51. Conti-Ramsden G, Botting N (1999) Characteristics of children attending language units in England: a national study of 7-year-olds. Int J Lang Commun Disord 34: 359–366.
52. Conti-Ramsden G, Crutchley A, Botting N (1997) The extent to which psychometric tests differentiate subgroups of children with SLI. J Speech Lang Hear Res 40: 765–777.
53. Francks C, Paracchini S, Smith SD, Richardson AJ, Scerri TS, et al. (2004) A 77-kilobase region of chromosome 6p22.2 is associated with dyslexia in families from the United Kingdom and from the United States. Am J Hum Genet 75: 1046–1058.
54. Scerri TS, Paracchini S, Morris A, MacPhie IL, Talcott J, et al. (2010) Identification of candidate genes for dyslexia susceptibility on chromosome 18. PLoS One 5: e13712.
55. Elliot C, Murray D, Pearson L (1983) British Abilities Scales Windsor, UK: NFER-Nelson.
56. Newnham JP, Evans SF, Michael CA, Stanley FJ, Landau LI (1993) Effects of frequent ultrasound during pregnancy: a randomised controlled trial. Lancet 342: 887–891.
57. Dunn L, Dunn L (1981) Peabody Picture Vocabulary Test-Revised: Manual. Circle Pines, MN: American Guidance Services.
58. Raven JC (1976) Ravens Coloured Progressive Matrices. London: Oxford Psychologists Press.
59. Dumontheil I, Roggeman C, Ziermans T, Peyrard-Janvid M, Matsson H, et al. (2011) Influence of the COMT genotype on working memory and brain activity changes during development. Biol Psychiatry 70: 222–229.
60. Soderqvist S, McNab F, Peyrard-Janvid M, Matsson H, Humphreys K, et al. (2010) The SNAP25 gene is linked to working memory capacity and maturation of the posterior cingulate cortex during childhood. Biol Psychiatry 68: 1120–1125.
61. Whitehouse AJ, Bishop DV, Ang QW, Pennell CE, Fisher SE (2011) CNTNAP2 variants affect early language development in the general population. Genes Brain Behav.
62. Purcell S, Neale B, Todd-Brown K, Thomas L, Ferreira MA, et al. (2007) PLINK: a tool set for whole-genome association and population-based linkage analyses. Am J Hum Genet 81: 559–575.
63. Abecasis GR, Cardon LR, Cookson WO (2000) A general test of association for quantitative traits in nuclear families. Am J Hum Genet 66: 279–292.
64. Hayasaka S, Phan KL, Liberzon I, Worsley KJ, Nichols TE (2004) Nonstationary cluster-size inference with random field and permutation methods. Neuroimage 22: 676–687.

5

Children with ADHD Symptoms Have a Higher Risk for Reading, Spelling and Math Difficulties in the GINIplus and LISAplus Cohort Studies

Darina Czamara[1,2], Carla M. T. Tiesler[3,4], Gabriele Kohlböck[3], Dietrich Berdel[5], Barbara Hoffmann[6], Carl-Peter Bauer[7], Sibylle Koletzko[8], Beate Schaaf[9], Irina Lehmann[10], Olf Herbarth[11], Andrea von Berg[5], Bertram Müller-Myhsok[1,2], Gerd Schulte-Körne[12], Joachim Heinrich[3]*

1 Max Planck Institute of Psychiatry, Munich, Germany, **2** Munich Cluster for Systems Neurology (SyNergy), Munich, Germany, **3** Helmholtz Zentrum München, German Research Center for Environmental Health, Institute of Epidemiology I, Neuherberg, Germany, **4** Ludwig-Maximilians-University of Munich, Dr. von Hauner Children's Hospital, Division of Metabolic Diseases and Nutritional Medicine, Munich, Germany, **5** Marien-Hospital Wesel, Department of Pediatrics, Wesel, Germany, **6** IUF Leibniz Research Institute for Environmental Medicine and Medical Faculty, Heinrich Heine University of Düsseldorf, Düsseldorf, Germany, **7** Technical University of Munich, Department of Pediatrics, Munich, Germany, **8** Ludwig-Maximilians-University of Munich, Dr. von Hauner Children's Hospital, Division of Paediatric Gastroenterology and Hepatology, Munich, Germany, **9** Medical Practice for Pediatrics, Bad Honnef, Germany, **10** Helmholtz Centre for Environmental Research - UFZ, Department for Environmental Immunology, Leipzig, Germany, **11** University of Leipzig, Faculty of Medicine, Environmental Medicine and Hygiene, Leipzig, Germany, **12** Department of Child and Adolescent Psychiatry, Psychosomatics and Psychotherapy, Ludwig-Maximilians-University of Munich, Munich, Germany

Abstract

Attention-deficit/hyperactivity disorder (ADHD) and dyslexia belong to the most common neuro-behavioral childhood disorders with prevalences of around 5% in school-aged children. It is estimated that 20–60% of individuals affected with ADHD also present with learning disorders. We investigated the comorbidity between ADHD symptoms and reading/spelling and math difficulties in two on-going population-based birth cohort studies. Children with ADHD symptoms were at significantly higher risk of also showing reading/spelling difficulties or disorder (Odds Ratio (OR) = 2.80, $p = 6.59 \times 10^{-13}$) as compared to children without ADHD symptoms. For math difficulties the association was similar (OR = 2.55, $p = 3.63 \times 10^{-04}$). Our results strengthen the hypothesis that ADHD and learning disorders are comorbid and share, at least partially, the same underlying process. Up to date, it is not clear, on which exact functional processes this comorbidity is based.

Editor: Michel Baudry, Western University of Health Sciences, United States of America

Funding: The GINI Intervention study was funded for 3 years by grants of the Federal Ministry for Education, Science, Research and Technology (Grant No. 01 EE 9401-4) and Helmholtz Zentrum München, the 6 and 10 years follow-up of the GINIplus study was funded by Helmholtz Zentrum München and, in addition, partly by the Federal Ministry of Environment (IUF, FKZ 20462296). The LISAplus study was funded by Helmholtz Zentrum München, by grants of the Federal Ministry of Environment (BMU) (for IUF, FKZ 20462296), and Federal Ministry for Education, Science, Research, and Technology (No. 01 EG 9705/2 and 01EG9732). The funders had no role in study design, data collection and analysis, decision to publish, or preparation of the manuscript.

Competing Interests: The authors have declared that no competing interests exist.

* E-mail: heinrich@helmholtz-muenchen.de

Introduction

Attention-deficit/hyperactivity disorder (ADHD) belongs to the most common neuro-behavioural childhood disorders [1] with a world-wide prevalence of 5.3% [2]. According to DSM-IV (Diagnostic and Statistical Manual of Mental Disorders) [3] it is characterized by two core symptoms which co-occur: inattention and overactivity-impulsiveness at home as well as in school environment. 75% of affected children are male [4].

Several environmental factors were suggested to increase the risk for ADHD. Among them, time spent in front of the TV [5], single parent headed households [6], parental education [7], maternal age at birth [7], and maternal smoking were reported [8–10]. Up to now, genome-wide association studies suggested markers which exhibit only low effect sizes on ADHD susceptibility [1].

Interestingly, ADHD is associated with other neurological and psychiatric disorders. More than 60% of individuals suffering from ADHD present with one ore more comorbid disorders [11] like oppositional defiant disorder, conduct disorder, depression, anxiety and tic disorders. 20–60% of children exhibiting ADHD are also affected by learning disorders [12,13].

Two of the most common learning disorders are dyslexia and dyscalculia with prevalence rates of about 5% in school-aged children [14,15]. Whereas dyslexia is more frequent in boys than in girls [16], no sex differences in prevalence rates have been reported for dyscalculia [17]. Dyslexic children suffer from difficulties in learning to read and spell which are not caused by neurological deficits, impairments in general intelligence or inadequate education. Dyscalculia is characterized by deficits in the acquisition of numerical abilities and calculation skills which are not due to low intelligence, inadequate schooling or sensory impairments [15].

To date, only few studies have examined the comorbidity between ADHD symptoms and reading/spelling and math difficulties. Especially the relationship between ADHD and dyscalculia has not yet been studied in detail yet.

We therefore investigated whether children with ADHD symptoms have a higher risk for also being affected with reading/spelling and math difficulties in a large population-based sample of over 4,000 children aged 10 years, in which also possible confounding factors like maternal smoking had been collected.

Methods

Ethics Statement

The LISAplus (The Influence of Life-style factors on the development of the Immune System and Allergies in East and West Germany plus the influence of environment and genetics) and the GINIplus (German Infant Study on the influence of Nutrition Intervention plus environmental and genetic influences on allergy development) studies were approved by the local ethics committees (Ethikkommission der Bayrischen Landeärztekammer, Ethikkommission an der Medizinischen Fakultät der Universität Leipzig, Ärztekammer Nordrhein) and written consent was obtained from the parents of all study participants.

Study Design

LISAplus and GINIplus are ongoing population-based birth cohort studies.

For the LISAplus study, the parents of neonates admitted to maternity hospitals in four German cities (Munich, Leipzig, Wesel and Bad Honnef) were contacted and 3,097 healthy full-term neonates were recruited in the study between December 1997 and January 1999. Screening, recruitment and exclusion criteria were described elsewhere [18,19]. Follow-up time points were at the ages of 0.5, 1, 1.5, 2, 4, 6 and 10 years.

For the GINIplus study, a total of 5,991 healthy full-term infants born between September 1995 and June 1998 in two regions of Germany (urban Munich and rural Wesel) were recruited. The study population is subdivided into an interventional (n = 2,252) and an observational group (n = 3,739). Children with family history of allergy were assigned to the intervention group and the observational subgroup comprises children with no family history of allergic disease and children whose parents refused to participate in the intervention trial. A description of the study design has been published previously [20]. Follow-up questionnaires on child's health were administered to the parents at 1, 2, 4, 6 and 10 years after birth.

In both studies, reading/spelling disorders or problems were assessed by questionnaire at the 10-year follow-up. ADHD symptoms at the age of 10 years were measured by the German parent-reported version of the Strengths and Difficulties Questionnaire (SDQ) [21–24].

Questionnaire Data

In GINIplus, the presence of a reading/spelling disorder or reading/spelling problems was assessed by one question each. Children, whose parents answered that their child presented with reading/spelling problems as well as with reading/spelling disorder were grouped into the more severe category of reading/spelling disorder, i.e. both categories are disjunct. In LISAplus, parents were asked a single question, i.e. whether their child suffered from reading/spelling disorder or reading/spelling problems.

In GINIplus and in LISAplus, parents were also asked via a single question, whether their child suffered from dyscalculia or had problems in mathematics.

In order to adjust the multivariable regression models in the analysis for covariates that might lead to confounding of the results, we included gender, age, study (GINIplus or LISAplus) and study center (Munich, Leipzig, Bad Honnef or Wesel) as basic characteristics of the child. Parental education, single-headed households, maternal age at birth, time which the child spent in front of a screen and pre- and/or postnatal environmental tobacco smoke (ETS) exposure are effect modifiers which have already been reported [5–10] and which were also available in LISAplus and GINIplus. Parental educational level was measured on a scale of 'low' (both parents with less than 10 years of schooling) over 'medium' (at least one parent with 10 years of schooling) to 'high' (at least one parent with more than 10 years of schooling). We further included maternal age at birth (more or equal to 30 years or younger) and single parent status at the child's age of 10 years. The time which the child usually spent in front of a screen (e.g. television, computer, ...) during the tenth year of life was categorized in 'low' defined as less than one hour per day in summer and less than two hours per day in winter compared to 'high'. Pre- and/or postnatal ETS exposure of the child at home was assessed by a four-category variable ('never' 'only postnatal', 'only prenatal' and 'pre- and postnatal'). A child was defined to be prenatally exposed if the mother reported active smoking in at least one trimester during pregnancy. Children who were reported to be exposed to ETS at home up to 10 years were classified as postnatally exposed.

Current methylphenidate treatment of ADHD symptoms was assessed by questionnaire at the 10-year follow-up.

Outcome Measure

ADHD symptoms were assessed by the hyperactivity/inattention subscale of the SDQ [21–24], an internationally disseminated and validated screening questionnaire to assess mental and behavioral strengths and difficulties in 3- to 16-year-olds. The five items for the hyperactivity/inattention subscale are "restless, overactive, cannot stay still for long", "constantly fidgeting or squirming", "easily distracted, concentration wanders", "thinks things out before acting", "sees tasks through to the end, good attention span". Every item is rated on a three-point scale: 'not true' (0), 'somewhat true' (1) and 'certainly true' (2). Positively worded items are reverse-scored. The score for the 'hyperactivity/inattention' subscale is calculated as the sum of the ratings. The children were then categorized into "normal", "borderline" and "high" scores according to cut-off points recommended for German samples [24].

Statistical Analysis

Individuals from both studies, GINIplus and LISAplus, were pooled into one sample. Comorbidity of either reading/spelling difficulties or math difficulties and ADHD symptoms was assessed using logistic regression. Reading/spelling and math difficulties, respectively, were used as dependent and ADHD symptoms as independent variable. Children with normal SDQ hyperactivity/inattention levels were defined as reference category, thus the logistic regression model yielded odds ratios (ORs) and significance values for the comparisons high to normal and borderline to normal SDQ hyperactivity/inattention scores.

Three different models were applied: no adjustment for covariates (dyslexia crude/dyscalculia crude), adjustment for the covariates gender, age, study and study centre (dyslexia adjusted I/dyscalculia adjusted I), additional adjustment for possible modifiers as parental education, age of mother at birth, daily TV/PC use, single parent and ETS exposure (dyslexia adjusted II/dyscalculia adjusted II). Additionally, we conducted a stratified analysis for gender and study. Statistical significance was defined by a two-sided alpha level of 5%. The results are presented as OR with corresponding 95% confidence interval (CI) and p-value. All analyses were performed using R, version 2.13.1 (http://www.r-project.org/).

Results

Sample characteristics for the core phenotypes as well as for covariates are depicted in Table 1. 8.1% of all children presented with ADHD symptoms and 25% of those were also affected with reading/spelling difficulties. Children with ADHD symptoms were at higher risk of also being affected with reading/spelling difficulties as compared to children without ADHD symptoms (Table 2). Without adjustment for covariates, the OR for also having reading/spelling difficulties was 4.39 ($p = 2.50 \times 10^{-23}$) for children with borderline and 3.57 ($p = 1.48 \times 10^{-22}$) for children presenting with a high SDQ-score. After adjusting for gender, age, study, study center, parental education, age of mother at birth, daily TV/PC use, single parent and ETS exposure (adjusted II model), these values dropped to 3.95 ($p = 7.27 \times 10^{-17}$) and 2.80 ($p = 6.59 \times 10^{-13}$), respectively. Stratified analyses for GINIplus and LISAplus revealed the same results (data not shown).

As gender differences in the prevalence of ADHD [4] and reading/spelling problems [16] have been reported, we conducted a sex-stratified analysis in the combined GINIplus and LISAplus sample to test if comorbidity rates differed between boys and girls. The prevalence for being affected by reading/spelling difficulties was higher in males (14.1%) than in females (8.7%). Males presenting with borderline SDQ-score had a higher risk than corresponding females (adjusted II model- males: OR = 4.11, $p = 6.68 \times 10^{-12}$, females: OR = 3.69, $p = 3.25 \times 10^{-06}$). Unexpectedly, males presenting with high SDQ-score showed a lower risk for also being affected with reading/spelling difficulties than the female group (adjusted II model- males: OR = 2.36, $p = 9.15 \times 10^{-09}$, females: OR = 3.34, $p = 1.41 \times 10^{-05}$).

In GINIplus, reading/spelling problems and reading/spelling disorder were assessed separately. Therefore a sensitivity analysis on the severity of these symptoms for children included in the GINIplus study was performed (Figure 1). Children with borderline SDQ-score showed a higher OR for having reading/spelling problems (adjusted II model: OR = 3.46, $p = 2.32 \times 10^{-08}$) as compared to children with high SDQ-score (adjusted II model: OR = 1.58, $p = 3.26 \times 10^{-02}$). However, for the risk of showing reading/spelling disorder, results were vice versa: children with high SDQ-score presented with a higher risk for reading/spelling disorder (adjusted II model: OR = 4.00, $p = 3.83 \times 10^{-08}$) as compared to children with borderline SDQ-score (adjusted II model: OR = 2.41, $p = 1.94 \times 10^{-02}$). In the stratified analysis, boys with borderline SDQ-score were at higher risk for presenting with reading/spelling problems (adjusted II model: OR = 3.40, $p = 2.25 \times 10^{-05}$) as compared to boys with high SDQ-score (adjusted II model: OR = 1.55, $p = 8.60 \times 10^{-02}$, Figure 2). For the risk of showing reading/spelling disorder, effects were in the opposite direction: male children with high SDQ-score presented with nearly the same risk (adjusted II model: OR = 3.22, $p = 1.32 \times 10^{-04}$) as compared to males with borderline SDQ-score (adjusted II model: OR = 2.95, $p = 1.45 \times 10^{-02}$). For girls, differences between both groups were more striking (Figure 3): girls with high SDQ-score had a higher risk for showing reading/spelling difficulties (adjusted II model: OR = 6.61, $p = 3.10 \times 10^{-05}$) as compared to girls with borderline SDQ-score (adjusted II model: OR = 1.54, $p = 5.72 \times 10^{-01}$).

In addition to comorbidity between ADHD symptoms and reading/spelling difficulties, we also investigated association between ADHD symptoms and math difficulties. 6.8% of children with ADHD symptoms also presented with math difficulties. Children with ADHD symptoms showed a higher risk of also being affected with math difficulties as compared to children without ADHD symptoms (Table 3). Without adjustment for covariates, the OR was 2.67 ($p = 3.95 \times 10^{-04}$) for children with borderline and 2.87 ($p = 3.21 \times 10^{-06}$) for children presenting with a high SDQ-score. After adjusting for covariates these values were 2.82 ($p = 4.90 \times 10^{-04}$) and 2.55 ($p = 3.63 \times 10^{-13}$) respectively. Stratified analyses for GINIplus and LISAplus showed similar results in both studies (data not shown).

Concerning comorbidity between ADHD symptoms and math difficulties we observed high gender differences. While males with borderline SDQ-score were not significantly at higher risk for math difficulties as compared to males with normal SDQ-score (adjusted II model: OR = 1.82, $p = 2.39 \times 10^{-01}$), males with high SDQ-score had a significantly higher risk (adjusted II model: OR = 2.14, $p = 3.70 \times 10^{-02}$). In the female group, children with borderline SDQ-score as well as with high SDQ-score had a significantly higher risk for math difficulties (borderline SDQ-adjusted II model: OR = 3.75, $p = 3.67 \times 10^{-04}$; high SDQ-adjusted II model: OR = 3.06, $p = 3.00 \times 10^{-03}$).

In studies of comorbidity possible treatment effects have to be considered. Treatment might influence ADHD symptoms as well as reading/spelling and math skills. In the combined GINI/LISA sample, data on therapy with methylphenidate was available for 3,601 children. The substance was administered to 87 (2.4%) out of these individuals. However, including this information as covariate into the analysis did not change the statistical association results for reading/spelling difficulties or for math difficulties (data not shown).

Discussion

We investigated the association between ADHD symptoms and reading/spelling and math difficulties in a pooled sample consisting of children from the LISAplus and GINIplus studies. Children with ADHD symptoms showed a significantly higher risk for reading/spelling difficulties as well as for math difficulties as compared to children presenting with normal SDQ-scores. Observed effects seem to be triggered by gender: while the prevalence for reading/spelling difficulties was higher in males (14.1%) than in females (8.7%), stratification analysis revealed that females showing ADHD symptoms were at a higher risk for also having reading/spelling difficulties than males. Only males with high SDQ-score were at significantly higher risk for having math difficulties while in females both groups- with borderline and high SDQ- showed significantly higher risk. For interpretation of these results, it has to be noted that we do not have information on which symptoms children presented with first – ADHD or dyslexia/dyscalculia symptoms, i.e. we can neither infer causality nor the chronology of symptoms. To diagnose a child with comorbid ADHD ADHD-symptoms need to be present before reading/spelling or arithmetic problems arised [25]. For this, a thorough medical history is essential.

Up to date, few studies, partly population-based but with smaller sample sizes than our study, reported comorbidity between ADHD and dyslexia [11,26,27]. In a longitudinal twin study Greven et al. [28] showed that ADHD and reading significantly predicted each other over time and that this association was mainly due to shared genetic factors. Results on the relationship between ADHD and dyscalculia are less consistent. While Kaufmann et al. [29] report a link between ADHD and numerical processing, Monuteaux et al. [30] suggest that both disorders are distinct. Our results point to a relationship between ADHD and both – dyslexia and dyscalculia. We would assume that for children who suffer from both learning

Table 1. Study characteristics of children aged 10 years from GINIplus and LISAplus.

	SDQ hyperactivity/inattention category[1]			
	Normal	Borderline	High	Total
Gender				
Male	2027 (81.9%)	163 (6.6%)	285 (11.5%)	2475
Female	2180 (91.4%)	95 (4.0%)	111 (4.6%)	2386
Study				
GINIplus	2782 (86.7%)	163 (5.1%)	262 (8.2%)	3207
LISAplus	1425 (86.2%)	95 (5.7%)	134 (8.1%)	1654
Study center				
Munich	2219 (87.0%)	128 (5.0%)	204 (8.0%)	2551
Leipzig	334 (84.8%)	23 (5.8%)	37 (9.4%)	394
Bad Honnef	175 (87.9%)	13 (6.5%)	11 (5.6%)	199
Wesel	1479 (86.1%)	94 (5.5%)	144 (8.4%)	1717
Parental education				
Both parents <10 yrs	256 (78.1%)	27 (8.2%)	45 (13.7%)	328
At least one parent 10 yrs	1046 (82.9%)	85 (6.7%)	132 (10.4%)	1263
At least one parent >10 yrs	2747 (88.9%)	138 (4.4%)	206 (6.7%)	3091
Age of mother				
At birth <30 yrs	1251 (83.9%)	94 (6.3%)	146 (9.8%)	1491
At birth at least 30 yrs	2924 (87.8%)	159 (4.8%)	246 (7.4%)	3329
Daily TV/PC use				
<1 h in summer & <2 h in winter	2790 (87.7%)	162 (5.1%)	230 (7.2%)	3182
>=1 h in summer or >=2 h in winter	1361 (84.3%)	93 (5.7%)	161 (10.0%)	1615
Single parent				
No	3714 (87.9%)	199 (4.7%)	312 (7.4%)	4225
Yes	422 (76.6%)	52 (9.4%)	77 (14.0%)	551
Exposure to tobacco smoke at home				
Never	2220 (89.4%)	108 (4.3%)	156 (6.3%)	2484
Only postnatal	1197 (84.7%)	83 (5.9%)	133 (9.4%)	1413
Only prenatal	101 (85.6%)	7 (5.9%)	10 (8.5%)	118
Pre- and postnatal	391 (77.1%)	43 (8.5%)	73 (14.4%)	507
Special training in reading/spelling				
No	3553 (89.5%)	167 (4.2%)	249 (6.3%)	3969
Yes	521 (70.8%)	81 (11.0%)	134 (18.2%)	736
Reading/spelling difficulties[2]				
No	3699 (89.1%)	173 (4.2%)	280 (6.7%)	4152
Yes	365 (67.8%)	75 (14.0%)	98 (18.2%)	538
Severity of dyslexia[3]				
Reading/spelling problems	191 (72.0%)	37 (14.0%)	37 (14.0%)	265
Reading/spelling disorder	79 (65.8%)	10 (8.3%)	31 (25.9%)	120
Math difficulties				
No	4000 (87.1%)	235 (5.1%)	355 (7.8%)	4590
Yes	102 (70.8%)	16 (11.1%)	26 (18.1%)	144

given numbers indicate the number of individuals with available corresponding phenotypes.
[1]SDQ hyperactivity/inattention is categorized as normal (SDQ score lower than 6), borderline (SDQ score between 6 and 7) and high (SDQ score higher than 7).
[2]refers to children with reading/spelling disorder as well as to children with reading/spelling problems.
[3]distinction between reading/spelling problems and reading/spelling disorder was only made in GINIplus.

Table 2. Association results from logistic regression analysis between reading/spelling difficulties and ADHD symptoms measured by the SDQ-hyperactivity/inattention score.

SDQ hyperactivity/inattention score

Model	**Normal**			**Borderline**				**High**			
	dyslexic[1]	**non dyslexic[2]**	**OR**	**dyslexic[1]**	**non dyslexic[2]**	**OR [95% CI]**	**p-value**	**dyslexic[1]**	**non dyslexic[2]**	**OR [95% CI]**	**p-value**
Dyslexia crude	n = 365	n = 3699	1.00 (reference)	n = 75	n = 173	4.39 [3.28–5.88]	**2.50×10^{-23}**	n = 98	n = 280	3.57 [2.75–4.57]	**1.48×10^{-22}**
Dyslexia adjusted I[3]	n = 365	n = 3699	1.00 (reference)	n = 75	n = 173	4.30 [3.20–5.78]	**3.35×10^{-22}**	n = 98	n = 280	3.25 [2.51–4.21]	**5.07×10^{-19}**
Dyslexia adjusted II[4]	n = 333	n = 3298	1.00 (reference)	n = 65	n = 154	3.95 [2.86–5.45]	**7.27×10^{-17}**	n = 87	n = 253	2.80 [2.11–3.70]	**6.59×10^{-13}**

[1]refers to the number of individuals with reading/spelling difficulties for whom full phenotypic information was available and who were included in regression analysis.
[2]refers to the number of individuals without reading/spelling difficulties for whom full phenotypic information was available and who were included in regression analysis.
[3]adjusted for gender, age, study and study center.
[4]additional adjustment for parental education, age of mother at birth, daily TV/PC use, single parent and ETS exposure.
p-values <0.05 are depicted in bold.

disorders, estimated risk values would be even higher. However, in our sample, only 62 individuals with reading/spelling and math difficulties were available and this number does not allow for valid statistical conclusions.

We observed sex-specific differences in the association between ADHD and reading/spelling difficulties. The scale used for assessment of ADHD symptoms in our study combines hyperactivity and inattention symptoms and is not validated for a separate analysis of these two symptoms. When Willcutt et al. [27] investigated the ADHD core symptoms inattention and hyperactivity/impulsivity stratified by gender, they found that reading disability was significantly associated with inattention in both girls and boys, but with hyperactivity/impulsivity only in boys. Thus, in future studies a more detailed analysis of ADHD subscales might be helpful to enlighten possible gender effects of the comorbidity.

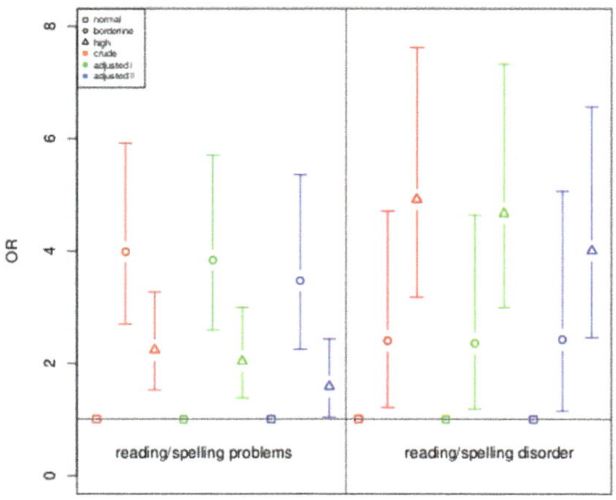

Figure 1. Sensitivity analysis for reading/spelling problems and reading/spelling disorder in GINIplus. ORs and 95% confidence intervals are depicted for reading/spelling problems and reading/spelling disorder in three investigated models (crude, adjusted for gender, age, study and study center and additional adjustment for parental education, age of mother at birth, daily TV/PC use, single parent and ETS exposure). Normal SDQ score was chosen as reference category.

We also found high differences in the effect sizes for associations between ADHD and math difficulties in girls and boys. To our knowledge, in the few studies on ADHD and dyscalculia that have already been published, sex-stratified analysis was not performed.

Our results are based on a large sample size in which prevalences for the different disorders are similar to already reported estimates. Further strengths are related to the population-based characteristic of both studies and to the consistency of results between GINIplus and LISAplus. In addition, we cautiously adjusted for several socio-economic factors such as parental education and TV/PC use to avoid confounding effects. However, there are also some flaws in the study design. First, ADHD symptoms are assessed by the parent-reported SDQ, a screening

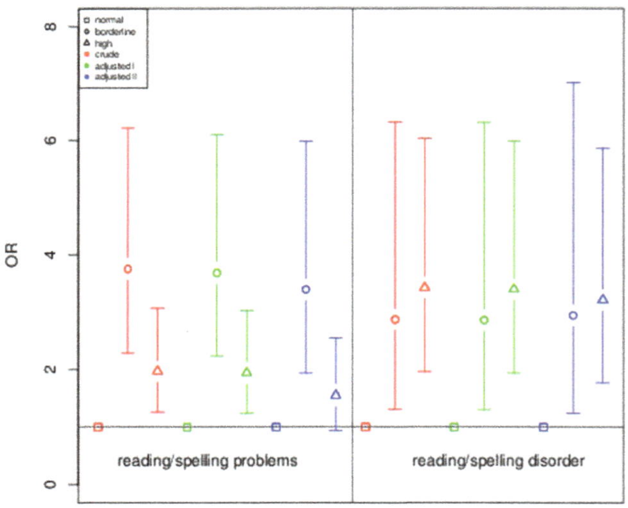

Figure 2. Sensitivity analysis for reading/spelling problems and reading/spelling disorder in males from GINIplus. ORs and 95% confidence intervals are depicted for reading/spelling problems and reading/spelling disorder in three investigated models (crude, adjusted for gender, age, study and study center and additional adjustment for parental education, age of mother at birth, daily TV/PC use, single parent and ETS exposure). Normal SDQ score was chosen as reference category.

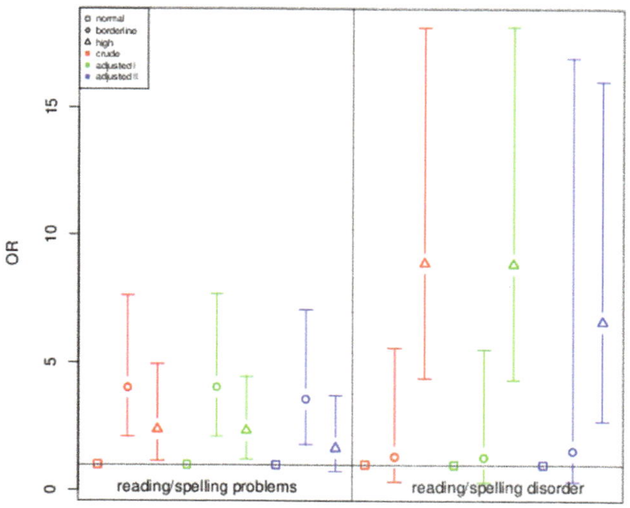

Figure 3. Sensitivity analysis for reading/spelling problems and reading/spelling disorder in females from GINIplus. ORs and 95% confidence intervals are depicted for reading/spelling problems and reading/spelling disorder in three investigated models (crude, adjusted for gender, age, study and study center and additional adjustment for parental education, age of mother at birth, daily TV/PC use, single parent and ETS exposure). Normal SDQ score was chosen as reference category.

instrument. No information on physician diagnosed ADHD was available. Furthermore, presence of dyslexia/dyscalculia symptoms is also based on parental questionnaires and validity of diagnosis may therefore exhibit uncertainness. However, self-reported data on spelling and reading have been reported to show high concordance rates with psychometric tests [31].

Only in GINIplus, reading/spelling problems and reading/spelling disorder were assessed separately. The overall results are based on the combined sample exhibiting both – therefore ORs might be overestimated. The same holds true for math difficulties as no distinction between problems in math and dyscalculia was made.

Unfortunately, no data on the psychopathology of the parents is available. We can therefore make no conclusions on a possible aggravation of symptoms in families or on a genetic component of the disorders.

LISAplus and GINIplus are ongoing longitudinal studies and the 15-year-follow up data will again include questions on reading/spelling and math difficulties. This will enable to analyse the long-term development of the disorders and if special training in reading/spelling lead to a decrease in literacy problems.

In our study ADHD symptoms and learning difficulties were comorbid, taking into account possible confounder variables. Several scenarios underlying this comborbidity are thinkable [32]: 1) ADHD implicates the development of learning disorders. 2) Genetic susceptibility factors for ADHD alone are different from risk variants for comorbid ADHD. ADHD alone and comorbid ADHD are thus genetically/environmentally distinct. 3) The comorbidity is due to environmental factors. In future studies it would be very interesting to conduct genome-wide association analyses in children with ADHD only, dyslexia/dyscalculia only as well as in comorbid children. This might enlighten what processes are causing the comorbidity on a genetic level.

From a diagnostic and therapeutic point of view, it is important to not only check for ADHD or learning disorders alone, but rather for ADHD and reading/spelling or math difficulties in parallel and to adapt the training and therapy accordingly.

Table 3. Association results from logistic regression analysis between math difficulties and ADHD symptoms measured by the SDQ-hyperactivity/inattention score.

Model	SDQ hyperactivity score: Normal			Borderline				High			
	dyscalculic[1]	non dyscalculic[2]	OR	dyscalculic[1]	non dyscalculic[2]	OR [95% CI]	p-value	dyscalculic[1]	non dyscalculic[2]	OR [95% CI]	p-value
Dyscalculia crude	n = 102	n = 4000	1.00 (reference)	n = 16	n = 235	2.67 [1.55–4.60]	**3.95×10^{-04}**	n = 26	n = 355	2.87 [1.84–4.48]	**3.21×10^{-06}**
Dyscalculia adjusted I[3]	n = 102	n = 4000	1.00 (reference)	n = 16	n = 235	3.03 [1.75–5.26]	**7.69×10^{-05}**	n = 26	n = 355	3.48 [2.20–5.50]	**9.91×10^{-08}**
Dyscalculia adjusted II[4]	n = 91	n = 3576	1.00 (reference)	n = 15	n = 207	2.82 [1.58–5.07]	**4.90×10^{-04}**	n = 21	n = 320	2.55 [1.52–4.26]	**3.63×10^{-04}**

[1]refers to the number of individuals with math difficulties for whom full phenotypic information was available and who were included in regression analysis.
[2]refers to the number of individuals without math difficulties for whom full phenotypic information was available and who were included in regression analysis.
[3]adjusted for gender, age, study and study center.
[4]additional adjustment for parental education, age of mother at birth, daily TV/PC use, single parent and ETS exposure.
p-values <0.05 are depicted in bold.

Children with learning disorders who also present with ADHD symptoms should receive different training as compared to children who present only with dyslexia and dyscalculia because ADHD itself can have an impact on the training methods and training success.

Conclusion

We found that children with ADHD symptoms are at higher risk for reading/spelling and math difficulties compared to children without ADHD symptoms. The exact functional process and causality pattern behind this comorbidity remains unknown.

Acknowledgments

GINIplus study group: Helmholtz Zentrum München, Institute of Epidemiology, München (Heinrich J, Wichmann HE, Schoetzau A, Mosetter M, Schindler J, Höhnke A, Franke K, Laubereau B, Gehring U, Sausenthaler S, Thaqi A, Zirngibl A, Zutavern A., Schnappinger M, Chen CM); Department of Pediatrics, Marien-Hospital, Wesel (Berdel D, von Berg A, Filipiak-Pittroff B, Albrecht B, Baumgart A, Beckmann C, Büttner S, Diekamp S, Groß I, Jakob T, Klemke K, Kurpiun S, Möllemann M, Varhelyi A,); Department of Pediatrics, Ludwig Maximilians University, Munich (Koletzko S, Reinhardt D, Weigand H, Antonie I, Bäumler-Merl B, Tasch C, Göhlert R, Mühlbauer D, Sönnichsen C, Sauerwald T, Kindermann A, Waag M, Koch M); Department of Pediatrics, Technical University, Munich (Bauer CP, Grübl A, Bartels P, Brockow I, Fischer A, Hoffmann U, Lötzbeyer F, Mayrl R, Negele K, Schill E-M, Wolf B, Paschke M); IUF – Leibniz Research Institute for Environmental Medicine, Düsseldorf (Krämer U, Link E, Ranft U, Schins R, Sugiri D, Cramer C); Centre for Allergy and Environment, Technical University, Munich (Behrendt H, Grosch J, Martin F)

LISAplus study group: Helmholtz Zentrum München, German Research Center for Environmental Health, Institute of Epidemiology, Munich (Heinrich J, Wichmann HE, Sausenthaler S, Chen CM, Schnappinger M); Department of Pediatrics, Municipal Hospital 'St.Georg', Leipzig (Borte M, Diez U), Marien-Hospital Wesel, Department of Pediatrics, Wesel (von Berg A, Beckmann C); Pediatric Practice, Bad Honnef (Schaaf B); Helmholtz Centre for Environmental Research - UFZ, Department of Environmental Immunology/Core Facility Studies, Leipzig (Lehmann I, Bauer M, Gräbsch C, Röder S, Schilde M); University of Leipzig, Institute of Hygiene and Environmental Medicine, Leipzig (Herbarth O, Dick C, Magnus J); IUF - Leibniz Research Institute for Environmental Medicine, Düsseldorf (Krämer U, Link E, Cramer C); Technical University Munich, Department of Pediatrics, Munich (Bauer CP, Hoffmann U); ZAUM - Center for Allergy and Environment, Technical University, Munich (Behrendt H).

We thank the families for participation in the studies; the obstetric units for allowing recruitment, the GINI and LISA study teams for excellent work.

Author Contributions

Conceived and designed the experiments: JH. Performed the experiments: GK DB BH C-PB SK BS IL OH AvB. Analyzed the data: DC CMTT BM-M GS-K JH. Wrote the paper: DC CMTT GK DB BH C-PB SK BS IL OH AvB BM-M GS-K JH.

References

1. Singh I (2008) Beyond polemics: science and ethics of ADHD. Nat Rev Neurosci 9: 957–964.
2. Polanczyk G, de Lima MS, Horta BL, Biederman J, Rohde LA (2007) The worldwide prevalence of ADHD: a systematic review and metaregression analysis. Am J Psychiatry 164: 942–948.
3. American Psychiatric Association (2004) Diagnostic and Statistical Manual of Mental Disorders (DSM-IV). Washington DC: American Psychiatric Publishing.
4. Schneider H, Eisenberg D (2006) Who receives a diagnosis of attention-deficit/hyperactivity disorder in the United States elementary school population? Pediatrics 117: e601–e609.
5. Lingineni RK, Biswas S, Ahmad N, Jackson BE, Bae S, et al. (2012) Factors associated with attention deficit/hyperactivity disorder among US children: Results from a national survey. BMC Pediatr 12: 50.
6. Biederman J, Milberger S, Faraone SV, Kiely K, Guite J, et al. (1995) Family-environment risk factors for attention-deficit hyperactivity disorder. A test of Rutter's indicators of adversity. Arch Gen Psychiatry 52: 464–470.
7. Sagiv SK, Epstein JN, Bellinger DC, Korrick SA (2012) Pre- and Postnatal Risk Factors for ADHD in a Nonclinical Pediatric Population. J Atten Disord 17: 47–57.
8. Rückinger S, Rzehak P, Chen CM, Sausenthaler S, Koletzko S, et al. (2010) Prenatal and postnatal tobacco exposure and behavioral problems in 10-year-old children: results from the GINI-plus prospective birth cohort study. Environ Health Perspect 118: 150–154.
9. Thapar A, Fowler T, Rice F, Scourfield J, van den BM, et al. (2003) Maternal smoking during pregnancy and attention deficit hyperactivity disorder symptoms in offspring. Am J Psychiatry 160: 1985–1989.
10. Tiesler CM, Chen CM, Sausenthaler S, Herbarth O, Lehmann I, et al. (2011) Passive smoking and behavioural problems in children: Results from the LISAplus prospective birth cohort study. Environ Res 111: 1173–1179.
11. Gillberg C, Gillberg IC, Rasmussen P, Kadesjo B, Soderstrom H, et al. (2004) Co-existing disorders in ADHD - implications for diagnosis and intervention. Eur Child Adolesc Psychiatry 13 Suppl 1: I80-I92.
12. Langberg JM, Vaughn AJ, Brinkman WB, Froehlich T, Epstein JN (2010) Clinical utility of the Vanderbilt ADHD Rating Scale for ruling out comorbid learning disorders. Pediatrics 126: e1033–e1038.
13. Pliszka SR (1998) Comorbidity of attention-deficit/hyperactivity disorder with psychiatric disorder: an overview. J Clin Psychiatry 59 Suppl 7: 50–58.
14. Shaywitz SE, Shaywitz BA, Fletcher JM, Escobar MD (1990) Prevalence of reading disability in boys and girls. Results of the Connecticut Longitudinal Study. JAMA 264: 998–1002.
15. von Aster MG, Shalev RS (2007) Number development and developmental dyscalculia. Dev Med Child Neurol 49: 868–873.
16. Rutter M, Caspi A, Fergusson D, Horwood LJ, Goodman R, et al. (2004) Sex differences in developmental reading disability: new findings from 4 epidemiological studies. JAMA 291: 2007–2012.
17. Shalev RS (2004) Developmental dyscalculia. J Child Neurol 19: 765–771.
18. Heinrich J, Bolte G, Holscher B, Douwes J, Lehmann I, et al. (2002) Allergens and endotoxin on mothers' mattresses and total immunoglobulin E in cord blood of neonates. Eur Respir J 20: 617–623.
19. Zutavern A, Brockow I, Schaaf B, Bolte G, von Berg A, et al. (2006) Timing of solid food introduction in relation to atopic dermatitis and atopic sensitization: results from a prospective birth cohort study. Pediatrics 117: 401–411.
20. von Berg A, Kramer U, Link E, Bollrath C, Heinrich J, et al. (2010) Impact of early feeding on childhood eczema: development after nutritional intervention compared with the natural course - the GINIplus study up to the age of 6 years. Clin Exp Allergy 40: 627–636.
21. Goodman R (1997) The Strengths and Difficulties Questionnaire: a research note. J Child Psychol Psychiatry 38: 581–586.
22. Goodman R, Meltzer H, Bailey V (2003) The Strengths and Difficulties Questionnaire: a pilot study on the validity of the self-report version. Int Rev Psychiatry 15: 173–177.
23. Woerner W, Becker A, Friedrich C, Klasen H, Goodman R, et al. (2002) Normal values and evaluation of the German parents' version of Strengths and Difficulties Questionnaire (SDQ): Results of a representative field study. Z Kinder Jugendpsychiatr Psychother 30: 105–112.
24. Woerner W, Becker A, Rothenberger A (2004) Normative data and scale properties of the German parent SDQ. Eur Child Adolesc Psychiatry 13 Suppl 2: II3–10.
25. Romanos M, Schwenck C, Walitza S (2008) Diagnosis of attention-deficit hyperactivity disorder in childhood and adolescence. Nervenarzt 79: 782–790.
26. Rommelse N, Altink M, Fliers E, Martin N, Buschgens C, et al. (2009) Comorbid Problems in ADHD: Degree of Association, Shared Endophenotypes, and Formation of Distinct Subtypes. Implications for a Future DSM. J Abnorm Child Psychol 37: 793–804.
27. Willcutt EG, Pennington BF (2000) Comorbidity of reading disability and attention-deficit/hyperactivity disorder: differences by gender and subtype. J Learn Disabil 33: 179–191.
28. Greven CU, Rijsdijk FV, Asherson P, Plomin R (2012) A longitudinal twin study on the association between ADHD symptoms and reading. J Child Psychol Psychiatry 53: 234–242.
29. Kaufmann L, Nuerk H (2008) Basic number processing deficits in ADHD: a broad examination of elementary and complex number processing skills in 9- to 12-year-old-children with ADHD-C. Dev Sci 11: 692–699.
30. Monuteaux M, Faraone S, Herzig K, Navsaria N, Biedermann J (2005) ADHD and dyscalculia: Evidence for independent familial transmission. J Learn Disabil 38: 86–93.
31. Schulte-Körne G, Deimel W, Remschmidt H (1997) Can self-reported data on deficits in reading and spelling predict spelling disability as defined by psychometric tests? Reading and Writing 9: 55–63.
32. Angold A, Costello EJ (1993) Depressive comorbidity in children and adolescents: empirical, theoretical, and methodological issues. Am J Psychiatry 150: 1779–1791.

History of Reading Struggles Linked to Enhanced Learning in Low Spatial Frequency Scenes

Matthew H. Schneps[1]*, James R. Brockmole[2], Gerhard Sonnert[1], Marc Pomplun[3]

1 Science Education Department, Harvard-Smithsonian Center for Astrophysics, Cambridge, Massachusetts, United States of America, **2** Department of Psychology, University of Notre Dame, Notre Dame, Indiana, United States of America, **3** Department of Computer Science, University of Massachusetts at Boston, Boston, Massachusetts, United States of America

Abstract

People with dyslexia, who face lifelong struggles with reading, exhibit numerous associated low-level sensory deficits including deficits in focal attention. Countering this, studies have shown that struggling readers outperform typical readers in some visual tasks that integrate distributed information across an expanse. Though such abilities would be expected to facilitate scene memory, prior investigations using the contextual cueing paradigm failed to find corresponding advantages in dyslexia. We suggest that these studies were confounded by task-dependent effects exaggerating known focal attention deficits in dyslexia, and that, if natural scenes were used as the context, advantages would emerge. Here, we investigate this hypothesis by comparing college students with histories of severe lifelong reading difficulties (SR) and typical readers (TR) in contexts that vary attention load. We find no differences in contextual-cueing when spatial contexts are letter-like objects, or when contexts are natural scenes. However, the SR group significantly outperforms the TR group when contexts are low-pass filtered natural scenes [$F(3, 39) = 3.15$, $p < .05$]. These findings suggest that perception or memory for low spatial frequency components in scenes is enhanced in dyslexia. These findings are important because they suggest strengths for spatial learning in a population otherwise impaired, carrying implications for the education and support of students who face challenges in school.

Editor: Satoru Suzuki, Northwestern University, United States of America

Funding: This work was supported by National Science Foundation Grant HRD-0930962 (http://www.nsf.gov/awardsearch/showAward.do?AwardNumber=0930962), and by the George E. Burch Foundation (http://www.si.edu/ofg/) that provided a fellowship to MS. The funders had no role in study design, data collection and analysis, decision to publish, or preparation of the manuscript.

Competing Interests: The authors have declared that no competing interests exist.

* E-mail: mschneps@cfa.harvard.edu

Introduction

It has long been recognized that memories for the structure and layout of a scene, whether real or imagined, can constitute a framework for housing decontextualized memories for discrete objects, numbers, or words that can powerfully augment abilities for episodic memory [1]. And thus, while scene memory is a vital life function in many applications for all individuals, it is perhaps especially important among those whose abilities for episodic memory are limited and who may depend on strengths for scene memory to compensate for impairments in other areas. Dyslexia is a neurological learning disability characterized by lifelong struggles with reading and spelling that are unexpected given a person's capabilities in other cognitive domains [2]. People with dyslexia exhibit phonological processing deficits, together with impairments in working memory and short term memory [3], that impair the episodic recall of words, dates, and numbers. Therefore, people with dyslexia stand to benefit from strategies that use spatial encoding to augment memory, and they may make use of such strategies to achieve at high levels despite struggles in various cognitive domains. Supporting this hypothesis, cases of nonverbal giftedness in dyslexia are documented [4], and those with dyslexia include numerous examples of highly successful individuals including the Nobel laureates Carol W. Greider and Baruj Benacerraf [5,6]. If such individuals use spatial learning strategies to compensate for difficulties encoding memories phonologically, we would expect to see evidence of exceptional facility for spatial learning in dyslexia.

Contextual cueing [7] is a research paradigm often used to provide a measure of spatial learning. In this task, participants search for a target hidden in a visual display, and the speed of search in spatial contexts that are novel is compared with the speed of search in contexts that have been previously searched. Response time is typically speeded up as repeated displays are learned, and this search benefit can be ascribed to spatial learning. Such learning has been demonstrated across a wide range of contexts, ranging from arrays of letters [7] to real-world scenes [8], and is driven by a variety of factors invoking processing in the central and peripheral visual fields [9–12]. However, when contextual cueing was used to investigate abilities for spatial learning in people with dyslexia [13–15], the expected advantages for spatial learning were not reliably observed.

We suggest that previous studies of contextual cueing in dyslexia failed to reveal advantages for spatial learning because these experiments were confounded by task-related demands for focal attention. People with dyslexia exhibit deficits in focal attention [16–18], which can even be observed in preschool children at risk of dyslexia prior to the acquisition of reading [19]. Hence, previous instantiations of contextual cueing paradigms have likely been ill suited tests of spatial abilities among individuals with dyslexia. Specifically, in the previous studies, letter-like objects were used for the spatial context. Subjects searched for a target while simultaneously performing a discrimination task to distinguish target objects (T shape) from similarly shaped background objects (L shapes) that were subtly doglegged to increase difficulty and slow the search. We suggest that the increased cognitive load at the fovea induced by this discrimination task evokes an inhibitory neurological response that diminishes sensitivity in the periphery [20]. Studies of contextual cueing during covert search show that the periphery plays an important role in spatial learning for contexts composed of letter-like forms [12]. Therefore, if peripheral sensitivity is inhibited in dyslexia by heightened cognitive demands during search, this effect could mask potential advantages for spatial learning and thereby account for the lack of reliable findings [14].

Here, we investigate the possibility that spatial learning advantages in dyslexia will be observed if the task is matched to strengths observed in this group. A number of authors stress a distinction between systems for focal attention and those for distributed spatial attention [21,22]. Distributed attention is thought to contribute to scene perception by enabling the extraction of a gist, a rapidly obtained initial hypothesis about the scene's identity and global layout [23] that is then refined through shifts of focal attention [24]. While focal attention is impaired in dyslexia [25,26], other evidence suggests that distributed attention is unimpaired and is perhaps even enhanced. For example, the recognition of impossible figures, which is thought to depend on the holistic integration of long-range spatial information, is faster among people with dyslexia, compared with typical readers [27]. Visuospatial advantages in dyslexia have also been suggested in letter identification tasks where letters are flashed simultaneously at fixation and in the periphery, a task that requires rapid deployment of spatially distributed attention. Recognition accuracy of letter pairs is enhanced in dyslexia when peripheral letters are presented at eccentricities $>7.5^\circ$ [28–34]. Similarly, those with dyslexia are reported to respond more rapidly to an unattended peripheral flash when the flash occurs at eccentricities $>8^\circ$ [35,36]. Collectively, these studies link dyslexia to advantages for distributed forms of spatial attention, typically in circumstances where peripheral information is important.

It has been suggested that these seemingly contradictory observations of co-occurring deficits and advantages in visual processing linked to dyslexia can be understood in a framework that considers the central and peripheral visual fields (here defined as divided at roughly 8° eccentricity) to be structurally segregated and differentiated by their anatomical and functional characteristics [37]. For example, while the center is helpful in searching for small objects [38], the periphery is better optimized for rapid discriminations [39]. Such functional differences can be traced to eccentricity dependent differences in cortical anatomy that originate at the retina [40,41] and that in turn project to the visual cortex so as to largely preserve the retinotopic organization. As a consequence, the functionalities of the center and the periphery remain grossly segregated throughout the brain [42]. If we take as an axiom that the center and periphery can be considered separate yet complementary visual systems, the degree to which individuals vary in their abilities to make use of each source of information can be characterized by using a semi-quantitative descriptor called the periphery-to-center ratio (PCR) [37]. In this perspective, PCR is high in many with dyslexia, which means that information in the peripheral visual field is favored over information in the center. This is consistent with accounts for focal attention deficits that impair search, but also with advantages for distributed attention that enhance spatial learning.

Keeping in mind deficits in focal attention and enhanced reliance on peripheral vision among individuals with dyslexia, we propose that advantages for spatial learning in dyslexia would be more likely evident if (a) a simple feature search replaced the previously used complex discrimination task to reduce cognitive load at the fovea, and (b) the contextual background to be learned made maximal use of long-range information sensitive to the periphery. While the periphery contributes to spatial learning when contexts are letter-like forms [12], in such contexts spatial learning is restricted to content local to the target [9]. In contrast, when contextual cueing is performed in natural scenes spatial learning is observed to be strongly influenced by long-range global information integrated across the scene [10]. Therefore, if contexts consisting of letter-like forms are replaced by natural scenes, and a simple feature search (to locate an L or T in the scene background) replaces the more complex discrimination task often used, spatial learning advantages in dyslexia may be more evident than they have been in previous studies [13–15]. These cases are explored in Experiments 1 and 2. Lastly, we suggest that spatial learning advantages in dyslexia are more likely to be detected if contexts are low-pass filtered scenes. While the center is exquisitely sensitive to high-spatial frequencies, the periphery is relatively blind to this information. Therefore, if natural scenes are low-pass filtered, the loss of high spatial frequency information would extract a greater toll on functionalities of the center. In the PCR framework, this would bias spatial learning in favor of those with dyslexia, a hypothesis explored in Experiment 3. (The experiments undertaken are schematically summarized in Figure 1.)

Experiment 1: Arrays of Letters

Methods

Ethics Statement. The Institutional Review Boards of Harvard University and Landmark College approved this study. All participants signed an informed consent form and were paid $20 for their participation in this experiment.

Participants. In this experiment a group of 10 struggling readers were randomly selected from a pool of 19 students recruited for these studies from Landmark College in Putney, VT. Landmark is a two-year liberal arts institution exclusively for students with learning impairments such as dyslexia. Students attend this school only if past instructional histories suggest severe learning impediments that were not remediated in previous grades and that would place these students at risk if enrolled directly in a traditional college environment without further support. All participants in our pool had childhood histories of serious reading impairments that persisted into adulthood, and had been assigned a diagnosis of dyslexia by the Landmark psychologist. Evidence of reading struggles consistent with dyslexia were ascertained by examining records of psychological testing on file at the school to verify that reading subtests from well-established achievement tests (WJ-III Achievement [43] or WIAT-II [44]) were significantly below ability tests (WAIS-III [45] or WJ-III Cognitive [46]), as is characteristic of dyslexia. Landmark students meeting these criteria were included in the study if no additional history of neurological disorders was evident. Table 1 summarizes behavioral data for each student in the pool who participated in these experiments, obtained from records on file at the school. Privacy conditions for access precluded our carrying out tests to obtain additional behavioral measures in this group. Hence, we have no information about effective subtypes of dyslexia represented in the sample and therefore refer to this group simply as "struggling readers" (SR). A control group of typical readers (TR) included 19 college students from Harvard

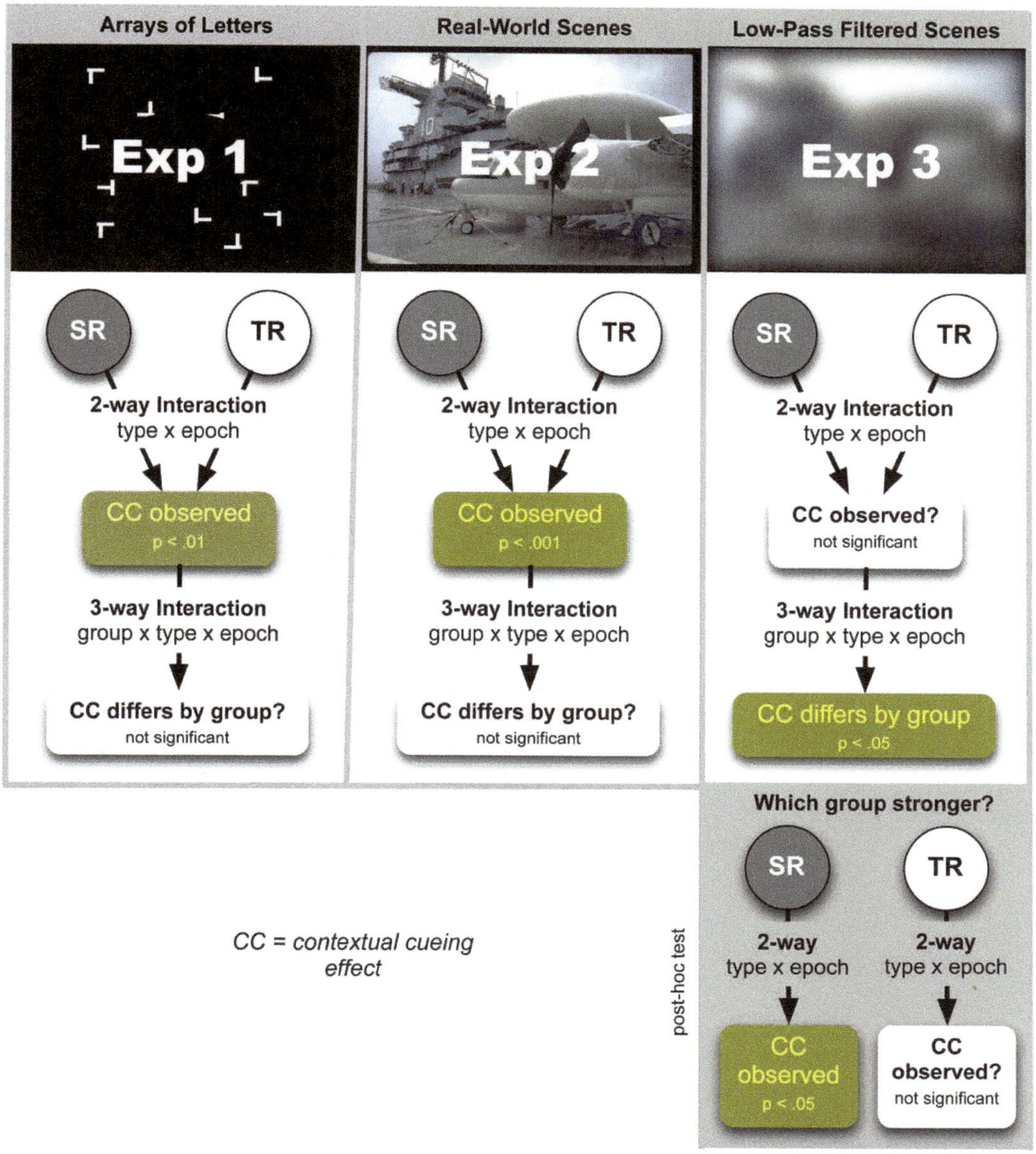

Figure 1. Schematic of experiments, analysis, and results. Contextual cueing is observed in both TR and SR groups when letter-like objects (Experiment 1) or natural scenes (Experiment 2) are used as spatial contexts. Here, the response in the two groups is indistinguishable. However, when low-pass filtered scenes are used as the spatial context (Experiment 3) a significant group interaction is observed. Further analysis reveals significant scene learning in the SR group not evident in the TR group.

University who had no history of dyslexia, attention deficit disorder (ADHD), or other neurological disorders. Harvard is ranked among the premier institutions of higher learning in the United States, and admission is highly competitive. Therefore, there is a strong selection bias in both the SR and TR groups, in that these are likely to represent the extremes in reading ability among college students. All Harvard recruits were administered questionnaires to check for possible histories of learning difficulties. The Adult Reading History Questionnaire (ARHQ), developed by Lefly and Pennington [47], based on [48], includes questions about learning letter names, learning to spell, reading speed, effort needed to succeed, and verbal short-term memory performance, etc. Lefly and Pennington (2000) reported the internal consistency (alpha) of the original ARHQ to be .94, and the test–retest reliability over a 2-year period to be .87. Volunteers were admitted to the study pool only if they scored above a cutoff of 0.30 on the ARHQ. In addition, the 6-question World Health Organization Adult ADHD Self-Report Scale (ASRS) was given to the Harvard recruits. This screener is a powerful tool used to discriminate DSM-IV cases from non-cases for screening purposes [49] and has been found to outperform much lengthier questionnaires for this purpose [50]. ASRS has been shown to be significantly related to the comparable clinical symptom ratings for inattention and impulsivity-hyperactivity, but to vary substantially in concordance (Cohen's k in the range 0.16–0.81). Harvard volunteers who scored above 3 on the ASRS were excluded from the study. All participants had vision that was normal or corrected to normal.

Apparatus. Stimuli were presented on a 20-inch Apple Cinema flat-screen LCD monitor viewed at a distance of 70 cm, with a resolution of 1680 by 1050 pixels and a refresh rate of

Table 1. Behavioral data for Landmark College participants (SR group).

	EXP			WAIS (or WISC)			READING					CTOPP
ID Code	**1**	**2**	**3**	**Full Scale IQ**	**Verbal IQ**	**Perfm IQ**	**Test Name**	**Spelling**	**Single word reading**	**Nonsense word reading**	**Reading Comprehension**	
A	X	X		85	91	78	WIAT II	64	54	58	64	
B	X	X		101	98	105	WIAT II	84	66	80	100	
C	X	X		86–90			WJIII	56	54	72		
D	X	X		94			WJIII		65		83	
E	X	X		97	94	100	WJIII	62	57	67	96	
F	X	X		97			KTEA		1	2	2	
G	X	X		117	100	125	WJIII	79	99	94		
H	X	X		**								
I	X			86	100	73	WJIII	Average	Average	Superior		
J		X			110	100	WJ-Munoz		86			
K	X		X	110	111	109	WIAT	102	108	94		PA:94 RAN:61
L			X	89	82	100	WRAT	80	75			
M			X	131	103	124	WRAT/*WJIII	99	86	91*	108*	
N			X	108	105	110	WIAT	63	76	84	100	PA: 85 PM:76 RAN:46
O			X	80	82	83	WIAT II	51	65	61	63	

Abbreviations:
WRAT Wide Range Achievement Test.
WIAT Wechsler Individual Achievement Test.
WJIII Woodcock Johnson Achievement Test III.
WJ-Munoz Woodcock Munoz Spanish Achievement Test.
KTEA Kaufman Test of Educational Achievement (percentiles).
WJR Woodcock Johnson Reading.
CTOPP Comprehensive Test of Phonological Processing.
PA Phonological Awareness.
PM Phonological Memory.
RAN Rapid Automatized Naming.
Perfm Performance IQ.
* Indicates Nonsense Word and Comprehension from WJIII (other scores from WRAT).
** French narrative report without numerical data.

60 Hz. Stimulus presentation and data acquisition were controlled by custom software using Matlab (The Mathworks, Natick, Massachusetts), and the Psychophysics Toolbox [51]. Participants used a chinrest with a forehead bar to stabilize the head.

Stimuli. Search displays consisted of twelve white objects (luminance: 360 cd/m^2) on a black background (3 cd/m^2), see Figure 2. One of these objects, which served at the search target, was the letter 'T', tilted by 90° either to the left or to the right. The direction of the tilt was randomly chosen, with the constraint that each direction occurred in exactly half of the displays. The other eleven objects were shaped like the letter 'L' in one of four randomly chosen orientations (0°, 90°, 180°, or 270°). Following Chun and Phelps [52], one leg of the L was offset to increase its similarity with the target. The objects had diameters of approximately 1.6° of visual angle and were randomly distributed on a display area of 22° by 22°. The minimum distance between the centers of neighboring objects was 3.8°.

Procedure. Twelve stimulus displays were chosen to serve as 'repeated displays' (repeated) and were presented to the subjects multiple times, while all other displays were 'new displays' (novel) that were shown only once. Each subject saw the same sets of repeated and new displays, but in individually randomized order. Subjects performed 30 blocks of 24 search trials. Each block consisted of a random sequence of the same twelve repeated displays that were shown in every block, plus twelve new displays. The subjects' task was to find the target and press the 'Z' button or the 'M' button on a computer keyboard if the target was tilted to the left or to the right, respectively. They were instructed to perform this task as quickly and as accurately as possible, but no time limit was imposed on their responses, and they were allowed to move their eyes freely throughout the experiment. After their manual response, subjects were presented with a sound informing them about whether their response was correct (800 Hz tone played for 20 ms) or incorrect (400 Hz tone played for 100 ms). Subsequently, a blank black screen was shown for 1 s, followed by the next trial. Subjects took short breaks after each block and started the next one with a mouse click. No information regarding block structure or scene repetition was given to participants. (The general principles underlying the experimental design are illustrated in Figure 3).

Results

Analysis. In terms of responses made, those in TR incorrectly identified the target on 1.5% of trials while those in SR incorrectly responded on 1.8% of trials [t (df) = 1.06, p = 0.30]. These trials were excluded from the analyses. Owing to the relatively low complexity of the task, no time cut-off was used, and none of the trials had a "no response."

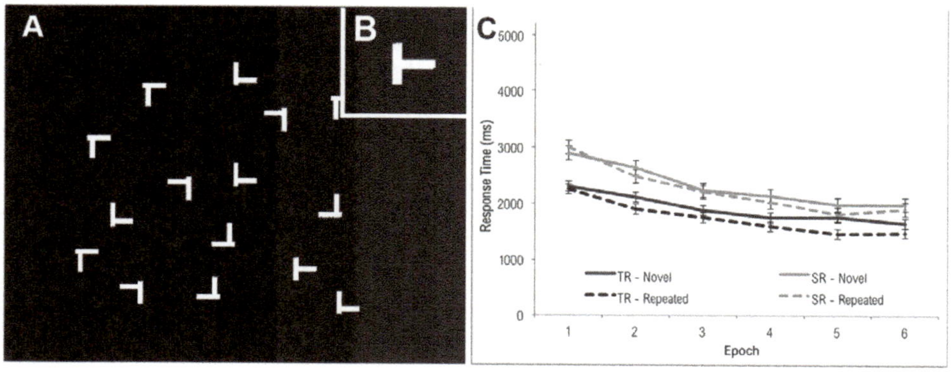

Figure 2. Example of stimulus used in Experiment 1. Participants search for and identify a side-facing T-shaped target, and indicate its direction left or right. The spatial context (A) is defined by a field of L-shaped objects, doglegged to resemble the target (B), inset. Manual response times for Experiment 1 are plotted in (C). Both typical readers and individuals with dyslexia show progressively faster search times in both the repeated and novel conditions, revealing a well-known practice effect associated with this task. Response times for repeated trials are generally shorter than for novel trials, and this difference grows as a function of epoch, indicative of a contextual cueing effect ascribed to spatial learning. The contextual cueing effect was equivalent for both SR and TR groups.

The dependent variable was Response Time (RT) in milliseconds. The 30 trial blocks were collapsed into 6 equal-sized epochs for analysis. A repeated-measures mixed model analysis of variance (ANOVA) was conducted to compare RTs across group (SR, TR), trial type (novel, repeated), and epoch (1–6). There were significant main effects of group, $F(1, 27) = 10.86$, $p<0.01$, trial type, $F(1, 27) = 39.51$, $p<0.0001$, and epoch, F $(5, 135) = 208$, $p<0.0001$. SR subjects had slower RTs ($M = 2278$ ms) than did TR subjects ($M = 1830$ ms); the repeated items were detected faster ($M = 1995$ ms) than the novel items ($M = 2114$ ms); and RTs generally decreased over the course of the experiment (epoch 1: $M = 2612$ ms; epoch 6: $M = 1762$ ms).

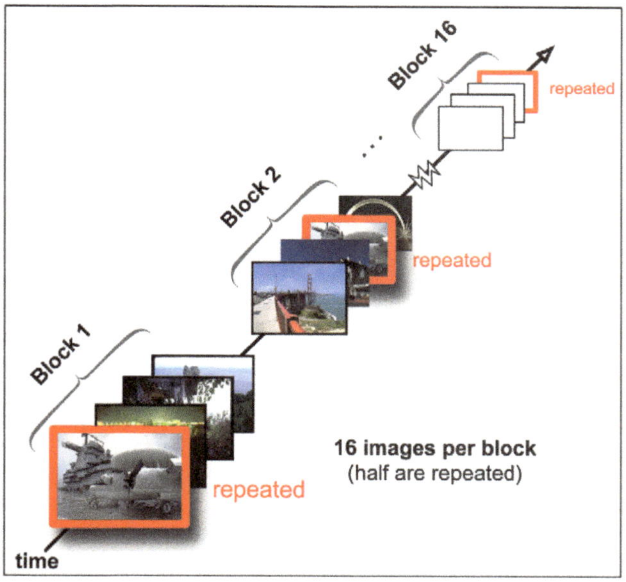

Figure 3. Contextual cueing paradigm. Participants search for a target in an image, and response times are observed. The paradigm assumes that spatial memory of the scene facilitates search for scenes that are repeated. A contextual cueing effect is observed if search is progressively speeded for repeated scenes compared to novel scenes as a function of block [7]. Here, the block design used in Experiments 2 and 3 is illustrated, consisting of 16 blocks, each containing 8 novel and 8 repeated images, randomly arrayed. (Blocking in Experiment 1 differed, employing 30 blocks of 24 trials, with 12 repeated images per block.).

A significant interaction between trial type and epoch, $F(5, 135) = 3.91$, $p<0.01$, indicated that the difference in response time between novel and repeated items became larger during the second and later epochs. This was to be expected—and is typical for a contextual cueing effect—because, at the outset, every item was novel, and the effect of repetition would grow more salient over the course of the experiment. A second significant interaction was found between group and trial type, $F(1, 27) = 5.96$, $p<0.05$. The response time difference between the novel and repeated items was more pronounced for the TR group than for the SR group. That is, the benefit of repetition was greater for the TR than for the SR group. Thirdly, group and epoch were found to interact significantly, $F(5, 135) = 8.88$, $p<0.0001$, indicating that the gap in response time between SR and TR subjects became narrower during the course of the experiment (i.e., the drop in response time was steeper for the SR than for the TR group, indicating a greater overall learning effect for the SR group). The three-way interaction, however, was not significant. This finding is consistent with previous observations in dyslexia [14].

The observation that the SR group is slower overall at visual search is consistent with prior studies suggesting focal visual attention deficits in dyslexia [26]. Impairments in visual search can lead to deficits in contextual cueing [53]. Therefore, it is perhaps surprising that we do not observe deficits for spatial learning in the SR group. Despite deficits for search, search benefits due to contextual cueing were observed in both groups, and the extent of this spatial learning benefit was indistinguishable in these groups, opening the possibility that scene perception and/or scene memory is enhanced in the SR group.

Experiment 2: Real-World Scenes

This experiment investigated the hypothesis that contextual cueing effects are enhanced in the SR group when spatial contexts are natural scenes. In Experiment 1, contextual cueing was investigated for contexts composed of letter-like objects. There, spatial learning was biased to information local to the target [9]. The situation is different when contextual cueing is performed in natural scenes. Here, long-range interactions are more important, and information global to the scene is integrated in spatial learning [10]. Long-range visuospatial processing is reported to be enhanced in dyslexia [27,29,36]. Therefore, we expect that contextual cueing is also likely to be enhanced in dyslexia for contexts that are natural scenes.

Methods

Participants. Two groups of subjects participated in Experiment 2. One group consisted of 9 students with histories of reading struggles randomly drawn from the pool of volunteers from Landmark College described in Experiment 1; the other consisted of 8 students with typical reading abilities at Harvard University as before. Other criteria were as in Experiment 1.

Stimuli and Apparatus. Stimuli consisted of photographs of real-world scenes previously used by Brockmole and Henderson [8]. Each scene (subtending a visual angle of 32° by 23°) contained a single gray T or L 0.18° in height (Figure 4b). Stimuli were displayed at a resolution of 800×600 pixels on a 19-inch CRT display at a constrained viewing distance of 70 cm. A video game controller was used to collect responses. Participants used a chinrest with a forehead bar to stabilize the head.

Procedure. Two types of trials were created. To measure baseline search speed, novel trials presented an image that had not been previously shown in the experiment. Any decrease in search speed on novel trials over the course of the experiment is therefore attributed to general practice effects. In contrast, repeated trials presented one of eight images that were previously displayed. With each repetition of an image, target location, but not target identity, was held constant. If this contingency is learned, search can be more efficient and response times on repeated trials should therefore decrease at a faster rate than observed on novel trials (i.e., an effect of learning over and above practice). The trial sequence was composed of 16 blocks, each containing 8 randomly selected novel trials and the 8 repeated trials (see Figure 3).

Trials were self-paced. Participants began each trial by fixating a dot in the center of the screen and pressed a button to initiate the onset of the stimulus. Targets were identified by pressing one of two buttons corresponding to the target (L or T). Trials were terminated if a response was not made within 20 s. No information regarding block structure or scene repetition was given to participants.

Results

Analysis. TR participants failed to respond on 3.8% of trials while those in the SR group did not respond on 9.6% of trials [$t(15) = 6.05$, $p<.001$]. However, this difference between groups was driven by the novel trials where the TR group failed to respond on 7.3% of trials and the SR group failed to respond on 16.4% of trials. This is a byproduct of overall slower search among SR participants (more below). By including an upper bound on response times in the study's design, the baseline rate of search for the SR group is likely to be underestimated in our data. Concerning the repeated trials (those subject to learning), however, both groups responded on more than 97% of trials. Thus, the impact of trial repetition on RTs is accurately described. The statistical consequence of these data patterns, if anything, is an underestimation of contextual cueing for the SR group. We are therefore at a disadvantage to support our hypothesis that SR participants will show bigger contextual cueing effects than TR participants. Accuracy was uniformly high with incorrect responses occurring on 1.2% of trials for the TR group and 2.1% of trials for the SR group [$t(15) = 1.96$, $p = .07$]. Trials on which a response was incorrect were excluded from the analyses.

The 16 trial blocks were collapsed into 4 equal-sized epochs for analysis. Search times were submitted to a 2 (group: TR vs. SR) ×2 (trial type: repeated vs. novel) ×4 (block) mixed model ANOVA (see Figure 4c). All three main effects were reliable [group: $F(1, 15) = 13.1$, $p<.01$; trial type: $F(1, 15) = 397$, $p<.001$; epoch: $F(3,45) = 14.7$, $p<.001$]. As in Experiment 1, SR observers took longer ($M = 3421$ ms) to find the target than those in TR ($M = 2701$ ms); faster responses were elicited on repeated trials ($M = 1997$ ms) compared with novel trials ($M = 4165$ ms), and RTs decreased over epochs (Ms = 3701 ms, 3057 ms, 2862 ms, and 2707 ms across epochs 1–4, respectively). The interaction between trial type and epoch was also observed [$F(3, 45) = 31.2$, $p<.001$]. Whereas search times for novel trials did not change over blocks (linear trend: $F(1, 16)<1$), responses to repeated trials progressively decreased over the course of the experiment (linear trend: $F(1, 16) = 66.1$, $p<.001$). Critically, the three-way interaction was not reliable [$F(3, 45) = 1.14$, $p = .34$], indicating equivalent contextual cueing among SR and TR groups. The hypothesis that contextual cueing is enhanced in the SR group for contexts composed of natural scenes was not supported, as the search benefit due to contextual cueing was indistinguishable between the two subject groups.

Search deficits (in terms of overall longer response times) are clearly evident in the SR group. This raises the question of whether search latencies observed in dyslexia result from deficits in visual attention [26], or visuomotor deficits that slow response [54]. Inspection of Figure 4 suggests that latencies in visual search (defined as the magnitude of the difference in RT between the SR and TR groups) that are clearly evident at the beginning of the

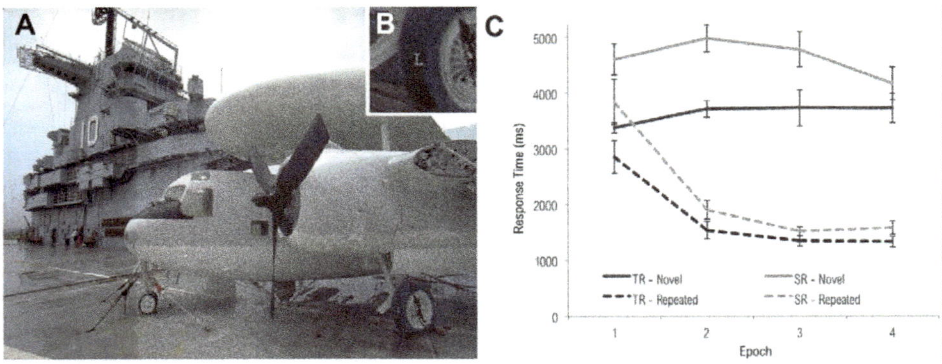

Figure 4. Example of stimulus used in Experiment 2. (A) Participants search for and identify a T or L target letter (here, a letter "L" on the aircraft tire, lower right). (B) Inset detail reveals target location. (C) Results of Experiment 2. Both typical readers and individuals with dyslexia show progressively faster search times for repeated trials, but not for novel trials. The magnitude of this difference was equivalent for both groups.

task are substantially reduced toward the end of the task, after practice and contextual cueing have had an effect. If contextual cueing reduces search latencies over the course of the experiment, this provides evidence that the slower response in dyslexia is likely the result of deficits in visual attention, and is not expressly due to a lag in visuomotor reaction as proposed, because such visuomotor deficits would not benefit from the memory-guided search.

To shed more light on this question, even though the corresponding overall interactions did not reach significance level, we employed a more focused approach and analyzed the RTs only at the end of the experiment (epochs 3 and 4), when contextual cueing, motor rehearsal, and practice with the task were expected to have had maximal effect. For novel trials in epochs 3 and 4, the main effect of group was significant, $F(1, 15) = 4.41$, $p = .05$. The repeated trials in the same blocks failed to show a similar effect of group, $F(1, 15) = 2.58$, $p = .13$ (see Table 2). This indicates that the SR group was still slower than the TR group at the end of the experiment when it came to searching through novel trials, but that, when it came to repeated trials, the differences between groups were so small at the end of the experiment that they failed to reach significance. This suggests some support for the hypothesis that, in the natural scene context, search latencies among struggling readers are largely eliminated by contextual cueing. It may, therefore, be that visuospatial deficits, and not motor response deficits, are the predominant factor accounting for search delays among struggling readers, when searching real-world scenes.

Experiment 3: Low-Pass Filtered Scenes

Here we explore contextual cueing in natural scenes that are low-pass filtered. Evidence suggests that dyslexia is linked to advantages, compared with the performance of typical readers, for visual cognition invoking long-range processing involving use of information the periphery [27,29,55]. Therefore, in this experiment, the application of a low-pass filter to natural scenes serves to limit the efficacy of foveal vision, and thereby biases visual processing toward peripheral visual content for which strengths are reported in dyslexia. This leads to the prediction that contextual cueing will be stronger in the SR group.

Methods

Participants. A group (SR) of 5 students with dyslexia was recruited from Landmark College, and a control group (TR) included 10 students from Harvard University, as previously described. None of the volunteers in this experiment participated in Experiment 2.

Table 2. Search latencies after contextual cueing and practice.

	Novel		Repeated	
Experiment	Latency	% of TR	Latency	% of TR
1	312	18	394	26
2	789	22	214	16
3	1223	72	583	51

Abbreviations: Latency = mean RTs for SR group minus mean RTs for TR group. % of TR = latency as a proportion of mean RTs for TR group, expressed as percentage. All means computed for the latter half of the experiment only (epochs 4–6 for Exp 1; blocks 9–16 for Exps 1 and 2).

Stimulus, Apparatus, and Procedure. Stimuli consisted of low-pass filtered color photographs of real-world scenes. Here, Adobe Photoshop CS3 was used to apply a Gaussian filter of radius 13.5 pixels (.54 degrees) to the image set used in Experiment 2. To understand the effect of the filter, a power spectrum was computed for each of the 162 images used, before and after the filter was applied. A two-sample Kolmogorov-Smirnov test (alpha = 5%) was used to compare the difference in median power before and after filtering in each of 800 spectral frequency bins. No significant difference was observed for spatial frequencies lower than 0.19 cycles/degree. However, as expected, the filtering produced significant effects in spatial frequency components higher than this, with 75% of the difference in median power accounted for in spatial frequencies lying between 0.20 and 0.67 cycles/degree (see Figure 5). Each scene contained a normal or mirror reversed C whose visual diameter was 1.67° (Figure 6b) that was blurred using a Gaussian filter with a radius of 4.4 pixels (.18 degrees). Thus, a subtle contrast difference was apparent between targets and backgrounds. All other aspects of the apparatus and design were the same as in Experiment 2.

Results

Analysis. TR participants failed to respond on <1% of trials while those in the SR group did not respond on 5.2% of trials [$t(13) = 2.22$, $p<.05$]. Once again, this difference between groups was driven by the novel trials where the TR group failed to respond on 1.4% of trials and the SR group failed to respond on 8.0% of trials. Concerning the repeated trials, both groups responded on more than 97% of trials. As in Experiment 2, therefore, we are at a disadvantage to support our hypothesis that SR participants will show bigger contextual cueing effects than TR participants. Accuracy was uniformly high with incorrect responses occurring on 2.2% of trials for the TR group and 2.6% of trials for the SR group [$t(13)<1$]. As before, trials on which a response was incorrect were excluded from the analyses.

As in Experiment 2, the 16 trial blocks were collapsed into 4 equal-sized epochs for analysis. Search times were submitted to a 2 (group: TR vs. SR) ×2 (trial type: repeated vs. novel) ×4 (epoch) mixed model ANOVA (see Figure 6c). As in Experiment 2, all three main effects were reliable [group: $F(1, 13) = 19.6$, $p<.001$; trial type: $F(1, 13) = 57.9$, $p<.001$; epoch: $F(3, 39) = 21.7$, $p<.001$]. Consistent with prior work, SR observers took longer to find the target ($M = 2660$ ms) than controls ($M = 1563$ ms); faster responses were elicited on repeated trials ($M = 1588$ ms) compared with novel trials ($M = 2270$ ms), and RTs decreased over epochs (M's = 2432 ms, 1842 ms, 1803 ms, and 1637 ms across epochs 1–4, respectively). The statistical hallmark of contextual cueing, an interaction between trial type and epoch, was marginally reliable [$F(3, 39) = 2.72$, $p = 0.58$]. However, a reliable three-way interaction [$F(3, 39) = 3.15$, $p<.05$] was observed indicating that contextual cueing differed by group. This prompted us to consider the TR and SR groups separately. To more precisely characterize the individual groups, we examined performance across all 16 experimental blocks and therefore conducted separate 2 (trial type) ×16 (block) repeated measures ANOVAs. (Observed mean search times (ms) by group, block, and trial type are shown in Table 3.) In these analyses, both groups displayed faster response times to the repeated trials and on the later blocks (all p's<.01). However, the critical interaction between trial type and block was not observed in TR [$F(15, 135) = 1.51$, $p = .11$] while it was observed for SR participants [$F(15, 60) = 1.92$, $p<.05$]. That said, because the differential effect of block on novel and repeated trials was marginal among typical readers, we also used linear regression analysis as a way to estimate the rate of learning in each group. For

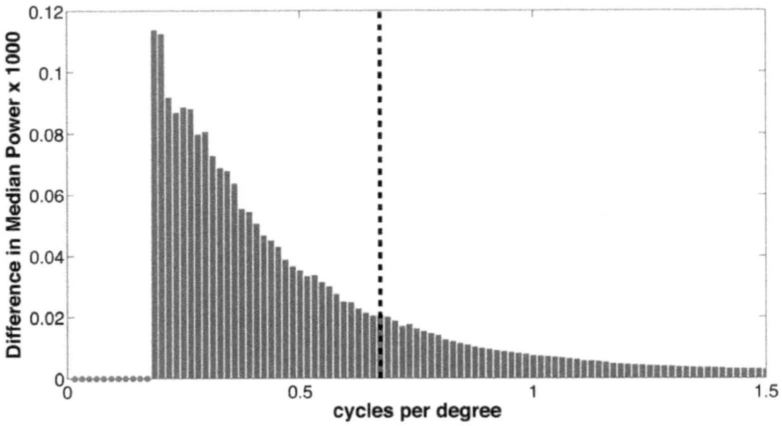

Figure 5. The effects of low-pass filtering on spectral power. Power spectra in 800 frequency bins were computed for the unfiltered images used in Experiment 2, and compared to power spectra of the Gaussian filtered images used in Experiment 3. The median difference in power per bin is plotted. This shows that seventy-five percent of the difference is accounted for in frequency bins between 0.2 and 0.67 cycles per degree (left of vertical dashed line). The power does not differ significantly in the range 0 to 0.19 cycles per degree (small red circles).

typical readers, linear models indicated a 42 ms decrease in RT per block within the repeated trial condition. Comparatively, for struggling readers, these models indicated a 144 ms decrease in RT per block, a rate of learning triple that of typical readers. From this analysis too, then, the hypothesis that contextual cueing is enhanced in struggling readers when scene contexts are low-pass filtered is supported.

Discussion

Implications for Dyslexia

Figure 1 schematically summarizes the results. While no group differences in contextual cueing were observed for letter-like contexts (Experiment 1) or natural scenes (Experiment 2), college students who face lifelong struggles with reading exhibited advantages in building scene memory when scenes are defined by natural images that are low-pass filtered (Experiment 3). This supports the peripheral-bias hypothesis [37]: When a low-pass filter is used in natural scenes to limit the efficacy of foveal vision and thereby biases visual processing toward long-range content for which strengths are reported in dyslexia [27,29,55], spatial learning is enhanced in struggling readers.

To what extent do these results in struggling readers apply to people with dyslexia in general? Those in the SR group, who are enrolled in special a remedial college for people with language-based learning disabilities, have had lifelong histories of struggles with reading that are typically characteristic of dyslexia. However, dyslexia is not a unitary phenomenon, but is instead described by subtypes that are as yet not well understood [56,57]. Given the generally small sample sizes used in our experiments, caution is therefore needed in generalizing our findings to all subtypes of dyslexia. Clearly, additional studies with large numbers of individuals, tracking factors indicative of subtypes within dyslexia, are needed. With this in mind, several explanations for our findings should be considered.

Given that the SR group consists of individuals who face unusual challenges with reading, it may not be dyslexia per se, but rather competition with reading that is the operant mechanism responsible for the effects observed. For example, tradeoffs between reading and visual cognition are reported in a functional magnetic resonance imaging study of illiterate adults who learn to read [58]. As acquisition of literacy strengthened activation in the left fusiform regions, activation for checkerboards and faces in the same location decreased. Similar effects of competition between reading and visual cognition are also observed in remediation

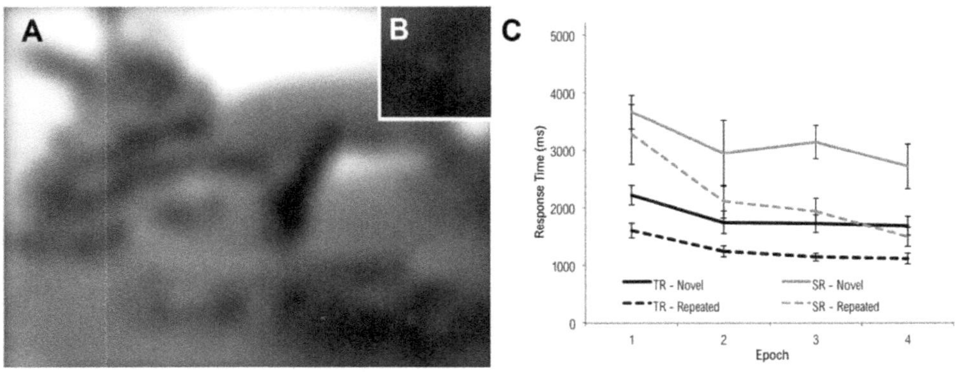

Figure 6. Example stimulus used in Experiment 3. (A) Participants search for a C or backwards C target (aircraft tire, lower right). Search times in novel and repeated contexts are compared to observe a contextual learning effect. (B) Inset detail reveals target location. (C) Results of reaction time analysis for Experiment 3. Individuals with dyslexia, but not typical readers, show evidence of contextual learning.

Table 3. Experiment 3 results: Mean RTs (ms) by group, block, and trial type.

	Block															
TrialType	**1**	**2**	**3**	**4**	**5**	**6**	**7**	**8**	**9**	**10**	**11**	**12**	**13**	**14**	**15**	**16**
	Typical Readers (TR)															
Novel	2564	1982	2435	1909	1617	1804	1725	1847	1581	1995	1383	1940	1462	1438	1797	2054
Repeated	2027	1697	1375	1324	1195	1385	1211	1203	1264	1119	1161	1045	1124	1140	1078	1130
	Struggling Readers (SR)															
Novel	3531	3286	3694	4132	3215	2717	1954	2912	2920	3788	2767	3086	2302	2541	2524	3503
Repeated	4127	3747	3296	1932	2388	2193	1883	1978	2188	2005	1757	1799	1333	1654	1591	1396

studies of people with dyslexia [29,31,59]. These reported that as struggling readers developed strategies that improved their reading, previously observed enhancements in peripheral sensitivity were observed to diminish. Therefore, similarly, it is possible that the effects we observe result from neural plasticity linked to lifelong experience with reading, differentiated in the SR and TR groups. If this were the case, then adults with dyslexia who struggled with reading throughout their lives would be expected to show enhanced peripheral sensitivity, when compared with people with dyslexia who had the benefit of a successful reading intervention early in life, and this effect would be independent of subtype classification.

If, on the other hand, we accept that the SR group is linked to dyslexia, then a possible alternate explanation for the findings in Experiment 3 is that contextual cueing is enhanced simply because those in the SR group take longer to find the target, affording this group more time to commit the scenes to memory during search. Dyslexia is linked to impaired sensitivity to low spatial frequencies [60], for briefly flashed sinusoidal gratings at ~4 cycles per degree. Diminished threshold sensitivity to low spatial frequency contrasts would make it difficult for these individuals to find the low spatial frequency targets, slowing their search and increasing their exposure to each scene. In Table 2 we summarize the mean search latencies in the last half of each Experiment, when contextual cueing and practice effects are the strongest. While in Experiments 1 and 2, the SR group spends on average about 20% more time searching each scene, in Experiment 3 the SR group spends 51% more time searching scenes that are repeated, and 72% more time searching those that are novel. The most pronounced latencies (observed in Experiment 3) are thus linked with enhanced contextual cueing (in that same experiment). Therefore it is plausible that the added time spent in search serves to facilitate scene learning, and future experiments should attempt to control for this effect.

Rapid semantic characterization of ambiguous scenes

It has been shown that, in real-world scenes, shifts of attention are initially based on scene identity, and subsequent shifts are guided by more detailed information regarding scene and object layout [8]. Semantic memory (e.g., "the L is on the tire") has been shown to play a causal and independent role in learning associations between objects in real-world scenes [61]. It has been demonstrated that many people with dyslexia are slower at retrieving names of letters, objects, and colors [62], deficits that are linked to a more generalized impediment in retrieving semantic labels from visual stimuli [63]. Difficulties retrieving verbal labels for objects and images are accompanied by a greater incidence of tip-of-the-tongue (TOT) responses, wherein the identity of the visual stimulus is familiar, understood, and known, but cannot be accurately named [64]. Anecdotally, people with dyslexia are observed to compensate for difficulties with semantic retrieval by making semantic substitutions in speech. Thus, if an individual is struggling to retrieve the verbal label for "tire," the idea "the L is on the tire" might be conceptualized instead as "the L is on the black blob," using a semantic substitution that is personal and meaningful to the individual, and that can be retrieved at speeds close to those seen in typical verbal retrieval.

We suggest that the compensatory practice individuals with dyslexia have with semantic substitution could account for the findings in Experiments 2 and 3. When natural scenes are low-pass filtered, object identity can become ambiguous. In this case, people in the SR group, who are adept at creating semantic labels for things that are difficult to describe will continue to use semantic substitution to generate meaningful semantic cues able to guide attention in contextual cueing. However, those in the TR group, who are likely expecting to apply accurate semantic labels for the low-pass filtered forms, would have difficulty doing so. Lacking semantic categories and object names to guide attention, the TR group would be at a disadvantage for contextual cueing when the scenes are low-pass filtered. But the two groups would be equivalent for the unfiltered contexts because semantic substitution used by the SR group and accurate verbal identification used by TR group would be equally effective for defining semantic cues able to guide attention. This hypothesis could therefore explain our findings indicating no significant group differences in contextual cueing for natural scenes (Experiment 2), but advantages for the SR group when scenes are low-pass filtered (Experiment 3). Empirically testing this semantic hypothesis should be the focus of future work.

Motor impairments cannot fully explain response latencies observed

All three experiments revealed a significant main effect of group indicating that the SR group was overall slower at search, compared with the typical readers. Search requires focal attention [22], and search impairments in dyslexia have been cited as evidence of a deficit in the magnocellular pathways [26], well explained by associated focal attention deficits [16–19,65,66]. Thus, to the extent that the SR group is representative of dyslexia, our findings are consistent with the observed deficits in focal attention. However, an alternate explanation is that the slower reaction times are a consequence of impaired motor response in dyslexia linked to cerebellar abnormalities [54], and not an effect of focal visual attention deficits.

To investigate these possibilities we separately analyzed search latencies in the latter half of Experiment 2, after contextual cueing, motor rehearsal, and practice with the task have had a chance to express their fullest benefit. We found that in repeated trials, where search is guided in part by memory, latencies were small (214 ms) and could not be reliably measured in our experiment. But in the novel condition the latencies were substantial (789 ms) and significant, persisting despite benefits of practice and motor rehearsal accrued in the first half of the experiment. We expected that motor deficits would have the same effect for both the novel and repeated conditions. However, the effects of focal attention deficits were expected to be different in the novel and repeated cases, because focal attention plays a small role when trials are repeated, and search is guided by memory.

The analysis of mean RT in the latter half of Experiment 2 (see Table 2, and Results described previously) showed that search times for struggling readers were indistinguishable in our experiments from the typical readers when the scenes were repeated, suggesting that once the task had been practiced, and motor actions had been learned, motor deficits no longer played a significant role in impeding search. However, in the novel trials, significant latencies remained evident even after motor rehearsal and task learning. Therefore, our observations lend support to the hypothesis that visual attention deficits, and not motor deficits, are the dominant mechanism acting to impede search in struggling readers in real scenes.

Spatial learning and distributed attention unaffected by attention deficits

In all cases, our experiments showed that, when search is performed in scenes that are novel, visual search was impaired in those who struggle to read. These observations support previous reports associating dyslexia with deficits for search [26,67], a finding that is in turn consistent with observations associating dyslexia with deficits for focal attention [16–19,65,66]. In contrast, none of our experiments revealed corresponding deficits for contextual cueing. The fact that contextual cueing was unaffected by deficits for focal attention in dyslexia is consistent with research that shows that the rapid categorization of natural scenes proceeds in parallel with attention, and is not affected by focal attention loads [68]. Contextual cueing has also been shown to be robust against interference from working memory loads [69,70], and thus working memory deficits in dyslexia [71] were not expected to interfere with processes important in scene learning. Consequently, visuospatial deficits characteristic of dyslexia were not expected to impair contextual cueing, and this was supported by our observations.

A number of authors stress a distinction between systems for focal attention and those for rapid distributed spatial attention, with both types of systems acting in concert to build the visual percept in a complex scene [21,22]. Distributed attention is thought to play a role in contextual cueing to form a rapid initial hypothesis about the global scene layout that is later refined through search [72]. Numerous studies point to findings that focal attention and slow sustained attention are impaired in dyslexia [25,26]. However, emerging research, including the findings here, suggests that rapidly deployed distributed attention is unimpaired in dyslexia, and if anything may be enhanced. For example, as mentioned before, recognition speed for impossible figures, a task that depends on the holistic integration of long-range spatial information across a scene, is observed to be enhanced in dyslexia without compromising speed [27]. Those with dyslexia have been observed to respond more rapidly to an unattended peripheral flash when the flash occurs at eccentricities $>8°$ [35,36]. Other studies found visuospatial advantages in dyslexia in letter identification tasks in cases where letters are flashed simultaneously at fixation and in the periphery, typically at eccentricities $>8°$ [28–34], a task that requires rapid deployment of spatially distributed attention. Collectively, these studies link dyslexia to advantages for distributed forms of spatial attention, typically in circumstances where peripheral (eccentricities $>\sim 8°$) information is important.

Implications for the magnocellular theory of dyslexia

The visual channels responsible for the processing of low spatial frequency information are thought to play a distinct role in the higher-order cognitive processing of visual information. Theories of visual recognition propose that visual scenes are processed in a temporal order that proceeds from coarse-to-fine [73]. Here, low spatial frequency information is thought to reach higher-order areas most rapidly to allow for an initial coarse parsing of the scene that precedes an analysis of high spatial frequency details [74–76]. An empirical test of this hypothesis showed that, when two spatial frequency-filtered natural scenes were presented in rapid succession during fMRI and ERP recording, low spatial frequencies increased activity in prefrontal and temporo-parietal areas first, before high spatial frequency detail produced an effect [77]. This demonstrates that low-pass signals can rapidly activate high-order areas to provide spatial, semantic, and attentional signals that together may promote perceptual organization and categorization of visual scenes.

Our findings that visual search is consistently impaired in the SR group are in line with reports of attention deficits and therefore support prior studies linking dyslexia to impairments in the magnocellular pathways [26]. However, if the findings of Experiment 3 are not simply consequences of longer exposure or rapid semantic characterization, as suggested earlier, but instead are a result of enhanced processing in dyslexia in the visual channels responsible for the coarse preprocessing of scenes, then our finding of enhanced spatial learning in low-pass filtered contexts presents a challenge for magnocellular theories of dyslexia. Low spatial frequencies are believed to be conveyed primarily by the magnocellular visual pathways [78,79] and dyslexia has been associated, albeit controversially, with deficits in functions conveyed by these channels [80,81]. Therefore, a magnocellular deficit cannot concurrently account for deficits in search and advantages for spatial processing unless each of these functions are sub-served by magnocellular neurologies that are distinct.

We suggest that a possible alternate perspective, consistent with the peripheral-bias hypothesis [37], is that, rather than an overall magnocellular deficit, there is a magnocellular *shift* in dyslexia toward the periphery. This is proposed to skew the distribution of magnocellular neurons (relative to parvocellular) retinotopically toward the periphery. This would have the effect of under-representing the magnocellular density near the fovea, but of over-representing the density toward the periphery. Such a pattern would thus concurrently account for magnocellular deficits near the fovea, including deficits for central-field tasks such as visual search [38], and for enhancements in spatial learning, conveyed by long-range interactions involving the periphery [10,12].

The proposal that magnocellular phenomena in dyslexia are better described in term of a retinotopic shift directed toward the periphery may be supported by emerging theories in the field of genetics [82,83]. These theories suggest that cytoarchitectonic abnormalities in dyslexia [80,84–87] are induced by heritable errors linked to 14 candidate genes thought to regulate neuronal migration (see review [88]). These errors are thought to disrupt the development of visual and auditory regions in the thalamus and elsewhere, including the magnocellular lamina in the LGN. Given that the fovea is magnified and highly over-represented in the LGN, even a minor redistribution of magnocellular neurons directed toward the retinotopic periphery, as proposed here, would have observable eccentricity-dependent consequences in dyslexia. Future tests of magnocellular phenomena should explicitly segregate visual contributions in the inner fields (inside 8°) from those at larger eccentricities.

Implications for education

The finding that college students with dyslexia are able to learn in some circumstances where typical readers cannot carries a number of important implications for education. It suggests that college students with dyslexia may benefit from encouragement in careers in which sensitivity to low spatial frequency scenes is valued. Radiology, astronomy, and cellular microscopy are all examples of domains making intensive use of spatial information in images that are blurred. Skills in processing blurred images may be beneficial also in other science-related fields. Furthermore, our findings show that contextual cueing is effective in counteracting latencies due to deficits in search, and therefore scene learning can serve as an effective compensatory technique for students with dyslexia. Practiced abilities for spatial learning can be used to spatially anchor memories for episodic information (such as names and dates). Such techniques have already been observed to effectively compensate for lapses in non-spatial memory in the elderly [89]. Similar gains can be expected in dyslexia.

Research in dyslexia has necessarily focused its greatest effort on phenomena pertinent to reading. Yet dyslexia has remained a puzzle for over a century. We suggest that efforts to investigate phenomena less relevant for reading, such as peripheral visual effects examined here, may be well rewarded. For not only do we believe that such research may help resolve questions that currently confound the interpretation of visual phenomena in dyslexia, but such research may lead to advancements in education that will increase support for children who otherwise struggle in school.

Acknowledgments

Amanda Heffner-Wong performed all experiments with assistance from Jamie O'Keeffe. Franklin Brown of Yale University performed the dyslexia evaluation at Landmark College. Alex D. Hwang and Hsueh-Cheng Wang wrote software used in the experiments. We acknowledge the helpful suggestions of anonymous reviewers. This work could not have been possible without extraordinary support provided by the staff and faculty of Landmark College. Special thanks to Linda Hecker, Manju Banerjee, and Jenny Thomson for helping prepare Table 1. We thank Kurt W. Fischer for pivotal contributions to the discussion, and his steadfast encouragement and support. This work is based upon work supported by NSF Grant HRD-0930962, and by a George E. Burch Foundation Fellowship (Smithsonian Institution) to MHS.

Author Contributions

Conceived and designed the experiments: MS JB MP. Performed the experiments: MS. Analyzed the data: JB GS. Contributed reagents/materials/analysis tools: JB MP. Wrote the paper: MS JB.

References

1. Kondo Y, Suzuki M, Mugikura S, Abe N, Takahashi S, et al. (2005) Changes in brain activation associated with use of a memory strategy: a functional MRI study. NeuroImage 24: 1154.
2. Shaywitz S, Shaywitz B (2005) Dyslexia (specific reading disability). Biological Psychiatry 57: 1301–1309.
3. Swanson HL, Zheng X, Jerman O (2009) Working memory, short-term memory, and reading disabilities: a selective meta-analysis of the literature. Journal of Learning Disabilities 42: 260–287.
4. Craggs J, Sanchez J, Kibby M, Gilger J, Hynd G (2006) Brain Morphology and Neuropsychological Profiles in A Family Displaying Dyslexia and Superior Nonverbal Intelligence. Cortex 42: 1107–1118.
5. Fink R (2006) Why Jane and John couldn't read - and how they learned: a new look at striving readers. 175 p.
6. Nuzzo R (2005) Biography of Carol W. Greider. Proceedings of the National Academy of Sciences, USA 102: 8077–8079.
7. Chun M, Jiang Y (1998) Contextual Cueing: Implicit Learning and Memory of Visual Context Guides Spatial Attention. Cognitive Psychology 36: 28–71.
8. Brockmole JR, Henderson JM (2006) Recognition and attention guidance during contextual cueing in real-world scenes: evidence from eye movements. Quarterly Journal of Experimental Psychology 59: 1177–1187.
9. Brady TF, Chun MM (2007) Spatial constraints on learning in visual search: modeling contextual cuing. Journal of Experimental Psychology Learning, Memory, and Cognition 33: 798–815.
10. Brockmole JR, Castelhano MS, Henderson JM (2006) Contextual cueing in naturalistic scenes: Global and local contexts. Journal of Experimental Psychology Learning, Memory, and Cognition 32: 699–706.
11. Jiang Y, Wagner L (2004) What is learned in spatial contextual cuing-configuration or individual locations? Perception and Psychophysics 66: 454–463.
12. van Asselen M, Castelo-Branco M (2009) The role of peripheral vision in implicit contextual cuing. Attention, Perception, and Psychophysics 71: 76–81.
13. Bennett IJ, Romano JC, Howard JH, Howard DV (2008) Two forms of implicit learning in young adults with dyslexia. Annals of the New York Academy of Sciences 1145: 184–198.
14. Howard J, Howard D, Japikse K, Eden G (2006) Dyslexics are impaired on implicit higher-order sequence learning, but not on implicit spatial context learning. Neuropsychologia 44: 1131–1144.
15. Jiménez-Fernández G, Vaquero JMM, Jiménez L, Defior S (2011) Dyslexic children show deficits in implicit sequence learning, but not in explicit sequence learning or contextual cueing. Annals of Dyslexia 61: 85–110.
16. Facoetti A, Ruffino M, Peru A, Paganoni P, Chelazzi L (2008) Sluggish engagement and disengagement of non-spatial attention in dyslexic children. Cortex 44: 1221–1233.
17. Ruffino M, Trussardi AN, Gori S, Finzi A, Giovagnoli S, et al. (2010) Attentional engagement deficits in dyslexic children. Neuropsychologia 48: 3793–3801.

18. Silva-Pereyra J, Bernal J, Rodríguez-Camacho M, Yáñez G, Prieto-Corona B, et al. (2010) Poor reading skills may involve a failure to focus attention. Neuroreport 21: 34–38.
19. Facoetti A, Corradi N, Ruffino M, Gori S, Zorzi M (2010) Visual spatial attention and speech segmentation are both impaired in preschoolers at familial risk for developmental dyslexia. Dyslexia (Chichester, England) 16: 226–239.
20. Schwartz S, Vuilleumier P, Hutton C, Maravita A, Dolan R, et al. (2005) Attentional Load and Sensory Competition in Human Vision: Modulation of fMRI Responses by Load at Fixation during Task-irrelevant Stimulation in the Peripheral Visual Field. Cerebral Cortex 15: 770–786.
21. Nakayama K (1990) The iconic bottleneck and the tenuous link between early visual processing and perception. Vision: Coding and efficiency. pp 411–422.
22. Treisman A, Gelade G (1980) A feature-integration theory of attention. Cognitive Psychology 12: 97–136.
23. Potter MC (1976) Short-term conceptual memory for pictures. Journal of Experimental Psychology: Human Learning and Memory 2: 509–522.
24. Oliva A (2005) Gist of the Scene. Neurobiology of attention. 696 p.
25. Facoetti A, Paganoni P, Turatto M, Marzola V, Mascetti G (2000) Visual-spatial attention in developmental dyslexia. Cortex 36: 109–123.
26. Vidyasagar TR, Pammer K (1999) Impaired visual search in dyslexia relates to the role of the magnocellular pathway in attention. Neuroreport 10: 1283–1287.
27. von Karolyi C, Winner E, Gray W, Sherman G (2003) Dyslexia linked to talent: Global visual-spatial ability. Brain and Language 85: 427–431.
28. Dautrich B (1993) Visual perceptual differences in the dyslexic reader: evidence of greater visual peripheral sensitivity to color and letter stimuli. Perceptual and Motor Skills 76: 755–764.
29. Geiger G, Lettvin J (1987) Peripheral vision in persons with dyslexia. New England Journal of Medicine 316: 1238–1243.
30. Geiger G, Lettvin J (2000) Developmental Dyslexia: a Different Perceptual Strategy and How to Learn a New Strategy for Reading. Saggi CD and D 26: 73–89.
31. Geiger G, Lettvin J, Fahle M (1994) Dyslexic children learn a new visual strategy for reading: a controlled experiment. Vision Research 34: 1223–1233.
32. Geiger G, Lettvin J, Zegarra-Moran O (1992) Task-determined strategies of visual process. Cognitive Brain Research 1: 39–52.
33. Lorusso M, Facoetti A, Pesenti S, Cattaneo C, Molteni M, et al. (2004) Wider recognition in peripheral vision common to different subtypes of dyslexia. Vision Research 44: 2413–2424.
34. Perry A, Dember W, Warm J, Sacks J (1989) Letter identification in normal and dyslexic readers: A verification. Bulletin of the Psychonomic Society 27: 445–448.
35. Facoetti A, Molteni M (2001) The gradient of visual attention in developmental dyslexia. Neuropsychologia 39: 352–357.
36. Facoetti A, Paganoni P, Lorusso M-L (2000) The spatial distribution of visual attention in developmental dyslexia. Experimental Brain Research 132: 531–538.
37. Schneps M, Rose L, Fischer K (2007) Visual learning and the brain: Implications for dyslexia. Mind, Brain, and Education 1: 128–139.
38. Carrasco M, Evert D, Chang I, Katz S (1995) The eccentricity effect: target eccentricity affects performance on conjunction searches. Percept Psychophys 57: 1241–1261.
39. Carrasco M, McElree B, Denisova K, Giordano A (2003) Speed of visual processing increases with eccentricity. Nature Neuroscience 6: 699–700.
40. Curcio C, Allen K (1990) Topography of ganglion cells in human retina. J COMP NEUROL 300: 5–25.
41. Dacey D (1994) Physiology, morphology and spatial densities of identified ganglion cell types in primate retina. Ciba Found Symp 184: 12–28 ; discussion 28–34, 63–70.
42. Gattass R, Nascimento-Silva S, Soares J, Lima B, Jansen A, et al. (2005) Cortical visual areas in monkeys: location, topography, connections, columns, plasticity and cortical dynamics. Philosophical Transactions Of The Royal Society Of London Series B, Biological Sciences 360: 709–731.
43. Woodcock RW, McGrew KS, Mather N (2001) Woodcock-Johnson III Tests of Achievemnent. Itasca, IL: Riverside Publishing.
44. (2002) Wechsler individual achievement test second edition. San Antonio, TX: Psychological Corporation: Harcourt Assessment.
45. (1997) Wechsler Adult Intelligence Scale-Third Edition. San Antonio, TX: Psychological Corporation.
46. Woodcock RW, McGrew KS, Mather N (2001) Woodcock-Johnson III Tests of Cognitive Abilities. Itasca, IL: Riverside Publishing.
47. Lefly D, Pennington B (2000) Reliability and validity of the adult reading history questionnaire. Journal of Learning Disabilities 33: 286–296.
48. Finucci JM, Whitehouse CC, Isaacs SD, Childs B (1984) Derivation and validation of a quantitative definition of specific reading disability for adults. Developmental Medicine and Child Neurology 26: 143–153.
49. Kessler RC, Adler LA, Gruber MJ, Sarawate CA, Spencer T, et al. (2007) Validity of the World Health Organization Adult ADHD Self-Report Scale (ASRS) Screener in a representative sample of health plan members. International Journal of Methods in Psychiatric Research 16: 52–65.
50. Kessler R, Adler L, Ames M, Demler O, Faraone S, et al. (2005) The World Health Organization Adult ADHD Self-Report Scale (ASRS): a short screening scale for use in the general population. Psychological Medicine 35: 245–256.
51. Brainard D (1997) The Psychophysics Toolbox. Spatial Vision 10: 433–436.
52. Chun MM, Phelps EA (1999) Memory deficits for implicit contextual information in amnesic subjects with hippocampal damage. Nature Neuroscience 2: 844–847.
53. Geringswald F, Pollmann S (2011) Impaired scene exploration causes deficits in visual learning. In: Thorpe S, ed. European Conference on Visual Perception 2011 Toulouse, France.
54. Stoodley C, Stein J (2005) A processing speed deficit in dyslexic adults? Evidence from a peg-moving task. Neuroscience Letters 399: 264–267.
55. Geiger G, Cattaneo C, Galli R, Pozzoli U, Luisa Lorusso M, et al. (2008) Wide and diffuse perceptual modes characterize dyslexics in vision and audition. Perception 37: 1745–1764.
56. McGrath LM, Pennington BF, Shanahan MA, Santerre-Lemmon LE, Barnard HD, et al. (2010) A multiple deficit model of reading disability and attention-deficit/hyperactivity disorder: searching for shared cognitive deficits. Journal of child psychology and psychiatry, and allied disciplines.
57. Katzir T, Kim Y-S, Wolf M, Morris R, Lovett MW (2008) The varieties of pathways to dysfluent reading: comparing subtypes of children with dyslexia at letter, word, and connected text levels of reading. Journal of learning disabilities 41: 47–66.
58. Dehaene S, Pegado F, Braga LW, Ventura P, Nunes Filho G, et al. (2010) How learning to read changes the cortical networks for vision and language. Science (New York, NY) 330: 1359–1364.
59. Luisa Lorusso M, Facoetti A, Toraldo A, Molteni M (2005) Tachistoscopic treatment of dyslexia changes the distribution of visual-spatial attention. Brain and Cognition 57: 135–142.
60. Lovegrove WJ, Bowling A, Badcock D, Blackwood M (1980) Specific reading disability: differences in contrast sensitivity as a function of spatial frequency. Science 210: 439–440.
61. Brockmole JR, Le-Hoa Võ M (2010) Semantic memory for contextual regularities within and across scene categories: evidence from eye movements. Attention, Perception, and Psychophysics 72: 1803–1813.
62. Denckla M, Rudel R (1976) Naming of Object-Drawings by Dyslexic and Other Learning Disabled Children. Brain and language 3: 1–15.
63. Jones MW, Branigan HP, Hatzidaki A, Obregón M (2010) Is the 'naming' deficit in dyslexia a misnomer? COGNITION 116: 56–70.
64. Faust M, Sharfstein-Friedman S (2003) Naming difficulties in adolescents with dyslexia: application of the tip-of-the-tongue paradigm. Brain and cognition 53: 211–217.
65. Facoetti A, Trussardi AN, Ruffino M, Lorusso ML, Cattaneo C, et al. (2010) Multisensory spatial attention deficits are predictive of phonological decoding skills in developmental dyslexia. Journal of Cognitive Neuroscience 22: 1011–1025.
66. Prado C, Dubois M, Valdois S (2007) The eye movements of dyslexic children during reading and visual search: impact of the visual attention span. Vision Research 47: 2521–2530.
67. Sireteanu R, Goebel C, Goertz R, Werner I, Nalewajko M, et al. (2008) Impaired serial visual search in children with developmental dyslexia. Annals of the New York Academy of Sciences 1145: 199–211.
68. Li FF, VanRullen R, Koch C, Perona P (2002) Rapid natural scene categorization in the near absence of attention. Proceedings of the National Academy of Science USA 99: 9596–9601.
69. Kessels RPC, Meulenbroek O, Fernández G, Olde Rikkert MGM (2010) Spatial working memory in aging and mild cognitive impairment: effects of task load and contextual cueing. Neuropsychology, Development, and Cognition Section B, Aging, Neuropsychology and Cognition 17: 556–574.
70. Vickery TJ (2010) Spatial context learning survives interference from working memory load. Journal of Experimental Psychology Human Perception and Performance 36: 1358–1371.
71. Smith-Spark J, Fisk J, Fawcett A, Nicolson R (2003) Investigating the central executive in adult dyslexics: Evidence from phonological and visuospatial working memory performance. European Journal of Cognitive Psychology 15: 567–587.
72. Huang T-R, Grossberg S (2010) Cortical dynamics of contextually cued attentive visual learning and search: spatial and object evidence accumulation. Psychological Review 117: 1080–1112.
73. Ahissar M, Hochstein S (2004) The reverse hierarchy theory of visual perceptual learning. Trends Cogn Sci 8: 457–464.
74. Bar M (2003) A cortical mechanism for triggering top-down facilitation in visual object recognition. Journal of Cognitive Neuroscience 15: 600–609.
75. Bullier J (2001) Integrated model of visual processing. Brain Research Reviews 36: 96–107.
76. Hegdé J (2008) Time course of visual perception: coarse-to-fine processing and beyond. Progress in Neurobiology 84: 405–439.
77. Peyrin C, Michel CM, Schwartz S, Thut G, Seghier M, et al. (2010) The neural substrates and timing of top-down processes during coarse-to-fine categorization of visual scenes: a combined fMRI and ERP study. Journal of Cognitive Neuroscience 22: 2768–2780.
78. Derrington A, Lennie P (1984) Spatial and temporal contrast sensitivities of neurones in lateral geniculate nucleus of macaque. Journal of Physiology 357: 219–240.
79. Ellemberg D, Hammarrenger B, Lepore F, Roy M-S, Guillemot J-P (2001) Contrast dependency of VEPs as a function of spatial frequency: the parvocellular and magnocellular contributions to human VEPs. Spatial Vision 15: 99–111.

80. Galaburda A, Livingstone M (1993) Evidence for a magnocellular defect in developmental dyslexia. Annals of the New York Academy of Sciences 682: 70–82.
81. Kevan A, Pammer K (2008) Making the link between dorsal stream sensitivity and reading. Neuroreport 19: 467–470.
82. Ramus F (2004) Neurobiology of dyslexia: a reinterpretation of the data. Trends in neurosciences 27: 720–726.
83. Rosen GD, Bai J, Wang Y, Fiondella CG, Threlkeld SW, et al. (2007) Disruption of Neuronal Migration by RNAi of Dyx1c1 Results in Neocortical and Hippocampal Malformations. Cerebral Cortex 17: 2562–2572.
84. Livingstone MS, Rosen GD, Drislane FW, Galaburda AM (1991) Physiological and anatomical evidence for a magnocellular defect in developmental dyslexia. Proceedings of the National Academy of Science USA 88: 7943–7947.
85. Galaburda AM, sherman GF, Rosen GD, Aboitiz F, Geschwind N (1985) Developmental dyslexia: Four consecutive patients with cortical anomalies. Annals of Neurology 18: 222–233.
86. Humphreys P, Kaufmann WE, Galaburda AM, MD (1990) Developmental dyslexia in women: neuropathological findings in three patients. Annals of Neurology 28: 727–738.
87. Kaufmann W, Galaburda A (1989) Cerebrocortical microdysgenesis in neurologically normal subjects: A histopathological study. Neurology 39: 238–244.
88. Poelmans G, Buitelaar JK, Pauls DL, Franke B (2011) A theoretical molecular network for dyslexia: integrating available genetic findings. Molecular Psychiatry 16: 365–382.
89. Verhaeghen P, Marcoen A (1996) On the Mechanisms of Plasticity in Young and Older Adults After Instruction in the Method of Loci: Evidence for an Amplification Model. Psychology and Aging 11: 164.

7

Atypical Balance between Occipital and Fronto-Parietal Activation for Visual Shape Extraction in Dyslexia

Ying Zhang[1,2]*, Susan Whitfield-Gabrieli[1], Joanna A. Christodoulou[1], John D. E. Gabrieli[1]

1 Department of Brain and Cognitive Sciences, McGovern Institute for Brain Research, Massachusetts Institute of Technology, Cambridge, Massachusetts, United States of America, **2** State Key Laboratory of Brain and Cognitive Science, Institute of Biophysics, Chinese Academy of Science, Beijing, China

Abstract

Reading requires the extraction of letter shapes from a complex background of text, and an impairment in visual shape extraction would cause difficulty in reading. To investigate the neural mechanisms of visual shape extraction in dyslexia, we used functional magnetic resonance imaging (fMRI) to examine brain activation while adults with or without dyslexia responded to the change of an arrow's direction in a complex, relative to a simple, visual background. In comparison to adults with typical reading ability, adults with dyslexia exhibited opposite patterns of atypical activation: decreased activation in occipital visual areas associated with visual perception, and increased activation in frontal and parietal regions associated with visual attention. These findings indicate that dyslexia involves atypical brain organization for fundamental processes of visual shape extraction even when reading is not involved. Overengagement in higher-order association cortices, required to compensate for underengagment in lower-order visual cortices, may result in competition for top-down attentional resources helpful for fluent reading.

Editor: Markus Lappe, University of Muenster, Germany

Funding: This work was supported by the Ellison Medical Foundation; MIT Class of 1976 Funds for Dyslexia Research; Bard and Julie Richmond through the Martin Richmond Memorial Fund; and NIH grants UL1RR025758 and F32EY014750-01. The funders had no role in study design, data collection and analysis, decision to publish, or preparation of the manuscript.

Competing Interests: The authors have declared that no competing interests exist.

* E-mail: yzhang00@mit.edu

Introduction

Developmental dyslexia is a significant impairment in reading, regardless of age, IQ, or educational opportunity [1,2], and it is associated with atypical brain function for reading [3,4]. The best understood cause for dyslexia is a weakness in phonological awareness [5,6]. Phonological training, however, is more effective in improving reading accuracy than reading speed [1,7], which suggests that other factors, such as visual deficits, may also play a causal role in preventing readers with dyslexia from efficiently extracting information from written language.

Visual deficits are frequently reported in dyslexia, although the nature and role of these deficits are less agreed upon. Using non-verbal visual stimuli such as gratings or simple geometric shapes, separate lines of evidence suggest dyslexic deficits in either sensory or attentional processes that are independent from language [8,9]. Visual sensory deficits associated with magnocellular functions have been suggested by anatomical, physiological, and behavioral studies [9,10,11], but the specificity of these deficits have been challenged [12,13,14,15,16,17]. The sensory deficit is further supported, however, by neuroimaging findings of reduced activation in individuals with dyslexia for visual motion in early visual areas [18,19]. Aside from sensory problems, visual attentional deficits in dyslexia are suggested by impaired performance on non-verbal covert attention or visual search tasks [20,21,22,23,24]. Indeed, children with dyslexia who also have reduced visual attention spans show reduced activation in parietal areas associated with visual attention [25].

Neuroimaging studies of basic visual processing in dyslexia have focused on motion or attention, but it is unknown as to whether individuals with dyslexia extract visual shapes differently in their brains than do typical readers. Fluent and skilled reading begins with shape extraction of letters from complex text and visual environments, and an altered brain basis of visual shape extraction could compromise reading. Here, we compared brain functions between adults with and without dyslexia for basic visual extraction of a non-verbal shape from a complex background. We used functional magnetic resonance imaging (fMRI) to investigate brain activations for a simple task in which a shape (an arrow) had to be extracted from a simple or a complex visual background. Behavioral studies have reported that individuals with dyslexia are impaired at extracting shape information from complex white noise backgrounds [16,26,27,28,29]. A fundamental question is whether visual shape extraction in dyslexia is associated with altered brain functions, and if so whether such alterations occur in occipital areas associated with sensory processes, in fronto-parietal areas associated with attentional processes, or in both sensory and attentional areas.

Materials and Methods

All participants were recruited from the Boston area and were provided written informed consent as approved by the Massachusetts Institute of Technology Institutional Review Board (IRB).

Participants and Testing Battery

Twenty-four healthy participants, between the ages of 18–37 years and having normal or corrected-to-normal vision were included. All participants were native English speakers, had no neurological or psychiatric disorders, were not on any medication, and had no contraindications for MRI. All participants were paid $20/hour for their participation.

For all participants, cognitive abilities, reading and related skills were assessed using a battery of standardized behavioral measures. The testing battery included indices of non-verbal cognitive ability (*Kaufman Brief Intelligence Test* (KBIT) [30], or *Wechsler Abbreviated Scale of Intelligence* (WASI) [31]. Untimed reading ability was measured by the total numbers of real words and pseudowords that were read correctly ("Word Identification" and "Word Attack" from the *Woodcock Reading Mastery Test-Revised, NU* (WRMT) [32]). Timed reading abilities were measured by the total numbers of words and pseudowords that were read correctly within a time limit ("Sight Word Efficiency" and "Phonemic Decoding Efficiency" from the *Test of Word Reading Efficiency* (TOWRE) [33]). Rapid naming scores were the time in seconds needed to name a series of letters as quickly and accurately as possible ("Rapid Letter Naming," *Comprehensive Test of Phonological Processing)* [34].

Participant Groups and Inclusion Criteria

Eleven participants with dyslexia and thirteen people with typical reading ability (i.e., the control group) were matched based on their non-verbal cognitive abilities (Performance IQ, Table 1). On measures of cognitive ability, all participants scored within 15 points or higher of the expected mean of 100. Criteria for dyslexia were met if participants reported a previous history of reading difficulty or a related diagnosis (e.g., reading disability, dyslexia), and also earned a current standard score below the 25th percentile rank based on norms from standardized tests, on at least two measures of single word or pseudoword timed or untimed reading.

Visual Stimulus and Shape Extraction Task

Visual stimuli consisted of a small arrow displayed at the center with either a background of a uniform gray display (simple condition) or a background of vertical gratings (complex condition) (Fig. 1A). The size of the center arrow was 0.47×0.95°; it was bright yellow with the red and the green luminance values at their maximal luminance. The background during the complex condition was a 0.47 cycle/degree, 100% contrast sinusoidal grating; it was 180° phase reversed every 1.5 seconds (0.33 Hz). The mean luminance of the gratings matched the luminance value of the gray background; the mean luminance values of the gray background and the mean luminance value of the gratings remained constant throughout the experiment. For gratings, the mean luminance value was 3.3 cd/m^2 with maximum and minimum luminance of 4.2 and 2.4/m^2, respectively. The low luminance level was used so as to be comparable to previous studies of basic visual perception in dyslexia [18,35]. Visual stimuli were programmed in Matlab using the Psychophysics Toolbox [36,37]. Visual stimuli were back-projected from an LCD projector on to a screen, and viewed through a prism mirror as participants were lying on their backs in the scanner. The screen was placed 1.2 meters away from the participants' eyes; the display subtended a visual angle of 17.8×17.8° and fully covered the opening of the scanner with some corners being concealed. The visual stimuli were simultaneously displayed on a PC monitor in the MRI control room so that they could be monitored continuously by the experimenter.

The shape extraction task required participants to detect the directional change of the arrow. Under both simple and complex conditions, participants were instructed to press a button as soon as they perceived the arrow changing direction, either from left to right or from right to left. Both complex and simple conditions were conducted in blocks of 12 seconds, with a 3-second fixation period between blocks during which participants were asked to look at a small red fixation dot displayed at the center of the screen. There were sixteen blocks per condition. The simple and complex conditions were pseudorandomized and counter-balanced. While there were four additional conditions not reported here, the sequences of the experimental conditions were the same

Table 1. Behavioral Profiles for Participants with and without Dyslexia.

	Control Readers	Dyslexic Readers	T-values: Control vs. Dyslexic Readers
	Mean±SD	Mean±SD	T p
N	13(8 female)	11 (7 female)	
Age	22.9±3.7	24.3±5.4	0.75.46
Behavioral Measure			
Performance IQ	108.9±8.4	107.2±13.9	0.38.71
Rapid Letter Naming	0.61±.50	−0.29±.86	3.19.004***
WRMT – Word Identification	107.1±7.2	92.9±8.9	4.32.000***
WRMT – Word Attack	107.9±8.8	92.0±12.6	3.63.001**
TOWRE – Sight Word Efficiency	109.1±6.9	91.3±13.5	4.16.000***
TOWRE – Phonemic Decoding Efficiency	106.2±7.3	82.8±5.0	9.02.000***

*$p<0.05$, two-tailed t-test;
**$p<0.01$, two-tailed t-test;
***$p<0.001$, two-tailed t-test.
Note: Standard scores are based on a mean of 100 and a standard deviation (SD) of 15. Note: Acronyms are as follows: WRMT for *Woodcock Reading Mastery Test – Revised NU*; TOWRE for *Test of Word Reading Efficiency. Note: Participants completed either the Kaufman Brief Intelligence Test (KBIT) (8 control; 8 dyslexic) or the Wechsler Abbreviated Scale of Intelligence (WASI) (5 control; 3 dyslexic) for Performance IQ; and either the CTOPP Rapid Letter Naming (10 control; 7 dyslexic) or the RAN/RAS Letter subtest (3 control; 4 dyslexic) [108]. Rapid Letter Naming scores are based on z scores to allow for comparison between different subtests used.*

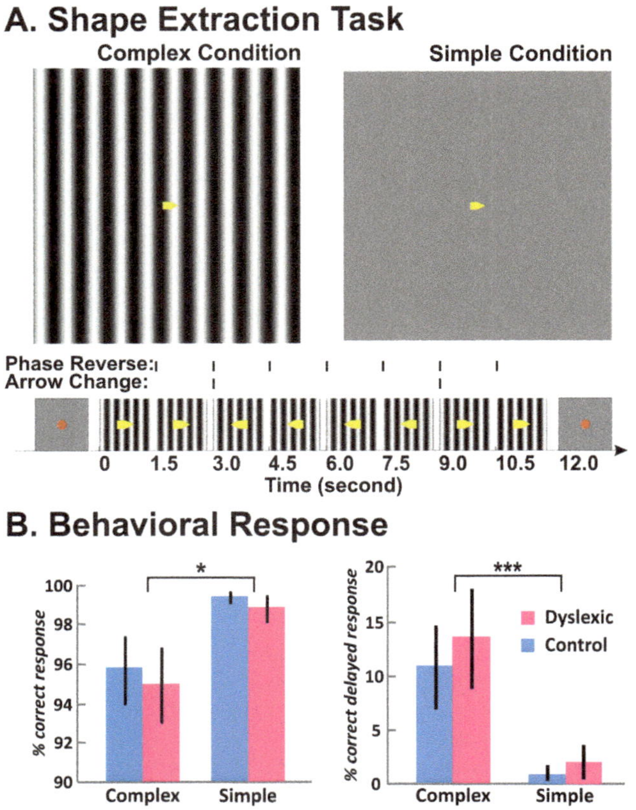

Figure 1. Task and performance. (*A*) The shape extraction task was performed under the complex condition with a large grating background (left panel) and the simple condition with a uniform gray background (right panel). The task had a 3-second fixation period and a 12-second block of stimulus period. During the stimulus period, participants were instructed to push the response button as soon as they saw a change in arrow direction. (*B*) The control and dyslexic groups performed similarly on the shape extraction task. The left panel shows that, for both groups, response accuracy was significantly lower for the complex condition than for the simple condition. The right panel shows that the percent of delayed, but correct, responses was significantly greater for the complex condition than for the simple condition. * $p<0.01$, ** $p<0.005$. Error bars indicate SEM within group.

for all participants. Arrow changes occurred randomly for durations in units of three seconds and there were three possible changes within each block of twelve seconds. The timing of the arrow change was synchronized with the phase reversal of the background grating as well as the onset of the time of repetition (TR time) in fMRI scanning. For the simple condition, there were 20 changes of arrow direction for the entire experiment duration: two blocks with no arrow change, ten with one arrow change, two with two changes and two with three changes. For complex condition, there were 28 changes of arrow direction: two blocks with no arrow change, four with one arrow change, six with two changes and four with three changes. During the complex condition, there were 112 phase reversals occurring periodically once every 1.5 seconds so that 25% of the phase reversals coincided with a change in arrow direction. Behavioral responses were recorded on the same laptop computer that was used for the stimulus presentation. The temporal resolution for behavioral responses was 1.5 seconds, the same as the TR. A response was considered correct if the button was pressed within a 3-second window after the arrow changed direction; a response was considered delayed but correct if the button was pressed between 1.5 and 3 seconds after the arrow changed direction.

Image Acquisition

MRI scans were performed on a 3T Siemens Magnetom Trio Tim system located at the Martinos Imaging Center at MIT. A T2*-weighted gradient-echo echo planar imaging (EPI) sequence was used for fMRI scans; slice thickness = 4 mm, in-plane resolution = 3.1×3.1 mm, repetition time/echo time/flip angle = 1,500 ms/30 ms/90° and the field of view of 200×200 mm^2. For all participants, a total of 128 images were collected for each experimental condition. At the beginning of each MRI experiment, high resolution ($1.3 \times 1.0 \times 1.3$ mm) anatomical images were also collected using a T1-weighted, three-dimensional gradient-echo sequence.

fMRI Data Analysis

Statistical parametric mapping software (SPM5) was used for image pre-processing and statistical analyses (Wellcome Department of Cognitive Neurology, London, http://www.fil.ion.ucl.ac.uk/spm). Functional images were realigned and normalized to an EPI template based on the ICBM152 stereotactic space (an approximation of canonical space). They were re-sampled into $2 \times 2 \times 2$-mm cubic voxels, and spatially smoothed by an isotropic Gaussian kernel (4 mm full width at half-maximum). The SPM5 canonical Hemodynamic Response Function (HRF), composed of two gamma functions, was used to predict responses. The predictor was obtained by convolving a time series of step function (box car) with this canonical HRF.

For second level within-group analysis, one sample t-test on contrast images (complex>simple) from first level images were computed separately for dyslexic and control groups. The voxelwise threshold was first set at $p<0.01$ uncorrected, and small volume corrected for multiple comparisons at level of $p<0.05$ for clusterwise correction for occipital, frontal and parietal lobes, respectively. For second-level between-group analyses, two sample t-tests on the contrast images (complex>simple) from first level images were computed. The statistical threshold for between-group contrasts was the same as the single group analysis ($p<0.01$, and $p<0.05$, small volume cluster corrected for occipital, frontal and parietal lobes). The masks used for occipital, frontal and parietal lobes were obtained from Talairach Daemon database atlases [38] in WFU PickAtlas [39].

All regions of interests (ROIs) used in the anatomical ROI analysis (Fig. 2B, 3B–C, 4C–D, 5B and 5D–E) were determined from cytoarchitectonically identified regions defined from the analysis of human post-mortem brains [38,39,40]. Specifically, the different cortical areas such as V1 and V2 were created from the anatomically normalized probabilistic cytoarchitectonic maps, a three-dimensional map in stereotaxic coordinate (the SPM Anatomy Toolbox, http://www.fz-juelich.de/inm/inm-1/spm_anatomy_toolbox, database: AllAreas_v16_MPM.mat). For every ROI, a binary mask was first made through the function of Create-Anatomical-ROIs in the SPM Anatomy Toolbox and all ROI analyses were then performed within this mask (http://www.fz-juelich.de/inm/inm-1/spm_anatomy_toolbox, database: AllAreas_v16_MPM.mat). In this study, the terms of visual areas V1 and V2 were interchangeably used with BA17 and BA18 [41]. V3, V4, and V5 [42,43,44,45] were used with the same naming system as shown in the toolbox. For regions in inferior parietal lobule, BA39 consisted of PGa and PGp; BA40 consisted of PFt, PF, PFm, Pfop, PFcm, OP1 and OP2; and BA43 consisted of OP3 and OP4 [46,47,48,49,50]. For regions in the superior parietal lobule, BA5 consisted of 5Ci, 5L, 5M, and BA7 consisted of 7A, 7M, 7P, and

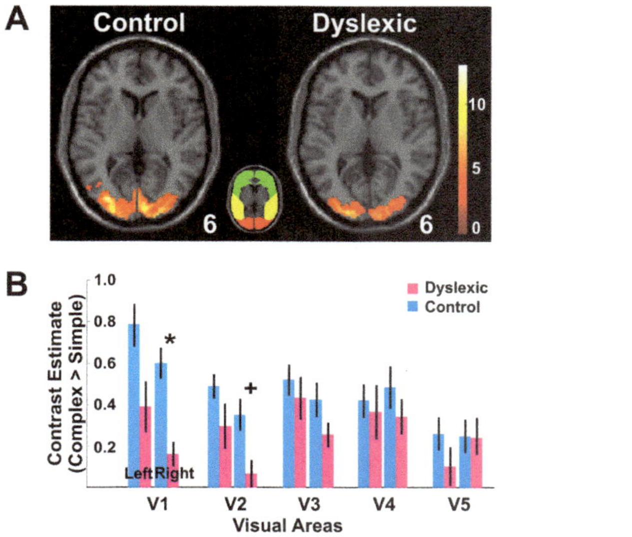

Figure 2. Activations in sensory regions. (*A*) The brain images illustrate occipital activation for control and dyslexic groups. For each image, the transverse slice shows voxels that exhibited a significantly greater activation for the complex condition than for the simple condition (Complex>Simple, $p<0.05$, cluster corrected for occipital lobe). The color bar depicts *t* values, and the color inset illustrates the subdivisions of occipital (red), temporal (yellow), and frontal (green) lobes. The number at the lower right corner of the transverse sections indicates that the images are taken at 6 mm above the AC–PC level. (*B*) Anatomically determined ROI analysis shows greater activation in visual areas V1, V2, V3, V4 and V5 for the control group (bars in blue) than for the dyslexic group (bars in red). $^{+}p<0.10$, $^{*}p<0.05$, Bonferroni corrected t-test between groups. Error bars represent SEM within group.

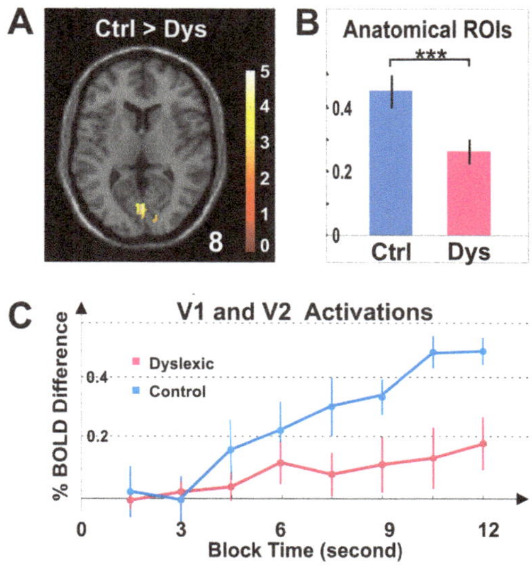

Figure 3. Hypoactivation for dyslexia in sensory regions. (*A*) The brain image illustrates occipital voxels that exhibited significantly greater activation for the control group than for the dyslexic group (Control>Dyslexic, $p<0.05$, cluster corrected for occipital lobe, shown at 8 mm above the AC-PC level). The difference in group activations was most evident at the posterior occipital lobe, around visual areas V1 and V2. (*B*) Occipital activation for the control group was significantly greater than for the dyslexic group. (*C*) The activation time course for anatomically determined visual areas in V1 and V2 shows greater occipital activation for the control group than for the dyslexic group. *** $p<10^{-6}$; main effect of group in two-way ANOVA for participant group and visual areas. Error bars indicate SEM within group.

7PC and hIP3 [51,52]. The intraparietal sulcus consisted of hIP1 and hIP2 [51,52,53].

The ROI images and the patterns of activation were reviewed visually, and presented through xjview8 (viewing program for SPM, Xu Cui, http://www.alivelearn.net/xjview/). For anatomically determined ROI analysis, the contrast estimates and the activation values were extracted with custom-made software rex.m (Susan Whitfield-Gabrieli, http://web.mit.edu/swg/software.htm) (Figs. 3B, 5B and 5D). For statistical analysis, the two-way ANOVAs, the two-tailed *t-tests* for groups with unequal variance, and the linear regression (Figs. 6D and 6E) were performed with custom-made Matlab scripts (MathWorks, Natick, MA). Bonferroni corrections were used to address the problems of multiple comparison [54] (Figs. 2B, 4C and 4D). With a threshold of $p_{threshold}$ and given n pairs of tests conducted, we would obtain an adjusted *threshold* of $p_{adjust} = p_{threshold}/n$. Respectively, the significance levels were adjusted to 0.005 for occipital (0.05/10, n = 10), 0.00625 for frontal (0.05/8, n = 8) and 0.00227 for parietal (0.05/22, n = 22) lobes.

For time course extractions, the mean BOLD signal in each ROI from the functional image time series was extracted with custom-made software rex.m; the difference in BOLD signal between simple and complex conditions was then used to evaluate the responses for shape extraction within the block time with values at each TR. To further normalize the results for all participants, a grand average value of $Resp_{avg\_all}$ was calculated by averaging the responses at the two fixation points between different experimental conditions for all participants included in this study. Respectively for dyslexic and control groups, the percentage BOLD difference shown in Figs. 3C and 5E was then calculated as $BOLD\_difference_{group}(t) = [Resp_{group}(t) - Resp_{avg\_all}] / Resp_{avg\_all} * 100\%$.

To examine the distribution of V1 activation along cortical representation of the visual field, we assumed that the retinotopic map of V1 was laid out across the folded cortical surface in the gray matter of the calcarine fissure. The central (foveal) part of the visual field is represented most posteriorly at the occipital pole, whereas the most peripheral regions of the visual field are located forward at the most anterior part of the calcarine fissure. To calculate the location of occipital activation along anterior-posterior direction of the calcarine fissure, we first obtained a mask of calcarine fissure from AAL atlases [55] in WFU PickAtlas [38] and found its most anterior and posterior locations. The most anterior point of calcarine structure was defined as the point with the largest y-value, and the most posterior point was the one with the smallest y value. We then divided the 3D structure of calcarine fissure into evenly distributed 1 mm thick coronal slices and calculated the number of activated voxels within the calcarine fissure mask.

Results

Behavioral Profile of Participants

The control and dyslexic groups performed similarly on measures of non-verbal cognitive ability (Table 1). The dyslexic group performed significantly worse than the control group for all reading measures for words and pseudowords under both untimed and timed conditions (i.e., for both accuracy and speed). The dyslexic group also performed significantly slower on the rapid letter naming task.

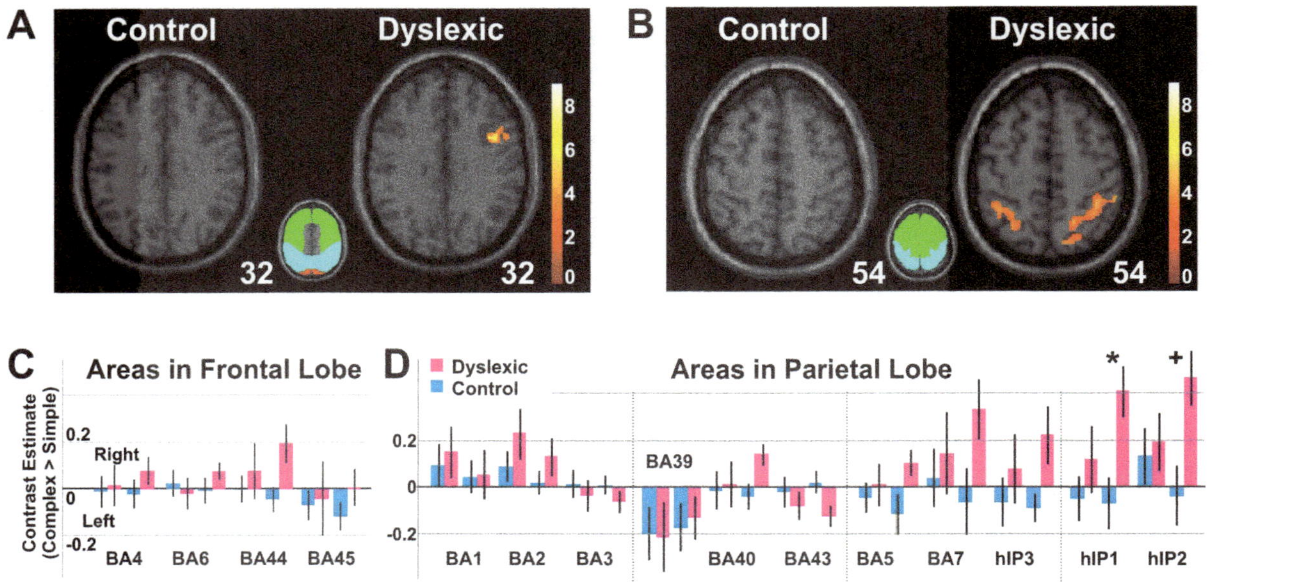

Figure 4. Activations in fronto-parietal regions. (*A*) Brain images illustrate frontal activations for control and dyslexic groups (Complex>Simple, $p<0.05$, cluster corrected for frontal lobe). There is one activation cluster for the dyslexic group, and none for the control group. (*B*) Brain images for parietal activations (Complex>Simple, $p<0.05$, cluster corrected for parietal lobe) indicates that in contrast to bilateral activation for the dyslexic group, there is none for the control group. In both **A** and **B**, the color bar depicts *t* values, and the color inset illustrates the subdivisions of occipital (red), frontal (green) and parietal (cyan) lobes. The transverse images are shown at 32 and 54 mm above the AC-PC level, respectively. (*C*) Anatomically determined ROI analysis shows activations for control and dyslexic groups. (*D*) Anatomically determined ROI analysis shows that the activation of area hIP1 in the dyslexic group is significantly greater than in the control group. From left to right, the parietal areas are shown in four groups: precentral gyrus (BA1, BA2, and BA3), inferior parietal lobule (BA39, BA40, and BA43), superior parietal lobule (BA5, BA7 and hIP3), and intraparietal sucus (hIP1 and hIP2). $^{+}p<0.10$; * $p<0.05$; Bonferroni corrected t-test. Error bars represent SEM within group.

Shape Extraction Task and In-Scanner Performance

For response accuracy (% correct), there were reliable differences between conditions, but not for groups or for any interaction (Fig. 1B, left panel; two-way ANOVA for condition, group and interaction between condition and group, $F_{condition}(1,42) = 7.68$, $p<0.01$; $F_{group,\ interaction}(1,42) = 0.22,\ 0.01$; p values >0.05). For response latency, we examined the rate of delayed but correct reaction times when the correct responses occurred not within but after 1.5s, and before the end of subsequent TR time. Similar to the response accuracy, response latencies were significantly longer for the complex than for the simple condition (Fig. 1B, right panel; main effect of condition, $F(1,42) = 11.79$, $p<0.005$). There was neither a main effect of group nor an interaction ($F(1,42) = 0.36,\ 0.06$; p values >0.05). These results indicated that, for both dyslexic and control groups, identifying the arrow change from the grating background at a low luminance were more difficult than from the uniform background at the same luminance level, but there was no difference behaviorally between the two groups on this simple perceptual task (Fig. 1B).

Hypoactivation in Sensory Regions in Dyslexia

For both groups, there was greater bilateral activation for the complex than for the simple condition in the occipital lobe (Fig. 2A and Table 2; Complex>Simple, $p<0.05$, cluster corrected for occipital lobe). For both groups, occipital activations included visual areas Brodmann area 17 (BA17), BA18, BA19, and cuneus (Table 2). The extent of occipital activation in the dyslexic group was 40.0 cm^3, somewhat smaller than the control group of 47.1 cm^3 (Table 2). Direct comparisons between the groups revealed significantly greater activation for the control than for the dyslexic group in occipital regions (Fig. 3A and Table 3; Control>Dyslexia, $p<0.05$, cluster corrected for occipital lobe). In contrast, no occipital region showed greater activation for the dyslexic than for the control group (Table 3; Dyslexia>Control, $p<0.05$, cluster corrected for occipital lobe).

For the dyslexic group, anatomically determined ROI analysis showed all activation values examined in the left and right visual areas V1, V2, V3, V4 and V5 were below the values in the control group (Fig. 2B). The average value of activation for the dyslexic group was significantly lower than the control group (Fig. 3B; two-way ANOVA of group and area, $F_{group}(1,220) = 23.89$, $p<10^{-6}$, $F_{area}(9,220) = 3.99$; $p<0.0005$ and $F_{interaction}(9,220) = 1.38$, $p>0.05$). The activation time course extracted from anatomical ROIs in occipital V1/V2 further verified the effect of dyslexic hypoactivation in visual sensory areas as indicated by mean differences in activation between conditions by TR (Fig. 3C).

Hyperactivation in Frontal and Parietal Lobes in Dyslexia

In contrast to occipital hypoactivation for the dyslexic group, we also found hyperactivation in both frontal and parietal lobes (Figs. 4, 5 and Table 2). In the frontal lobe, there was greater and more widespread activation in the dyslexic group than in the control group (Fig. 4A and Table 2; 3.2/0.0 cm^3; Complex>‴ Simple, $p<0.05$, cluster corrected for frontal lobe). For the control group, there was no activation found in the frontal lobes (Fig. 4A, left panel and Table 2). For the dyslexic group, activation in precentral, middle frontal, and inferior frontal gyri was found in the right hemisphere (Fig. 4A, right panel and Table 2). Direct comparisons between the groups revealed significantly greater activation for the dyslexic than the control group (Fig. 5A and Table 3; Dyslexia>Control, $p<0.05$, cluster corrected for frontal lobe). In comparison to frontal activations

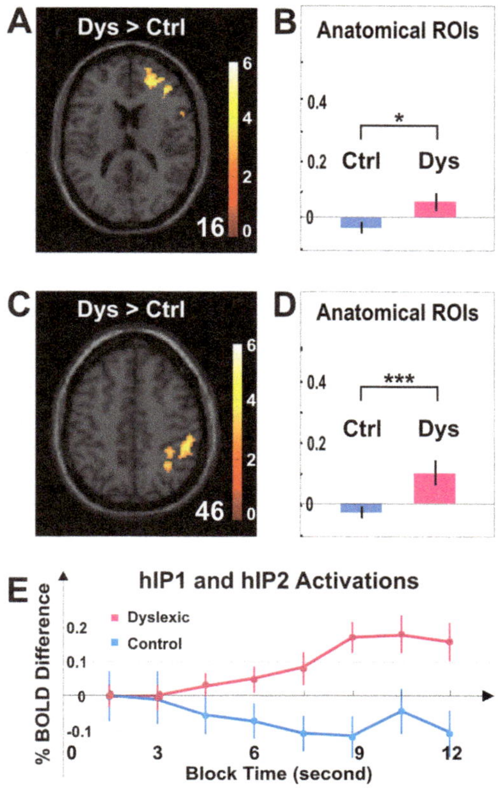

Figure 5. Hyperactivation for dyslexia in fronto-parietal regions. (*A*) The brain image illustrates frontal voxels that exhibited significantly greater activation for the dyslexic group than for the control group (Dyslexic>Control, $p<0.05$, cluster corrected for frontal lobe, shown at 16 mm above the AC-PC level). (*B*) Anatomically determined ROI analysis shows that frontal activation for the dyslexic group was significantly greater than for the control group. (*C*) The brain image illustrates parietal voxels that exhibited significantly greater activation for the dyslexic group than for the control group (Dyslexic>Control, $p<0.05$, cluster corrected for parietal lobe). (*D*) Parietal activation for dyslexic group was significantly greater than the control group. (*E*) The activation time course for anatomically determined areas hIP1 and hIP2 showed greater parietal activation for the dyslexic group than for the control group. * $p<0.05$; *** $p<10^{-6}$; main effect of group in two-way ANOVA for group and area. Error bars indicate SEM within group.

for dyslexic group alone (Fig. 4A), the hyperactivation obtained from the group contrast between the dyslexic and control participants included an additional cluster located more towards the anterior and ventral portion of the frontal lobe (Fig. 5A).

In the parietal lobe, there was bilateral activation in the dyslexic group, but no above-threshold activation in the control group (Fig. 4B and Table 2; 11.2/0.0 cm^3; Complex>Simple, $p<0.05$, cluster corrected for parietal lobe). The activation for the dyslexic group was bilateral, but substantially greater in the right than in the left hemisphere (Table 2; 8.8/2.4 cm^3). Greater activation in the dyslexic group than in the control group occurred in the right hemisphere; primarily in the inferior parietal lobule (Fig. 5C and Table 3; Dyslexia>Control, $p<0.05$, cluster corrected for parietal lobe). In contrast, no frontal or parietal region showed greater activation for the control than for the dyslexic group (Table 3; Control>Dyslexia, $p<0.05$, cluster corrected for frontal or parietal lobe).

Anatomically defined regions of interest (ROIs) analysis were used to further quantify the findings of increased frontal and parietal activation in dyslexia. The dyslexic group showed significantly greater activation than the control group in frontal regions (Figs. 4C and 5B; BA4, BA6, BA44, and BA45; two-way ANOVA, $F_{group}(1,176)=4.46$, $p<0.05$; $F_{area}(7,176)=0.74$, $p>0.05$; and $F_{interaction}(7,176)=0.61$, $p>0.05$) and parietal regions (Figs. 4D and 5D; BA1, BA2, BA3, BA5, BA7, BA39, BA40, BA43, and hIP1, hIP2, hIP3; two-way ANOVA, $F_{group}(1,484)=16.82$, $p<10^{-6}$; $F_{area}(21,484)=2.21$, $p<0.005$; and $F_{interaction}(21,484)=1.55$, $p>0.05$). The parietal hyperactivation for the dyslexic group was further confirmed by the activation time course extracted from parietal hIP1/hIP2 (Fig. 5E).

Pattern of Occipital Hypoactivation and Relation between Occipital and Parietal Activations in Dyslexia

The V1 activations distributed along the cortical representation of the visual field were measured by dividing the calcarine fissure into evenly distributed fine coronal slices (subdivisions along anterior/posterior dimension in the 3D volume) and counting the number of above-threshold voxels of activation. In unit of the maximal length of calcarine fissure along the anterior/posterior direction, activation for the control group extended from 0.03 to 0.55, with a median distance of 0.22 from the most posterior end of the cortex, the occipital pole (Fig. 6A). The distribution for the dyslexic group extended from 0.02 to 0.38, with a median distance of 0.17 (Fig. 6B). Unlike the activation distribution for the control or dyslexic groups, the occipital hypoactivation extended more anteriorly from 0.13 to 0.58, with a median distance of 0.36 (Fig. 6C). The dyslexic hypoactivation occurring in visual cortex appeared to occur in more anterior calcarine cortex, likely representing peripheral visual areas, and to reflect a deactivation (more activation for the simple than the complex conditions) in the dyslexic group (Fig. 6A–C).

To understand the relation between occipital hypoactivation and parietal hyperactivations in the dyslexic group, linear regression analysis between occipital and parietal activations were performed for the dyslexic and the control groups respectively. There was no significant correlation between occipital V1/V2 activation (values for individual participants in Fig. 3B) and parietal hIP1/hIP2 activation (values for individual participants in Fig. 5D) in the control group (Fig. 6D, N = 13, $R^2=0.015$, and $p>0.05$). In contrast, occipital activations were significantly correlated with the parietal activations in the dyslexic group (Fig. 6E, N = 11, $R^2=0.526$, and $p<0.05$).

Discussion

We used fMRI to examine the underlying neural mechanisms for visual shape extraction from a complex relative to a simple visual background, and found occipital hypoactivation accompanied with fronto-parietal hyperactivation in adults with persistent dyslexia. The brain organization for basic visual shape extraction from a complex background appears to be fundamentally different in people with or without dyslexia. Because this atypical balance of activation occurred in a simple visual task without the involvement of reading or language, these findings support the view that visual differences, in addition to well-documented phonological differences, contribute to reading difficulty, on average, in dyslexia. Prior neuroimaging studies of basic visual processing had examined motion and only reported decreased posterior activations in dyslexia (18, 19), but here we found differences related to shape extraction. These differences involved opposite patterns of atypical activation in dyslexia with decreased activation in posterior visual areas associated with basic visual processing and

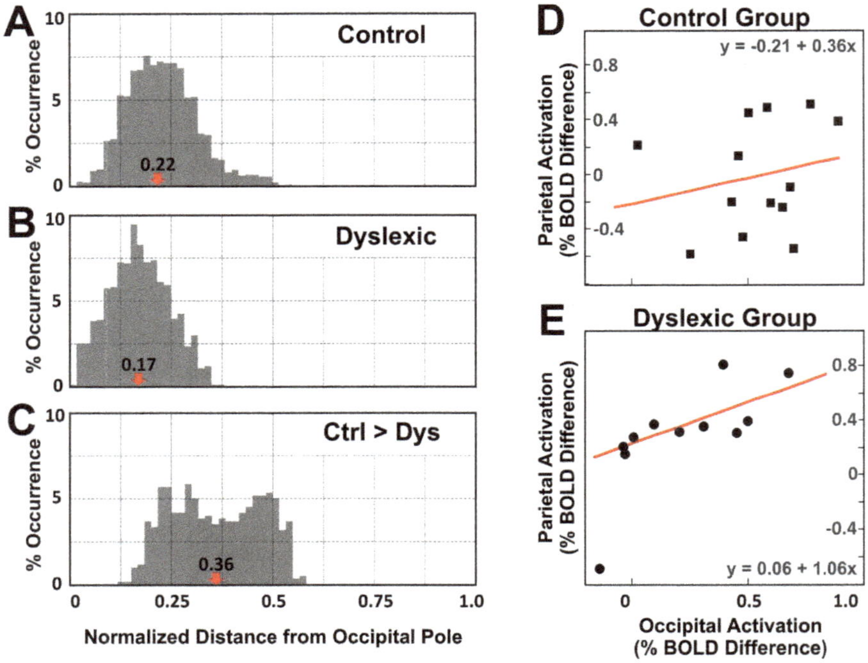

Figure 6. Occipital activation and its relation to parietal activation. (*A*) Frequency histogram shows the distribution of calcarine activation for the control group, along the posterior and anterior direction. The x-axis shows the distance between the intersected coronal section and the occipital pole, normalized to maximal length of calcarine fissure along the posterior and anterior direction. The y-axis shows the percent occurrence of activation within a coronal section over all activation within the calcarine structure. The red arrow indicates the median distance and the number above shows the value of the median distance. (*B*) The distribution of calcarine activation for the dyslexic group is similar to the one for the control group. (*C*) The distribution of dyslexic calcarine hypoactivation differs from A or B: it evades areas around the occipital pole. (*D*) For participants in the control group, parietal activations in areas hIP1 and hIP2 were not not correlated with occipital activations in areas V1 and V2 ($N = 13$, $R^2 = 0.015$, and $p > 0.05$). The line in red shows the linear regression line. (*E*) In contrast, for participants in the dyslexic group, the parietal activations were positively correlated with occipital activations ($N = 11$, $R^2 = 0.526$, and $p < 0.05$).

increased activation in fronto-parietal areas associated with attentional and cognitive processes. The regions of increased activation suggest a mechanism by which weaknesses in lower-order perceptual cortices may interfere with reading-relevant processes in higher-order cortices.

Shape Extraction Task and Behavioral Performance in Dyslexia

In this experiment, we chose the term "shape extraction" to contrast with prior imaging studies of basic visual processing in

Table 2. Activation for Dyslexic and Control Groups.

	Control Group (Complex>Simple)							Dyslexic Group (Complex>Simple)					
	Cluster	Voxel						Cluster	Voxel				
	p_cor	*k*	*(x y z)*	*Z Score*	Brain Region			p_cor	*k*	*(x y z)*	*Z Score*	Brain Region	
Occipital	0	5883	−30 −84 8	*5.73*	MOG	BA18		0	4995	−20 −98 6	*5.28*	MOG	BA18,
			8 −94 −6	*5.56*	Cuneus	BA19				−24 −98 −6	*5.08*	Cuneus	BA19
			2 −80 −2	*5.45*	LinG	BA17				−26 −94 0	*5.01*	LinG	BA17
Frontal								0	396	46 6 32	*4.66*	PrecentralG	BA6
										52 4 34	*4.15*	IFG	BA9
										50 28 18	*3.47*	MFG	
Parietal								0	1096	58 −22 32	*4.33*	IPL	BA7
										50 −42 50	*3.96*	SupMG	BA40
										30 −56 62	*3.77*	PostcentralG	BA2
								0	298	−26 −54 58	*3.77*	IPL	BA40
										−36 −44 46	*3.18*	PostcentralG	BA7
										−40 −44 56	*3.1*	SPL	

Table 3. Differential Activation between Groups.

	Hypoactivation (Control>Dyslexic)						Hyperactivation (Dyslexic>Control)					
	Cluster	**Voxel**					**Cluster**	**Voxel**				
	p_cor	*k*	*(x y z)*	*Z Score*	**Brain Region**		**p_cor**	*k*	*(x y z)*	*Z Score*	**Brain Region**	
Occipital	0	494	2 −78 6	*3.72*	Cuneus	BA18						
			2 −80 −2	*3.71*	Calcarine	BA17						
			10 −86 −2	*3.18*								
Frontal							0	404	40 6 32	*4.22*	IFG	BA9
									46 4 32	*4.12*	PreCentralG	BA44
									52 4 36	*3.42*	MFG	
							0	418	24 48 20	*3.99*	SFG	BA10
									38 30 22	*3.98*	MFG	BA46
									38 36 18	*3.77*	IFG	
Parietal							0	783	60 −22 30	*4.57*	IPL	BA40
									54 −24 32	*4.46*	SupMG	BA2
									50 −38 44	*3.94*	PostcentralG	

p-cor values are corrected for multiple comparisons at the level of occipital, frontal and parietal lobes (except for Z Scores reported in italics). *k* is the number of voxels in each cluster. (x y z) represents the location of maximal response in MNI coordinates. The brain regions listed are obtained from the Talairach Daemon database, and they are the first three largest brain areas that are at or above 10% of the total area. F = Frontal; G = Gyrus; I = Inferior; L = Lobule; Lin = Lingual; M = Middle; O = Occipital; P = Parietal; S = Superior; and SupM = SupraMarginal.

dyslexia that focused on motion, and to offer a relatively theoretically neutral term describing the task demand. Following the notion that "the human visual system efficiently extracts and identifies shapes and forms, including letters, digits, signs, and line drawings" [56], we have conceptualized the primary task contrast as one of shape extraction rather than shape identification. Participants had to separate the shape of the arrow from the background grating in one condition but not the other, but identifying the altered shape of the simple arrow was constant across conditions.

The task of shape extraction involves both foveal processes related to analysis of the arrow and peripheral processes related to the full screen background. The finding that group differences were greatest in calcarine cortex associated with peripheral rather than foveal visual processing suggests that the hypocativation in dyslexia was not simply stimulus-driven by the arrow. Instead, the hypoactivation may reflect processes that integrated the effect of the task, the full screen background, and the processing of the target arrow.

The brain differences for individuals with dyslexia occurred despite no group differences in task performance. On the one hand, this means that the brain differences were not a consequence of or secondary to behavioral difficulties; on the other hand, functional brain differences are of interest primarily to the extent that they are relevant to behaviors, such as reading. One possible interpretation relates to the ease of the task on which most participants performed nearly perfectly. On such an easy task, individuals with dyslexia may have been able to fully compensate behaviorally, and the frontoparietal hyperactivation for dyslexia may reflect the recruitment of additional neural resources that supported such compensation. It is also possible that the limited temporal resolution of our behavioral measure obscured subtle group differences in latency. In either case, there is evidence from other studies with non-verbal tasks that individuals with dyslexia tend to exhibit behavioral deficits as a function of task difficulty for both verbal [57,58] and non-verbal stimuli [21,59,60,61,62,63]. Therefore, it may be that the minimal challenge of the task in the present study revealed functional brain differences that could lead to impaired behavioral performance in more demanding experimental conditions or during the reading of letters in the context of other letters or words. Future studies can examine conditions under which individuals with dyslexia perform both similarly and also less well than typical readers to further relate the patterns of brain activation to intact and impaired visual performance in dyslexia.

Interpretations for Occipital Hypoactivation and Fronto-Parietal Hyperactivation

Occipital hypoactivation accompanied with fronto-parietal hyperactivation in dyslexia demonstrates that both sensory and attentional visual processes may be altered in dyslexia. These findings may be interpreted in several ways because sensory and attentional processes interact in many ways [64,65,66,67,68,69,70]. Occipital hypoactivation and fronto-parietal hyperactivation could reflect separable visual sensory and attentional deficits in dyslexia. Alternatively, occipital hypoactivation may cause fronto-parietal hyperactivation in dyslexia. Typical readers may be able to extract visual shape information based largely on early subcortical and cortical processes. Greater activation of early visual areas in typical readers may reflect this active visual shape extraction processing that alleviates the need for higher-order cortices to support focused attention on this relatively simple task. In contrast, reduced activation of early visual areas in readers with dyslexia may signal impaired visual perceptual process that causes the recruitment of compensatory attentional resources supported by fronto-parietal regions. The idea that higher-order brain regions are recruited when lower-order regions cannot support perception of stimuli is supported by studies reporting greater activation in fronto-parietal regions when sensory information is degraded either by presenting degraded words to typical readers or the blurring of vision in patients with macular degeneration [71,72].

The finding that occipital activation was significantly correlated with parietal activation in the dyslexic group, but not in the typically reading group, suggests that the atypical occipital and parietal activations were associated rather than dissociated in dyslexia. Perhaps greater top-down attentional processes supported by parietal cortex enhanced, or attempted to enhance, bottom-up visual processes supported by occipital cortex.

Magnocellular Pathway Hypothesis of Dyslexia

Visual deficit hypotheses for dyslexia can be divided broadly into two categories that focus on either bottom-up sensory deficits or top-down attentional problems. Among the sensory hypotheses, the most studied is the magnocellular visual pathway hypothesis positing that dyslexia is partially due to a disorder of the fast processing magnocellular (M) sub-system, a visual pathway extending from the retina to the occipital and parietal areas of the brain. The magnocellular hypothesis of dyslexia has also been extended to proposals of weaknesses in functionally analogous auditory and tactile modalities [73,74,75,76,77]. Because the visual stimuli in this study were not designed to selectively involve the magnocellular system, our findings cannot directly support or challenge the magnocellular hypothesis of dyslexia. Our finding of hypoactivation for the dyslexic group in sensory regions is consistent with previous neuroimaging studies reporting reduced activations to moving stimuli in early visual areas [18,19,78]. The present study extends those prior findings in two ways. First, those studies examined brain responses to visual motion, whereas we examined brain responses to stationary visual shape extraction. Second, prior studies focused on verifying the magnocellular hypothesis in early visual areas, and did not examine the frontal and parietal regions associated with visual attention. The present study, therefore, demonstrates that altered brain activations in dyslexia are not limited to early visual areas involved in visual motion, but rather are accompanied by altered responses in higher-order cortical regions as well.

Noise-exclusion Hypothesis and Visuo-spatial Attention Hypothesis in Dyslexia

Instead of emphasizing bottom-up sensory deficits, the noise-exclusion and the visuo-spatial attention hypotheses of dyslexia focus on deficits in top-down cognitive processes. Psychophysical studies have reported that individuals with dyslexia have a deficit for perceiving simple non-verbal stimuli presented in white noise, in both vision and audition [16,26,27,28,29,79,80,81]. There has not been prior evidence about a potential brain basis for the noise exclusion deficit in dyslexia. Because the complex condition in the current study can be considered as the extraction of arrow shape information from the background noise of a grating, our results suggest that the underlying neural mechanism for noise exclusion in dyslexia could be that weakened early visual processes fail to discriminate useful signals from background noise, and such weakened sensory processes are compensated for by the recruitment of higher-order attentional processes.

We found parietal hyperactivation that may be associated with the visuo-spatial attention hypothesis of dyslexia. The visuo-spatial attention hypothesis of dyslexia has been motivated by behavioral studies reporting impairments on visual attentional tasks, such as identifying a target that was spatially or temporally distinguished from distractors in the background or masks [21,22,23,24,82,83,84]. In the brain, the effect of visual attention is often associated with activations in fronto-parietal regions [85,86,87,88,89,90,91,92,93,94,95]. The attentional hypothesis of dyslexia is supported by the present finding of hyperactivation in frontal-parietal regions and a prior finding of parietal hypoactivation [25]. The difference in hyper- vs. hypoactivation in the parietal lobe may be due to differences in participant selection, visual stimuli involved in tasks, or both. The present study recruited people with poor reading only whereas the prior study recruited people with both reading and visual attention span deficits; thus, the discrepancy in parietal activation might be due to the fact that people with and without attention deficits have different neural mechanisms for attentional modulation. In addition, whereas the present study used simple nonverbal visual stimuli without any involvement of language or reading, the visual stimuli in the prior study consisted of a mixture of geometric shape and letters. Prior studies employing reading-related tasks have shown reduced activation in parietal regions of people with dyslexia [96,97,98], so it may be that individuals with dyslexia can compensate via parietal hyperactivation for simple tasks (as in the present study), but not for more demanding reading tasks. Given the evidence of right-hemisphere specialization for visuo-spatial functions from both lesion studies [99] and imaging studies (e.g., [100]), the visuo-spatial nature of the present study may also explain why activation differences between groups were predominantly right-lateralized.

Limitations of Study

Two limitations of the present study may be addressed in future studies. First, the present study lacked a resting baseline, precluding separate analyses of the complex and simple conditions relative to baseline of fixation. Therefore, we cannot determine if the group differences arose from only the complex or simple conditions or both conditions. A previous study reported no activation difference in inferior occipital-temporal cortex between dyslexic and normal children in a contrast between identifying a shape in isolation versus looking at a blank screen with only a fixation point [25]. This supports the idea that the present difference may arise from the complex condition. A resting or fixation baseline condition, however, may not be definitive, because resting-state functional connectivity appears to differ in typical and dyslexic readers [101,102]). Second, this study was performed with adults who had a childhood diagnosis of dyslexia and continued to demonstrate behavioural manifestations of dyslexia in adulthood. It is unknown whether this atypical pattern of brain activation for visual shape extraction is present in children with dyslexia, and therefore a potential cause for dyslexia, or whether it emerges through development as a type of adaptation, and therefore is a consequence of dyslexia (e.g., the consequence of far less reading practice). In prior studies, core brain differences observed in adults with dyslexia have resembled brain differences observed in children with dyslexia, such as temporo-parietal hypoactivation for phonological analysis in adults [103,104] and in children [4,98], and reduced frontal activation for rapid auditory non-verbal stimuli in adults [4] and in children [105]. These prior similarities between children and adults suggest that a similar atypical balance may be found in children with dyslexia, but only studies conducted with children can determine whether this atypical balance is present before reading or early in reading in children who progress to dyslexia.

Relation of Atypical Balance of Activation to Reading and Dyslexia

The present study extends knowledge about the neural correlates of visual processing in adult dyslexia in three fundamental ways. First, prior imaging studies of basic visual processing with non-verbal stimuli in dyslexia focused on *motion* (18, 19, 73), and here we focused on *shape extraction*, a process that is important in reading letters and words embedded in text. Second, in addition to prior imaging findings of reduced activations in occipito-temporal brain areas specialized for vision, we found altered brain responses in higher-order brain regions associated with top-down attentional network. Our finding in the higher-order brain regions is consistent with multiple imaging studies of dyslexia employing reading-related tasks [96,97,98]. Third, the concurrent and correlated hypoactivation and hyperactivation in different brain regions in a simple visual task in dyslexia raises a possible direct link between lower-order visual weaknesses and higher-order reading weaknesses.

Reading is understood to be an interaction between perceptual processes involved in the extraction of letter shape in the complex visual environment of the printed page and cognitive processes involved in comprehension, interpretation, and prediction. Previous reading studies have demonstrated that phonological recoding involves central attention processes as shown by the effect of other ongoing mental events that also require central attention [106,107]. Although future studies will be needed to directly link a basic brain alteration of visual shape extraction to the specific processes used to read print, the finding of an atypical balance between occipital and fronto-parietal functions suggests how a difference in visual shape extraction may impede reading through a shared central attentional mechanism. The underengagement of sensory processes supported by early visual areas may fail to support effective shape extraction during reading, and the consequent overengagement of attentional areas may compete for cognitive resources and thus further undermine fluent reading.

Acknowledgments

We thank the participants who made this work possible; Pamela Hook and Charlie Haynes for advice on the behavioral experiment design; Zuxiang Liu for help on MRI experiment design; Mayme Hostetter, Carlos Cardenas, Patricia Chang, Steve Shannon, and Sheeba Arnold Anteraper (Athinoula A. Martinos Imaging Center at McGovern Institute for Brain Research, MIT) for technical assistance.

Author Contributions

Conceived and designed the experiments: YZ JG. Performed the experiments: YZ JC. Analyzed the data: YZ SG. Wrote the paper: YZ JG.

References

1. Gabrieli JD (2009) Dyslexia: a new synergy between education and cognitive neuroscience. Science 325: 280–283.
2. Shaywitz SE, Shaywitz BA (2005) Dyslexia (specific reading disability). Biol Psychiatry 57: 1301–1309.
3. Lyon GR, Shaywitz, S E., & Shaywitz, B A. (2003) a definition of dyslexia.. Annals ofDyslexia, 53: 1–14.
4. Temple E, Poldrack RA, Salidis J, Deutsch GK, Tallal P, et al. (2001) Disrupted neural responses to phonological and orthographic processing in dyslexic children: an fMRI study. Neuroreport 12: 299–307.
5. Bradley L, Bryant PE (1978) Difficulties in auditory organisation as a possible cause of reading backwardness. Nature 271: 746–747.
6. Wagner RKT, J.K. (1987) The nature of phonological processing and its causal role in the acquisition of reading skills. Psychological Bulletin 101: 192–212.
7. Shaywitz SE, Shaywitz BA, Fulbright RK, Skudlarski P, Mencl WE, et al. (2003) Neural systems for compensation and persistence: young adult outcome of childhood reading disability. Biol Psychiatry 54: 25–33.
8. Facoetti A, Zorzi M, Cestnick L, Lorusso ML, Molteni M, et al. (2006) The relationship between visuo-spatial attention and nonword reading in developmental dyslexia. Cogn Neuropsychol 23: 841–855.
9. Lovegrove WJ, Bowling A, Badcock D, Blackwood M (1980) Specific reading disability: differences in contrast sensitivity as a function of spatial frequency. Science 210: 439–440.
10. Stein J, Walsh V (1997) To see but not to read; the magnocellular theory of dyslexia. Trends Neurosci 20: 147–152.
11. Livingstone MS, Rosen GD, Drislane FW, Galaburda AM (1991) Physiological and anatomical evidence for a magnocellular defect in developmental dyslexia. Proc Natl Acad Sci U S A 88: 7943–7947.
12. Evans BJ, Drasdo N, Richards IL (1994) An investigation of some sensory and refractive visual factors in dyslexia. Vision Res 34: 1913–1926.
13. Amitay S, Ben-Yehudah G, Banai K, Ahissar M (2002) Disabled readers suffer from visual and auditory impairments but not from a specific magnocellular deficit. Brain 125: 2272–2285.
14. Skottun BC (2000) The magnocellular deficit theory of dyslexia: the evidence from contrast sensitivity. Vision Res 40: 111–127.
15. Barnard N, Crewther SG, Crewther DP (1998) Development of a magnocellular function in good and poor primary school-age readers. Optom Vis Sci 75: 62–68.
16. Sperling AJ, Lu ZL, Manis FR, Seidenberg MS (2005) Deficits in perceptual noise exclusion in developmental dyslexia. Nat Neurosci 8: 862–863.
17. Olson R, Datta H (2002) Visual-temporal processing in reading-disabled and normal twins. Reading and Writing: An Interdisciplinary Journal 127–149.
18. Demb JB, Boynton GM, Heeger DJ (1998) Functional magnetic resonance imaging of early visual pathways in dyslexia. J Neurosci 18: 6939–6951.
19. Eden GF, VanMeter JW, Rumsey JM, Maisog JM, Woods RP, et al. (1996) Abnormal processing of visual motion in dyslexia revealed by functional brain imaging. Nature 382: 66–69.
20. Vidyasagar TR, Pammer K Dyslexia: a deficit in visuo-spatial attention, not in phonological processing. Trends Cogn Sci 14: 57–63.
21. Vidyasagar TR, Pammer K (1999) Impaired visual search in dyslexia relates to the role of the magnocellular pathway in attention. Neuroreport 10: 1283–1287.
22. Facoetti A, Paganoni P, Lorusso ML (2000) The spatial distribution of visual attention in developmental dyslexia. Exp Brain Res 132: 531–538.
23. Vidyasagar TR, Pammer K (2010) Dyslexia: a deficit in visuo-spatial attention, not in phonological processing. Trends Cogn Sci 14: 57–63.
24. Waldie KE, Hausmann M (2010) Right fronto-parietal dysfunction in children with ADHD and developmental dyslexia as determined by line bisection judgements. Neuropsychologia 48: 3650–3656.
25. Peyrin C, Demonet JF, N'Guyen-Morel MA, Le Bas JF, Valdois S (2011) Superior parietal lobule dysfunction in a homogeneous group of dyslexic children with a visual attention span disorder. Brain Lang 118: 128–138.
26. Sperling AJ, Lu ZL, Manis FR, Seidenberg MS (2006) Motion-perception deficits and reading impairment: it's the noise, not the motion. Psychol Sci 17: 1047–1053.
27. Beattie RL, Lu ZL, Manis FR (2011) Dyslexic adults can learn from repeated stimulus presentation but have difficulties in excluding external noise. PLoS One 6: e27893.
28. Conlon EG, Lilleskaret G, Wright CM, Power GF (2012) The influence of contrast on coherent motion processing in dyslexia. Neuropsychologia 50: 1672–1681.
29. Dole M, Hoen M, Meunier F (2012) Speech-in-noise perception deficit in adults with dyslexia: effects of background type and listening configuration. Neuropsychologia 50: 1543–1552.
30. Kaufman AS, Kaufman NL (1997) Kaufman Brief Intelligence Test, 2nd Edition (KBIT2) Minneapolis, MN: NCS Pearson, Inc.
31. Wechsler D (1999) *The Wechsler Abbreviated Scale of Intelligence* (WASI) San Antonio, TX: PsychCorp.
32. Woodcock RW (1998) Woodcock Reading Mastery Tests – Revised/Normative Update (WRMT-R/NU) Circle Pines, MN: American Guidance Service.
33. Wagner R, Torgesen JK, Rashotte C (1999) Comprehensive Test of Phonological Processing (CTOPP) Austin, TX: Pro-Ed.
34. Wagner Torgesen, Rashotte (1999) Comprehensive Test of Phonological Processing (CTOPP). Austin, TX: Pro-Ed.
35. Lovegrove W, Martin F, Bowling A, Blackwood M, Badcock D, et al. (1982) Contrast sensitivity functions and specific reading disability. Neuropsychologia 20: 309–315.
36. Brainard DH (1997) The Psychophysics Toolbox. Spat Vis 10: 433–436.
37. Pelli DG (1997) The VideoToolbox software for visual psychophysics: transforming numbers into movies. Spat Vis 10: 437–442.
38. Lancaster JL, Woldorff MG, Parsons LM, Liotti M, Freitas CS, et al. (2000) Automated Talairach atlas labels for functional brain mapping. Hum Brain Mapp 10: 120–131.
39. Maldjian JA, Laurienti PJ, Kraft RA, Burdette JH (2003) An automated method for neuroanatomic and cytoarchitectonic atlas-based interrogation of fMRI data sets. Neuroimage 19: 1233–1239.
40. Eickhoff SB, Stephan KE, Mohlberg H, Grefkes C, Fink GR, et al. (2005) A new SPM toolbox for combining probabilistic cytoarchitectonic maps and functional imaging data. Neuroimage 25: 1325–1335.
41. Amunts K, Malikovic A, Mohlberg H, Schormann T, Zilles K (2000) Brodmann's areas 17 and 18 brought into stereotaxic space-where and how variable? Neuroimage 11: 66–84.
42. Wilms M, Eickhoff SB, Homke L, Rottschy C, Kujovic M, et al. Comparison of functional and cytoarchitectonic maps of human visual areas V1, V2, V3d, V3v, and V4(v). Neuroimage 49: 1171–1179.

43. Rottschy C, Eickhoff SB, Schleicher A, Mohlberg H, Kujovic M, et al. (2007) Ventral visual cortex in humans: cytoarchitectonic mapping of two extrastriate areas. Hum Brain Mapp 28: 1045–1059.
44. Malikovic A, Amunts K, Schleicher A, Mohlberg H, Eickhoff SB, et al. (2007) Cytoarchitectonic analysis of the human extrastriate cortex in the region of V5/MT+: a probabilistic, stereotaxic map of area hOc5. Cereb Cortex 17: 562–574.
45. Wilms M, Eickhoff SB, Specht K, Amunts K, Shah NJ, et al. (2005) Human V5/MT+: comparison of functional and cytoarchitectonic data. Anat Embryol (Berl) 210: 485–495.
46. Caspers S, Eickhoff SB, Geyer S, Scheperjans F, Mohlberg H, et al. (2008) The human inferior parietal lobule in stereotaxic space. Brain Struct Funct 212: 481–495.
47. Caspers S, Geyer S, Schleicher A, Mohlberg H, Amunts K, et al. (2006) The human inferior parietal cortex: cytoarchitectonic parcellation and interindividual variability. Neuroimage 33: 430–448.
48. Eickhoff SB, Grefkes C, Zilles K, Fink GR (2007) The somatotopic organization of cytoarchitectonic areas on the human parietal operculum. Cereb Cortex 17: 1800–1811.
49. Eickhoff SB, Schleicher A, Zilles K, Amunts K (2006) The human parietal operculum. I. Cytoarchitectonic mapping of subdivisions. Cereb Cortex 16: 254–267.
50. Eickhoff SB, Amunts K, Mohlberg H, Zilles K (2006) The human parietal operculum. II. Stereotaxic maps and correlation with functional imaging results. Cereb Cortex 16: 268–279.
51. Scheperjans F, Eickhoff SB, Homke L, Mohlberg H, Hermann K, et al. (2008) Probabilistic maps, morphometry, and variability of cytoarchitectonic areas in the human superior parietal cortex. Cereb Cortex 18: 2141–2157.
52. Scheperjans F, Hermann K, Eickhoff SB, Amunts K, Schleicher A, et al. (2008) Observer-independent cytoarchitectonic mapping of the human superior parietal cortex. Cereb Cortex 18: 846–867.
53. Choi HJ, Zilles K, Mohlberg H, Schleicher A, Fink GR, et al. (2006) Cytoarchitectonic identification and probabilistic mapping of two distinct areas within the anterior ventral bank of the human intraparietal sulcus. J Comp Neurol 495: 53–69.
54. Glantz SA (1992) Primer of BioStatistics. McGray-Hill: 309–310.
55. Tzourio-Mazoyer N, Landeau B, Papathanassiou D, Crivello F, Etard O, et al. (2002) Automated anatomical labeling of activations in SPM using a macroscopic anatomical parcellation of the MNI MRI single-subject brain. Neuroimage 15: 273–289.
56. Ben-Shachar M, Dougherty RF, Deutsch GK, Wandell BA (2007) Differential sensitivity to words and shapes in ventral occipito-temporal cortex. Cereb Cortex 17: 1604–1611.
57. Marinus E, de Jong PF (2010) Variability in the word-reading performance of dyslexic readers: effects of letter length, phoneme length and digraph presence. Cortex 46: 1259–1271.
58. Durrwachter U, Sokolov AN, Reinhard J, Klosinski G, Trauzettel-Klosinski S (2010) Word length and word frequency affect eye movements in dyslexic children reading in a regular (German) orthography. Ann Dyslexia 60: 86–101.
59. Moores E, Cassim R, Talcott JB (2011) Adults with dyslexia exhibit large effects of crowding, increased dependence on cues, and detrimental effects of distractors in visual search tasks. Neuropsychologia 49: 3881–3890.
60. Roach NW, Hogben JH (2008) Spatial cueing deficits in dyslexia reflect generalised difficulties with attentional selection. Vision Res 48: 193–207.
61. Roach NW, Hogben JH (2004) Attentional modulation of visual processing in adult dyslexia: a spatial-cuing deficit. Psychol Sci 15: 650–654.
62. Spinelli D, De Luca M, Judica A, Zoccolotti P (2002) Crowding effects on word identification in developmental dyslexia. Cortex 38: 179–200.
63. Iles J, Walsh V, Richardson A (2000) Visual search performance in dyslexia. Dyslexia 6: 163–177.
64. Brefczynski JA, DeYoe EA (1999) A physiological correlate of the 'spotlight' of visual attention. Nat Neurosci 2: 370–374.
65. Gandhi SP, Heeger DJ, Boynton GM (1999) Spatial attention affects brain activity in human primary visual cortex. Proc Natl Acad Sci U S A 96: 3314–3319.
66. O'Craven KM, Rosen BR, Kwong KK, Treisman A, Savoy RL (1997) Voluntary attention modulates fMRI activity in human MT-MST. Neuron 18: 591–598.
67. Twomey T, Kawabata Duncan KJ, Price CJ, Devlin JT Top-down modulation of ventral occipito-temporal responses during visual word recognition. Neuroimage 55: 1242–1251.
68. Cieslik EC, Zilles K, Kurth F, Eickhoff SB Dissociating bottom-up and top-down processes in a manual stimulus-response compatibility task. J Neurophysiol 104: 1472–1483.
69. Twomey T, Kawabata Duncan KJ, Price CJ, Devlin JT (2011) Top-down modulation of ventral occipito-temporal responses during visual word recognition. Neuroimage 55: 1242–1251.
70. McMains S, Kastner S (2011) Interactions of top-down and bottom-up mechanisms in human visual cortex. J Neurosci 31: 587–597.
71. Cohen L, Dehaene S, Vinckier F, Jobert A, Montavont A (2008) Reading normal and degraded words: contribution of the dorsal and ventral visual pathways. Neuroimage 40: 353–366.
72. Szlyk JP, Little DM (2009) An FMRI study of word-level recognition and processing in patients with age-related macular degeneration. Invest Ophthalmol Vis Sci 50: 4487–4495.
73. Mody M, Studdert-Kennedy M, Brady S (1997) Speech perception deficits in poor readers: auditory processing or phonological coding? J Exp Child Psychol 64: 199–231.
74. Tallal P, Miller S, Fitch RH (1993) Neurobiological basis of speech: a case for the preeminence of temporal processing. Ann N Y Acad Sci 682: 27–47.
75. Van Ingelghem M, van Wieringen A, Wouters J, Vandenbussche E, Onghena P, et al. (2001) Psychophysical evidence for a general temporal processing deficit in children with dyslexia. Neuroreport 12: 3603–3607.
76. Tallal P, Piercy M (1973) Defects of non-verbal auditory perception in children with developmental aphasia. Nature 241: 468–469.
77. Walker KM, Hall SE, Klein RM, Phillips DP (2006) Development of perceptual correlates of reading performance. Brain Res 1124: 126–141.
78. Demb JB, Boynton GM, Heeger DJ (1997) Brain activity in visual cortex predicts individual differences in reading performance. Proc Natl Acad Sci U S A 94: 13363–13366.
79. Chandrasekaran B, Hornickel J, Skoe E, Nicol T, Kraus N (2009) Context-dependent encoding in the human auditory brainstem relates to hearing speech in noise: implications for developmental dyslexia. Neuron 64: 311–319.
80. Ziegler JC, Pech-Georgel C, George F, Lorenzi C (2009) Speech-perception-in-noise deficits in dyslexia. Dev Sci 12: 732–745.
81. Brown JM (2009) Visual streams and shifting attention. Prog Brain Res 176: 47–63.
82. Facoetti A, Lorusso ML, Paganoni P, Cattaneo C, Galli R, et al. (2003) Auditory and visual automatic attention deficits in developmental dyslexia. Brain Res Cogn Brain Res 16: 185–191.
83. Facoetti A, Turatto M, Lorusso ML, Mascetti GG (2001) Orienting of visual attention in dyslexia: evidence for asymmetric hemispheric control of attention. Exp Brain Res 138: 46–53.
84. Lobier M, Zoubrinetzky R, Valdois S (2011) The visual attention span deficit in dyslexia is visual and not verbal. Cortex.
85. Snyder LH, Batista AP, Andersen RA (1997) Coding of intention in the posterior parietal cortex. Nature 386: 167–170.
86. McMains SA, Fehd HM, Emmanouil TA, Kastner S (2007) Mechanisms of feature- and space-based attention: response modulation and baseline increases. J Neurophysiol 98: 2110–2121.
87. Kastner S, De Weerd, P Desimone, R., and Ungerleider, L.G. (1998) Mechanisms of directed attention in the human extrastriate tems. In Analysis of Visual Behavior, D.J. Ingle, M.A. Goodale, and cortex as revealed by functional MRI. Science 282: 108–111.
88. Kastner S, Pinsk MA, De Weerd P, Desimone R, Ungerleider LG (1999) Increased activity in human visual cortex during directed attention in the absence of visual stimulation. Neuron 22: 751–761.
89. Gottlieb JP, Kusunoki M, Goldberg ME (1998) The representation of visual salience in monkey parietal cortex. Nature 391: 481–484.
90. Hopfinger JB, Buonocore MH, Mangun GR (2000) The neural mechanisms of top-down attentional control. Nat Neurosci 3: 284–291.
91. Corbetta M (1998) Frontoparietal cortical networks for directing attention and the eye to visual locations: identical, independent, or overlapping neural systems? Proc Natl Acad Sci U S A 95: 831–838.
92. Corbetta M, Shulman GL (2002) Control of goal-directed and stimulus-driven attention in the brain. Nat Rev Neurosci 3: 201–215.
93. Callaway EM (2005) Structure and function of parallel pathways in the primate early visual system. J Physiol 566: 13–19.
94. Buschman TJ, Miller EK (2007) Top-down versus bottom-up control of attention in the prefrontal and posterior parietal cortices. Science 315: 1860–1862.
95. Saalmann YB, Pigarev IN, Vidyasagar TR (2007) Neural mechanisms of visual attention: how top-down feedback highlights relevant locations. Science 316: 1612–1615.
96. Hoeft F, Meyler A, Hernandez A, Juel C, Taylor-Hill H, et al. (2007) Functional and morphometric brain dissociation between dyslexia and reading ability. Proc Natl Acad Sci U S A 104: 4234–4239.
97. Temple E, Deutsch GK, Poldrack RA, Miller SL, Tallal P, et al. (2003) Neural deficits in children with dyslexia ameliorated by behavioral remediation: evidence from functional MRI. Proc Natl Acad Sci U S A 100: 2860–2865.
98. Shaywitz BA, Shaywitz SE, Pugh KR, Mencl WE, Fulbright RK, et al. (2002) Disruption of posterior brain systems for reading in children with developmental dyslexia. Biol Psychiatry 52: 101–110.
99. Mesulam MM (1981) A cortical network for directed attention and unilateral neglect. Ann Neurol 10: 309–325.
100. Oleksiak A, Postma A, van der Ham IJ, Klink PC, van Wezel RJ (2010) A review of lateralization of spatial functioning in nonhuman primates. Brain Res Rev 67: 56–72.
101. Koyama MS, Di Martino A, Zuo XN, Kelly C, Mennes M, et al. (2011) Resting-state functional connectivity indexes reading competence in children and adults. J Neurosci 31: 8617–8624.
102. Koyama MS, Kelly C, Shehzad Z, Penesetti D, Castellanos FX, et al. (2010) Reading networks at rest. Cereb Cortex 20: 2549–2559.
103. Rumsey JM (1992) The biology of developmental dyslexia. JAMA 268: 912–915.

104. Shaywitz SE, Shaywitz BA, Pugh KR, Fulbright RK, Constable RT, et al. (1998) Functional disruption in the organization of the brain for reading in dyslexia. Proc Natl Acad Sci U S A 95: 2636–2641.
105. Gaab N, Gabrieli JD, Deutsch GK, Tallal P, Temple E (2007) Neural correlates of rapid auditory processing are disrupted in children with developmental dyslexia and ameliorated with training: an fMRI study. Restor Neurol Neurosci 25: 295–310.
106. Reynolds MG, Besner D (2011) There goes the neighbourhood: Contextual control over the breadth of lexical activation when reading aloud. Q J Exp Psychol (Hove) 64: 2405–2424.
107. Reynolds M, Besner D (2006) Reading aloud is not automatic: processing capacity is required to generate a phonological code from print. J Exp Psychol Hum Percept Perform 32: 1303–1323.
108. Nassi JJ, Lyon DC, Callaway EM (2006) The parvocellular LGN provides a robust disynaptic input to the visual motion area MT. Neuron 50: 319–327.

8

Cortical Signatures of Dyslexia and Remediation: An Intrinsic Functional Connectivity Approach

Maki S. Koyama[1,2]*, Adriana Di Martino[2], Clare Kelly[2], Devika R. Jutagir[2], Jessica Sunshine[2], Susan J. Schwartz[3], Francisco X. Castellanos[2,4], Michael P. Milham[3,4]

1 Rutgers University Center for Molecular and Behavioral Neuroscience, Newark, New Jersey, United States of America, **2** Phyllis Green and Randolph Cowen Institute for Pediatric Neuroscience, New York University Child Study Center, NYU Langone Medical Center, New York, New York, United States of America, **3** Center for the Developing Brain, Child Mind Institute, New York, New York, United States of America, **4** Nathan Kline Institute for Psychiatric Research, Orangeburg, New York, United States of America

Abstract

This observational, cross-sectional study investigates cortical signatures of developmental dyslexia, particularly from the perspective of behavioral remediation. We employed resting-state fMRI, and compared intrinsic functional connectivity (iFC) patterns of known reading regions (seeds) among three dyslexia groups characterized by (a) no remediation (current reading and spelling deficits), (b) partial remediation (only reading deficit remediated), and (c) full remediation (both reading and spelling deficits remediated), and a group of age- and IQ-matched typically developing children (TDC) (total N = 44, age range = 7–15 years). We observed significant group differences in iFC of two seeds located in the left posterior reading network – left intraparietal sulcus (L.IPS) and left fusiform gyrus (L.FFG). Specifically, iFC between L.IPS and left middle frontal gyrus was significantly weaker in all dyslexia groups, irrespective of remediation status/literacy competence, suggesting that persistent dysfunction in the fronto-parietal attention network characterizes dyslexia. Additionally, relative to both TDC and the no remediation group, the remediation groups exhibited stronger iFC between L.FFG and right middle occipital gyrus (R.MOG). The full remediation group also exhibited stronger negative iFC between the same L.FFG seed and right medial prefrontal cortex (R.MPFC), a core region of the default network These results suggest that behavioral remediation may be associated with compensatory changes anchored in L.FFG, which reflect atypically stronger coupling between posterior visual regions (L.FFG-R.MOG) and greater functional segregation between task-positive and task-negative regions (L.FFG-R.MPFC). These findings were bolstered by significant relationships between the strength of the identified functional connections and literacy scores. We conclude that examining iFC can reveal cortical signatures of dyslexia with particular promise for monitoring neural changes associated with behavioral remediation.

Editor: Nanyin Zhang, University of Massachusetts Medical School, United States of America

Funding: This study was supported by grants from NIMH [R01MH081218, K23MH087770], the Stavros Niarchos Foundation, and the Leon Levy Foundation. The funders had no role in study design, data collection and analysis, decision to publish, or preparation of the manuscript.

Competing Interests: The authors have declared that no competing interests exist.

* E-mail: makisophiakoyama@gmail.com

Introduction

Although the phonological deficit hypothesis (e.g., [1–2]) is the dominant explanatory theory of developmental dyslexia (a reading disorder), impaired phonological processing alone cannot explain the entirety of clinical symptomatology in the disorder. The majority of individuals with dyslexia suffer from multiple deficits in addition to or independent of phonological deficits [3–7]. Beyond abnormalities in phonological processing systems, emerging models of dyslexia highlight the potential contributions of dysfunction within systems supporting visual perceptual processing [8], auditory perceptual processing [9–11], rapid naming [12], and attention control [13–15]. In recent years, speculation has increased regarding cerebellar dysfunction in dyslexia [16–17]. Yet, with few exceptions [18–20], imaging studies of dyslexia have primarily focused on phonological deficits.

To help individuals with dyslexia improve literacy performance, substantial remediation efforts have been made, such as those targeting phonological deficits. These efforts have generally resulted in successful behavioral remediation (For review, see [21]). Recent task-based fMRI studies, using mainly phonological tasks, provide evidence of cortical activation changes associated with such behavioral changes (i.e., differences between before and after intervention) in individuals with dyslexia. Broadly, two cortical patterns appear to characterize behavioral remediation: 1) normalized (e.g., increased) activity detected in the known left hemisphere reading network (e.g., left temporoparietal and frontal regions) and 2) compensatory activity detected outside known reading networks (e.g., in right frontal regions) [22–26].

The goals of the present work are twofold. First, we aimed to conduct a broader examination of the cortical signatures of dyslexia by employing task-independent "resting-state" fMRI (R-fMRI). While task-based fMRI is of undoubted value, R-fMRI enables bypassing some of the limitations inherent to task-based developmental fMRI studies on reading and dyslexia (e.g., difficulties in developing reading tasks that can be equivocally performed by children in different age/grade groups). Second, we sought to obtain preliminary insights into the cortical signatures of behavioral remediation for reading and spelling deficits in individuals with dyslexia, using an observational, cross-sectional design. Specifically, we recruited individuals with documented evidence of a previous diagnosis of dyslexia, irrespective of the presence of prior remediation efforts or the current level of literacy competence. Consequently, participants varied substantially in literacy profiles, with some continuing to exhibit deficient reading and spelling, whereas others had apparently remediated reading difficulties and, in some cases, spelling deficiencies as well. To investigate the cortical signatures of this well-documented heterogeneity in dyslexia outcomes [27–28], we subdivided participants with a previous diagnosis of dyslexia into three groups: (a) children with current literacy deficits (no remediation), (b) children who remediated their reading deficits (partial remediation), and (c) children who remediated both reading and spelling deficits (full remediation).

Primary analyses focused on the examination of intrinsic functional connectivity (iFC) [29] in the aforementioned three dyslexia groups (i.e., no remediation, partial remediation, full remediation) and a matched typically developing comparison (TDC) group. Intrinsic functional connectivity is detected by examining inter-regional correlations in spontaneous low-frequency (<0.1 Hz) fluctuations in the R-fMRI signal [30]. This approach has delineated iFC patterns representing distinct functional networks [31–36] including reading networks [37–39]. Resting-state fMRI is increasingly being applied to studies of developmental disorders, including autism (e.g., [40–43]), attention deficit hyperactivity disorder (e.g., [44–47]), and Tourette syndrome [48]. In dyslexia, only one R-fMRI study has been conducted, focusing on the inter-hemispheric functional connectivity of inferior frontal regions [49].

In our previous work, we employed seed-based correlation analyses to assess iFC of regions commonly implicated in word reading [50–51] and demonstrated the utility of this approach for mapping reading networks in children and adults [38–39]. These reading circuits encompass regions previously identified as being dysfunctional in dyslexia (For review, see [52]). Here, we aimed to detect differences in iFC patterns of known reading regions as a function of the presence or absence of history of dyslexia (i.e., dyslexia vs. typically developing), as well as remediation status (i.e., no remediation, partial remediation, full remediation, typically developing). Accordingly, we predicted that we would detect three types of outcomes: 1) atypical iFC associated with a history of dyslexia (e.g., iFC common to all dyslexia groups and distinct from that of the TDC group), 2) altered iFC reflecting cortical compensation associated with behavioral remediation (e.g., iFC distinguishing the remediation groups from both the TDC group and the no remediation group), and 3) altered iFC reflecting cortical normalization associated with behavioral remediation (e.g., iFC distinguishing the remediation groups only from the no remediation group but not from the TDC group). These hypothetical iFC profiles are illustrated in Figure 1.

Materials and Methods

Participant Characteristics

Participants were native English-speaking children with (n = 33) and without (n = 11) a history of dyslexia (i.e., documented prior diagnosis of dyslexia). We recruited children with a history of dyslexia through referrals from the clinical services at the New York University Child Study Center and the New York International Dyslexia Association. Inclusion in dyslexia groups was based upon parental report of prior diagnosis of reading disorder in accord with DSM-IV or ICD-10, accompanied by prior written documentation. We enrolled a total of 33 children with a history of dyslexia. Among them, 22 exhibited partial (n = 11) or full (n = 11) literacy remediation based on standardized subtests of the Wechsler Individual Achievement Test – Second Edition (WIAT) [53]. Specifically, children with a history of dyslexia were classified as remediated if their current standard scores were above 85, corresponding to one standard deviation below the norm, on the WIAT Word Reading subscale (partial remediation), or on both the WIAT Word Reading and the WIAT Spelling subscales (full remediation). The remaining 11 individuals with current standard scores lower than 85 on both the WIAT Word Reading and the WIAT Spelling subscales constituted the no remediation group. Accordingly, there were 3 dyslexia groups: (1) children with current deficits in both reading and spelling ("Dys-N": Dyslexia with no remediation), (2) children with a previous diagnosis of dyslexia but exhibiting no current reading deficit ("Dys-R": Dyslexia with reading remediation), and (3) children with a previous diagnosis of dyslexia but exhibiting no current deficits in either reading or spelling ("Dys-RS": Dyslexia with reading and spelling remediation).

According to parental report (and supporting documentation for some cases), children in the remediation groups had a history of one or more targeted interventions prior to the current study (e.g., the Orton Gillingham approach; http://www.ortonacademy.org, Wilson Language Training; http://www.wilsonlanguage.com, or miscellaneous school intervention efforts). In contrast, none of the children with current literacy deficits (no remediation group) had a history of targeted dyslexia intervention training. This pattern suggests that behavioral remediation is related, at least in part, to targeted intervention training, although the specific forms of intervention varied and are not a focus of examination here due to limited sample size. Importantly, prior written documentation served to verify literacy impairment in the two remediation groups (standard scores lower than 85 on any type of standardized literacy test prior to remediation). Similarly, the written documentation provided evidence that the majority of these children had exhibited deficits in phonological skills (e.g., phonological awareness), consistent with the phonological deficit hypothesis (e.g., [54]).

For a control group, eleven typically developing children (TDC) were selected from a larger pool of children participating in ongoing studies at NYU Child Study Center. In the TDC group, all children's standard scores were above 85 on both WIAT Word Reading and WIAT Spelling, confirming lack of impairments in either reading or spelling. They had no previous or current DSM-IV-TR diagnoses of psychiatric disorders based on the Schedule for Affective Disorders and Schizophrenia for School-Age Children–Present and Lifetime Version [KSADS-PL: 55], which was administered to parents and child participants separately. The KSADS-PL was not administered to children with a history of dyslexia and/or their parents. Nevertheless, we ascertained whether these children had received a previous diagnosis of disorders other than dyslexia, such as attention deficit hyperactivity disorder (ADHD), through informal interviews with parents of dyslexic children and by reviewing documentation of prior clinical evaluations whenever available (Three out of 33 children with a history of dyslexia had been previously diagnosed with ADHD).

Children in each of the 4 groups were group-matched on age (overall mean age = 12.2±2.3 years: range = 7.7–15.7 years), sex, estimated full-scale IQ, and handedness. The Wechsler Abbreviated Scale of Intelligence (WASI) [56] provided full-scale IQ estimates, and all participants had full-scale IQ estimates above 85. We also administered two subtests of the Test of Word Reading Efficiency (TOWRE) [57]) – Sight Word Efficiency (SWE) and Phonemic Decoding Efficiency (PDE). Further literacy-related

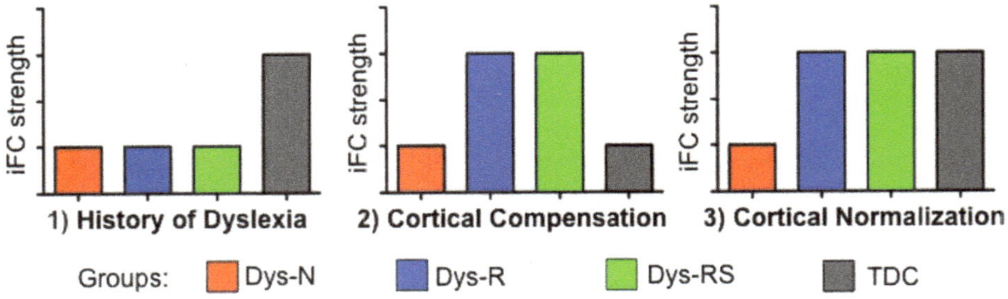

Figure 1. Hypothetical profiles of intrinsic functional connectivity. iFC = intrinsic Functional Connectivity, Dys-N = Dyslexia with No Remediation, Dys-R = Dyslexia with Reading Remediation, Dys-RS = Dyslexia with Reading and Spelling Remediation, TDC = Typically Developing Children.

measures were administered to children in the dyslexia groups, including two subtests of the Comprehensive Test of Phonological Processing (CTOPP) [58] – Elision (a phonological awareness test) and Nonword Repetition (a phonological short-term memory test), as well as WIAT Reading Comprehension. Additionally, given the increased incidence of ADHD symptomatology in individuals with dyslexia (e.g., [59–60]), we asked all parents to complete the Conners Parent Rating Scales–Revised Long Version (CPRS-R-L: [61]) which addresses ADHD symptoms. Table 1 provides demographic and cognitive measures for each group, and Figure 2 illustrates their literacy profiles.

To help anchor the results of the current study, we performed a secondary analysis that aimed to verify that iFC patterns derived from the TDC group represent normative/typical iFC profiles. We examined iFC in an age- and IQ-matched, independent group of TDC (n = 25, mean age = 11.7±1.5 years), as well as in a group of typical adults (TA; n = 25, mean age: 31.6±8.2), both of which were studied previously [39]. This enabled us to examine whether iFC strength for regions showing significant group effects was normative in the two additional typical groups. The current study was approved by the institutional review board of New York University (NYU) School of Medicine, and all parents and children provided written informed consent and assent.

Table 1. Demographic and cognitive profiles (means and standard deviation) for each group.

	Dyslexia-N	Dyslexia-R	Dyslexia-RS	TDC	F or X^2
Age (years)	12.4 (2.1)	11.8 (2.2)	12.6 (2.9)	12.2 (2.3)	N.S.
Gender (n)	6M/5F	5M/6F	5M/6F	6M/5F	N.S.
Handedness	0L/11R	0L/11R	0L/11R	0L/11R	N.S.
WASI Full IQ (ss)	108.1 (6.9)	101.3 (9.8)	108.1 (5.1)	106.5 (5.8)	N.S.
WIAT Read (ss)	74.2 (11.3)	96.3 (7.3)	103.8 (9.3)	110.1 (7.0)	F = 34.1***
WIAT Spell (ss)	78.0 (10.2)	82.3 (5.9)	96.7 (7.9)	115.6 (5.76)	F = 61.3***
WIAT RC (ss)	94.6 (9.9)	97.4 (8.3)	113.5 (14.2)	N.A.	F = 9.4***
TOWRE SWE (ss)	77.1 (12.7)	92.8 (9.9)	94.6 (9.2)	101.5 (11.0)	F = 10.0***
TOWRE PDE (ss)	78.8 (11.4)	90.9 (5.9)	94.0 (10.0)	109.0 (12.6)	F = 15.8***
CTOPP Elision (ss) †	7.9 (2.7)	12.4 (1.9)	11.6 (2.8)	N.A.	F = 13.5***
CTOPP NWR (ss)†	6.9 (2.4)	7.7 (2.2)	9.4 (2.5)	N.A.	F = 3.6*
CPRS-IA (ts)	57.1 (11.3)	62.6 (15.2)	53.4 (9.4)	44.8 (5.1)	F = 5.3**
CPRS-HI (ts)	56.0 (6.5)	55.4 (13.4)	50.8 (9.9)	45.5 (4.1)	F = 3.1*

n = 11 for each group, *p<0.05, **p<0.01, ***p<0.001: N.A. = Not Available, N.S. = Not Significant; Dys-N = Dyslexia with No Remediation, Dys-R = Dyslexia with Reading Remediation, Dys-RS = Dyslexia with Reading and Spelling Remediation, TDC = Typically Developing Children, ss = standard score (mean = 100, standard deviation = 15), ts = t score, M = Male, F = Female, L = Left, R = Right, WASI = *Wechsler Abbreviated Scale of Intelligence*, WIAT = Wechsler Individual Achievement Test – Second Edition, RC = Reading Comprehension, TOWRE = Test of Word Reading Efficiency, SWE = Sight Word Reading Efficiency, PDE = Phonemic Decoding Efficiency, CTOPP = Comprehensive Test of Phonological Processing, NWR = NonWord Repetition, CPRS-IA = *Conners' Parent Rating Scales DSM-IV Symptom Inattentive index, CPRS-HI = Conners' Parent Rating Scales DSM-IV Symptom Hyperactive-Impulsive index:* † Standard scores for CTOPP measures are based on a mean of 10 with standard deviation of 3.

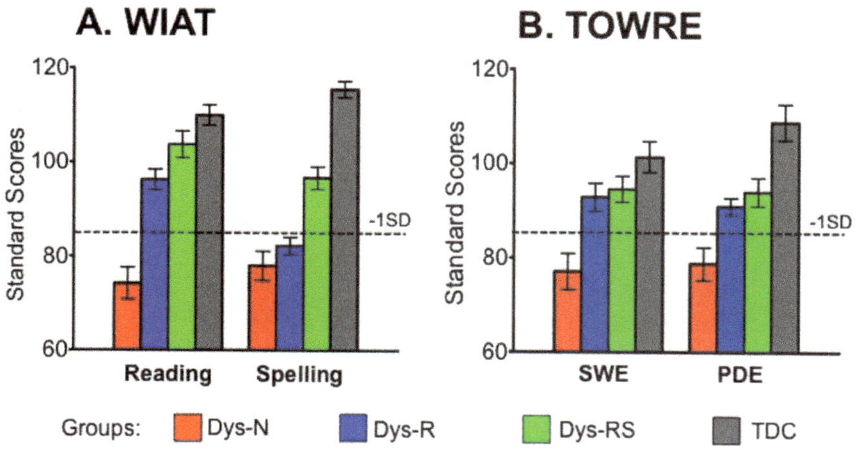

Figure 2. Group mean and standard deviation of literacy performance. (A) WIAT = Wechsler Individual Achievement Test and (B) TOWRE = Test of Word Reading Efficiency, n = 11 for each group. SWE = Sight Word Reading Efficiency, PDE = Phonemic Decoding Efficiency, SD = Standard Deviation, Dys-N = Dyslexia with No Remediation, Dys-R = Dyslexia with Reading Remediation, Dys-RS = Dyslexia with Reading and Spelling Remediation, TDC = Typically Developing Children: -1SD represents a standard score of 85, one standard deviation below the norm.

MRI Data Acquisition

MRI data were collected on a Siemens Allegra 3.0 T scanner at the NYU Center for Brain Imaging. We collected resting-state fMRI data in an oblique plane using a customized multi-echo planar imaging (EPI): 180 whole-brain volumes; TR = 2000 ms; effective TE = 33 ms; flip angle = 90°; 33 contiguous 4 mm slices, matrix = 80×64; acquisition voxel size = 3×3×4 mm. This sequence uses the dead time that precedes the readout in EPI sequences with normal TEs (~33 ms) to collect additional images at several echo times. However, the information from these additional echo times in not used in our reconstruction of the data. For spatial normalization and localization, we also acquired a high-resolution T1-weighted magnetization prepared gradient echo sequence (TR = 2530 ms; TE = 3.25 ms; TI = 1100 ms; flip angle = 7°; 128 slices; field of view = 256 mm).

Data Preprocessing

For each participant, image preprocessing was carried out using a combination of AFNI (http://afni.nimh.nih.gov) [62] and FSL (http://www.fmrib.ox.ac.uk/fsl/). Scripts containing data processing steps similar to those employed here have been released as part of the '1000 Functional Connectomes Project [63] (http://www.nitrc.org/projects/fcon_1000). Preprocessing comprised: 1) discarding the first 4 EPI volumes from each scan to allow for signal equilibration, 2) slice timing correction for interleaved acquisitions, 3) 3D motion correction with Fourier interpolation, 4) time series despiking (detection and reduction of extreme time series outliers), 5) spatial smoothing (6 mm FWHM Gaussian kernel), 6) mean-based intensity normalization of all volumes by the same factor, 7) temporal band-pass filtering (0.009–0.11 Hz), and 8) linear and quadratic detrending. Registration of each participant's high-resolution anatomical image to standard 2×2×2 mm MNI space was accomplished in two steps [64]. First, a 12-degrees-of-freedom linear affine transformation was computed using FLIRT [65–66]. This transformation was then refined using FNIRT nonlinear registration [64]. Linear registration of each participant's functional time series to the high-resolution structural image was performed using FLIRT. This functional-to-anatomical co-registration was improved by intermediate registration to a low-resolution image and b0 warping. To control for potential effects of physiological processes (e.g., fluctuations related to cardiac and respiratory cycles) [67–68], motion and large-scale neural signals present throughout the brain [69], each participant's preprocessed data was regressed on nine nuisance covariates (signals from white matter, cerebrospinal fluid, the global signal, and six motion parameters). Each participant's resultant 4D residual volume was spatially normalized by applying the previously computed transformation to 2 mm MNI space.

Table 2. MNI coordinates of the regions of interest.

Regions-of-Interest			MNI (x, y, z)
Occipital			
	IOG	Inferior Occipital Gyrus (posterior)	−25 −87 −10
	FFG	Fusiform Gyrus (posterior)	−48 −57 -20
Temporal			
	STG	Superior temporal gyrus (posterior)	−53 −31 9
	TPJ	Temporoparietal Junction	−59 −45 15
Parietal			
	IPL	Inferior parietal lobule	−40 −48 42
	IPS	Intraparietal sulcus (posterior)	−30 −58 48
Motor			
	PCG	Precentral gyrus (dorsal)	−48 −12 45
	SMA	Supplementary motor area	−4 10 58
Frontal			
	IFGop	Inferior frontal gyrus (opercularis)	−51 10 10
	IFGtr	Inferior frontal gyrus (triangularis)	−48 32 6
	MFG	Middle frontal gyrus (ventral)	−44 10 30
Subcortical			
	THAL	Thalamus	−10 −14 8

The seeds were selected based on meta-analyses of reading in typical adults [50] and typically developing children [51], as well as dyslexic children [52].

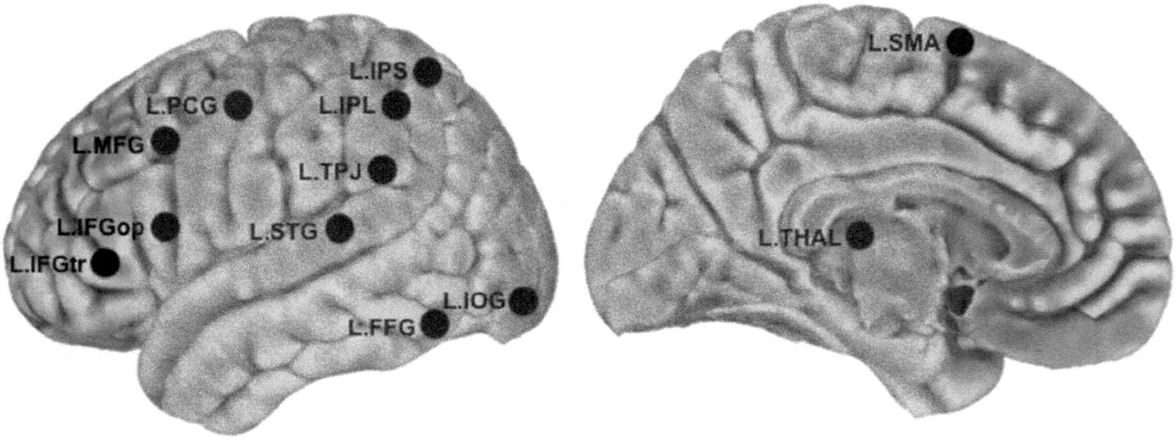

Figure 3. Locations of seed ROIs. Seeds are presented as overlaid black circles. MNI coordinates of these seeds are provided in Table 2. L.IOC = Left Inferior Occipital Gyrus, L.FFG = Left Fusiform Gyrus, L.STG = Left Superior Temporal Gyrus, L.TPJ = Left Temporoparietal Junction, L.IPS = Left Inferior Parietal Lobule, L.IPS = Left Intraparietal Sulcus, L.PCG = Left Precentral Gyrus, L.SMA = Left Supplementary Motor Area, L.IFGop = Left Inferior Frontal Gyrus pars Opercularis, L.IFGtr = Left Inferior Frontal Gyrus pars Triangularis, L.MFG = Left Middle Frontal Gyrus, L.THAL = Left Thalamus.

Seed Regions-of-interest (ROIs)

We examined functional connectivity associated with 12 regions of interest (ROIs), including 11 regions that had been derived from meta-analyses of reading in children [51] and adults [50] and validated in a previous R-fMRI study [39]. One additional region, the left inferior parietal lobule (L.IPL), was added based on the most recent meta-analysis of children with dyslexia [52]; the remainder of the regions in the meta-analysis were already included in our previous work [39]. The 12 ROIs in the current study were: 1) left inferior occipital gyrus (L.IOG), 2) left posterior fusiform gyrus (L.FFG), 3) left posterior superior temporal gyrus (L.STG), 4) left temporoparietal junction (L.TPJ), 6) left inferior parietal lobule (L.IPL), 7) left intraparietal sulcus (L.IPS), 8) left dorsal precentral gyrus (L.PCG), 9) left supplementary motor area (L.SMA), 8) left inferior frontal gyrus pars opercularis (L.IFGop), 10) left inferior frontal gyrus pars triangularis (L.IFGtr), 11) left middle frontal gyrus (L.MFG), and 12) left thalamus (L.THAL). Each ROI was a spherical seed (6 mm radius in 2 mm standard space) [39], centered on the MNI coordinates listed in Table 2. Figure 3 shows the spatial locations of the seeds.

Participant-level iFC Analyses

For each participant, the representative time series for each seed ROI was extracted from their 4D residuals volume in standard space by averaging the time series across all voxels within the ROI. This step ensured, to as great an extent as possible, that the mean time series were extracted from the same regions across participants. Calculation of the correlation between each seed ROI time series and that of every other brain voxel was performed in native space to minimize computational and storage demands. This procedure is consistent with our prior publications [70–72]. The resultant participant-level correlation maps were Fisher-r-to-z transformed, then transformed into MNI152 2 mm standard space for group-level analyses.

Group-level iFC Analyses

For each seed ROI, group-level analyses were carried out using a random-effects ordinary least squares model. Whole-brain correction for multiple comparisons was performed using Gaussian Random Field Theory (min $Z > 2.3$; cluster significance: $p < 0.05$, corrected). To test the effect of group on iFC, we performed a one-way ANOVA, treating group as a 4-level factor (Dyslexia-N, Dyslexia-R, Dyslexia-RS, and TDC). Subsequently, regions exhibiting significant main effects of group on iFC were interrogated by post hoc analysis using unpaired t-tests to determine significant pair-wise differences between groups.

To account for the effects of head motion [73–76], we calculated frame-by-frame changes in head position, referred to as framewise displacement (FD), for each participant, and included mean FD values as a covariate in the group-level model. As detailed elsewhere [73], FD is calculated from the derivatives of the rigid body realignment estimates produced by the motion correction algorithm during fMRI preprocessing. Statistically, mean FD values neither differed among the four groups, $F(3, 40) = 1.06$, $p = 0.38$, (Figure S1.A), nor correlated with age ($R^2 = 0.01$, $p = 0.49$) (Figure S1.B).

In addition to the primary group analysis, which included both global signal regression (GSreg) at the individual level and mean FD regression (FDreg) at the group level (i.e., +GSreg+FDreg), we performed several additional confirmatory group analyses. These were carried out in response to recent debates regarding R-fMRI analytic methods, particularly concerning the effects of micro-movements (e.g., [73]) and global signal regression [77–78]. Four confirmatory group analyses were conducted: 1) with GSreg at the individual level but no mean FDreg at the group level (+GSreg-FDreg), 2) with GSreg and removal ("scrubbing") of volumes with FD larger than 0.5 mm at the individual level, without FDreg at the group level (+GSreg+Scrub), 3) without GSreg at the individual level but with mean FDreg at the group level (-GSreg+FDreg), 4) without GSreg at the individual level or mean FDreg at the group level (-GSreg-FDreg).

Brain-behavior Relationships

We explored relationships between the strength of iFC among regions showing group effects and literacy performance (i.e., accuracy on WIAT Word Reading and WIAT Spelling subtests) as well as ADHD symptom scores (two CPRS DSM-IV Symptoms Subscales: Inattention and Hyperactivity-Impulsivity). Multiple regression analyses were performed to investigate whether individual differences in literacy performance (and ADHD symptoms) were associated with individual differences in the strength of iFC associated with each seed in each group, across dyslexia groups, and/or across all groups.

Secondary Analysis

n the current study, the sample size for each group was equal but relatively small (n = 11 for each group). In order to verify that iFC patterns derived from the TDC group are representative of normative/typical iFC profiles, we performed unpaired t-tests comparing the strength of iFC between regions exhibiting significant group effects between all pairs of the following three groups; 1) the current TDC group (n = 11), 2) an age- and IQ-matched, independent TDC group (n = 25), and 3) a typical adult (TA) group (n = 25). The latter two groups were described previously [39]. We expected that the two TDC groups would not differ from one another. Group differences between each of the two TDC groups and the TA group would only be expected if the networks exhibiting significant dyslexia-related differences were also developmentally sensitive.

Results

Dyslexia Sample Characterization

One-way ANOVA showed that the four groups (i.e., TDC, Dys-N, Dys-R, and Dys-RS) did not differ significantly with respect to age, sex, estimated full-scale IQ, or handedness, but differed significantly on the literacy measures (i.e., WIAT Reading, WIAT Spelling, TOWRE SWE, and TOWRE PDE), as expected (Table 1 and Figure 2). Post-hoc analysis using unpaired t-tests revealed significant differences on these measures between each pair of groups; as expected, the Dys-N group performed significantly worse on all these measures than the TDC group (Supplementary Material1).

On other literacy-related measures (i.e., WIAT Reading Comprehension, CTOPP Elision, and CTOPP Nonword Repetition) specifically administered to children with a history of dyslexia, the three dyslexia groups also differed significantly (Table 1). Significant post-hoc differences between each pair of groups were noted (Supplementary Material1). Of note, all dyslexic children's performance (except for one child in the Dys-N group) fell within the normal range on WIAT Reading Comprehension. However, some dyslexic children, particularly those in the Dys-N group, showed impairments (i.e., standard scores <8) on the CTOPP phonological measures.

When reading and spelling errors were examined, some children with a history of dyslexia, even in the remediation groups, made errors such as substitution of visually similar words (e.g., 'useless' pronounced as 'unless'), omission (e.g., 'climb' spelled as 'clim'), transposition (e.g., 'receive' spelled as 'recieve'), and sounding out silent letters (e.g., 'b' pronounced in 'subtle'). These errors, typically made by individuals with dyslexia, are considered to reflect inadequate phonological and/or orthographic representations of words [79].

Among the 33 children with dyslexia, a previously established diagnosis of ADHD was reported for only three participants. However, as expected for individuals with dyslexia [80], elevated levels of inattention and hyperactivity-impulsivity, indexed as T scores higher than 60 on the Conners' Inattentive and Hyperactive-Impulsive subscales, respectively, were noted in these children: One-way ANOVA showed a significant main effect of group for both inattention and hyperactivity-impulsivity scores (Table 1), and post-hoc analysis revealed that both ADHD symptom domains were significantly elevated in the dyslexia groups relative to the TDC group (Material S1 and Figure S2.A). Consistent with recent evidence emphasizing the importance of attention in reading (For review, see [81]), inattention scores were negatively correlated with reading scores across all groups ($R^2 = 0.24$, $p<0.001$), and across dyslexia groups ($R^2 = 0.12$, $p<0.05$), particularly in Dys-R ($R^2 = 0.65$, $p<0.01$) (Figure S2.B.1). A significant correlation between hyperactivity-impulsivity and reading scores was also observed across all groups ($R^2 = 0.13$, $p<0.05$) (Figure S2.B.2). Accordingly, in addition to our primary analyses, we examined the association between each of these two measures of ADHD symptoms and iFC within the reading network (details below).

Group Effects

One-way ANOVA, with group as level (4 levels: no remediation, partial remediation, full remediation, and TDC), identified a significant main effect of group ($Z > 2.3$; $p<0.05$, corrected) on iFC associated with two seeds in the posterior reading network – the left intraparietal sulcus (L.IPS) and left fusiform gyrus (L.FFG). Specifically, we observed a main effect of group on iFC between the L.IPS seed and left middle frontal gyrus (L.MFG, BA9; $x = -34$, $y = 4$, $z = 40$; see Figure 4), and on iFC between the L.FFG seed and the right middle occipital gyrus, extending towards the right intraparietal sulcus (R.MOG, BA19; $x = 34$, $y = -70$, $z = 4$; see Figure 5.A), as well as between the L.FFG seed and the right medial prefrontal cortex (R.MPFC, BA33; $x = 14$, $y = 46$, $z = 10$; see Figure 5.B), a region corresponding to the anterior region of the dorsal MPFC [82].

Of note, our findings were generally robust to the particular micro-movement correction strategy employed (i.e., regression of mean FD, "FDreg"; scrubbing at FD >0.5 mm, "Scrub"; see Figure S3). In contrast, dependencies on global signal regression (GSreg) were noted for iFC of the L.FFG seed but not that of the L.IPS seed: In the absence of GSreg, the L.FFG findings failed to survive multiple comparison correction, but were significant only at uncorrected $p<0.05$. Figure S4 illustrates such region-specific effects of GSreg on the group differences in these intrinsic functional connections. These findings suggest that GSreg served to account for unexplained variation in these connections, although resolution of this issue is beyond the scope of the current study. Accordingly, the remainder of the results section focuses on findings revealed by the analysis conducted with GSreg.

Interrogation of Pairwise Group Differences

Statistical interrogation (i.e., pairwise comparisons via unpaired t-test) of regions exhibiting a main effect of group revealed two profiles – one associated with the historical diagnosis of dyslexia, regardless of remediation status (L.IPS-L.MFG), and one reflecting cortical compensation associated with behavioral remediation (L.FFG-R.MOG, L.FFG-R.MPFC).

Atypical Connectivity Associated with Historical Diagnosis of Dyslexia

Post-hoc analysis showed that the iFC between the L.IPS seed and L.MFG was weaker in all dyslexia groups relative to TDC (Figure 4): Dys-N ($t = 8.44$, $p<0.001$), Dys-R ($t = 4.42$, $p<0.001$), and Dys-RS ($t = 3.75$, $p<0.01$). Among dyslexia groups, iFC between L.IPS and L.MFG was significantly weaker in Dys-N relative to both Dys-R ($t = 2.69$, $p<0.05$) and Dys-RS ($t = 4.06$, $p<0.001$). That is, amongst dyslexia groups, iFC between L.IPS and L.MFG was weakest in the no remediation group. Notably, all children in TDC group exhibited positive L.IPS-L.MFG connectivity, as contrasted with negative connectivity exhibited by the majority of children in the no remediation group.

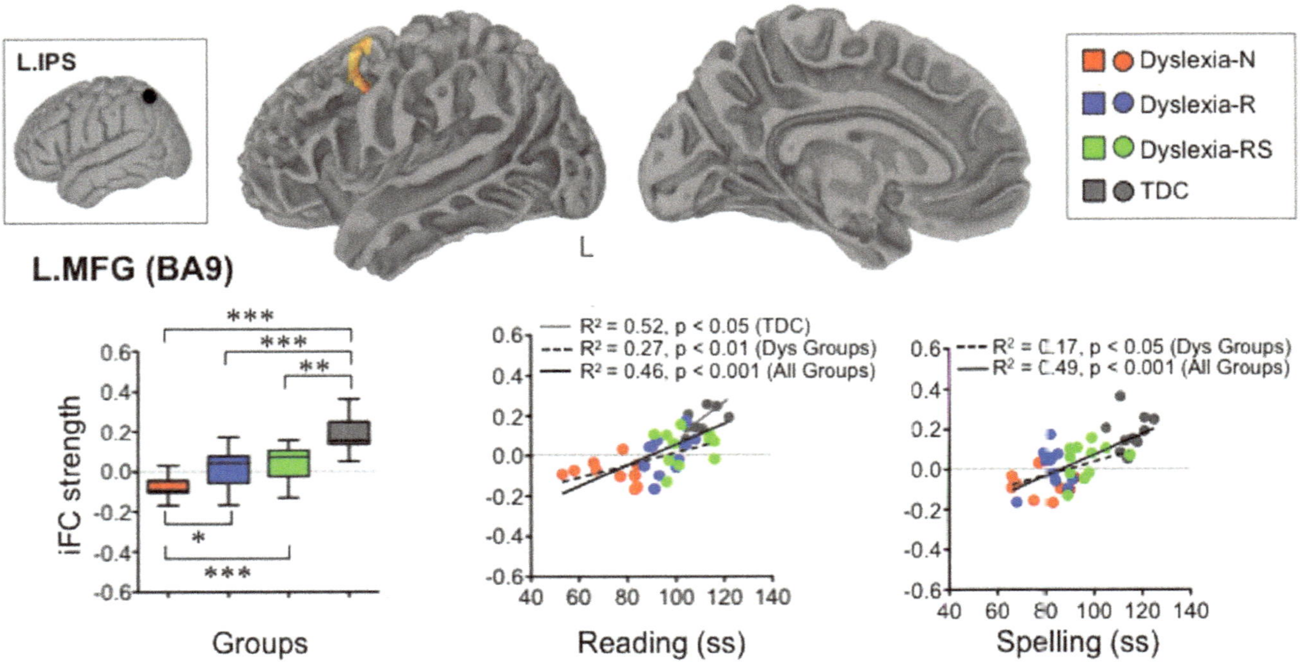

Figure 4. Atypical iFC between the left intraparietal sulcus (L.IPS) and left middle frontal gyrus (L.MFG) associated with historical diagnosis of dyslexia. The box-and-whisker plot depicts L.IPS-L.MFG iFC for each group and group differences, whereas the two scatterplots represent the relationships between the strength of this connection and reading as well as spelling scores. iFC = intrinsic Functional Connectivity, Dys-N = Dyslexia with No Remediation, Dys-R = Dyslexia with Reading Remediation, Dys-RS = Dyslexia with Reading and Spelling Remediation, TDC = Typically Developing Children, Dys = Dyslexia, ss = standard scores: ***$p<0.001$, **$p<0.01$, *$p<0.05$ (corrected): L.IPS-L.MFG iFC was weaker in all dyslexia groups relative to TDC.

Examination of dimensional relationships between iFC and literacy competence (i.e., reading and spelling) further highlighted the contributions of L.IPS-L.MFG functional connectivity to literacy. Specifically, multiple regression analyses revealed that iFC between L.IPS and L.MFG was positively correlated with literacy performance across all groups (Reading, $R^2 = 0.46$, $n = 44$, $p<0.001$; Spelling, $R^2 = 0.49$, $n = 44$, $p<0.001$; scatter plots in Figure 4). That is, children who exhibited stronger positive iFC between L.IPS and L.MFG tended to have higher scores in literacy performance. Such brain-behavior relationships were also noted across all dyslexia groups (Reading, $R^2 = 0.27$, $n = 33$, $p<0.01$; Spelling, $R^2 = 0.17$, $n = 33$, $p<0.05$). When examining individual groups, only the relationship between L.IPS-L.MFG iFC and reading performance within the TDC group reached statistical significance ($R^2 = 0.52$, $n = 11$, $p<0.05$).

Cortical Changes Associated with Behavioral Remediation

Post-hoc analysis revealed that the iFC patterns associated with the L.FFG seed differed significantly between the remediation groups and the remaining groups (i.e., the TDC group and the no remediation group) (Figure 5). First, the two remediation groups (the partial and full remediation groups) exhibited significantly stronger positive iFC between L.FFG and R.MOG, relative to TDC (Dys-R, $t = 6.15$, $p<0.001$; Dys-RS, $t = 4.84$, $p<0.01$), and relative to Dys-N (Dys-R, $t = 5.30$, $p<0.001$; Dys-RS, $t = 3.39$, $p<0.01$). No group difference was observed either between Dys-R and Dys-RS ($t = 1.31$) or between TDC and Dys-N ($t = 0.85$) (Figure 5.A). Second, Dys-RS (the full remediation group) exhibited stronger negative iFC between L.FFG and R.MPFC, relative to TDC ($t = 4.61$, $p<0.001$), Dys-N ($t = 5.73$, $p<0.001$), and Dys-R ($t = 3.41$, $p<0.01$). Among the latter three groups, no differences were observed (Figure 5.B). This pattern of results – the remediation groups(s) (Dys-R and Dys-RS for L.FFG-R.MOG iFC; Dys-RS for L.FFG-R.MPFC) being different from both TDC and the no remediation groups – is suggestive of compensatory cortical changes associated with remediation, rather than cortical normalization.

Examination of dimensional relationships between iFC and literacy competence further highlighted the contributions of these two L.FFG connections to literacy (scatter plots in Figure 5). First, iFC between L.FFG and R.MOG was positively correlated with literacy performance across dyslexia groups (Reading, $R^2 = 0.49$, $n = 33$, $p<0.001$; Spelling $R^2 = 0.14$, $n = 33$, $p<0.05$; Figure 5.A). When examining groups individually, iFC was positively correlated with reading scores in each remediation group (Dys-R, $R^2 = 0.55$, $n = 11$, $p<0.01$; Dys-RS, $R^2 = 0.77$, $p<0.001$), and with spelling scores within Dys-RS ($R^2 = 0.40$, $p<0.05$). Such brain-behavior relationships were absent in the Dys-N and TDC groups. That is, children who exhibited stronger positive iFC between L.FFG and R.MOG tended to have higher scores in literacy performance across dyslexia groups, and this trend was particularly prominent in the remediation groups.

Second, iFC between L.FFG and R.MPFC was negatively correlated with literacy skills across dyslexia groups (Reading, $R^2 = 0.52$, $n = 33$, $p<0.001$; Spelling, $R^2 = 0.33$, $n = 33$, $p<0.001$; Figure 5.B). That is, children with dyslexia who exhibited more strongly negative iFC between L.FFG and R.MPFC tended to have higher literacy scores. When looking at groups individually, such brain-behavior relationships were present only within the full remediation group (Reading, $R^2 = 0.61$, $n = 11$, $p<0.01$; Spelling, $R^2 = 0.50$, $n = 11$, $p<0.05$), and absent in the TDC group and

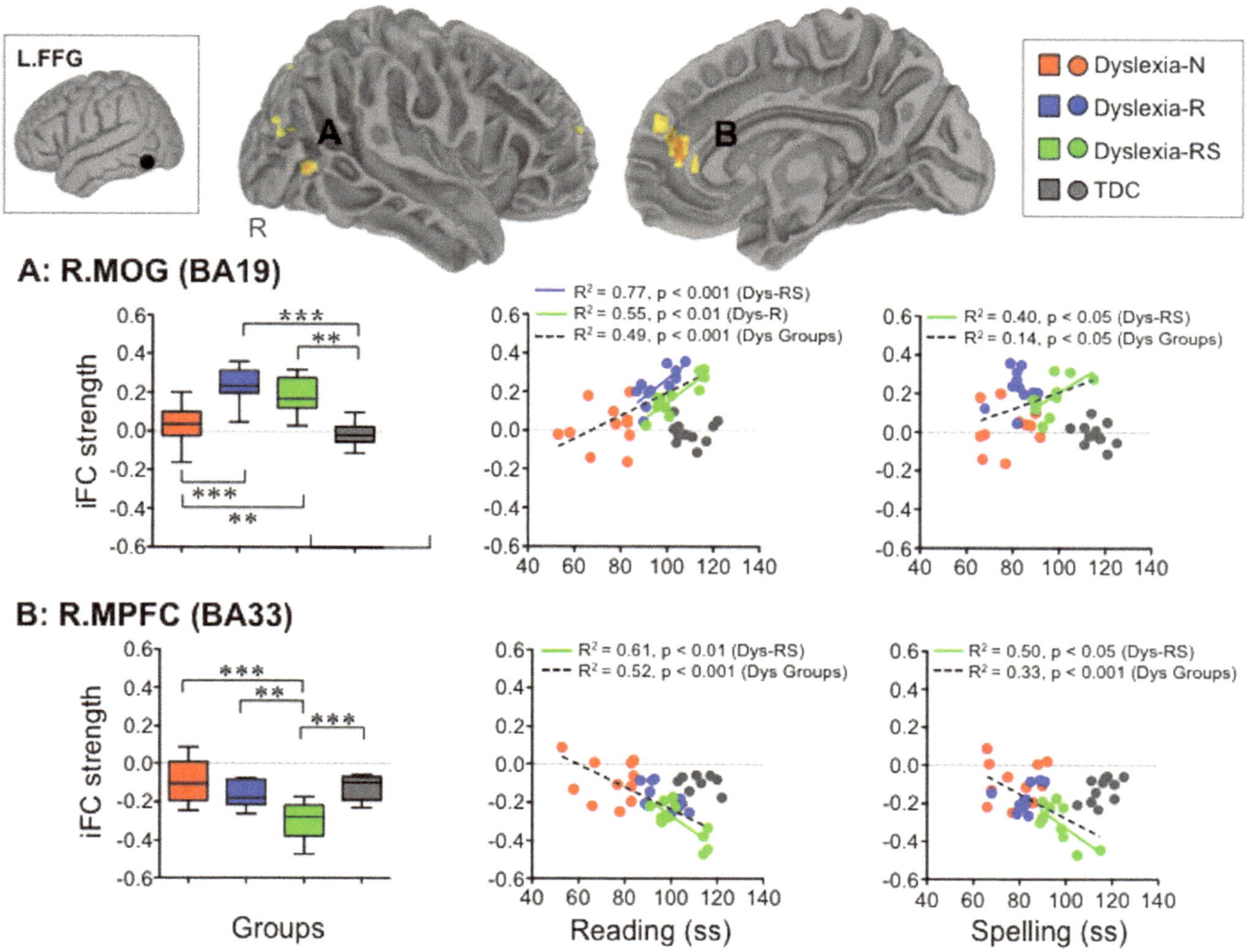

Figure 5. Compensatory changes in iFC of the left fusiform gyrus (L.FFG) in the remediation groups. The box-and-whisker plots depict (A) L.FFG-R.MOG iFC and (B) L.FFG-R.MPFC iFC for each group and group differences, whereas the scatterplots represent the relationships between the strength of these connections and reading as well as spelling scores. iFC = intrinsic Functional Connectivity, R.MOG = Right Middle Occipital Gyrus, R.MPFC = Right Medial Prefrontal Cortex, Dys-N = Dyslexia with No Remediation, Dys-R = Dyslexia with Reading Remediation, Dys-RS = Dyslexia with Reading and Spelling Remediation, TDC = Typically Developing Children, Dys = Dyslexia, ss = standard scores: ***p<0.001, **p<0.01 (corrected): Both the partial and full remediation groups exhibited stronger L.FFG-R.MOG iFC, relative to both DTC and Dys-N, whereas the full remediation group exhibited stronger negative L.FFG-R.MPFC iFC, relative to TDC, Dys-N, and Dys-R.

other dyslexia groups. This result with respect to the TDC group is consistent with our previous work, in which iFC between L.FFG and the medial prefrontal cortex negatively correlated with literacy performance in typical adults, but not in typically developing children [39].

Given that L.FFG is involved in both functional connections (L.FFG-R.MOG, L.FFG-R.MPFC) associated with compensatory changes, an obvious question regards the relationship between these two sets of L.FFG connections. We examined their relationship (Figure 6). The correlation between L.FFG iFC with R.MOG and with R.MPFC was significantly negative across all groups ($R^2 = 0.39$, $n = 44$, $p<0.001$) as well as across dyslexia groups ($R^2 = 0.38$, $n = 33$, $p<0.001$). When examining groups individually, this relationship was significant in the full remediation group (Dys-RS, $R^2 = 0.61$, $n = 11$, $p<0.01$). That is, children with stronger positive L.FFG-R.MOG connectivity were characterized by stronger negative iFC for the L.FFG-R.MPFC circuit, and this was particularly true in children in the full remediation group.

Consideration of ADHD Symptomology as a Confound

To investigate potential effects of inattention and hyperactivity-impulsivity on the identified iFC of reading regions, we plotted relationships between iFC strength and scores of the inattentive and hyperactive-impulsive scores (CPRS DSM-IV), respectively. The iFC between L.IPS and L.MFG, within the dorsal attention network (e.g., [83]), was negatively correlated with inattention scores across all groups ($R^2 = 0.18$, $n = 44$, $p<0.01$) (Figure S5.A.1). This brain-behavior relationship remained significant even after hyperactivity-impulsivity scores were covaried ($R^2 = 0.11$, $n = 44$, $p<0.05$). Similarly, iFC between these regions was negatively correlated with hyperactivity-impulsivity scores across all groups ($R^2 = 0.26$, $n = 44$, $p<0.001$) and across dyslexia groups ($R^2 = 0.20$, $n = 33$, $p<0.01$) (Figure S5.A.2). These brain-behavior relationships remained significant after inattention scores were covaried (across all groups; $R^2 = 0.20$, $n = 44$, $p<0.01$: across dyslexia groups; $R^2 = 0.18$, $n = 33$, $p<0.05$). In examining brain-behavior correlations for L.IPS-L.MFG iFC in each group individually, only one significant correlation was observed:

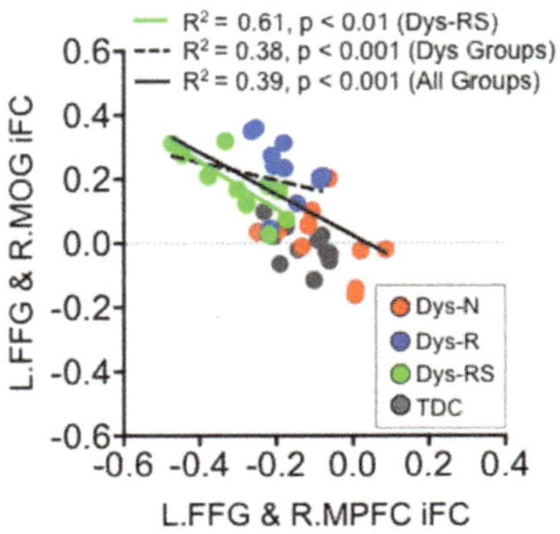

Figure 6. Relationship between the two putatively compensatory functional connections of the left fusiform gyrus (L.FFG) seed. The scatterplot represents the relationships between the two L.FFG connections (one with R.MOG and another with R.MPFC). iFC = intrinsic Functional Connectivity, R.MOG = Right Middle Occipital Gyrus, R.MPFC = Right Medial Prefrontal Cortex, Dys-N = Dyslexia with No Remediation, Dys-R = Dyslexia with Reading Remediation, Dys-RS = Dyslexia with Reading and Spelling Remediation, TDC = Typically Developing Children, Dys = Dyslexia: The correlation between these two L.FFG connections was significantly negative across all groups, across dyslexia groups, and in the full remediation group.

between L.IPS-L.MFG iFC and inattention scores in the Dys-R group, both before ($R^2 = 0.37$, n = 11, $p<0.05$) (Figure S5.A.1) and after ($R^2 = 0.45$, n = 11, $p<0.05$) covarying hyperactivity-impulsivity. For the two L FFG-based connections that differed among groups, neither exhibited a significant correlation with ADHD symptoms across all groups, although iFC between L.FFG and R.MOG was significantly correlated with inattention scores in the Dys-RS group before ($R^2 = 0.51$, n = 11, $p<0.05$) (Figure S5.B.1) and after ($R^2 = 0.56$, n = 11, $p<0.05$) covarying hyperactivity-impulsivity.

Secondary Analysis

A secondary analysis aimed to verify that the iFC patterns observed in the current TDC group are representative of normative/typical iFC profiles. As expected, pair-wise comparisons using unpaired t-tests revealed that, for all identified connections (L.IPS-L.MFG, L.FFG-R.MOG, and L.FFG-R.MPFC), there were no significant differences between the two TDC groups (Figure 7). This allows us to assert that the group differences observed in the present study reflect atypical/altered iFC patterns associated with dyslexia. In addition, for all identified connections, there were no significant differences between the TDC groups and the TA group (Figure 7), indicating that either they are not developmentally sensitive, or they are mature prior to age 7 (but see [39] for developmental differences for brain-behavior relationships with respect to L.FFG-R.MPFC iFC).

Discussion

We identified group differences in the strength of intrinsic functional connectivity (iFC) of known reading regions among TDC and three dyslexia groups (i.e., no remediation, partial remediation, full remediation), with a particular focus on discerning potential effects of remediation. The findings are consistent with our first two predictions: 1) atypical iFC was associated with a history of dyslexia and 2) altered iFC consistent with cortical compensation associated with behavioral remediation. Specifically, the first finding suggests that dyslexia-related atypicality (i.e., reduced positive connectivity strength) in the L.IPS persists following remediation, even in fully remediated individ-

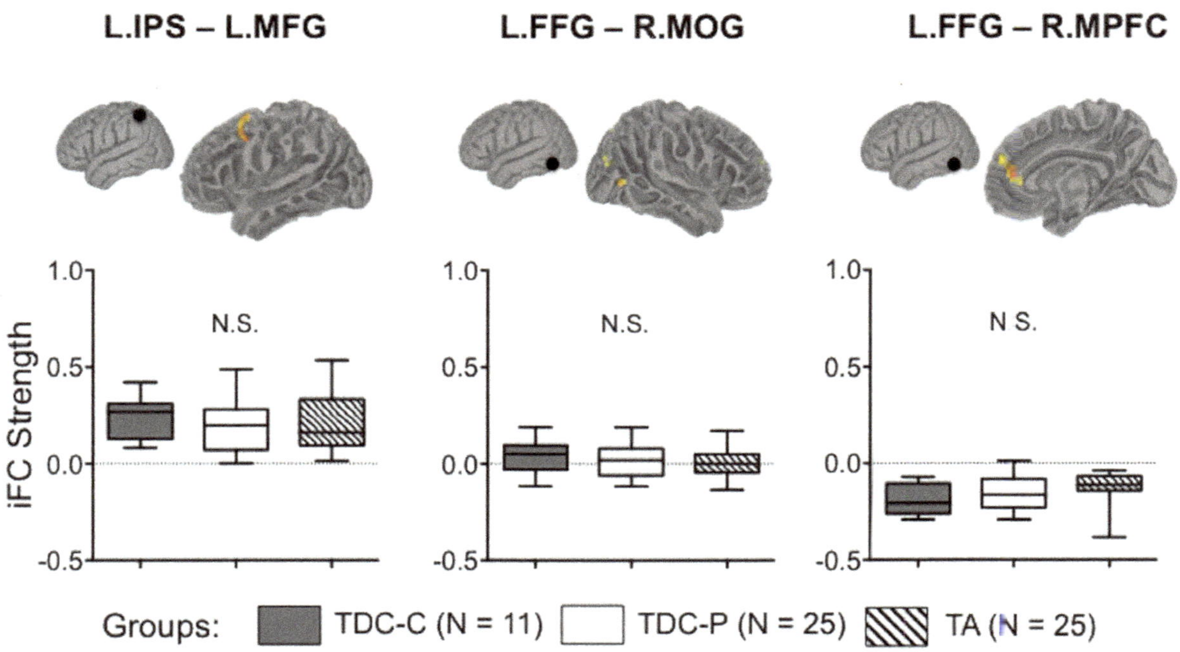

Figure 7. The strength of the identified iFC in two typically developing child groups and a typical adult group. iFC = Intrinsic Functional Connectivity, L.IPS = Left Intraparietal Sulcus, L.MFG = Left Middle Frontal Gyrus, L. FFG = Left Fusiform Gyrus, R.MOG = Right Middle Occipital Gyrus, R.MPFC = Right Medial Prefrontal Cortex, N.S. = Not Significant, TDC-C = Typically Developing Children in the Current work (n = 11), TDC-P = Typically Developing children in the Previous work (n = 25) [39], TA = Typical Adults (n = 25): Group differences were observed neither between the two TDC groups nor between TDC and TA groups.

uals. The second finding suggests that successful remediation of literacy deficits is associated with the emergence of compensatory changes in L.FFG iFC. Confidence in these results was bolstered by observing relationships between iFC strength and dimensional assessments of literary competence. However, we found no evidence supporting our third prediction, namely that we would find altered iFC reflecting cortical normalization. As discussed below, our findings, which complement those of task-based fMRI studies (e.g., [84–86]), should motivate the pursuit of longitudinal, multimodal (e.g., resting-state fMRI, task-based fMRI) studies with adequate sample size and systematic treatment of interventions.

Atypical Connectivity Associated with Historical Diagnosis of Dyslexia

Our findings highlight the presence of dyslexia-related differences in iFC within the dorsal attention network [31,83,87–88]. Specifically, our analyses revealed reduced iFC between the left intraparietal sulcus (L.IPS) and left middle frontal gyrus (L.MFG) for all dyslexia groups, irrespective of remediation status. Notably, all children in the TDC group exhibited positive L.IPS-L.MFG connectivity, whereas the majority of the Dys-N group exhibited negative L.IPS-L.MFG connectivity (and thus this group had the weakest L.IPS-L.MFG iFC). Considering that brain regions involved in similar functions (i.e., co-activated by similar tasks) typically exhibit positive iFC [31], this result suggests that dysfunctional iFC between frontal and parietal regions within the attention network characterizes a history of dyslexia.

Consistent with its hypothesized role in attentional function, weaker iFC in this circuit was also associated with higher parental ratings of inattention and of hyperactivity-impulsivity, both of which were negatively correlated with children's reading competence (i.e., the more elevated the ADHD-related symptoms, the poorer the reading performance). Persistence of weaker L.IPS-L.MFG iFC, even among highly remediated individuals, suggests that interventions do not directly address alterations within the dorsal attention network. This is not surprising, as current interventions tend to exclusively focus on phonetics and word processing and ignore attentional function. Our findings support recent calls for an increased focus on attention as a potential target for intervention [81,89–90].

Cortical Compensation Associated with Behavioral Remediation

A key question in the dyslexia literature is the extent to which intervention efforts "cure" the underlying deficit or invoke alternative, compensatory processing strategies capable of overcoming innate deficiencies [23,91–94]. Our findings suggest the latter with respect to the iFC between the left fusiform gyrus (L.FFG) and regions in the right hemisphere outside the known reading network. L.FFG, part of the ventral visual pathway and known as the Visual Word Form Area [95–96], exhibits reduced activity (e.g., [86,97–98]) and reduced functional connectivity with other language regions [85,99–100] in individuals with dyslexia. Our findings indicate that L.FFG may exhibit compensatory changes associated with behavioral remediation (i.e., normalized literacy skills). Specifically, we observed two patterns of change that may reflect these compensatory effects. First, iFC between the L.FFG and the right middle occipital gyrus (R.MOG), a component of the dorsal visual pathway [101–102], was increased in both remediation groups. Second, the full remediation group (Dys-RS) exhibited stronger negative iFC between the L.FFG and the right medial prefrontal cortex (R.MPFC), a core region of the default network [103–105]. This pattern – the remediation groups (i.e., only in the Dys-RS group for L.FFG-R.MPFC iFC) being different from the TDC group and Dys-N group – is more likely to reflect cortical compensation than normalization. Of note, the strength of these two functional connections based in the L.FFG was strongly correlated within the full remediation group, further supporting the suggestion that L.FFG serves as a hub region for compensatory changes in the dyslexic brain.

Importantly, the two observed connections of L.FFG are relevant to literacy competence. First, stronger coupling between posterior visual regions (L.FFG-R.MOG) was associated with better literacy performance across dyslexic children, particularly those in the remediation groups. This atypically increased functional coupling within the visual network may suggest greater reliance on visual reading strategies to compensate for weak phonological processing skills (i.e., phonological weakness was documented in prior psychoeducational evaluations for children in the two remediation groups, although the majority of them showed no phonological deficits in the current assessment). Our interpretation is supported by reading errors made by children in the remediation groups, such as misreading of visually similar words (e.g., "useless" pronounced as "unless"). Of note, reading errors for visually similar words are reported to be common in dyslexic individuals [79], even in those who exhibit good reading comprehension [106].

The second observation with respect to L.FFG's behavioral relevance is that stronger negative connectivity or functional segregation between task-positive and task-negative default networks/regions (L.FFG and R.MPFC) was associated with better literacy performance across dyslexic children, particularly those in the full remediation group. This brain-behavior relationship – the more negative the iFC, the better the literacy performance – is characteristic of typical adult readers [39]. Given that functional segregation from the default network is thought to support efficient cognitive processing in typical adults [107], stronger negative iFC between L.FFG-R.MPFC and its adult-like relationships with literacy competence in the full remediation group may reflect increased behavioral efficiency, as a compensatory mechanism, following effective remediation. This finding suggests the merits of expanding models of dyslexia to include interactions between task-positive or reading networks and the default network [39]. Although negative iFC has been reported by a number of studies (e.g., [108]), its underlying physiological mechanisms remain a topic of research. Thus, longitudinal studies are required to test our interpretations and to further clarify the roles of negative iFC/functional segregation between task-active and task-negative default regions/networks in clinical populations, particularly with respect to remediation effects.

Limitations

The results of this study must be interpreted in light of its limitations. First, we employed an observational, cross-sectional design, rather than a longitudinal approach. This raises the question of whether there were differences in literacy performance between the dyslexia groups that preceded their intervention training, potentially explaining the patterns observed in the present study. Although we cannot rule out the presence of subtle pre-existing differences between the groups, the level of literacy performance prior to any intervention in children of the remediation groups was grossly similar to that of the current literacy performance in children of the no remediation group. That is, we obtained evidence that children in both remediation groups had standard scores lower than 85 on a standardized literacy test at the time of their prior assessment and diagnosis; children in the no remediation group (i.e., no experience of intervention training) currently had standard scores lower than 85 on both the WIAT Word Reading and the WIAT Spelling subscales when assessed as part of this study. Nevertheless, cortical changes associated with remediation would best be captured by longitudinal studies involving coordinated interventions for dyslexia, as remediation is not instantaneous, but instead occurs over time. Still, our findings should motivate continued examination of cortical signatures of different dyslexia profiles, assessed by multiple approaches, including R-fMRI, before, during, and after remediation efforts. The second limitation derives from the modest size of the individual dyslexia groups. Despite the modest sample size, we were able to stratify individuals with dyslexia on the basis of remediation status. This enhanced our statistical power to detect group differences [109]. Third, this study lacked one type of dyslexia group: children with a history of dyslexia diagnosis, who completed intervention training but remained deficient in reading skills [110]. Although a few children screened in the current study exhibited literacy deficits after having intervention training (confirmed by a previous clinical documentation and/or informal interview with parents), they were excluded due to their low IQ scores, which typically preclude diagnosis of dyslexia. It is worth noting that this widely applied diagnostic criterion based on the IQ-reading discrepancy has been criticized and remains a topic of investigation [111–112]. Future research is urgently needed to elucidate potential differences in reading-related iFC patterns between responders and non-responders (including those with low IQ) to intervention training. Finally, the present investigation was limited to R-fMRI data. Although this approach has been fruitful, the combination of task-based and task-independent modalities holds the greatest potential for the further characterization and interpretation of deficits, compensatory responses, and functional normalization in dyslexia.

Conclusions

Using task-independent R-fMRI, we delineated candidate cortical signatures of distinct dyslexia profiles. Reduced intrinsic functional connectivity within the dorsal attention network is associated with a history of dyslexia, calling for further focus on the role of attention in dyslexia and on targeted interventions, whereas the left fusiform gyrus in the ventral visual pathway appears to be a hub for compensatory mechanisms in dyslexia remediation. Intrinsic functional connectivity approaches appear to provide a firm basis for investigating the cortical correlates of dyslexia, for monitoring dynamic changes associated with behavioral remediation in individuals with dyslexia, and eventually for evaluating the effectiveness of dyslexia remediation.

Supporting Information

Figure S1 Mean Framewise Displacement (FD). The box-and-whisker plot (A) depicts mean FC for each group and no group differences, whereas the scatter plot (B) depicts no relationship between age and mean FD. Dys-N = Dyslexia with No Remediation, Dys-R = Dyslexia with Reading Remediation, Dys-RS = Dyslexia with Reading and Spelling Remediation, TDC = Typically Developing Children.

Figure S2 Conners' Parent Rating Scales of DSM-IV Symptoms of Inattention and Hyperactivity-Impulsivity. The box-and-whisker plots depict (A.1) inattention and (A.2) hyperactivity-impulsivity scores for each group and group differences. The scatterplots represent relationships of WIAT Word Reading scores with (B.1) inattention and (B.2.) hyperactivity-impulsivity scores. Dys-N = Dyslexia with No Remediation, Dys-R = Dyslexia with Reading Remediation, Dys-RS = Dyslexia with Reading and Spelling Remediation, TDC = Typically Developing Children, ss = standard scores, $**p<0.01$, $*p<0.05$: The mean scores in Inattention and Hyperactivity-Impulsivity subscales were significantly lower in TDC than the dyslexia groups, and significant negative correlations between attention (i.e., both inattention and hyperactivity-impulsivity) and reading scores were observed across all groups.

Figure S3 Effects of five different statistical models with respects to global signal regression (GSreg), framewise displacement regression (FDreg), and data scrubbing (Scrub). +GSreg = analyzed with GSreg, -GSreg = analyzed without GSreg, +FDreg = analyzed with FDreg, -FDreg = analyzed without FDreg, +Scrub = frames larger than 0.5FD were Scrubbed from the dataset, iFC = Intrinsic Functional Connectivity, L.IPS = Left Intraparietal Sulcus, L.FFG = Left Fusiform Gyrus, R.MOG = Right Middle Occipital Gyrus, R.MPFC = Right Medial Prefrontal Cortex, Dys-N = Dyslexia with No Remediation, Dys-R = Dyslexia with Reading Remediation, Dys-RS = Dyslexia with Reading and Spelling Remediation, TDC = Typically Developing Children: The results from the primary analysis (+GSreg+FDreg were replicated in other analyses, although those yielded from the model where the global signal was not regressed (i.e., -GSreg+FDreg and -GSreg-FDreg) were significant only at uncorrected $p<0.05$.

Figure S4 Region-specific effects of global signal regression on the group difference in intrinsic functional connectivity. L.IPS = left intraparietal suclus, L.FFG = left fusiform gyrus, R. MOG = right middle occipital gyrus, R.MPFC = right medial prefrontal cortex, +GSreg+FDreg = analyzed with both GSreg and FDreg, -GSreg+FDreg = analyzed without GSreg but with FDreg: $Z > 2.3$, cluster significance, $p<0.05$, corrected; With no global signal regression, the L.FFG seed failed to show the group differences identified in the primary analysis where global signal was regressed (A: R.MOG and B: R.MPFC).

Figure S5 Relationships between each iFC and ADHD-symptoms (Conners' Parent Rating Scales; DSM-IV Symptoms of Inattention and Hyperactivity-Impulsivity). The upper scatterplots depict relationships between iFC and inattention scores (A.1, B.1, and C.1), whereas the lower ones depict relationships between iFC and hyperactivity-impulsivity scores (A.2, B.2, and C.2). iFC = intrinsic Functional Connectivity, L.IPS = Left Intraparietal Sulcus, L.FFG = Left Fusiform Gyrus, R.MOG = Right Middle Occipital Gyrus, R.MPFC = Right Medial Prefrontal Cortex, Dys-N = Dyslexia with No Remediation, Dys-R = Dyslexia with Reading Remediation, Dys-RS = Dyslexia with Reading and Spelling Remediation, TDC = Typically Developing Children, Dys = Dyslexia: The iFC between L.IPS and L.MFG was negatively correlated with inattention scores as well as hyperactivity-impulsivity scores across all groups.

Materials and Methods S1 Dyslexia sample characterization.

Acknowledgments

We thank the New York branch of the International Dyslexia Association for helping us to recruit participants with dyslexia, as well as J.M. Fletcher for providing valuable insights into behavioral evaluations of dyslexia.

Author Contributions

Conceived and designed the experiments: MSK MPM FXC CK. Performed the experiments: MSK DRJ JS. Analyzed the data: MSK. Wrote the paper: MSK MPM. Contributed reagents/materials/analysis tools: CK AD SJS.

References

1. Bradley L, Bryant PE (1978) Difficulties in auditory organisation as a possible cause of reading backwardness. Nature 271: 746–747.
2. Stanovich KE (1988) Explaining the differences between the dyslexic and the garden-variety poor reader: the phonological-core variable-difference model. Journal of learning disabilities 21: 590–604.
3. Ramus F, Rosen S, Dakin SC, Day BL, Castellote JM, et al. (2003) Theories of developmental dyslexia: insights from a multiple case study of dyslexic adults. Brain : a journal of neurology 126: 841–865.
4. Pennington BF, Santerre-Lemmon L, Rosenberg J, MacDonald B, Boada R, et al. (2012) Individual prediction of dyslexia by single versus multiple deficit models. Journal of abnormal psychology 121: 212–224.
5. Georgiou GK, Papadopoulos TC, Zarouna E, Parrila R (2012) Are auditory and visual processing deficits related to developmental dyslexia? Dyslexia 18: 110–129.
6. Valdois S, Bidet-Ildei C, Lassus-Sangosse D, Reilhac C, N'Guyen-Morel MA, et al. (2011) A visual processing but no phonological disorder in a child with mixed dyslexia. Cortex; a journal devoted to the study of the nervous system and behavior 47: 1197–1218.
7. Peyrin C, Lallier M, Demonet JF, Pernet C, Baciu M, et al. (2012) Neural dissociation of phonological and visual attention span disorders in developmental dyslexia: FMRI evidence from two case reports. Brain and Language 120: 381–394.
8. Stein J (2001) The magnocellular theory of developmental dyslexia. Dyslexia 7: 12–36.
9. Goswami U, Thomson J, Richardson U, Stainthorp R, Hughes D, et al. (2002) Amplitude envelope onsets and developmental dyslexia: A new hypothesis. Proceedings of the National Academy of Sciences of the United States of America 99: 10911–10916.
10. Tallal P (1980) Auditory temporal perception, phonics, and reading disabilities in children. Brain and Language 9: 182–198.
11. Hämäläinen JA, Salminen HK, Leppänen PHT (2012) Basic Auditory Processing Deficits in Dyslexia: Systematic Review of the Behavioral and Event-Related Potential/Field Evidence. Journal of Learning Disabilities.
12. Wolf M, Bowers PG, Biddle K (2000) Naming-speed processes, timing, and reading: a conceptual review. Journal of learning disabilities 33: 387–407.
13. Bosse ML, Tainturier MJ, Valdois S (2007) Developmental dyslexia: the visual attention span deficit hypothesis. Cognition 104: 198–230.
14. Vidyasagar TR, Pammer K (2010) Dyslexia: a deficit in visuo-spatial attention, not in phonological processing. Trends in Cognitive Sciences 14: 57–63.
15. Facoetti A, Trussardi AN, Ruffino M, Lorusso ML, Cattaneo C, et al. (2010) Multisensory spatial attention deficits are predictive of phonological decoding skills in developmental dyslexia. Journal of cognitive neuroscience 22: 1011–1025.
16. Stoodley CJ, Stein JF (2011) The cerebellum and dyslexia. Cortex; a journal devoted to the study of the nervous system and behavior 47: 101–116.
17. Nicolson RI, Fawcett AJ (2005) Developmental dyslexia, learning and the cerebellum. Journal of neural transmission Supplementum: 19–36.
18. Demb JB, Boynton GM, Heeger DJ (1998) Functional magnetic resonance imaging of early visual pathways in dyslexia. The Journal of neuroscience : the official journal of the Society for Neuroscience 18: 6939–6951.
19. Eden GF, VanMeter JW, Rumsey JM, Zeffiro TA (1996) The visual deficit theory of developmental dyslexia. NeuroImage 4: S108–117.
20. Peyrin C, Demonet JF, N'Guyen-Morel MA, Le Bas JF, Valdois S (2011) Superior parietal lobule dysfunction in a homogeneous group of dyslexic children with a visual attention span disorder. Brain and Language 118: 128–138.
21. Duff FJ, Clarke PJ (2011) Practitioner Review: Reading disorders: what are the effective interventions and how should they be implemented and evaluated? Journal of Child Psychology and Psychiatry 52: 3–12.
22. Sarkari S, Simos PG, Fletcher JM, Castillo EM, Breier JI, et al. (2002) Contributions of magnetic source imaging to the understanding of dyslexia. Semin Pediatr Neurol 9: 229–238.
23. Simos PG, Fletcher JM, Sarkari S, Billingsley RL, Denton C, et al. (2007) Altering the brain circuits for reading through intervention: a magnetic source imaging study. Neuropsychology 21: 485–496.
24. Gaab N, Gabrieli JD, Deutsch GK, Tallal P, Temple E (2007) Neural correlates of rapid auditory processing are disrupted in children with developmental dyslexia and ameliorated with training: an fMRI study. Restor Neurol Neurosci 25: 295–310.
25. Shaywitz BA, Shaywitz SE, Blachman BA, Pugh KR, Fulbright RK, et al. (2004) Development of left occipitotemporal systems for skilled reading in children after a phonologically- based intervention. Biol Psychiatry 55: 926–933.
26. Eden GF, Jones KM, Cappell K, Gareau L, Wood FB, et al. (2004) Neural Changes following Remediation in Adult Developmental Dyslexia. Neuron 44: 411–422.
27. Davis N, Barquero L, Compton DL, Fuchs LS, Fuchs D, et al. (2011) Functional correlates of children's responsiveness to intervention. Developmental neuropsychology 36: 288–301.
28. Torgesen JK, Alexander AW, Wagner RK, Rashotte CA, Voeller KK, et al. (2001) Intensive remedial instruction for children with severe reading disabilities: immediate and long-term outcomes from two instructional approaches. Journal of learning disabilities 34: 33–58, 78.
29. Kelly C, Biswal BB, Craddock RC, Castellanos FX, Milham MP (2012) Characterizing variation in the functional connectome: promise and pitfalls. Trends in Cognitive Sciences 16: 181–188.
30. Biswal B, Yetkin FZ, Haughton VM, Hyde JS (1995) Functional connectivity in the motor cortex of resting human brain using echo-planar MRI. Magnetic resonance in medicine : official journal of the Society of Magnetic Resonance in Medicine/Society of Magnetic Resonance in Medicine 34: 537–541.
31. Fox MD, Corbetta M, Snyder AZ, Vincent JL, Raichle ME (2006) Spontaneous neuronal activity distinguishes human dorsal and ventral attention systems. Proceedings of the National Academy of Sciences 103: 10046–10051.
32. Cordes D, Haughton VM, Arfanakis K, Wendt GJ, Turski PA, et al. (2000) Mapping Functionally Related Regions of Brain with Functional Connectivity MR Imaging. American Journal of Neuroradiology 21: 1636–1644.
33. Greicius MD, Krasnow B, Reiss AL, Menon V (2003) Functional connectivity in the resting brain: A network analysis of the default mode hypothesis. Proceedings of the National Academy of Sciences 100: 253–258.
34. Margulies DS, Kelly AMC, Uddin LQ, Biswal BB, Castellanos FX, et al. (2007) Mapping the functional connectivity of anterior cingulate cortex. NeuroImage 37: 579–588.
35. Di Martino A, Scheres A, Margulies DS, Kelly AMC, Uddin LQ, et al. (2008) Functional Connectivity of Human Striatum: A Resting State fMRI Study. Cerebral Cortex 18: 2735–2747.
36. Krienen FM, Buckner RL (2009) Segregated Fronto-Cerebellar Circuits Revealed by Intrinsic Functional Connectivity. Cerebral Cortex 19: 2485–2497.
37. Hampson M, Tokoglu F, Sun Z, Schafer RJ, Skudlarski P, et al. (2006) Connectivity'Äìbehavior analysis reveals that functional connectivity between left BA39 and Broca's area varies with reading ability. NeuroImage 31: 513–519.
38. Koyama MS, Kelly C, Shehzad Z, Penesetti D, Castellanos FX, et al. (2010) Reading Networks at Rest. Cerebral Cortex 20: 2549–2559.
39. Koyama MS, Di Martino A, Zuo X-N, Kelly C, Mennes M, et al. (2011) Resting-State Functional Connectivity Indexes Reading Competence in Children and Adults. The Journal of Neuroscience 31: 8617–8624.
40. Di Martino A, Kelly C, Grzadzinski R, Zuo X-N, Mennes M, et al. (2011) Aberrant Striatal Functional Connectivity in Children with Autism. Biological psychiatry 69: 847–856.
41. Cherkassky VL, Kana RK, Keller TA, Just MA (2006) Functional connectivity in a baseline resting-state network in autism. NeuroReport 17: 1687–1690.
42. Kennedy DP, Courchesne E (2008) The intrinsic functional organization of the brain is altered in autism. NeuroImage 39: 1877–1885.
43. von dem Hagen EA, Stoyanova RS, Baron-Cohen S, Calder AJ (2012) Reduced functional connectivity within and between 'social' resting state networks in Autism Spectrum Conditions. Social cognitive and affective neuroscience.
44. Cao X, Cao Q, Long X, Sun L, Sui M, et al. (2009) Abnormal resting-state functional connectivity patterns of the putamen in medication-na√Øve children with attention deficit hyperactivity disorder. Brain Research 1303: 195–206.
45. Fair DA, Posner J, Nagel BJ, Bathula D, Dias TGC, et al. (2010) Atypical Default Network Connectivity in Youth with Attention-Deficit/Hyperactivity Disorder. Biological psychiatry 68: 1084–1091.
46. Castellanos FX, Margulies DS, Kelly C, Uddin LQ, Ghaffari M, et al. (2008) Cingulate-Precuneus Interactions: A New Locus of Dysfunction in Adult Attention-Deficit/Hyperactivity Disorder. Biological psychiatry 63: 332–337.
47. Chabernaud C, Mennes M, Kelly C, Nooner K, Di Martino A, et al. (2012) Dimensional brain-behavior relationships in children with attention-deficit/hyperactivity disorder. Biological psychiatry 71: 434–442.
48. Church JA, Fair DA, Dosenbach NU, Cohen AL, Miezin FM, et al. (2009) Control networks in paediatric Tourette syndrome show immature and anomalous patterns of functional connectivity. Brain : a journal of neurology 132: 225–238.
49. Farris EA, Odegard TN, Miller HL, Ring J, Allen G, et al. (2011) Functional connectivity between the left and right inferior frontal lobes in a small sample of children with and without reading difficulties. Neurocase: 1–15.
50. Bolger DJ, Perfetti CA, Schneider W (2005) Cross-cultural effect on the brain revisited: universal structures plus writing system variation. Human Brain Mapping 25: 92–104.

51. Houde O, Rossi S, Lubin A, Joliot M (2010) Mapping numerical processing, reading, and executive functions in the developing brain: an fMRI meta-analysis of 52 studies including 842 children. Developmental Science 13: 876–885.
52. Richlan F, Kronbichler M, Wimmer H (2011) Meta-analyzing brain dysfunctions in dyslexic children and adults. NeuroImage 56: 1735–1742.
53. Wechsler D (2001) Wechsler Individual Achievement Test–Second Edition (WIAT-II) San Antonio: The Psychological Corporation.
54. Snowling M (1998) Dyslexia as a Phonological Deficit: Evidence and Implications. Child and Adolescent Mental Health 3: 4–11.
55. Kaufman J, Birmaher B, Brent D, Rao U, Ryan N (1996) The schedule for affective disorders and schizophrenia for school-age children Pittsburgh: University of Pittsburgh Medical Center.
56. Wechsler D (1999) Wechsler Abbreviated Scale of Intelligence (WASI). San Antonio: The Psychological Corporatio.
57. Torgesen J, Wagner R, Rashotte C (1999) Test of Word Reading Efficiency (TOWRE). Austin, TX: Pro-ED Inc.
58. Wagner RK, Torgesen JK, Rashotte CA (1999) CTOPP, Comprehensive Test of Phonological Processing. Austin, Tex.: PRO-ED. 1 case. p.
59. Willcutt EG, Pennington BF, Olson RK, DeFries JC (2007) Understanding comorbidity: a twin study of reading disability and attention-deficit/hyperactivity disorder. American journal of medical genetics Part B, Neuropsychiatric genetics : the official publication of the International Society of Psychiatric Genetics 144B: 709–714.
60. Willcutt EG, Pennington BF (2000) Comorbidity of Reading Disability and Attention-Deficit/Hyperactivity Disorder. Journal of learning disabilities 33: 179–191.
61. Conners CK (1997) Conners' Rating Scales-Revised: Technical manual. North Tonawanda, NY:: Multi-Health Systems.
62. Cox RW (1996) AFNI: software for analysis and visualization of functional magnetic resonance neuroimages. Computers and biomedical research, an international journal 29: 162–173.
63. Biswal BB, Mennes M, Zuo XN, Gohel S, Kelly C, et al. (2010) Toward discovery science of human brain function. Proceedings of the National Academy of Sciences of the United States of America 107: 4734–4739.
64. Andersson J, Jenkinson M, Smith S (2007) Non-linear registration, aka spatial normalisation. Oxford, UK: FMRIB.
65. Jenkinson M, Bannister P, Brady M, Smith S (2002) Improved optimization for the robust and accurate linear registration and motion correction of brain images. NeuroImage 17: 825–841.
66. Jenkinson M, Smith S (2001) A global optimisation method for robust affine registration of brain images. Med Image Anal 5: 143–156.
67. Bianciardi M, Fukunaga M, van Gelderen P, Horovitz SG, de Zwart JA, et al. (2009) Sources of functional magnetic resonance imaging signal fluctuations in the human brain at rest: a 7 T study. Magn Reson Imaging 27: 1019–1029.
68. Shmueli K, van Gelderen P, de Zwart JA, Horovitz SG, Fukunaga M, et al. (2007) Low-frequency fluctuations in the cardiac rate as a source of variance in the resting-state fMRI BOLD signal. NeuroImage 38: 306–320.
69. Schölvinck ML, Maier A, Ye FQ, Duyn JH, Leopold DA (2010) Neural basis of global resting-state fMRI activity. Proceedings of the National Academy of Sciences 107: 10238–10243.
70. Margulies DS, Kelly AM, Uddin LQ, Biswal BB, Castellanos FX, et al. (2007) Mapping the functional connectivity of anterior cingulate cortex. NeuroImage 37: 579–588.
71. Castellanos FX, Margulies DS, Kelly C, Uddin LQ, Ghaffari M, et al. (2008) Cingulate-precuneus interactions: a new locus of dysfunction in adult attention-deficit/hyperactivity disorder. Biol Psychiatry 63: 332–337.
72. Di Martino A, Shehzad Z, Kelly C, Roy AK, Gee DG, et al. (2009) Relationship between cingulo-insular functional connectivity and autistic traits in neurotypical adults. Am J Psychiatry 166: 891–899.
73. Power JD, Barnes KA, Snyder AZ, Schlaggar BL, Petersen SE (2012) Spurious but systematic correlations in functional connectivity MRI networks arise from subject motion. NeuroImage 59: 2142–2154.
74. Van Dijk KR, Sabuncu MR, Buckner RL (2012) The influence of head motion on intrinsic functional connectivity MRI. NeuroImage 59: 431–438.
75. Satterthwaite TD, Wolf DH, Loughead J, Ruparel K, Elliott MA, et al. (2012) Impact of in-scanner head motion on multiple measures of functional connectivity: relevance for studies of neurodevelopment in youth. NeuroImage 60: 623–632.
76. Carp J (2011) Optimizing the order of operations for movement scrubbing: Comment on Power et al. NeuroImage.
77. Murphy K, Birn RM, Handwerker DA, Jones TB, Bandettini PA (2009) The impact of global signal regression on resting state correlations: are anti-correlated networks introduced? NeuroImage 44: 893–905.
78. Saad ZS, Gotts SJ, Murphy K, Chen G, Jo HJ, et al. (2012) Trouble at rest: how correlation patterns and group differences become distorted after global signal regression. Brain connectivity 2: 25–32.
79. Moats LC (1996) Phonological spelling errors in the writing of dyslexic adolescents. Reading and Writing 8: 105–119.
80. Willcutt EG, Pennington BF (2000) Comorbidity of reading disability and attention-deficit/hyperactivity disorder: differences by gender and subtype. J Learn Disabil 33: 179–191.
81. Shaywitz SE, Shaywitz BA (2008) Paying attention to reading: the neurobiology of reading and dyslexia. Development and psychopathology 20: 1329–1349.
82. Amodio DM, Frith CD (2006) Meeting of minds: the medial frontal cortex and social cognition. Nat Rev Neurosci 7: 268–277.
83. Corbetta M, Shulman GL (2002) Control of goal-directed and stimulus-driven attention in the brain. Nature reviews Neuroscience 3: 201–215.
84. Hoeft F, Hernandez A, McMillon G, Taylor-Hill H, Martindale JL, et al. (2006) Neural Basis of Dyslexia: A Comparison between Dyslexic and Nondyslexic Children Equated for Reading Ability. The Journal of Neuroscience 26: 10700–10708.
85. Pugh KR, Mencl WE, Shaywitz BA, Shaywitz SE, Fulbright RK, et al. (2000) The angular gyrus in developmental dyslexia: task-specific differences in functional connectivity within posterior cortex. Psychological science 11: 51–56.
86. Shaywitz BA, Shaywitz SE, Pugh KR, Mencl WE, Fulbright RK, et al. (2002) Disruption of posterior brain systems for reading in children with developmental dyslexia. Biological psychiatry 52: 101–110.
87. Corbetta M (1998) Frontoparietal cortical networks for directing attention and the eye to visual locations: Identical, independent, or overlapping neural'Äâ-systems? Proceedings of the National Academy of Sciences 95: 831–838.
88. Pessoa L, Rossi A, Japee S, Desimone R, Ungerleider LG (2009) Attentional control during the transient updating of cue information. Brain Research 1247: 149–158.
89. Zorzi M, Barbiero C, Facoetti A, Lonciari I, Carrozzi M, et al. (2012) Extra-large letter spacing improves reading in dyslexia. Proceedings of the National Academy of Sciences of the United States of America.
90. Franceschini S, Gori S, Ruffino M, Pedrolli K, Facoetti A (2012) A Causal Link between Visual Spatial Attention and Reading Acquisition. Current biology : CB 22: 814–819.
91. Gaab N, Gabrieli JD, Deutsch GK, Tallal P, Temple E (2007) Neural correlates of rapid auditory processing are disrupted in children with developmental dyslexia and ameliorated with training: an fMRI study. Restorative neurology and neuroscience 25: 295–310.
92. Eden GF, Jones KM, Cappell K, Gareau L, Wood FB, et al. (2004) Neural changes following remediation in adult developmental dyslexia. Neuron 44: 411–422.
93. Shaywitz SE, Shaywitz BA, Fulbright RK, Skudlarski P, Mencl WE, et al. (2003) Neural systems for compensation and persistence: young adult outcome of childhood reading disability. Biological psychiatry 54: 25–33.
94. Temple E, Deutsch GK, Poldrack RA, Miller SL, Tallal P, et al. (2003) Neural deficits in children with dyslexia ameliorated by behavioral remediation: Evidence from functional MRI. Proceedings of the National Academy of Sciences 100: 2860–2865.
95. Dehaene S, Le Clec'H G, Poline J-B, Le Bihan D, Cohen L (2002) The visual word form area: a prelexical representation of visual words in the fusiform gyrus. NeuroReport 13: 321–325.
96. Dehaene S, Cohen L (2011) The unique role of the visual word form area in reading. Trends in Cognitive Sciences 15: 254–262.
97. Blau V, Reithler J, van Atteveldt N, Seitz J, Gerretsen P, et al. (2010) Deviant processing of letters and speech sounds as proximate cause of reading failure: a functional magnetic resonance imaging study of dyslexic children. Brain : a journal of neurology 133: 868–879.
98. van der Mark S, Bucher K, Maurer U, Schulz E, Brem S, et al. (2009) Children with dyslexia lack multiple specializations along the visual word-form (VWF) system. NeuroImage 47: 1940–1949.
99. van der Mark S, Klaver P, Bucher K, Maurer U, Schulz E, et al. (2011) The left occipitotemporal system in reading: disruption of focal fMRI connectivity to left inferior frontal and inferior parietal language areas in children with dyslexia. NeuroImage 54: 2426–2436.
100. Horwitz B, Rumsey JM, Donohue BC (1998) Functional connectivity of the angular gyrus in normal reading and dyslexia. Proceedings of the National Academy of Sciences of the United States of America 95: 8939–8944.
101. Wandell BA, Dumoulin SO, Brewer AA (2007) Visual field maps in human cortex. Neuron 56: 366–383.
102. Renier LA, Anurova I, De Volder AG, Carlson S, VanMeter J, et al. (2010) Preserved functional specialization for spatial processing in the middle occipital gyrus of the early blind. Neuron 68: 138–148.
103. Andrews-Hanna JR, Reidler JS, Sepulcre J, Poulin R, Buckner RL (2010) Functional-Anatomic Fractionation of the Brain's Default Network. Neuron 65: 550–562.
104. Buckner RL, Andrews-Hanna JR, Schacter DL (2008) The brain's default network: anatomy, function, and relevance to disease. Annals of the New York Academy of Sciences 1124: 1–38.
105. Raichle ME, MacLeod AM, Snyder AZ, Powers WJ, Gusnard DA, et al. (2001) A default mode of brain function. Proceedings of the National Academy of Sciences 98: 676–682.
106. McCloskey M, Rapp B (2000) Attention-referenced visual representations: evidence from impaired visual localization. Journal of experimental psychology Human perception and performance 26: 917–933.
107. Kelly AM, Uddin LQ, Biswal BB, Castellanos FX, Milham MP (2008) Competition between functional brain networks mediates behavioral variability. NeuroImage 39: 527–537.

108. Fox MD, Zhang D, Snyder AZ, Raichle ME (2009) The global signal and observed anticorrelated resting state brain networks. Journal of Neurophysiology 101: 3270–3283.
109. Kraemer HC (1991) To increase power in randomized clinical trials without increasing sample size. Psychopharmacology bulletin 27: 217–224.
110. Odegard T, Ring J, Smith S, Biggan J, Black J (2008) Differentiating the neural response to intervention in children with developmental dyslexia. Annals of Dyslexia 58: 1–14.
111. Ferrer E, Shaywitz BA, Holahan JM, Marchione K, Shaywitz SE (2010) Uncoupling of reading and IQ over time: empirical evidence for a definition of dyslexia. Psychol Sci 21: 93–101.
112. Tanaka H, Black JM, Hulme C, Stanley LM, Kesler SR, et al. (2011) The brain basis of the phonological deficit in dyslexia is independent of IQ. Psychol Sci 22: 1442–1451.

9

Brain Bases of Reading Fluency in Typical Reading and Impaired Fluency in Dyslexia

Joanna A. Christodoulou[1,2,3]*, Stephanie N. Del Tufo[1], John Lymberis[1], Patricia K. Saxler[1,3], Satrajit S. Ghosh[1], Christina Triantafyllou[1,4], Susan Whitfield-Gabrieli[1,4], John D. E. Gabrieli[1,3,4]

1 McGovern Institute for Brain Research and Department of Brain and Cognitive Sciences, Massachusetts Institute of Technology, Cambridge, Massachusetts, United States of America, **2** MGH Institute of Health Professions, Boston, Massachusetts, United States of America, **3** Harvard Graduate School of Education, Cambridge, Massachusetts, United States of America, **4** Athinoula A. Martinos Imaging Center, McGovern Institute for Brain Research, Massachusetts Institute of Technology, Cambridge, Massachusetts, United States of America

Abstract

Although the neural systems supporting single word reading are well studied, there are limited direct comparisons between typical and dyslexic readers of the neural correlates of reading fluency. Reading fluency deficits are a persistent behavioral marker of dyslexia into adulthood. The current study identified the neural correlates of fluent reading in typical and dyslexic adult readers, using sentences presented in a word-by-word format in which single words were presented sequentially at fixed rates. Sentences were presented at slow, medium, and fast rates, and participants were asked to decide whether each sentence did or did not make sense semantically. As presentation rates increased, participants became less accurate and slower at making judgments, with comprehension accuracy decreasing disproportionately for dyslexic readers. In-scanner performance on the sentence task correlated significantly with standardized clinical measures of both reading fluency and phonological awareness. Both typical readers and readers with dyslexia exhibited widespread, bilateral increases in activation that corresponded to increases in presentation rate. Typical readers exhibited significantly larger gains in activation as a function of faster presentation rates than readers with dyslexia in several areas, including left prefrontal and left superior temporal regions associated with semantic retrieval and semantic and phonological representations. Group differences were more extensive when behavioral differences between conditions were equated across groups. These findings suggest a brain basis for impaired reading fluency in dyslexia, specifically a failure of brain regions involved in semantic retrieval and semantic and phonological representations to become fully engaged for comprehension at rapid reading rates.

Editor: Lawrence M. Ward, University of British Columbia, Canada

Funding: This work was supported by Ellison Medical Foundation; MIT Class of 1976 Funds for Dyslexia Research Bard and Julie Richmond through the Martin Richmond Memorial Fund; Clinical Research Center (CRC) at the Massachusetts Institute of Technology, Grant Number UL1 RR025758- Harvard Clinical and Translational Science Center, from the National Center for Research Resources. The funders had no role in study design, data collection and analysis, decision to publish, or preparation of the manuscript.

Competing Interests: The authors have declared that no competing interests exist.

* Email: jchristo@mit.edu

Introduction

Reading fluency, the ability to read accurately and at a rate that enables comprehension [1,2], is a cornerstone of skilled reading. Developmental dyslexia, defined as a specific learning disability with a neurological basis, manifests as difficulty in reading accurately or fluently at the single word level [3]. The ability to extract the meaning of text requires the coordination of multiple processing demands [4], and readers with dyslexia can struggle with reading comprehension due to impaired decoding and/or through a slow reading rate [5,6]. Despite consensus that reading fluency is essential for efficient reading and that reading dysfluency is a severe problem encountered by adolescents and adults with a history of dyslexia, there is little direct evidence regarding the neural systems critical for reading fluency and disruptions of those neural systems in dyslexia. Our aim was to identify the neural systems associated with fluent reading in typical adult readers, and discover how those systems differed in adults with dyslexia.

Reading fluency deficits are persistent and widespread in both adolescents and adults with a history of dyslexia [7,8]. In contrast to effective interventions focusing on phonological deficits [9–11], dysfluent reading is especially difficult to remediate [6,12–14]. Particularly beyond elementary school, remediation attempts to boost reading fluency yield only minimal improvements for dyslexic readers [15]. Challenges with reading fluency are not restricted to readers of English, but rather play a prominent role across languages [8,16–20].

The brain basis of single word reading has been the focus of many functional magnetic resonance imaging (fMRI) and magnetoencephalography (MEG) reading studies, but the brain basis of reading connected text has been investigated less often [21–24]. In typical readers, brain regions associated with sentence reading include greater left-hemisphere than right-hemisphere activation in the inferior frontal gyrus, posterior superior and middle temporal gyri, as well as left occipito-temporal cortex, bilateral occipital cortex, left cerebellar declive, and dorsolateral prefrontal cortex [25]. Studies using fMRI to examine the neural correlates of sentence reading indicate that semantic processing is associated with activation in the temporal lobes, greater on the left, and left inferior frontal gyrus (BA47) [25,26], and that processing accelerated text presentation is associated with activation in left occipito-temporal cortex [27]. For typically developing readers, higher scores on single-word reading tests are associated with increased activation during sentence reading in left temporo-parietal and ventral occipito-temporal regions [28]. Studies comparing readers with dyslexia to typical readers on whole-sentence reading have found relative hypo-activation in bilateral parietal cortices [24] and left occipito-temporal gyrus [17], but hyper-activation in left inferior frontal gyrus [17]. A MEG study of silent passage reading with each word presented individually at a constant rate (700 ms) found that, compared to typical readers, dyslexic readers exhibited hypo-activation bilaterally in the temporo-parietal and occipital cortices [28].

To date, fMRI studies of reading fluency using sentence stimuli have not examined and compared directly fluency per se in typical and atypical reading development (i.e., by varying and comparing fluency demands). One indirect approach involved correlating out-of-scanner standardized scores on tests of reading fluency with brain activations measured during scanning on tasks that did not vary fluency demands (reading sentences versus noun strings) [29]. In typical readers, higher fluency scores were associated positively with activations in left occipitotemporal cortex (BA18) and negatively with activations in right superior temporal gyrus, left insula, and left cerebellum. In a study that varied presentation rate on a word-by-word sentence reading judgment task in Hebrew with slower and faster rates, activation differences based on rate comparisons were not reported. However, typical adult readers showed greater activation in left premotor, left anterior insula/inferior frontal gyrus, right anterior insula, left middle temporal gyrus, and bilateral extrastriate visual cortex for each rate compared to fixation [30]. Readers with dyslexia showed less activation than typical readers during the relatively fast rate condition (versus fixation) in the posterior right temporal regions. Although these imaging studies considered fluency and involved reading sentences, as opposed to isolated words, none of the studies directly examined brain systems underlying reading fluency in readers with and without dyslexia.

Impaired reading fluency could arise from several sources. First, dyslexia has often been associated with impaired phonological awareness, even before the onset of reading instruction, that is thought to slow single-word decoding and, in turn, connected text composed of single words [31]. Second, dyslexia has also been associated with impaired naming speed for lists of stimuli, even for nonverbal material [32], and such slowness in processing for a series of stimuli may slow the reading of a series of words that constitute a sentence. Third, dyslexia has been associated with other temporal processing impairments for both linguistic and non-linguistic stimuli, such as deficits in general auditory processing [33], speech-specific processing [34], rise-time discrimination [35], or auditory sampling at optimal frequencies for analyzing language sounds [36]. Slowed temporal processing could impede reading fluency.

The major impediment for direct identification of neural systems important for reading fluency is that the kinds of educational and clinical tests used to measure fluency are not easily translated for fMRI experimentation. Further, it is not obvious what task would serve as an informative baseline for fluent reading. Therefore, the current study investigated the neural correlates of reading fluency by parametrically varying the rate at which sentences were presented one word at a time that were read silently. Accuracy and speed of comprehension, as indicated by plausibility judgments, verified reading performance. There were three rates of word presentation that corresponded to typical silent reading rates in 3rd or 4th grades (150 words per minute (wpm) (*slow rate*)), in 8th or 9th grades (240 wpm) (*medium rate*), and surpassing typical college reader expectations (600 wpm) (*fast rate*).

We examined neural systems that may be important for fluency by identifying brain regions that changed activation in response to changes in presentation rate in typical young adult readers and readers with dyslexia. The use of three different reading rates allowed for a comparison of typical readers and readers with dyslexia with performance differences equated by examination of a faster rate in the typical readers compared to a slower rate in readers with dyslexia. Such performance-equated comparisons permit consideration of whether activation differences between typical readers and readers with dyslexia are simply a consequence of performance differences or are related more directly to the cause of reduced fluency in dyslexia [37]. We hypothesized that brain regions showing increasing activation with increasing rates of presentation would be important for reading fluency, and that activation patterns would differ in readers with and without dyslexia.

Methods

Ethics statement

Written informed consent for participation in the study, approved by the Massachusetts Institute of Technology (MIT) and Harvard University Institutional Review Boards, was obtained from all participants.

Participants

Participants recruited from online recruitment in the local community of urban and suburban areas met inclusion criteria of: between 18–35 years of age; native English speakers; completion of high school or higher levels of formal education; right handedness as indicated by responses to a questionnaire adapted from the *Edinburgh Handedness Inventory* [38]; no contraindications to MRI; and absence of neurological or psychiatric impairments or associated medications. Participants completed a behavioral testing session at MIT and an MR scanning session at the Athinoula A. Martinos Imaging Center, McGovern Institute for Brain Research at MIT.

Behavioral assessment

Standardized measures of cognitive, reading, and reading-related abilities were administered to participants by trained researchers at MIT. The testing battery included measures of cognitive ability, *Wechsler Abbreviated Scale of Intelligence, 3rd Ed.* (WASI) [39]; phonological processing, *Comprehensive Test of Phonological Processing* (CTOPP) [40]; and rapid naming, "Letters," "Numbers," and "2-set" from the *Rapid Automatized Naming and Rapid Alternating Stimulus Tests* (RAN/RAS) [41]. Untimed reading ability was indexed by accuracy for reading real words and pseudowords, "Word Identification" and "Word Attack" from the *Woodcock Reading Mastery Test-Revised, NU* (WRMT) [42]. Timed reading ability was indexed by accuracy for reading real words and pseudowords within time limits, "Sight Word Efficiency" and "Phonemic Decoding Efficiency" from the *Test of Word Reading Efficiency* (TOWRE) [43]. Untimed and timed measures of connected text reading were used to index reading comprehension ability by using cloze sentences, which are sentences in which a reader is asked to supply a word that has been removed from a passage in order to assess comprehension. These measures were "Passage Comprehension" from the WRMT, text passages from the *Nelson-Denny Reading Test* (NDRT) [44], and sentences that required a semantic plausibility judgment within a time limit, "Reading Fluency" from the *Woodcock-Johnson III* (WJ) [45]. Reading rate was recorded as the number of words in a text passage read silently at a typical pace within a time limit, "Reading Rate," NDRT. Participants completed a background questionnaire regarding developmental history of language and literacy skills.

Participant groups

Two participant groups were included in this study. Typical readers (n = 12; 5 female) were between 18–28 years of age ($M = 22.5$; $SD = 3.1$) and earned a score at or above the 25th percentile on four measures of untimed or timed single word reading (TOWRE, WRMT; Table 1). Readers with dyslexia (n = 12; 8 female) were between 18–31 years of age ($M = 23.3$; $SD = 4.1$) and had both a history and a clinical diagnosis of reading disability, and were also currently scoring below the 25th percentile rank on at least two subtests of timed or untimed single word or pseudoword reading measures (TOWRE, WRMT; Table 1). All participants demonstrated cognitive performance at or above the expected mean range of 100±15 (WASI). The two groups did not differ significantly on age or nonverbal cognitive ability (Table 1). Among participants who reported ethnicity, 100% of adults in the control group reported having a Caucasian background. Among participants with dyslexia, 75% reported having a Caucasian background, one identified as Black, and 2 elected not to respond. There were no between group differences in education level attained.

Task design and materials

The sentence reading paradigm consisted of five words presented sequentially, followed by a question mark, for each trial. Participants were asked to indicate via button press whether each sentence was semantically plausible (e.g., *Bulls charge with great ferocity*) or semantically nonplausible (e.g., *Kangaroos type for their jobs*). Participants practiced the paradigm with unique stimuli prior to the scanning session to ensure understanding of task directions and mastery of task demands.

Words in each sentence trial were presented at one of three speeds: Slow (400 milliseconds/word), Medium (250 milliseconds/word), or Fast (100 milliseconds/word). The slow sentence presentation rate, corresponding to 150 words per minute, was commensurate with a silent reading rate for typical readers in grade three or four [46,47]. The medium sentence presentation rate, corresponding to 240 words per minute, was consistent with typical grade eight or nine silent reading rates [44,46]. The fast sentence presentation rate, corresponding to a rate of 600 words per minute, was selected to be challenging for typical adult readers by surpassing the typical college-level silent reading rate of about 280 words per minute and efficient reading rates of about 500 words per minute [46,47].

The nouns and verbs in sentence sets were matched for written frequency and number of syllables in three ways: between runs (run 1, run 2), between conditions (Slow, Medium, Fast), and between sentence types (plausible, nonplausible). One-way analysis of variance (ANOVA) was used to compare stimuli characteristics, which were compiled using the MRC Psycholinguistic Database (www.psy.uwa.edu.au/mrcdatabase/uwa_mrc.htm). First, sentences were balanced across run 1 and run 2 for written frequency [nouns: $F(1, 295) = 1.08, p = .30$; verbs: $F(1, 150) = 1.30, p = .26$] and for number of syllables [nouns: $F(1, 318) = 0.02, p = .90$; verbs: $F(1, 154) = 1.65, p = .20$]. Second, sentences were matched across the three conditions (Slow, Medium, Fast) for written frequency [nouns: $F(2, 294) = 1.27, p = .28$; verbs: $F(2, 149) = 1.37, p = .26$] and for number of syllables [nouns: $F(2, 317) = 0.94, p = .39$; verbs: $F(2, 153) = 0.08, p = .93$] to minimize effects of reading time that could be impacted by longer or less frequent words. Third, sentences were matched across the two types, plausible and nonplausible, for written frequency [nouns: $F(1, 295) = 0.90, p = .34$; verbs: $F(1, 150) = 0.17, p = .68$] and for number of syllables [nouns: $F(1, 318) = 2.35, p = .13$; verbs: $F(1, 154) = 0.92, p = .34$]. The sequence of sentence and rest trials was based on the output from a randomization program (OPTSEQ2) that generated three equivalent versions of the fluency task. Each version used the same sentence stimuli, but balanced the rate of presentation so that each sentence was presented in each condition across the three versions.

A jittered event-related design was used in which sentence conditions and a rest condition were randomly intermixed. The duration between trials, which constituted the rest condition, varied (i.e., was jittered). For the rest condition, participants were asked to stare at a fixation cross; this condition served as a low-level baseline. Rest trials were interspersed at random between sentence trials (i.e., jittered time periods), and the duration of the rest trials ranged from 200–2200 milliseconds at increments of 200 (e.g., 200 ms, 400 ms, 600 ms, ... , 2200 ms). The total presentation time of each sentence condition was equal to the total duration of rest trials. Each sentence trial totaled four seconds and consisted of a sentence and a question mark. The question mark duration made up for the varying length of the sentence duration to total 4 seconds (i.e., 3500 ms for Fast, 2750 ms for Medium, and 2000 ms for Slow).

Each participant completed two consecutive runs (10.4 minutes each) of the sentence-reading fMRI task. Each run consisted of 78 sentences, with 13 semantically plausible and 13 nonplausible sentences at each of the three rates. Thus, there were 156 sentences in total across both runs. Stimuli were presented on a rear projection screen in white on a black background via PsychToolBox software [48]. The screen size, zoom, and focus were calibrated for each participant to ensure that the entire visual field of the projected images was visible through the mirror mounted on the head coil.

Imaging data acquisition

Imaging was performed using a Siemens 3T MAGNETOM Trio, a Tim System, (Siemens Medical Solutions, Erlangen, Germany) and a commercial 12-Channel Matrix head coil (Siemens Medical Solutions, Erlangen, Germany). To minimize head movement, tetrahedron-shaped foam pads were placed between the head coil and either side of the participant's head. Sagittal localizer scans were aligned to a multi-subject atlas to derive automatic slice prescription for consistent head position across participants. At the beginning of each functional scan, five images (10 second duration) were discarded to allow for T1 equilibration. High-resolution structural whole-brain images were acquired using a T1-weighted anatomical scan (128 slices per slab; 256×256 matrix; 256 mm FOV; 1.33 mm slice thickness; 0.63 mm interslice gap; TR = 2530 ms; TI = 1100 ms; TE = 3.39 ms; flip angle = 7°).

Functional data were collected using a gradient echo T2*-weighted EPI sequence sensitive to the BOLD contrast. The gradient-echo EPI images were acquired with PACE [49], an online motion correction algorithm that minimizes movement-related artifacts by adjusting the system gradients and the acquisition field of view between one whole brain acquisition and another for participant movement. Thirty-two sagittal slices parallel to the anterior commissure-posterior commissure (AC-PC)

Table 1. Participant Scores for Typical Readers and Readers with Dyslexia.

		Typical Reader Group	Dyslexic Group	p-values: Typical vs. Dyslexic
N		12	12	–
Age		22.5±3.1	23.3±4.1	.61
Construct	**Behavioral Measure**			
Cognitive Abilities	WASI – Verbal	121.17±13.04	109.00±7.31	.010
	WASI – Performance	114.67±8.2	110.58±6.05	.181
Phonological Processing	CTOPP – Elision	11.00±0.85	8.27±1.62	.0005
	CTOPP – Blending Words	11.00±1.41	8.83±2.76	.024
	CTOPP – Memory For Digits	12.33±2.71	12.27±1.49	.948
	CTOPP – Nonword Repetition	9.33±1.92	7.42±1.51	.013
Sublexical Fluenc	RAN – Numbers	112.83±5.28	105.00±6.84	.005
	RAN – Letters	112.00±3.24	102.00±7.39	.0005
	RAN – RAS	112.33±5.85	101.67±11.20	.008
Word Reading Accurac	WRMT – Word Identification	108.83±10.07	90.25±8.97	.0005
	WRMT – Word Attack	111.00±12.23	93.92±6.99	.0005
Word Reading Fluency	TOWRE – Sight Word Efficiency	103.58±8.24	85.00±6.36	.0005
	TOWRE – Phonemic Decoding Efficiency	100.17±6.83	80.83±8.94	.0005
Connected Text Reading Fluency	WJ – Reading Fluency	118.55±8.65	93.92±10.03	.0005
Connected Text Reading Comprehension	WRMT – Passage Comprehension	115.00±11.10	106.07±6.90	.031
	NDRT – Reading Comprehension	241.00±11.34	209.75±14.64	.0005
Connected Text Reading Rate	NDRT – Reading Rate	224.58±23.83	186.33±11.60	.0005
In-Scanner Task Performance				
Accuracy (% correct)	Fast	81±10	64±11	.001
	Medium	94±6	83±9	.002
	Slow	95±3	92±6	.150
Reaction Time (ms)	Fast	975.39±254.72	1230.13±312.70	.040
	Medium	629.88±187.12	954.92±259.49	.002
	Slow	512.65±218.92	755.73±168.58	.006

Mean ± SD; *p* values below .05 are statistically significant based on two-tailed t-tests. Note: Standard scores are based on a mean of 100 and a standard deviation of 15 (average range of 85-115) except for the CTOPP (based on mean of 10 and a standard deviation of 3; average range of 7-13) and NDRT (based on mean of 200 and a standard deviation of 25; average range of 175-225). SD = Standard deviation.

line were imaged (voxel size of 3.1×3.1×4.0 mm, 64×64 mm matrix, 200 mm field-of-view, 4 mm slice thickness, 0.8 mm inter-slice gap). Other imaging acquisition parameters included: TR = 2000 ms, TE = 30 ms, flip angle = 90°, bandwidth = 2298 Hz/Px, echo spacing = 0.5 ms.

In-Scanner recording of performance

Accuracy and reaction time in judging semantic plausibility were recorded when participants responded via button press for each trial. The scanner paradigm was programmed to take one response from the time that the trial began (first word in the sentence) to the end of the trial (question mark).

fMRI data analysis

The neural correlates associated with increasing reading fluency demands were measured using a within-subjects design and a parametric modulation analysis, which creates a statistical parametric mapping of the significance of the correlation between cognitive parameters and physiology [50]. Preprocessing and statistical analysis were performed using statistical parametric mapping software (SPM8; Wellcome Department of Cognitive Neurology, London, UK; http://www.fil.ion.ucl.ac.uk/spm). During preprocessing, data were realigned to the first functional volume and spatially normalized using the mean functional volume to the Montreal Neurological Institute (MNI) template. Normalized images were smoothed using a Gaussian filter (6-mm full width at half maximum) to decrease spatial noise.

Analysis included individual and group level statistics. For the individual level analysis, the stimuli (defined as the start of the first word and the end of the last word) were modeled as box-car functions aligned with the onset of each stimulus, the width of which corresponded to the duration of each stimulus. The expected BOLD responses to the stimuli were obtained by convolving a canonical hemodynamic response function with the modeled stimuli. A high-pass filter (cutoff = 128 s) was used on both the data and the model to reduce impact of physiological noise. The mean voxel value was used for the global calculation. Grand mean scaling was based on session specific parameters. Global normalization was not used.

Outlier image volumes in the BOLD time series were identified based on either the mean intensity of image volume greater than 3 standard deviations from the mean intensity of the time series or the largest voxel movement of the image volume greater than .5 mm, based on scan-to-scan movement. Image volumes were masked by a binary image created from the functional time series (using the same procedure as that used to create the SPM analysis mask). Outlier images were included as nuisance regressors in the first-level analysis per person. The typical reader group (M = 11.7, SD = 11.3) and the dyslexic group (M = 7.0, SD = 5.5) did not differ in the number of outlier images ($t(22) = 1.27$, $p = .22$).

A random effects model [51] was used to characterize group level effects (second-level analysis). Brain regions were identified using a threshold of $p<.001$ cluster-level FDR corrected for multiple comparisons and using a cluster extent threshold (ET) of 10 voxels or more. We used the Topological False Discovery Rate (FDR) calculations from SPM8. SPM8 computes FDR by assigning corrected p-values to the local maxima. Peak-wise FDR has fewer false positives than conventional voxel-wise FDR [52,53].

The comparison between the typical reader group and the dyslexic group was based on differences between mean parameter estimates in a linear parametric modulation contrast (Fast > Medium > Slow) using a threshold of $p<.01$ cluster-level FDR corrected for multiple comparisons. An independent samples t-test was used to characterize clusters showing significant difference between groups. Within and between group comparisons were also completed for Medium > Slow to ensure that the parametric comparison was not driven by aberrant activations elicited by the fast rate, which exceeded expectations for even typical adult readers. For these analyses, all trials (correct and incorrect) were used to maximize power and not bias data-points in favor of the typical reader group, who answered more items correctly compared to readers with dyslexia. In addition, the Fast > Slow contrast for typical readers was compared to Medium > Slow for dyslexic readers because these contrasts yielded comparable behavioral performance between the groups. For this comparison, in-scanner accuracy changes in performance between presentation rates did not significantly differ between groups.

We also examined as an *a priori* region of interest the putative visual word form area (VWFA), which has been associated with rapid visual analysis of text for typical readers [54]. The ROI was defined as a 10 mm sphere with the location taken from the imaging literature (Standard Talairach Coordinates: $x = -43$, $y = -54$, $z = -12$; [55]).

Results

Behavioral measures

The typical reader group performed significantly better than the dyslexic group on standardized measures of verbal cognitive abilities, phonological processing (with the exception of Memory for Digits, an index of phonological memory), rapid naming (letters, numbers, 2-set), timed and untimed single word reading, timed and untimed text comprehension, and reading rate (Table 1; independent samples t-tests, two-tailed, all $p<.05$). The typical reader group and the dyslexic group did not differ significantly on non-verbal cognitive abilities ($p = .18$).

Scanner task performance

In-scanner performance (Table 1) for the typical reader group and the dyslexic group was analyzed with a 3×2 repeated measures ANOVA, with Condition (Fast, Medium, Slow) as a within-subjects factor and Group (typical readers vs. readers with dyslexia) as a between-subjects factor. The typical reader group was more accurate than the dyslexic group as indicated by a significant main effect for Group [$F(1,22) = 14.16$, $p<.001$]. Accuracy declined with greater rates of presentation as indicated by a significant main effect of Condition [$F(2,21) = 61.34$, $p< .0005$]. Accuracy differences between groups varied as a function of presentation rate as shown by a significant Group X Condition interaction [$F(2,21) = 8.46$, $p<.002$], with the dyslexic group performing significantly worse on Fast [$t(22) = 4.05$, $p<.001$] and Medium [$t(22) = 3.59$, $p<.002$] conditions, but not on the Slow condition [$t(22) = 1.49$, $p = .15$]. Groups did not differ on rates of response across conditions [$t(22) = 1.77$, $p = .09$], indicating that both groups of participants had sufficient time to respond to items.

The typical reader group was faster to respond than the dyslexic group as indicated by a significant main effect for Group [$F(1,22) = 9.76$, $p<.005$]. Responses were slower as presentation rates increased as shown by a significant main effect of Condition [$F(2,21) = 49.06$, $p<.0001$]. The Group X Condition interaction was not significant [$F(2,21) = 2.10$, $p = .15$].

In-scanner performances for the typical reader group and the dyslexic group were compared to determine if performance was comparable at the Fast rate for the typical reader group and at the Medium rate for the dyslexic group. Independent samples t-tests showed that performance for the typical reader group during the Fast-rate condition did not differ significantly from performance for the dyslexic group during the Medium-rate condition for accuracy [$t(22) = 1.04$, $p = .31$] or reaction time [$t(22) = 0.49$, $p = .63$]. Thus, we included these conditions as a performance-equated group comparison. Further analysis indicated that the difference between Slow and Fast conditions for the typical reader group and the difference between Slow and Medium conditions for the group with dyslexia was not statistically significant for accuracy [$t(22) = 1.58$, $p = .13$], but was for reaction time, with the typical reader group exhibiting a larger difference than dyslexic group [$t(22) = 2.99$, $p<.05$].

Relation of in-scanner performance with standardized measures of reading fluency and phonological awareness

We examined the relationship between behavioral performance in the scanner and a standardized test of reading fluency on which the task was based ("Reading Fluency," WJ) across participants in both groups using correlation analysis (uncorrected for multiple comparisons). There were significant negative correlations between age-standardized Reading Fluency scores and in-scanner reaction time at all three reading rates: Slow (standard scores: $r = -.69$, $p<.01$); Medium (standard scores: $r = -.68$, $p<.01$), and Fast (standard scores: $r = -.54$, $p<.01$). There were significant positive correlations between Reading Fluency scores and accuracy at the Medium and Fast rates, which did not show ceiling effects for accuracy: Medium (standard scores: $r = .47$, $p< .05$); Fast (standard scores: $r = .63$, $p<.01$). These correlations reflected group differences between the typical reader and dyslexic groups, because the correlations were not significant within either group alone.

We also examined the relationship between phonological processing and in-scanner performance. Standard scores from a measure of phonological awareness ("Elision," CTOPP) showed significant correlations with in-scanner reaction time for Medium ($r = -.49$, $p<.05$) and Slow ($r = -.43$, $p<.05$) rates, and accuracy for Fast ($r = .44$, $p<.05$) and Medium ($r = .47$, $p<.05$) rates. Other measures of phonological awareness and phonological memory were not significantly correlated with in-scanner performance ($p> .05$). Once again, these correlations reflected group differences between the typical reader and dyslexic groups, because the correlations were not significant within either group alone.

fMRI Activation for Typical Readers

Fast > Medium > Slow. Typical readers showed greater activation for faster rates of word presentation in a distributed cortical network including peak activations in left superior frontal gyrus, left middle temporal gyrus, right superior temporal and insular regions, left inferior occipital gyrus, right middle occipital gyrus, and cerebellar and subcortical regions (Table 2 & Figure 1, top panel).

Medium > Slow. In typical readers, comparisons excluding the fastest rate continued to demonstrate robust activations in networks including frontal systems with peaks in the superior frontal gyrus that was situated medially and extending to both hemispheres; right middle and inferior frontal gyrus; and right precentral gyrus. Activations also included clusters with peaks in the right middle temporal gyrus, left postcentral gyrus extending to inferior frontal gyrus, right inferior parietal lobule and precuneus, and a cluster with a peak in right lingual gyrus that included bilateral fusiform gyri and left cuneus (Table 2).

fMRI Activation for Dyslexic Readers

Fast > Medium > Slow. Dyslexic readers showed greater activation for faster rates of word presentation in a distributed cortical network including left superior frontal gyri, right middle frontal gyrus, bilateral insular and middle temporal regions, left postcentral gyrus, left superior parietal lobule, bilateral inferior parietal lobule, right precuneus, and cerebellar and subcortical regions (Table 3 and Figure 1, middle panel).

Medium > Slow. Comparing the medium to slow rates of sentence presentation, readers with dyslexia showed activations with peaks in right superior, middle, and inferior frontal gyri and left inferior frontal gyrus; left middle temporal gyrus and insula, superior parietal lobule and postcentral gyrus; bilateral middle occipital gyrus and right cuneus; and cerebellar regions (Table 3).

Comparing Typical and Dyslexic Readers: Fast > Medium > Slow

Compared to readers with dyslexia on the parametric analysis (Fast > Medium > Slow), typical readers showed greater activation in a cluster with a peak in left middle frontal gyrus that extended into the inferior frontal gyrus, insula, and precentral gyrus; a cluster with a peak in left superior temporal gyrus that extended into the supramarginal gyrus, inferior parietal lobule, middle temporal gyrus, and cingulate cortex; and a cluster with a peak in the brainstem that extended into bilateral brainstem regions, medulla, and right cerebellum (Table 4; Figure 1, bottom panel). Readers with dyslexia did not show any activation greater than typical readers (Table 4).

In order to characterize the nature of these group differences in activation, we extracted parameter estimate values for each reading rate, relative to the fixation baseline, from peaks of activation in regions showing greatest group differences (10 mm spheres around activation peaks in left middle ($x = -54$, $y = 22$, $z = 26$) and inferior ($x = -44$, $y = 24$, $z = 6$) frontal gyri and left superior temporal gyrus ($x = -60$, $y = -46$, $z = 16$)). In left middle frontal gyrus, typical readers showed significantly more activation than dyslexic readers at all rates ($p = .01$) (Figure 2a). In left inferior frontal (Figure 2b) and left superior temporal (Figure 2c) regions, there were no significant differences for the Slow condition ($p > .05$), but typical readers exhibited greater activation in the Medium [left middle frontal gyrus, $t(22) = 2.47$, $p = .02$; left

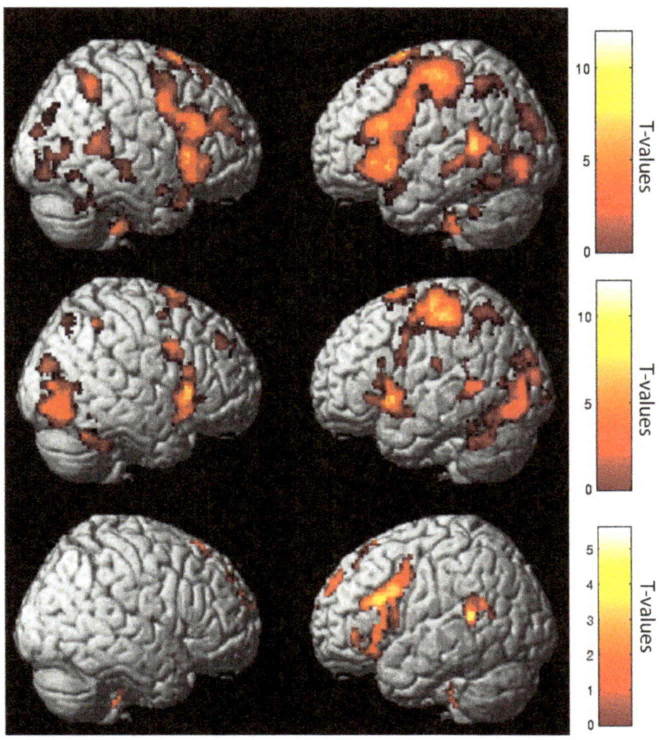

Figure 1. Sentence presentation rate differentially impacts brain activation by group. Fast > Medium > Slow parametric modulation (cluster level FDR corrected) for a) Typical Reader Group (p<.001) (top panel); b) Dyslexic Group (p<.001) (middle panel); c) Typical > Dyslexic Groups (p<.01) (bottom panel). Color bar indicates T-values.

Table 2. Activations for Fast > Medium > Slow contrasts for Typical Readers.

Region (peak activation)	BA	x	y	z	Cluster extent	p	Z score
Fast > Medium > Slow							
Frontal Lobe							
L. Superior frontal gyrus	6	−2	8	70	5008	<.0001	6.61
Temporal Lobe							
R. Insula	13	30	26	0	3841	<.0001	6.11
L. Middle temporal gyrus	21	−50	−46	8	1270	<.0001	5.53
R. Superior temporal gyrus	22	54	−46	14	666	<.0001	5.47
Parietal Lobe							
N/A							
Occipital Lobe							
L. Inferior occipital gyrus	19	−34	−76	−4	1082	<.0001	5.32
R. Middle occipital gyrus	19	36	−88	18	81	.017	4.52
R. Middle occipital gyrus	19	48	−78	4	327	<.0001	4.04
Cerebellum							
L. Cerebellum	N/A	−38	−46	−38	199	<.0001	4.42
L. Cerebellum	N/A	−8	−78	−38	83	.017	4.30
Sub-lobar							
Thalamus	N/A	−8	−16	4	16152	<.0001	6.22
R. Caudate	N/A	12	12	8	115	.006	4.11
Brainstem	N/A	4	−34	−46	577	<.0001	4.98
Medium > Slow							
Frontal Lobe							
L. Superior frontal gyrus	6	−2	8	60	2605	<.0001	6.42
R. Middle frontal gyrus	46	48	26	26	216	.001	5.24
R. Inferior frontal gyrus	47	34	32	−2	324	<.0001	4.43
R. Precentral gyrus	6	38	−4	38	90	.028	4.42
Temporal Lobe							
R. Middle temporal gyrus	22	50	−40	6	104	.021	4.39
Parietal Lobe							
L. Postcentral gyrus	3	−40	−24	48	6078	<.0001	5.98
R. Inferior parietal lobule	40	36	−46	50	132	.009	3.89
R. Precuneus	19	30	−68	36	87	.028	3.66
Occipital Lobe							
R. Lingual gyrus	18	18	−80	−2	6923	<.0001	5.46

$p < .001$, cluster level FDR corrected (T = 3.50); ET = 10. N/A = Not applicable. L.= Left hemisphere. R.= Right hemisphere. Coordinates reported in Talairach space.

Table 3. Activations for Fast > Medium > Slow contrasts for Readers with Dyslexia.

Region (peak activation)	BA	x	y	z	Cluster extent	*p*	Z score
Fast > Medium > Slow							
Frontal Lobe							
L. Superior frontal gyrus	8	6	16	50	3902	<.0001	6.06
R. Middle frontal gyrus	9	36	44	36	94	.023	4.42
R. Middle frontal gyrus	6	28	4	46	84	.029	4.16
Temporal Lobe							
L. Insula	13	−36	12	2	1432	<.0001	5.93
R. Insula	13	30	24	2	1866	<.000	6.15
L. Middle temporal gyrus	21	−62	−46	8	324	<.0001	4.29
R. Middle temporal gyrus	21	48	−34	−4	69	.049	3.41
Parietal Lobe							
L. Postcentral gyrus	3	−36	−30	52	2626	<.0001	5.77
L. Superior parietal lobule	7	−30	−52	52	817	<.0001	4.65
L. Inferior parietal lobule	40	−54	−20	24	90	.025	3.75
R. Inferior parietal lobule	40	46	−50	52	96	.023	3.71
R. Precuneus	7	26	−68	50	223	.001	3.81
Occipital Lobe							
N/A							
Cerebellum							
Anterior lobe	N/A	0	−54	−30	216	.001	3.96
Sub-lobar							
L. Thalamus	N/A	−10	−20	0	11851	<.0001	5.93
Cingulate gyrus	23	8	−22	26	99	.023	4.53
Medium > Slow							
Frontal Lobe							
R. Superior frontal gyrus	8	6	16	52	1744	<.0001	6.15
R. Middle frontal gyrus	9	48	8	34	146	.002	4.17
R. Inferior frontal gyrus	47	34	32	0	279	<.0001	5.11
L. Inferior frontal gyrus	44	−46	10	20	961	<.0001	4.45
Temporal Lobe							
L. Middle temporal gyrus	21	−50	−48	4	157	.002	4.17
L. Insula	13	−48	−22	20	101	.01	4.02
Parietal Lobe							
Postcentral gyrus	3	−38	−22	52	2095	<.0001	5.71
Superior parietal lobule	7	−30	−50	58	260	<.0001	4.22

Table 3. Cont.

Region (peak activation)	BA	x	y	z	Cluster extent	p	Z score
Occipital Lobe							
R. Cuneus	17	8	−78	10	4909	<.0001	5.44
L. Middle occipital gyrus	18	−22	−92	16	572	<.0001	4.83
R. Middle occipital gyrus	18	26	−90	10	187	.001	4.09
Cerebellum							
L. Anterior culmen	N/A	−8	−28	−10	476	<.0001	4.68

$p<.001$, cluster level FDR corrected (T = 3.50); ET = 10. N/A = Not applicable. L. = Left hemisphere. R. = Right hemisphere. Coordinates reported in Talairach space.

superior temporal gyrus, $t(22) = 2.73$, $p = .01$] and Fast conditions [left middle frontal gyrus, $t(22) = 4.78$, $p<.0005$; left superior temporal gyrus, $t(22) = 2.67$, $p = .02$; left inferior frontal gyrus, $t(22) = 2.67$, $p = .02$]. In addition, the putative visual word form area (VWFA; left fusiform gyrus) region of interest exhibited greater activation as a function of rate ($p<.0001$), but there was neither an effect of group nor a group x rate interaction ($p = .41$) (Figure 2d).

Comparing conditions matched for in-scanner performance

Typical readers (Fast > Slow) and readers with dyslexia (Medium > Slow) were compared based on matched in-scanner performance (Table 4). Typical readers showed significantly greater activation in almost all brain regions engaged by the task (Figure 3). Readers with dyslexia showed greater activations compared to typical readers in left anterior cingulate regions.

Discussion

We compared the neural correlates of reading fluency in adult readers with and without dyslexia using an fMRI sentence reading paradigm that parametrically varied fluency demands by increasing the rate at which sentences were presented for semantic plausibility judgments. Faster presentation rates resulted in slower responses and reduced judgment accuracy in both groups. Readers with dyslexia were slower and less accurate across rates than typical readers, and their accuracy declined disproportionately as rates increased. In-scanner behavioral performance correlated with standardized measures of reading fluency, indicating that the scanner task explored the same underlying fluency processes, and also standardized measures of phonological awareness. For both typical and dyslexic readers, a large bilateral network of cortical, subcortical, and cerebellar systems supported fluent sentence reading. Readers with dyslexia showed less of an increase in activation, as a function of reading rate, in left prefrontal and left superior temporal cortices, anterior cingulate, and brainstem/cerebellar regions. The relationship between performance levels did not account for the differences in activation, because equating performance at different rates between the typical and dyslexic readers enhanced, rather than reduced, group differences. These findings point to brain regions that are associated with reading fluency in typical reading and with reading dysfluency in dyslexia.

Defining and measuring fluent reading

The current study overcame several challenges in defining and measuring reading fluency directly using fMRI. Reading fluency was measured by using silent sentence reading in a word-by-word presentation format with the rate of word presentation manipulated on a sentence-by-sentence basis. Presentation rate was chosen as the independent variable because reading rate is a core aspect of reading fluency [56], and it can be manipulated in an fMRI task. Attention to the task was required as participants were asked to make semantic plausibility judgments following each sentence.

Silent reading of sentences was feasible for use in an fMRI study and similar to real world reading experiences. Implicit, or silent, word reading is effective in eliciting activations from brain areas associated with language processing [57]. Furthermore, for most adult readers, reading connected text silently is the most frequent interaction with written language, and predominantly involves decoding strings of words to extract meaning as opposed to reading isolated single words. Previous studies using word reading tasks have provided a basis for understanding the brain networks

Table 4. Activations for Typical Reader > Dyslexic Groups.

Region (peak activation)	BA	x	y	z	Cluster extent	*p*	Z score
***Typical**$_{(Fast > Medium > Slow)}$ > **Dyslexic**$_{(Fast > Medium > Slow)}$*							
L. Middle frontal gyrus	9	−54	22	26	1319	<.0001	4.01
L. Superior temporal gyrus	22	−60	−46	16	324	.048	4.29
Cingulate gyrus	32	14	20	44	772	<.001	4.38
Brainstem/Cerebellum		−2	−32	−38	380	<.0001	4.01
***Dyslexic**$_{(Fast > Medium > Slow)}$ > **Typical**$_{(Fast > Medium > Slow)}$*							
N/A							
***Typical**$_{(Fast > Slow)}$ > **Dyslexic**$_{(Medium > Slow)}$*							
L. Superior frontal gyrus	6	−4	10	66	7165	<.0001	6.65
L. Inferior frontal gyrus	45	−44	24	6	38925	<.0001	6.39
***Dyslexic**$_{(Medium > Slow)}$ > **Typical**$_{(Fast > Slow)}$*							
L. Anterior cingulate gyrus	24	−6	24	−4	2159	<.0001	4.45
Sub-lobar		34	−34	−6	470	.006	3.94
Sub-lobar		−22	−8	26	699	.001	3.88
Sub-lobar		32	−8	−4	324	.025	3.65

$p<.01$, cluster level FDR corrected ($T = 2.51$); ET = 10. N/A = Not applicable. L. = Left hemisphere.

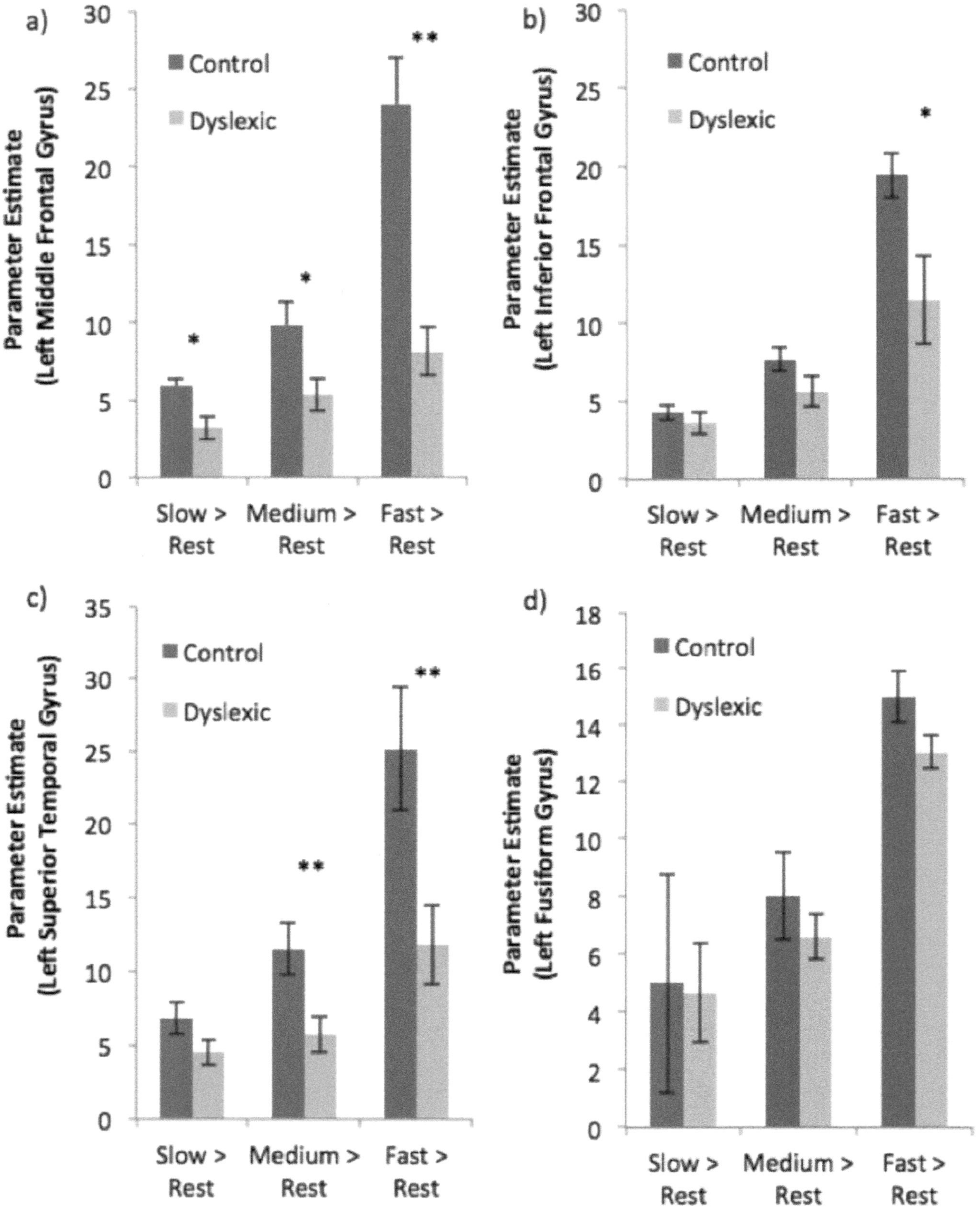

Figure 2. Comparison between Typical Reader and Dyslexic Groups (with standard error bars) showing region-of-interest activations for a) left middle frontal gyrus; b) left inferior frontal gyrus; c) left superior temporal gyrus; and d) left fusiform gyrus (visual word form area, VWFA). Note: *p<.05; **p<.01.

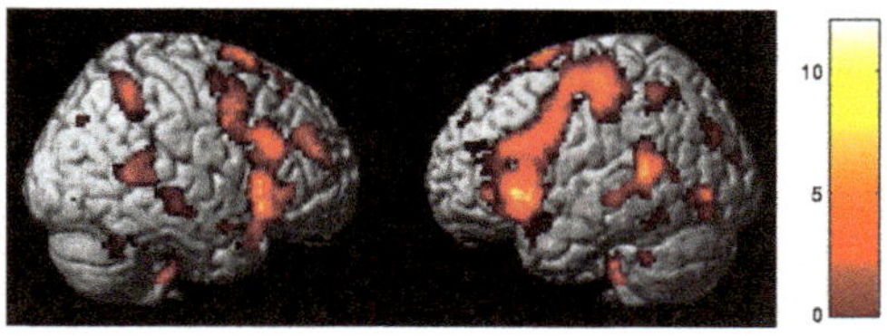

Figure 3. The Dyslexic Group showed reduced activation relative to the Typical Reader Group even when accuracy differences across conditions were equated between the groups. Greater activation for Fast > Slow contrast for Typical Readers versus Medium > Slow contrast for the Dyslexic Group (cluster level FDR corrected results displayed at $p<.001$). Color bar indicates T-values.

recruited for decoding and recognizing single words (i.e., isolated text), and studies using sentence reading tasks have identified brain regions recruited to process semantic or syntactic properties of sentences instantiated by relations among words. Sentence reading tasks can provide the additional advantage of localizing cognitive functions pertaining specifically to reading fluency - a dynamic aspect of reading behavior.

Limitations

We presented sentences one word at a time to control reading rate. A limitation of this approach is that some sentence-reading processes that are typically engaged during the reading of text, such as the voluntary allocation of different viewing times for different words, or looking back at words, were not invoked in this design. Several behavioral observations indicate, however, that this task probed reading fluency processes. First, faster rates reduced judgment accuracy and latency across all participants. Second, the dyslexic group exhibited the expected deficits in accuracy and latency, and accuracy decreased disproportionately as a function of increasing reading rate. Third, when reading was examined across participants from typical and dyslexic groups, in-scanner performance correlated with scores from a standardized reading fluency test that is widely used in educational and clinical testing. These behavioral findings support the validity of the reading rate manipulation as a test of reading fluency.

Brain regions associated with typical or impaired reading fluency

In typical readers, increased rates of word presentation likely influence many perceptual, phonological, semantic, syntactic, and pragmatic processes, and, correspondingly, resulted in increased activation in a large bilateral network of cortical, subcortical, and cerebellar regions. This activation pattern included brain regions implicated in processing visual (ventral occipital regions), phonological (inferior frontal gyrus, posterior superior temporal gyrus), and semantic (middle temporal gyrus, posterior superior temporal gyrus) information [58,59].

The group with dyslexia showed many similarities to the typical group in regards to increased activation as a function of word presentation rate in a large bilateral network. The dyslexic group showed significantly less gain in activation relative to the control group in primarily left hemisphere regions, including left middle and inferior frontal gyri and left superior temporal gyrus. The left posterior superior temporal gyrus supports processing of semantic judgments, and shows greater activation as a function of greater semantic analysis [59]. The left inferior frontal gyrus has been implicated in semantic working memory [60], unrelated to general task difficulty [61], but related to competition between or selection among related semantic response options [62]. Although the current study did not directly investigate the distinct contributions of phonological and semantic processing, left inferior frontal gyrus activation in this study closely approximates the location identified in previous research ($x = -37$, $y = 28$, $z = -9$) showing greater activation for semantic versus phonological processing [63]. The left inferior frontal gyrus is also activated for extracting a coherent meaning from individual words in a sentence [64] and semantic processing of sentences [65]. At the same time, there is considerable overlap in brain regions associated with semantic and phonological analysis of language (e.g., the left posterior superior temporal gyrus) [58,59]. To further characterize the relevant roles of the left inferior frontal gyrus and superior temporal gyrus in fluent reading, future analyses can compare activations for semantically appropriate and inappropriate sentences, or vary phonological demands.

Thus, some of the regions that showed significantly less activation in readers with dyslexia, which differed most at the fastest rate, are implicated in the control (left inferior frontal gyrus) or representation (left superior temporal gyrus) of semantic verbal knowledge. Weak responses in these regions associated with semantic processes during rapid or fluent reading could diminish comprehension during reading, as occurred for readers with dyslexia in the medium and fast conditions.

There was also greater activation in the group of typical readers in the cerebellum. Some studies have pointed to cerebellar anatomical differences in dyslexia [66], and it has been hypothesized that automaticity deficits in dyslexia may be associated with atypical cerebellar function [67]. The cerebellum, in addition to supplemental motor area (SMA) and primary motor cortex, shows increased recruitment for increasing rate (faster) and shorter duration when naming visually presented words [68], and for semantic and phonological processing [69]. The right cerebellar declive in particular has been implicated in automaticity in reading [70]. Functional connectivity between the cerebellum and inferior frontal and lateral temporal regions during reading suggests a coordinated cortico-cerebellar system that facilitates fluent reading [71]. The present findings are consistent with the impairment of the cerebellar component of this reading network in dyslexia.

Although activation was found in the purported visual word form area (VWFA) in the left temporo-occipital cortex and increased with reading rate, it did so similarly for both groups. This region has been associated with rapid processing of text for typical readers. Previously, this region has been found to show reduced activation in children with developmental dyslexia [72,73]. Due to previous findings, we had expected to observe reduced activation in dyslexic adults as a function of reading rate. Perhaps the increasing intensity of visual processing across the faster rates of word presentation was such a strong manipulation that it dominated activation in the VWFA.

The most striking group differences occurred in left-hemisphere cortical regions implicated in semantic processing and required to perform the semantic analyses of the sentences. The present study, however, cannot determine what kinds of processing bottlenecks in the brain restricted the flow of information to brain regions involved in semantic analysis and judgment. Such bottlenecks may have been due to slow phonological decoding of single words, or impaired temporal processing that limited coordination of reading processes across words. The absence of a group difference in VWFA suggests the dyslexic group may not have been limited by the rate of orthographic processing per se, but only more targeted experiments can better elucidate the bases of the fluency impairment.

The activation differences between the groups could reveal the cause or the consequence of impaired fluency in dyslexia (or both). One approach towards this issue of interpretation is to compare typical and dyslexic groups under conditions where behavioral performance or comprehension is equated. This analytic approach was possible by comparing the difference between slow and medium rates in the dyslexic group to the difference between slow and fast rates in the typical reading group, because these comparisons did not show significant accuracy differences between the groups. When reading accuracies across conditions were equated, however, there remained large brain activation differences between the groups. Therefore, the activation differences between groups were not simply the consequence of worse performance by the group with dyslexia. Rather, weakened engagement of brain regions associated with semantic processing and automated reading may reflect the cause of the fluency deficits that make reading comprehension so challenging for many readers with dyslexia.

Acknowledgments

We thank the participants, A. A. Martinos Imaging Center at McGovern Institute for Brain Research (MIT) for making this research possible, as well as Tyler Perrachione, Bianca Levy, Alison Bloomfield, Rebecca Winter, Carlos Cardenas, Omar Hadzipasic, Sara Beach, for assistance with data collection. We thank Steve Shannon and Sheeba Arnold for data collection technical support.

Author Contributions

Conceived and designed the experiments: JAC JDEG. Performed the experiments: JAC SNDT PKS JL. Analyzed the data: JAC SNDT JL. Contributed reagents/materials/analysis tools: JAC SNDT PKS JL SSG SWG CT. Wrote the paper: JAC SNDT JDEG.

References

1. Wolf M, Katzir-Cohen T (2001) Reading fluency and its intervention. Scientific Studies of Reading 5: 211–239.
2. National Institute of Child Heath and Human Development (2000) Report of the National Reading Panel. Teaching children to read: An evidence-based assessment of the scientific research literature on reading and its implications for reading instruction: Reports of the subgroups (NIH Publication No. 00–4754). Washington, DC: U.S. Government Printing Office. Available: www.nichd.nih.gov/publications/nrp/smallbook.cfm.
3. Lyon GR, Shaywitz SE, Shaywitz BA (2003) A definition of dyslexia. Annals of Dyslexia 53: 1–14.
4. Hudson RF, Pullen PC, Lane HB, Torgesen JK (2008) The complex nature of reading fluency: A multidimensional view. Reading & Writing Quarterly 25: 4–32.
5. Meyer MS, Felton RH (1999) Repeated reading to enhance fluency: Old approaches and new directions. Annals of Dyslexia 49: 283–306.
6. Torgesen JK, Alexander AW, Wagner RK, Rashotte CA, Voeller KK, et al. (2001) Intensive remedial instruction for children with severe reading disabilities: Immediate and long-term outcomes from two instructional approaches. Journal of Learning Disabilities 34: 33–58.
7. Leinonen S, Müller K, Leppänen PH, Aro M, Ahonen T, et al. (2001) Heterogeneity in adult dyslexic readers: Relating processing skills to the speed and accuracy of oral text reading. Reading and Writing 14: 265–296.
8. Ziegler JC, Perry C, Ma-Wyatt A, Ladner D, Schulte-Körne G (2003) Developmental dyslexia in different languages: Language-specific or universal? Journal of Experimental Child Psychology 86: 169–193.
9. Share DL, Stanovich KE (1995) Cognitive processes in early reading development: Accommodating individual differences into a model of acquisition. Issues in Education: Contributions from educational psychology 1: 1–58.
10. Snowling MJ (1981) Phonemic deficits in developmental dyslexia. Psychological Research 43: 219–234.
11. Gabrieli JDE (2009) Dyslexia: a new synergy between education and cognitive neuroscience. Science 325: 280–283.
12. Roberts G, Torgesen JK, Boardman A, Scammacca N (2008) Evidence-based strategies for reading instruction of older students with learning disabilities. Learning Disabilities Research & Practice 23: 63–69.
13. Torgesen JK, Hudson RF (2006) Reading fluency: Critical issues for struggling readers. In S. J. Samuels & A. E. Farstrup (Eds.), What research has to say about fluency instruction (pp.130–158). Newark, DE: International Reading Assocation.
14. Lovett MW, Steinbach KA, Frijters JC (2000) Remediating the core deficits of developmental reading disability: A double-deficit perspective. Journal of Learning Disabilities 33: 334–358.
15. Wexler J, Vaughn S, Edmonds M, Reutebuch CK (2008) A synthesis of fluency interventions for secondary struggling readers. Reading and Writing 21: 317–347.
16. Katzir T, Shaul S, Breznitz Z, Wolf M (2004) The universal and the unique in dyslexia: A cross-linguistic investigation of reading and reading fluency in Hebrew-and English-speaking children with reading disorders. Reading and Writing 17: 739–768.
17. Kronbichler M, Hutzler F, Staffen W, Mair A, Ladurner G, et al. (2006) Evidence for a dysfunction of left posterior reading areas in German dyslexic readers. Neuropsychologia 44: 1822–1832.
18. Landerl K, Wimmer H (2008) Development of word reading fluency and spelling in a consistent orthography: An 8-year follow-up. Journal of Educational Psychology 100: 150–161.
19. Thaler V, Ebner EM, Wimmer H, Landerl K (2004) Training reading fluency in dysfluent readers with high reading accuracy: Word specific effects but low transfer to untrained words. Annals of Dyslexia 54: 89–113.
20. Wimmer H, Mayringer H (2002) Dysfluent reading in the absence of spelling difficulties: A specific disability in regular orthographies. Journal of Educational Psychology 94: 272.
21. Capek CM, Bavelier D, Corina D, Newman AJ, Jezzard P, et al. (2004) The cortical organization of audio-visual sentence comprehension: An fMRI study at 4 Tesla. Cognitive Brain Research 20: 111–119.
22. Constable RT, Pugh KR, Berroya E, Mencl WE, Westerveld M, et al. (2004) Sentence complexity and input modality effects in sentence comprehension: An fMRI study. NeuroImage 22: 11–21.
23. Gernsbacher MA, Kaschak MP (2003) Neuroimaging studies of language production and comprehension. Annual Review of Psychology 54: 91–114.
24. Meyler A, Keller TA, Cherkassky VL, Gabrieli JDE, Just MA (2008) Modifying the brain activation of poor readers during sentence comprehension with extended remedial instruction: A longitudinal study of neuroplasticity. Neuropsychologia 46: 2580–2592.
25. Cutting L, Clements A, Courtney S, Rimrodt S, Schafer J, et al. (2006) Differential components of sentence comprehension: Beyond single word reading and memory. NeuroImage 29: 429–438.
26. Glaser YG, Martin RC, Van Dyke JA, Hamilton AC, Tan Y (2013) Neural basis of semantic and syntactic interference in sentence comprehension. Brain and Language 126: 314–326.
27. Benjamin CF, Gaab N (2012) What's the story? The tale of reading fluency told at speed. Human Brain Mapping 33: 2572–2585.
28. Simos PG, Rezaie R, Fletcher JM, Juranek J, Papanicolaou AC (2011) Neural correlates of sentence reading in children with reading difficulties. NeuroReport 22: 674–678.
29. Rimrodt S, Clements-Stephens A, Pugh K, Courtney S, Gaur P, et al. (2009) Functional MRI of sentence comprehension in children with dyslexia: Beyond word recognition. Cerebral Cortex 19: 402–413.
30. Karni A, Morocz I, Bitan T, Shaul S, Kushnir T, et al. (2005) An fMRI study of the differential effects of word presentation rates (reading acceleration) on dyslexic readers' brain activity patterns. Journal of Neurolinguistics 18: 197–219.
31. Wagner RK, Torgesen JK (1987) The nature of phonological processing and its causal role in the acquisition of reading skills. Psychological Bulletin 101: 192–212.
32. Wolf M, Bowers PG (1999) The double-deficit hypothesis for the developmental dyslexias. Journal of Educational Psychology 91: 415–438.
33. Tallal P (1980) Auditory temporal perception, phonics, and reading disabilities in children. Brain and Language 9: 182–198.
34. Mody M, Studdert-Kennedy M, Brady S (1997) Speech perception deficits in poor readers: Auditory processing or phonological coding. Journal of Experimental Child Psychology 64: 199–231.
35. Goswami U, Thomson J, Richardson U, Stainthorp R, Hughes D, et al. (2002) Amplitude envelope onsets and developmental dyslexia: A new hypothesis. Proceedings of the National Academy of Sciences 99: 10911–10916.
36. Lehongre K, Ramus F, Villiermet N, Schwartz D, Giraud A-L (2011) Altered low-gamma sampling in auditory cortex accounts for the three main facets of dyslexia. Neuron 72: 1080–1090.
37. Hoeft F, Hernandez A, McMillon G, Taylor-Hill H, Martindale JL, et al. (2006) Neural basis of dyslexia: A comparison between dyslexic and nondyslexic children equated for reading ability. The Journal of Neuroscience 26: 10700–10708.
38. Oldfield RC (1971) The assessment and analysis of handedness: The Edinburgh inventory. Neuropsychologia 9: 97–113.
39. Wechsler D (1999) Manual for the Wechsler Abbreviated Intelligence Scale. San Antonio, TX: The Psychological Corporation.
40. Wagner R, Torgesen J, Rashotte C (1999) Comprehensive Test of Phonological Processing. Austin, TX: Pro-Ed.

41. Wolf M, Denckla MB (2005) RAN/RAS: Rapid Automatized Naming and Rapid Alternating Stimulus Tests. Austin, TX: Pro-Ed.
42. Woodcock RW (1998) Woodcock Reading Mastery Tests, Revised Normative Update. Circle Pines, MN: American Guidance Service.
43. Torgesen J, Wagner R, Rashotte C (1999) Test of Word Reading Efficiency. Austin, Texas: Pro-Ed. Inc.
44. Brown JI, Fishco VV, Hanna G (1993) Nelson-Denny Reading Test. Itasca, IL: Riverside Publishing Company.
45. Woodcock RW, McGrew KS, Schrank FA, Mather N (2007) Woodcock-Johnson III Normative Update. Rolling Meadows, IL: Riverside Publishing.
46. Cioffi G (2010) Fluency. University of New Hampshire, Durham, NH.
47. Taylor SE, Frackenpohl H, Pettee JL (1960) Grade level norms for the components of the fundamental reading skill. NY: Educational Developmental Laboratories.
48. Brainard DH (1997) The psychophysics toolbox. Spatial Vision 10: 433–436.
49. Thesen S, Heid O, Mueller E, Schad LR (2000) Prospective acquisition correction for head motion with image-based tracking for real-time fMRI. Magnetic Resonance in Medicine 44: 457–465.
50. Friston KJ, Holmes AP, Worsley KJ, Poline JP, Frith CD, et al. (1994) Statistical parametric maps in functional imaging: a general linear approach. Human Brain Mapping 2: 189–210.
51. Friston KJ, Holmes AP, Price C, Büchel C, Worsley K (1999) Multisubject fMRI studies and conjunction analyses. NeuroImage 10: 385–396.
52. Chumbley J, Worsley K, Flandin G, Friston K (2010) Topological FDR for neuroimaging. NeuroImage 49: 3057–3064.
53. Chumbley JR, Friston KJ (2009) False discovery rate revisited: FDR and topological inference using Gaussian random fields. NeuroImage 44: 62–70.
54. Mechelli A, Friston KJ, Price CJ (2000) The effects of presentation rate during word and pseudoword reading: A comparison of PET and fMRI. Journal of Cognitive Neuroscience 12: 145–156.
55. McCandliss BD, Cohen L, Dehaene S (2003) The visual word form area: Expertise for reading in the fusiform gyrus. Trends in Cognitive Sciences 7: 293–299.
56. Breznitz Z (2001) The determinants of reading fluency: A comparison of dyslexic and average readers. In M.Wolf (Ed.), Dyslexia, Fluency and the Brain (pp.245–276) Cambridge, MA: York Press.
57. Price CJ, Wise R, Frackowiak R (1996) Demonstrating the implicit processing of visually presented words and pseudowords. Cerebral Cortex 6: 62–70.
58. Jobard G, Crivello F, Tzourio-Mazoyer N (2003) Evaluation of the dual route theory of reading: A metanalysis of 35 neuroimaging studies. NeuroImage 20: 693–712.
59. Ruff I, Blumstein SE, Myers EB, Hutchison E (2008) Recruitment of anterior and posterior structures in lexical–semantic processing: An fMRI study comparing implicit and explicit tasks. Brain and Language 105: 41–49.
60. Gabrieli JD, Poldrack RA, Desmond JE (1998) The role of left prefrontal cortex in language and memory. Proceedings of the National Academy of Sciences 95: 906–913.
61. Demb JB, Desmond JE, Wagner AD, Vaidya CJ, Glover GH, et al. (1995) Semantic encoding and retrieval in the left inferior prefrontal cortex: A functional MRI study of task difficulty and process specificity. Journal of Neuroscience 15: 5870–5878.
62. Thompson-Schill SL, D'Esposito M, Kan IP (1999) Effects of repetition and competition on activity in left prefrontal cortex during word generation. Neuron 23: 513–522.
63. Poldrack RA, Wagner AD, Prull MW, Desmond JE, Glover GH, et al. (1999) Functional specialization for semantic and phonological processing in the left inferior prefrontal cortex. NeuroImage 10: 15–35.
64. Zhu Z, Zhang JX, Wang S, Xiao Z, Huang J, et al. (2009) Involvement of left inferior frontal gyrus in sentence-level semantic integration. NeuroImage 47: 756–763.
65. Dapretto M, Bookheimer SY (1999) Form and content: Dissociating syntax and semantics in sentence comprehension. Neuron 24: 427–432.
66. Pernet C, Poline J, Demonet J, Rousselet G (2009) Brain classification reveals the right cerebellum as the best biomarker of dyslexia. BMC Neuroscience 10: 67.
67. Nicolson RI, Fawcett AJ (2011) Dyslexia, dysgraphia, procedural learning and the cerebellum. Cortex 47: 117–127.
68. Price C, Moore C, Frackowiak R (1996) The effect of varying stimulus rate and duration on brain activity during reading. NeuroImage 3: 40–52.
69. Fulbright RK, Jenner AR, Mencl WE, Pugh KR, Shaywitz BA, et al. (1999) The cerebellum's role in reading: A functional MR imaging study. American Journal of Neuroradiology 20: 1925–1930.
70. Pernet C, Andersson J, Paulesu E, Demonet JF (2009) When all hypotheses are right: A multifocal account of dyslexia. Human Brain Mapping 30: 2278–2292.
71. Booth JR, Wood L, Lu D, Houk JC, Bitan T (2007) The role of the basal ganglia and cerebellum in language processing. Brain Research 1133: 136–144.
72. Shaywitz BA, Skudlarski P, Holahan JM, Marchione KE, Constable RT, et al. (2007) Age-related changes in reading systems of dyslexic children. Annals of Neurology 61: 363–370.
73. Van der Mark S, Bucher K, Maurer U, Schulz E, Brem S, et al. (2009) Children with dyslexia lack multiple specializations along the visual word-form (VWF) system. NeuroImage 47: 1940–1949.

Spherical Lenses and Prisms Lead to Postural Instability in Both Dyslexic and Non Dyslexic Adolescents

Zoi Kapoula*, Chrystal Gaertner, Eric Matheron

IRIS Group, Centre d'Etudes SensoriMotrices UMR8194, CNRS, Université Paris Descartes, Paris, France

Abstract

There is controversy as to whether dyslexic children present systematic postural deficiency. Clinicians use a combination of ophthalmic prisms and proprioceptive soles to improve postural performances. This study examines the effects of convergent prisms and spherical lenses on posture. Fourteen dyslexics (13–17 years-old) and 11 non dyslexics (13–16 years-old) participated in the study. Quiet stance posturography was performed with the TechnoConcept device while subjects fixated a target at eye-level from a distance of 1_m. Four conditions were run: normal viewing; viewing the target with spherical lenses of −1 diopter (ACCOM1) over each eye; viewing with −3 diopters over each eye (ACCOM3); viewing with a convergent prism of 8 diopters per eye. Relative to normal viewing, the −1 lenses increased the surface of body sway significantly whereas the −3 diopter lenses only resulted in a significant increase of antero-posterior body sway. Thus, adolescents would appear to cope more effectively with stronger conflicts rather than subtle ones. The prism condition resulted in a significant increase in both the surface and the antero-posterior body sway. Importantly, all of these effects were similar for the two groups. Wavelet analysis (time frequency domain) revealed high spectral power of antero-posterior sway for the prism condition in both groups. In the ACCOM3 condition, the spectral power of antero-posterior sway decreased for non dyslexics but increased for dyslexics suggesting that dyslexics encounter more difficulty with accommodation. The cancelling time for medium range frequency (believed to be controlled by the cerebellum), was shorter in dyslexics, suggesting fewer instances of optimal control. We conclude that dyslexics achieve similar postural performances albeit less efficiently. Prisms and lenses destabilize posture for all teenagers. Thus, contrary to adults, adolescents do not seem to use efferent, proprioceptive ocular motor signals to improve their posture, at least not immediately when confronted to convergence accommodation conflict.

Editor: Andrea Serino, University of Bologna, Italy

Funding: This study is funded by CNRS (www.cnrs.fr). The funders had no role in study design, data collection and analysis, decision to publish, or preparation of the manuscript.

Competing Interests: The authors have declared that no competing interests exist.

* E-mail: zoi.kapoula@egp.aphp.fr

Introduction

Postural control during quiet stance involves continuous multisensory central integration of visual, vestibular and proprioceptive inputs in order to produce motor commands controlling the body's position in space. Kapoula and Bucci [1] measured postural control in 13 year-old dyslexic adolescents during both closed and opened eye conditions while they were instructed to fixate a target at distances of 25 cm and 150 cm. Dyslexics were more unstable during such fixation tasks regardless of the distance at which the target was placed, be it proximal or distal. Nevertheless, when they were asked to make active vergence eye movements between the proximal and the distal target (convergence-divergence), their postural stability improved and became almost normal, while no significant change was observed in the non dyslexic control group. Moreover, a separate eye movement study [1] performed with the aid of video-oculography demonstrated marked fixation instability for dyslexics in the simple task requiring prolonged fixation. This was in keeping with single posturography testing conditions. Thus, Kapoula and Bucci [1] concluded that rather than suffering from a primary postural syndrome, dyslexic adolescents exhibit ocular fixation instability coupled with a particularly reduced capacity to maintain the angle of vergence at the required depth, resulting in the putative postural instability observed in this patient population. Unstable fixation may be due to attention fluctuation. Actively performing vergence eye movements engages their visual attention thus leading to improved postural stability. Rochelle et al. [2] also proposed that postural instability in dyslexics might be due to their diminished capacity to maintain attention.

Such interpretations are at variance with studies which suggest a postural deficiency in dyslexics. For example, Quercia et al. [3], and Pozzo et al. [4] suggested that there is a postural deficiency syndrome in dyslexia, that is an alteration of postural equilibrium accompanied by a deficit in the sensory processing of proprioceptive afferences from the legs and feet, and a deficit of visual information and extraocular proprioceptive input (see [3,4]). Vieira et al. [5] used a double task (reading words of different colors) inspired from the well known Stroop test, introduced in 1935. They studied both dyslexics (age range of 8–16, mean age 12) before and after wearing prisms and proprioceptive soles for a period of 3 months as well as a control group of non dyslexics. The authors reported no difference between groups with respect to postural stability in the fixation control task. In contrast, for the double task, postural instability was greater in dyslexics than in controls; moreover, after the 3-month period of prismatic treatment combined with soles, this difference was resolved. Consequently, the Viera study [5] suggests that postural deficits in dyslexics are task specific and that prisms combined with soles are useful for improving postural stability. Note that posture recordings were performed without prisms and soles, both before and after the 3-month trial period. We will return to the use of prisms later. As far as the double task is concerned, another study from our group [6] combining posturography with the Stroop task was run on older adolescents. We used a series of words of different colors presented on a page. The participants had to keep themselves from reading the word and instead name the color of the ink in which the word was written – the task was similar but not identical to that used by Vieira et al [5]. The mean age of the adolescents studied by Kapoula et al. [6] was 15 years-old (14–17). The results demonstrated no deficit for the dyslexic versus the control group relative to basic postural parameters i.e. surface area of the center of pressure (CoP) excursions, the standard deviations of lateral and antero-posterior excursions, and its variance of speed. Subtle differences were found in the time frequency domain (wavelet analysis) suggesting relative inefficiency, yet without deterioration of stability. Thus, the existence of a postural deficit in dyslexics remains controversial.

We will now return to the prisms. One of the many hypotheses advanced in order to account for the origin of developmental dyslexia points toward a possible dysfunction of the cerebellum (e.g., see [7,8]). To test this hypothesis, Brookes et al. [9] studied prism adaptation and showed that in most cases of dyslexia impairment of such adaptation does indeed occurs. The use of prisms as a tool for reducing some of the difficulties associated with reading has been studied by several research teams [10–14]. Motivated by the clinical use of prisms on postural behavior in dyslexia, the present laboratory study aims to assess the immediate effects of convergent prisms on posture in dyslexic and non-dyslexic teenagers. Prisms deviate the images and require a change in the ocular motor vergence angle. In healthy adults, use of convergent prisms is known to improve postural stability [15]. Whether a similar effect can be seen in adolescents (dyslexic or non-dyslexic) is not yet known. As mentioned in the study conducted by Vieira et al. [5], prisms were not used during posture recordings; prisms and proprioceptive soles were used as clinical treatment for 3 months. The present study aims to respond to the theoretical question of the immediate effects produced by convergent prisms and does not apply the prism configuration used in the Vieira study [5] even though the clinical configuration of the prisms used might also exhibit a convergent component. Other relevant laboratory studies on prisms and posture concern vertical prisms. Matheron et al. [16] and Matheron and Kapoula [17] used small vertical prisms in adults and reported that the effects on posture are complex, improving or deteriorating posture, depending on the eye wearing the prism (dominant *versus* non dominant). Indeed, while recording eye movements, Matheron et al. [18] showed that the quality of vergence eye movements that reduce more or less efficiently the disparity induced by the prism depends on the eye wearing the vertical prism: eye movements being more appropriate when the dominant eye wears the prism. Vertical prisms in children and their effect on posture were not examined in these above mentioned studies.

It should be noted that prisms modify the vergence angle thereby creating a conflict with the accommodation of the eyes. Accordingly, in the present study we therefore examined the effects of accommodation. To this end we used a negative spherical lense over each eye (-1 or -3 diopters). A change of accommodation produced by the lenses causes conflict with the vergence angle. The conflict technique used here aims to test the potential of each of these two initial catalysts (prism-induced vergence and lense-induced accommodation) in modifying postural stability in adolescents. One such methodology has been used in the past by our group (see [19]). It should be noted that because of reciprocal interactions between vergence and accommodation, the use of a prism will ultimately result in a slight modification in accommodation, and conversely a spherical lens accommodative change will also modify the vergence angle. These two interactions are described by the well known ratios of accommodative convergence to accommodation – AC/A – or convergent accommodation to convergence – CA/C – (e.g. [20,21]). The results show that due to such conflicts, both prisms and spherical lenses, particularly those of small power, reduce postural stability and they do so similarly in both dyslexic and non-dyslexic adolescents. Wavelet analysis in the time frequency domain reveals increased spectral power for the prisms in both groups and suggests more difficulty with accommodation lenses in dyslexics as well as less efficient control of medium range frequencies hypothetically depending on the cerebellum. Taken together the results provide evidence for the importance of vergence and accommodation, such that when dyslexic and non-dyslexic teenagers are confronted by the conflict induced by prisms and lenses, a demonstrable deterioration in posture can be found.

Materials and Methods

Ethics Statement

The postural control investigation complied with the tenets of the Declaration of Helsinki and was approved by the local human experimentation committee, the "Comité de Protection des Personnes" (CPP) Ile de France VI (No: 07035), Necker Hospital in Paris, France. Written, informed consent was obtained from the participant's parents after the nature of the procedure had been explained.

Subjects

Twenty-five emmetropic adolescents (5 females) were recruited from the College of Saint Sulpice in Paris, France. Fourteen were dyslexics (3 females, 11 males) in the age range of 13–17 years (15.6±0.9), and 11 non dyslexics (2 females, 9 males) in the age range of 13–16 years (15.1±1.0).

Dyslexics were admitted to this college precisely because they were known to be dyslexic. They underwent extensive examination, including neurological/psychological and phonological tests which were conducted during the course of the current year of the present study. For each participant, their rate of reading, text comprehension, as well as their capacity to read word/pseudo words was evaluated by using the L2MA battery [22]. This is the standard test developed by the applied psychology centre of Paris, and is used extensively in France. Inclusion criteria were: scores in these tests beyond two standard deviations; a normal mean intelligence quotient (IQ, evaluated with WISC III), i.e., between 85 and 115. Attention and concentration problems in the absence of hyperactivity were present in 6 of the dyslexics (3 with severe dyslexia and 3 with moderate); no teenager had dyspraxia. Such a population, including a few cases of teenagers with attention problems, is representative of the general dyslexic population. At secondary school, dyslexics followed the same educational program as the other pupils with the exception of additional classes for improving reading and orthographic skills. In parallel, they followed individual training with an orthophonist. However, reading difficulties persisted and were especially severe for 5 of the students. Problems with orthography were also present in 4 of the dyslexics.

Non-dyslexic adolescents had to satisfy the following criteria: no known neurological or psychiatric abnormalities, no history of reading difficulty, no visual stress or any difficulties with near vision. IQ and reading measurements could not be applied to these teenagers. It should be noted that there is no evidence that postural control depends on intelligence. Non dyslexics were selected by the director of their school on the basis of their overall school performance which includes their score in French (reading, understanding, and orthography), mathematics and foreign languages all of which were above the mean score of the class. It should also be noted that the reading score for non dyslexics was higher than that of dyslexics. Recruitment of non dyslexics adolescents based entirely on academic performance alone has been done previously by others [23–25].

Platform characteristics

To measure postural stability, we used a force platform (principle of strain gauge) consisting of two dynamometric clogs (Standards by Association Française de Posturologie; produced by TechnoConcept, Céreste, France). Body sway was evaluated by computing the excursions of the center of pressure (CoP) measured over a period of 51.2 seconds; the equipment contained an Analog–Digital converter of 16 bits and the sampling frequency of the CoP was 40 Hz.

Visual target

The visual target was placed at eye level for each subject in upright stance on the force platform. A white wall was used to display the target along the vertical midline. The visual target was a picture with a little cross "x" (see Figure 1).

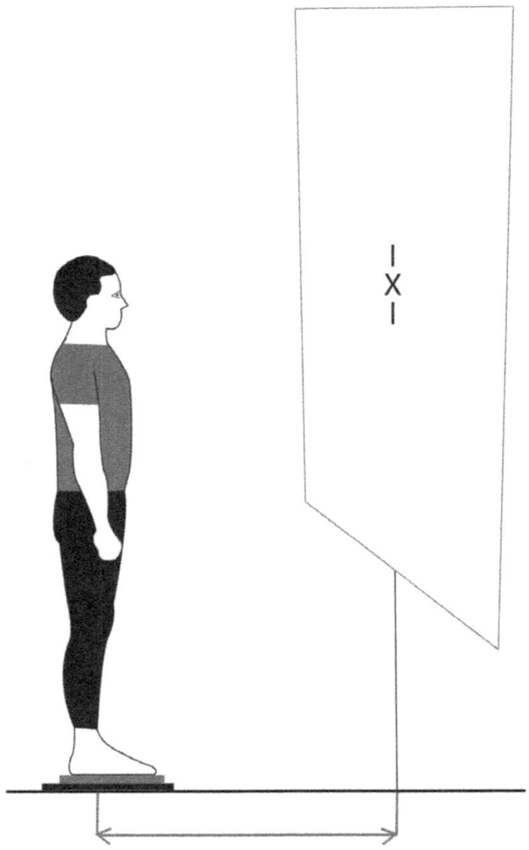

Figure 1. Illustrations of posturographic testing conditions. The subject viewed the "X" target on the screen at eye-level and from distance of 1 m.

Testing conditions

Subjects were placed on the force platform and were asked to fixate the "x" target in the straight ahead position for 51.2 seconds. The target was positioned at eye-level and at a distance of 100 cm (see Figure 1). There were four conditions: normal viewing (NV), accommodation with a negative spherical lens of −1 diopter in front of each eye (ACCOM1), accommodation with a negative spherical lens of −3 diopters in front of each eye (ACCOM3), vergence with a convergent prism of 8 diopters in front of each eye (PRISM).

For the condition ACCOM3, the use of a −3 diopter spherical lens in front of each eye was aimed at bringing the accommodation to 33 cm, conflicting with the accommodation required by the physical distance of the target on the screen (1 m i.e., −1 spherical diopter). Such spherical negative lenses caused blur and stimulated accommodation, and subsequently accomodative convergence. The normal AC/A ratio [Accommodative/Convergence (in prism Diopters)/Accommodation (in spherical diopters)] is 3–4 (see [26]). Mutti et al. [27] showed that the AC/A ratio does not change significantly with age between 6 to 14 years. Therefore, given the −3 diopters lenses we used, the expected accommodation would be −4 spherical diopters, and the expected accommodative convergence would be 10–12 prisms diopters, which approximately corresponds to 5–6° of convergence (1 prism diopter = 0.57°). Note that the vergence angle while fixating the target naturally at a distance of 1_m should be about 3.4° and at a distance of 33 cm around 9°. Thus, the modified vergence angle will also be in conflict with the vergence angle required by the physical distance (3.4° for 1_m viewing distance).

For the condition ACCOM1, the required accommodation for vergence at 1_m is −1 spherical diopter. By inserting a −1 spherical diopter lens in front of each eye we induce an accommodative requirement of 2 diopters. Thus, the accommodation requirement and the potential conflict with the vergence angle were less than in the ACCOM3 condition; considering the accommodation vergence interaction and the hypothetical AC/A ratio of 3–4, one would expect the vergence angle to also be modified to 6–8 prism diopters (corresponding to 3–4°), which is close but not identical to the vergence angle required by the physical distance of 1 m. This conflict is also smaller for the ACCOM1 than for the ACCOM3 condition.

The prism condition was performed as follows: the target on the screen was always positioned at a distance of 1 m. An 8 diopter convergent prism was placed in front of each eye. Such a prism should stimulate convergence of the eyes by 16 prism diopters approximately corresponding to the vergence required by a target presented at a distance of 33 cm (9°). The initial conflict here was between the vergence angle induced by the prism and the vergence angle required by the physical distance; also a conflict between the convergence angle induced by the prism and the accommodation corresponding to the physical distance of 1_m. Again, because of the reciprocal interaction between convergence and accommodation, the prism induced convergence could modify the accommodation. The normal CA/C ratio being 0.1, i.e., 10 prismatic diopters of convergence would cause approximatively 1 spherical diopter of accommodation; one would expect that prisms bring accommodation to −2.6 diopters, i.e., a level still different from that required by the 1_m physical distance. Thus, for all conditions except the NV, there was a mismatch between both vergence and accommodation as they are related to each other, as well as between vergence and accommodation and conflicts relative to values required by the physical distance.

Throughout the experiment the participants wore an ophthalmologic spectacle frame upon which were inserted the spherical lenses or the prisms. The Fresnel prisms used did not alter visibility of the fixation target. The order of the conditions was counterbalanced. Between conditions, the participants sat on a chair and one minute rest period was provided. We asked the participants to close their eyes before standing up. Then, upon a "go" signal given by the investigator, the children opened their eyes and the posturographic recordings were initiated. No preliminary training was necessary, as all teenagers readily performed the sequence of conditions.

Basic postural parameters

We analyzed the surface of the CoP excursions, the standard deviations of lateral (SDx) and anteroposterior (SDy) body sways and the variance of speed. The surface area was measured with the confidence ellipse including 90% of the CoP positions sampled eliminating the extreme points [28].

Frequency analysis

We also applied a wavelet non linear analysis to study frequency in the time domain. Applied to CoP displacements, the wavelet transform elaborates a time-frequency chart of body sway [29,30]. The wavelet analysis used by the software is a continuous one. The mother wavelet used is Morlet. The time-frequency plane's principle advantage is its double resolution (time and frequency). Thus, the fact that the spectrum of the body sway is not constant over time is shown. The wavelet analysis was applied on the anteroposterior and mediolateral sway data. The spectral power was calculated for the frequency bands 0.05–0.5 Hz (F1), 0.5–1.5 Hz (F2), higher than 1.5 Hz (F3) on the anteroposterior and mediolateral sways as power indices (PIy and PIx, respectively). The hypothetical physiological significance of the spectral power of different bands is as follows: 0–0.5 Hz visual-vestibular [31,32,33], 0.5–1.5 Hz cerebellar [33], >1.5 Hz reflexive loops [30,34]. As a rule, power in the higher band (F3) is minimal in healthy subjects during quiet standing, but it can be observed with aging, and postural pathology, or in dynamic postural conditions [30]. Moreover, the canceling time (CT) of each frequency band was also calculated for the antero-posterior (CTy) and mediolateral (CTx) sway, i.e., the total time during which the spectral power of the body sway for the frequency range was cancelled by the posture control mechanisms; the longer the canceling time of a frequency band, the better the posture control [29,30]. The fact that a certain frequency has its power reduced to zero over a period of time shows that there has been a successful action of the postural control system since the overall entropy of the sway is reduced. While most healthy subjects exhibit these zero power instances in their postural sway spectrum, the pathological subjects cannot. How the cancelled frequencies are "chosen" by the postural control system is not known, but it may be assumed that the choice criterion is the minimization of muscular effort required for controlling the sway. The postural instability index (PII) which quantifies the postural performance by taking into account the two precedent indices (PI and CT), was also calculated [29,30] and yielded the following results: PII = SxSyPI(F1, F2, F3)/CT(F1, F2, F3). In healthy adults and during the single quiet stance task, the PII is close to unity (see [30]). This additional analysis and associated parameters were obtained with the software PosturoPro (Framiral, Cannes, France, www.framiral.fr).

Statistical analysis

After the log transformation of the data (due to differences in variance), a mixed ANOVA design was used, with a main factor, the different viewing conditions with 4 levels (NV, ACCOM1, ACCOM3 and PRISM), and one inter-subject factor with 2 levels, subjects with dyslexia or not. The post hoc comparisons were done by Fischer's PLSD test. $P<0.05$ was considered significant.

Results

Results for basic posture parameters

Means and standard errors are shown in Table 1 for each group of subjects (Dyslexics and Controls) and for each condition (NV, ACCOM1, ACCOM3 and PRISM) for all basic postural parameters, i.e. the surface area of CoP excursions, the standard deviation of lateral and anterior-posterior body sway, and the variance of speed.

There was no group effect or interaction between the inter-subject factor and the viewing conditions for all parameters. In contrast, there was a main effect of the viewing conditions on the surface area of CoP ($F(3,69) = 3.72$, $p = .015$), and on the standard deviation of anterior-posterior body sway ($F(3,69) = 5.85$, $p = .001$), but not on the standard deviation of lateral body sway ($F(3,69) = 1.05$, $p = .376$), nor on the variance of speed ($F(3,69) = 2.60$, $p = .060$). Next will be presented the post-hoc analysis for the accommodation and prisms conditions.

Effects of accommodation

The Fischer's PLSD post hoc showed significant increase of the surface area of the CoP for the ACCOM1 compared with the NV ($p = .046$). Interestingly, lenses of −3 diopters in the ACCOM3 condition did not induce significant increase of surface of the body sway (see Figure 2-A).

In contrast, the ACCOM3 condition caused a significant increase of the standard deviation of anterior-posterior body sway compared to NV ($p = .048$), see Figure 2-B.

Effects of prisms

The PRISM condition increased the surface significantly compared to the NV condition ($p = .001$); moreover it also increased the standard deviation of anterior-posterior body sway relative to NV ($p = .0001$). See Figure 2-A.

Comparison Accommodation vs. Prism conditions

The standard deviation of anterior-posterior body sways for the PRISM was higher than that for either of the accommodation conditions (respectively $p = .008$ and $p = .037$, see Figure 2-B).

To summarize, both, the lenses and the prisms modified spatial but not temporal parameters of postural control and they did so similarly for dyslexic and non dyslexic teenagers.

Results for frequency analysis

This section presents the results of the wavelet analysis applied on the CoP displacements (see Methods). Table 2 shows the group means and the standard errors of the postural instability index (PII), the canceling time of each frequency band and the spectral power for different frequency bands for anteroposterior and medio-lateral sways. Results are shown for each of the four conditions and for each group of subjects.

Effect of prisms

There was a main effect of the condition on the power index for the low frequency band (PIy 1, $F(3,69) = 3.03$, $p = .035$) and for the

Table 1. Postural stability measurements in quiet stance (51.2 seconds duration) for basic parameters.

	Conditions			
	Normal Viewing	**Accommodation 1**	**Accommodation 3**	**Convergent Prisms 8**
Surface of CoP (mm^2)				
Dyslexics	164.35±26.06	272.84±35.50	251.95±40.72	282.27±39.66
Controls	223.91±39.23	295.61±79.92	216.77±27.76	337.49±52.46
Standard deviation of lateral sway (mm)				
Dyslexics	2.84±0.33	3.80±0.38	3.54±0.43	3.29±0.31
Controls	3.81±0.49	3.85±0.55	3.14±0.30	3.95±0.44
Standard deviation of A/P sway (mm)				
Dyslexics	4.28±0.34	5.68±0.83	5.28±0.35	6.15±0.58
Controls	4.35±0.24	4.96±0.79	4.99±0.37	6.51±0.62
Speed variance (mm^2/s^2)				
Dyslexics	44.93±8.49	58.58±10.94	46.78±8.11	63.94±8.93
Controls	62.33±12.43	66.85±10.11	67.28±9.02	76.05±11.27

Means and standard errors of the surface of CoP, standard deviations of lateral and of anteroposterior body sway, and variance of speed for each conditions i.e., normal viewing (NV), accommodation with a negative spherical lens of −1 diopter in front of each eye (ACCOM1), accommodation with a negative spherical lens of −3 three diopters in front of each eye (ACCOM3), and with convergent prism of 8 diopters in front of each eye (PRISM) for 14 dyslexics and 11 non dyslexic adolescents.

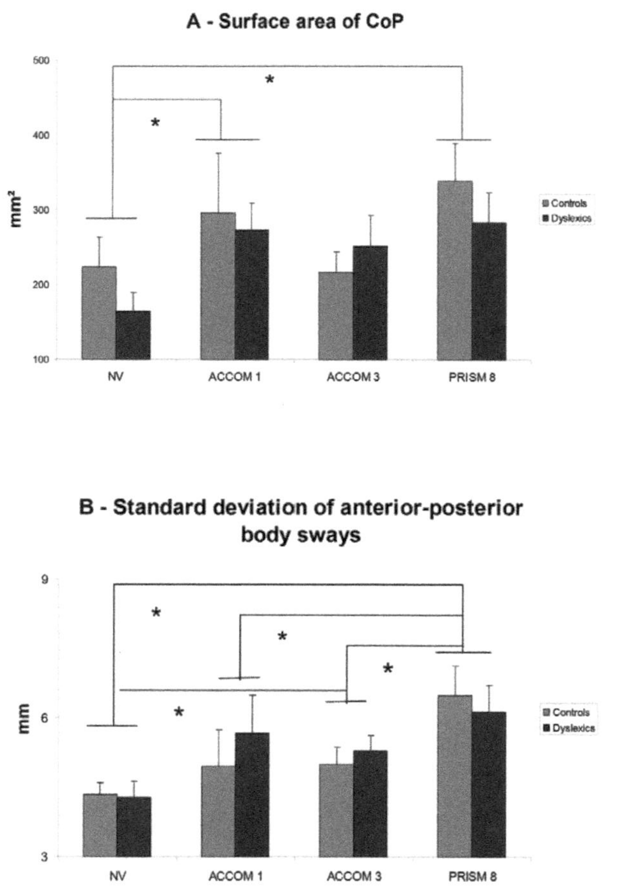

Figure 2. Effects of spherical lenses and prisms on postural parameters. Means of the surface area of CoP (**A**) and of the standard deviations of anteroposterior (SDy) body sway (**B**) for both, Dyslexic and Control adolescents. Error bars represent the standard error. Asterisks indicate significant differences ($p<0.05$).

high frequency band (PIy 3, $F(3,69) = 2.87$, $p = .043$) on the antero-posterior sway. The Fisher's PLSD post hoc showed significant increase of PIy 1 and of PIy 3 for the PRISM condition compared to the NV condition (p = . 011 and p = .019, respectively), also compared to the ACCOM1 condition (p = .013 and p = .033, respectively) and to the ACCOM3 condition (p = .017 and p = .019, respectively (see Figure 3A,B).

Effect of group

There was a main effect of group for two of the parameters elaborated from the wavelet analysis: the canceling time of medium frequency band (0.5–1.5 Hz, hypothetically controlled by the cerebellum) was shorter for dyslexics than non dyslexics; this was the case for both the antero-posterior (CTy) and the mediolateral (CTx) sway (respectively, $F(1,23) = 7.16$, $p = .014$ and $F(1,23) = 5.94$, $p = .023$, see Figure 4).

Group condition interaction

A significant interaction between group and condition was found on the parameter PIy 1, i.e., the power index for the low frequency band on the antero-posterior sway (PIy 1, $F(3,69) = 4.02$, $p = .011$ (see Figure 5). The Fisher's PLSD post hoc showed significant increment of the PIy 1 in dyslexics *versus* controls for the ACCOM3 condition ($p<0.05$). Comparisons within each group show the following. In dyslexics, the PIy 1 is higher in ACCOM3 and in the PRISM conditions compared to the NV (p = . 014 and $p = .0009$, respectively), and also compared to the ACCOM1 condition (p = .022 and p = .001, respectively). In contrast, for the controls, this parameter is lower in the ACCOM3 condition relative to the PRISM condition (p = .046).

To summarize, the main effects revealed by wavelet analysis are for antero-posterior sway: the PRISM condition shows the highest spectral power for both groups, in the ACCOM3 condition the power index is higher in dyslexics than non dyslexics; canceling time of the medium range frequency of both, antero-posterior or mediolateral sway are shorter for dyslexics than for non dyslexics. The statistically significant effects from both sections are summarized in Table 3.

Table 2. Values of postural parameters from wavelet analysis.

		Controls	Dyslexics
Wavelets PII	*NV*	1.85±0.19	1.40±0.17
	ACCOM1	1.63±0.18	1.46±0.11
	ACCOM3	1.62±0.20	1.67±0.12
	PRISM	1.80±0.15	1.82±0.10
Ply (mm^2*10^6) 0–0.5 Hz	*NV*	73.58±1.80	70.91±1.04
	ACCOM1	73.46±1.93	71.17±1.28
	ACCOM3	70.70±1.69	74.82±1.41
	PRISM	74.26±2.15	76.33±1.24
0.5–1.5 Hz	*NV*	61.40±2.15	58.39±1.70
	ACCOM1	61.26±2.03	59.25±1.10
	ACCOM3	59.60±1.60	60.77±1.46
	PRISM	62.50±1.61	63.27±1.17
>1.5 Hz	*NV*	45.46±2.08	41.73±1.63
	ACCOM1	44.36±1.71	42.73±1.20
	ACCOM3	42.99±1.88	44.2±1.36
	PRISM	46.51±1.56	46.70±1.11
Plx (mm^2*10^6) 0–0.5 Hz	*NV*	68.80±2.88	63.61±2.55
	ACCOM1	67.05±2.98	64.10±1.84
	ACCOM3	67.09±2.35	67.67±2.02
	PRISM	67.16±2.20	68.12±1.15
0.5–1.5 Hz	*NV*	58.56±2.48	52.77±2.41
	ACCOM1	56.40±2.80	53.32±1.88
	ACCOM3	56.56±2.19	55.29±1.59
	PRISM	55.30±1.98	56.39±1.04
>1.5 Hz	*NV*	41.21±2.81	35.22±2.33
	ACCOM1	38.73±2.76	35.72±1.87
	ACCOM3	39.60±2.67	39.00±1.88
	PRISM	39.00±1.88	39.75±1.10
CTy (s) 0–0.5 Hz	*NV*	0.41±0.07	0.56±0.09
	ACCOM1	0.64±0.19	0.57±0.08
	ACCOM3	0.71±0.15	0.51±0.12
	PRISM	0.50±0.09	0.45±0.09
0.5–1.5 Hz	*NV*	1.33±0.20	0.92±0.12
	ACCOM1	1.48±0.22	0.94±0.09
	ACCOM3	1.66±0.28	0.89±0.14
	PRISM	1.59±0.23	1.11±0.14
>1.5 Hz	*NV*	0.01±0.00	0.01±0.01
	ACCOM1	0.01±0.00	0.01±0.01
	ACCOM3	0.01±0.01	0.00±0.00
	PRISM	0.01±0.00	0.01±0.01
CTx (s) 0–0.5 Hz	*NV*	0.92±0.29	1.33±0.21
	ACCOM1	1.46±0.76	0.99±0.15
	ACCOM3	1.04±0.33	0.94±0.17
	PRISM	0.73±0.16	0.86±0.19
0.5–1.5 Hz	*NV*	0.97±0.12	0.53±0.12
	ACCOM1	0.84±0.18	0.66±0.18
	ACCOM3	1.22±0.28	0.50±0.10
	PRISM	1.19±0.21	0.78±0.12
>1.5 Hz	*NV*	0.01±0.00	0.01±0.01
	ACCOM1	0.01±0.01	0.00±0.00
	ACCOM3	0.02±0.01	0.00±0.00
	PRISM	0.01±0.00	0.01±0.01

Means and standard errors of PII, and PI and CI for each plane (Ply, Plx, Cly and Clx, respectively) for each frequency band (0.05–0.50 Hz, 0.50–1.50 Hz, 1.50–10.00 Hz) and for each condition, i.e. normal viewing (NV), accommodation with a negative spherical lens of −1 diopter in front of each eye (ACCOM1), accommodation with a negative spherical lens of −3 three diopters in front of each eye (ACCOM3), and with convergent prisms of 8 diopters in front of each eye (PRISM); data from 14 dyslexics and 11 non dyslexic adolescents.

Discussion

The study provides several new results:

(1) Spherical lenses modifying accommodation decrease postural stability (increase of standard deviation of anteroposterior body sway and/or of the surface); paradoxically lenses of weaker power are more disturbing.

(2) Convergent prisms also destabilize posture, increasing the surface of body sway and of standard deviation of anteroposterior body sway.

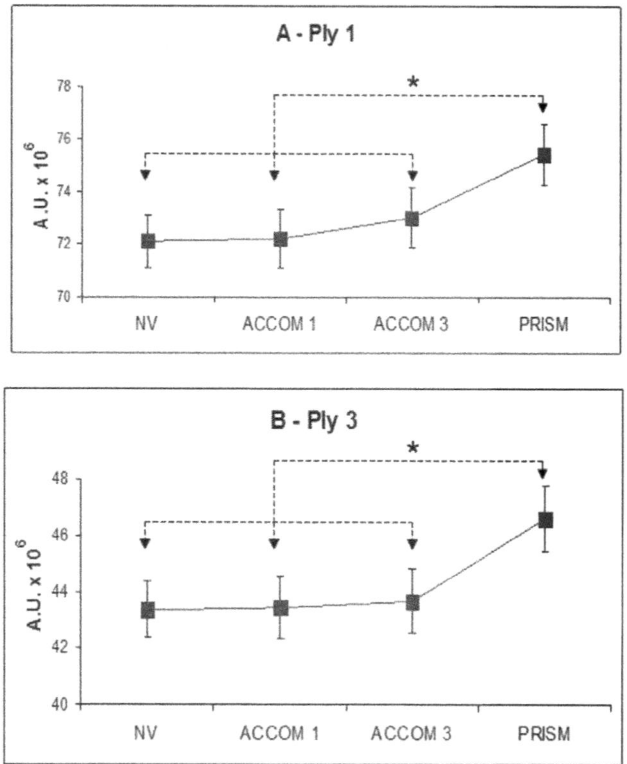

Figure 3. Effects of prisms. The power index of the anteroposterior body sway for the low frequency band (A) and for the high frequency band (B) is higher for the PRISM condition relative to all other conditions. Bars represent the standard error, asterisks indicate significant difference ($p<0.05$).

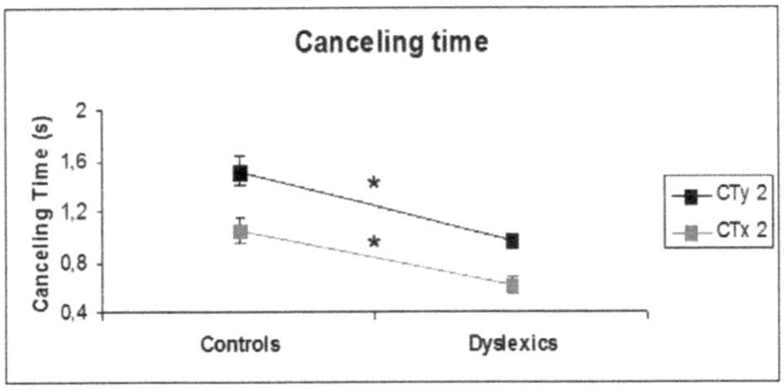

Figure 4. Effects of group in dyslexics vs. controls on the canceling time. Cancelling time of the medium frequency band (0.5–1.5 Hz) for the anteroposterior (CTy 2) and the mediolateral (CTx 2) body sway is shorter for dyslexics. Bars represent the standard error, asterisks indicate significant difference ($p<0.05$).

(3) All effects on basic parameters of posture are similar for the two groups of teenagers and there is no significant difference between dyslexics and non dyslexics.

(4) In the frequency domain, the spectral power for the antero-posterior body sway (low and high frequency bands), is higher for the PRISM condition relative to all other conditions, again with no difference between dyslexics and non dyslexics.

(5) Modification of accommodation with the three diopter spherical lenses decreases the power index of antero-posterior sway for non dyslexics but increases it for dyslexics to a level as high as that for the prism condition.

(6) The canceling time of medium frequency range, believed to be controlled by the cerebellum, is shorter in dyslexics, indicating shorter periods of optimal control.

Each of these results will be discussed below.

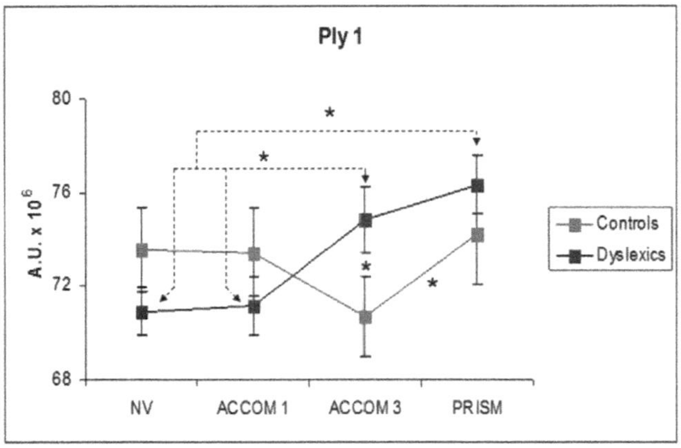

Figure 5. Interaction between groups and tasks for the Ply 1. Power index of anteroposterior body sway for the low frequency band (0–0.5 Hz) believed to be control by vision. Bars represent the standard error, asterisks indicate significant difference ($p<0.05$). Spherical lenses of −3 diopters used in ACCOM3 condition to induce strong accommodation increases considerably Ply 1 for dyslexics but decreases for non dyslexics. On the other hand, non dyslexics show similar Ply for all other viewing conditions while dyslexics show increase Ply for frequency also for the PRISM condition.

Table 3. P-values from ANOVA.

	p Group	*p* Task	*p* Task*Group
Surface mm²	0.675	0.015*	0.366
Sdy (mm)	0.830	0.001*	0.643
Sdx (mm)	0.411	0.376	0.213
Speed Variance (mm²/s)	0.146	0.059°	0.699
Wavelets PII	0.370	0.194	0.177
Ply 1	0.855	0.035*	0.011*
Ply 2	0.646	0.069°	0.269
Ply 3	0.538	0.043*	0.224
Plx1	0.489	0.618	0.261
Plx2	0.277	0.921	0.239
Plx3	0.313	0.591	0.264
CTy1	0.673	0.406	0.385
CTy2	0.014*	0.246	0.432
CTy3	0.471	0.834	0.685
CTx1	0.987	0.237	0.240
CTx2	0.023*	0.197	0.227
CTx3	0.166	0.948	0.105

On the studied postural parameters for group (dyslexics vs. controls), task (normal viewing task, accommodation with a negative spherical lens of −1 and −3 diopters, vergence with a convergent prism of 8 diopters) and group-task interaction effects. Asterisk indicates significant difference ($p<0.05$) and circle indicates marginally significant effects.

Spherical lenses - accommodation and posture instability

As mentioned in the introduction, the spherical lenses used cause blur stimulating accommodation changes by 2 or 4 spherical diopters in the ACCOM1 and ACCOM3 conditions respectively. Such change of accommodation creates a conflict with the vergence angle corresponding to the physical distance (1_m). Due to reciprocal interaction, accommodation changes will induce some changes in the vergence angle, but some conflict will always remain. Although neither the accommodation nor the vergence angle were objectively measured in the study, it is certain that such changes occurred. Here we objectivised the consequences of such changes on postural control. The results showed that changes of the accommodation and to a less degree of vergence have a direct effect on the basic parameters of posture of teenagers. To our knowledge, prior studies of the impact of accommodation on posture are scarse. Early in the 1980's, some studies reported effects of blurring of the images (corresponding to accommodation cues) on postural control (see [35,36]). Our observations in teenagers expand this conclusion.

By what mechanism does the accommodation driver act on postural control? The most relevant study is that of Han and Lennerstrand [37]. These authors reported that vibration of cervical muscles changed the dynamics of accommodative vergence. Therefore, we propose that accommodation, and accommodative vergence induced by the lenses could modify activity in the neck muscles that are known to be a major relay for postural control. Visual, oculomotor and somatosensory inputs are all integrated in the superior colliculus, the cerebellum and the vestibular nuclei (see [38]), and influence the vestibuloocular, vestibulospinal and reticulospinal systems that are involved in postural control (see [39]). At the perceptual level, accommodation provides a cue related to depth. Thus, it is interesting that the major effect on posture in the ACCOM3 condition is seen on the standard deviation of anteroposterior body sway. This effect is plausible physiologically and occurs for the strong power lenses (−3 spherical diopters). Next, we will discuss the paradoxical observation of increase of the surface of body sway for the weaker spherical lenses relative to the control condition.

We propose that posture instability (increase of surface) results when the accommodative response to spherical lenses is inappropriate, e.g., too high or too weak relative to the power of the lens. A similar mechanism has been proposed by Matheron et al. [16,18] in their adult studies dealing with small vertical prisms. We suggest that with spherical lenses of −3 diopters, teenagers can mobilize robust compensatory accommodative responses. Indeed their accommodative abilities are robust [26]. High gain accommodative ability is perhaps reinforced by dense, every day activities such as watching movies, play stations (on PCs, I-Pod, I-Phone). The condition ACCOM1, using 1 diopter lenses, requires a subtle, moderate, modification of the accommodation. Most likely teenagers fail to perform such adjustments; perhaps they over accommodate and this increased the conflict thereby leading to more posture instability. As mentioned in the Introduction, the studies of Mutti et al. [27] show that the AC/A ratio does not change significantly with the age of children from 6 to 14 years old. Yet, the AC/A ratio can increase if the interpupillary distance of the subjects increases (see [40]). To our knowledge, objective measures of the accommodation and of vergence are missing in the literature as well as in the present study. The frequency analysis results to be discussed later indicate significant differences between dyslexics and non dyslexics for the ACCOM3 condition even though the two groups did not differ in terms of basic parameters; presumably the same stability can be obtained via different mechanisms, and accommodation could be more highly demanding for dyslexics.

Moreover, if, as we suggest, accommodative vergence induced by the lenses could modify activity in the neck muscles (see [37]) that are known to be a major relay for postural control, a kinematic analysis using a motion tracking system, instead of simple posturography recordings, would be of interest. Kinematic analysis has been used in children and adolescents, providing accurate descriptions of inter-segmental orientation in multiple postural tasks, an important analysis not possible with posturography platforms (see [41]).

Effects of prisms

The convergent prisms used called the eyes to converge significantly, as if they were fixating at 33_cm, creating a conflict with the vergence required by the physical distance which was 1_m. Convergence of the eyes (even though not measured) occurred. A conflict also exists between the vergence angle and accommodation. Here again, because of the reciprocal interaction between convergence and accommodation, convergence induced by the prisms would modify the accommodation by an amount determined by the AC/A ratio of the teenagers (see Methods). A prior study in healthy adults [15] showed improvement of posture stability with convergent prisms of 5 diopters per eye, despite conflicts. Note that the study in adults compared 200_cm versus 40_cm distances, while in the present study we used 100_cm versus 33_cm for which conflict is perhaps more intense. Kapoula and Lê [15] attributed the improvement of the posture in adults to the benefit from efferent and afferent oculomotor signals related to convergence of the eyes, improving the stability despite conflicts. The observations for teenagers show a different opposite pattern indeed, as the surface of body sway increased as well as the anteroposterior body sway. Perhaps teenagers do not produce well matched vergence accommodation responses when wearing the prisms. Another complementary possibility is that teenagers do not yet rely as much as adults on internal ocular motor signals and thus cannot yet benefit from the convergence to stabilize posture. In other words, the conflict between vergence and accommodation prevails relative to the benefit from strong convergence described in adults by Kapoula and Lê [15]. Furthermore, vision has an important effect in adolescents' body stabilization, and adolescents do not use proprioceptive inputs optimally; Viel et al. [42] suggested that the mechanisms underlying postural control are still maturing during adolescence, which might constitute a transient period of proprioceptive neglect in sensory integration of postural control. Further studies with objective measures of accommodation and of vergence combined with posturography would be of interest. In conclusion, the study shows that convergent prisms have destabilizing immediate effects on posture of teenagers. The frequency analysis in the time domain showed increased spectral power for both low and high frequency ranges in the PRISM condition relative to all other conditions. This additional analysis clearly indicates that prisms are highly demanding, requiring increased energy to maintain postural stability for all teenagers.

No differences in basic posture parameters between dyslexic and non dyslexic teenagers

The comparison between groups for all conditions shows irrevocably no differences between dyslexic and non dyslexic teenagers on the basic parameters of posture control. The evidence provided here is in line with our prior studies [1,6] and argues for no systematic deficits on posture in dyslexics teenagers. As discussed by Kapoula et al. [6] a recruiting bias (school versus clinic) might explain controversies in the literature, as well as differences in age of subjects studied [42] and differences of categories/comorbidity with dyslexia (see [2,43–47]). Other authors have proposed that evaluating postural control in challenging postures, instead of during a simple "standing upright" condition, may be necessary to detect alterations of postural control (e.g. [34,48]). This point was beyond our aim, i.e. to test first the effects of convergent prisms and spherical lenses during quiet upright stance, nevertheless reminds of interest. Other controversies are based mostly on the study of basic parameters of posture. As other studies point to the need to examine further parameters including frequency analysis and diffusion analysis (see [6,49,50], we also studied frequency aspects with wavelets analysis. The subtle differences that were found will be discussed later.

Prisms induce higher spectral power

The major effect of the present study is that the PRISM condition increases the power indices for the low and high frequency ranges for the antero-posterior body-sway (see Figure 3A and 3B). This global effect which concerns both groups provides further evidence, in keeping with the basic posture parameters, that prisms for teenagers are highly demanding. They deteriorate postural stability (increase of surface) and amplify the spectral power for both the low and high frequency ranges that are believed to be controlled by vision, and rapid sensorimotor loops, respectively.

Strong accommodation increases power frequency for dyslexics

For the −3 diopters spherical lens condition, the basic posture parameters showed increase of antero-posterior body sway relative to other conditions similarly for both groups. Yet, the wavelet analysis indicates that such an increase is subtended by different physiologic mechanisms for the two groups of teenagers: for non dyslexics the power index decreases (e.g., relative to normal viewing condition) while for dyslexics it increases. Thus, dyslexics require greater energy expenditure in order to achieve similar postural behaviors in terms of antero-posterior sway. These results indicate that dyslexics might have more difficulty with strong accommodative requirements than non dyslexics. This is congruent with recent studies of children with reading difficulties who were found to have reduced accommodative amplitude assessed by optometric tests (see [51,52]).

Time of optimal posture control is shorter for dyslexics

The wavelet analysis revealed shorter cancellation times for dyslexics with respect to the medium frequency band which is hypothesized to be controlled by the cerebellum; cancellation time was shorter for both lateral and antero-posterior body sways. This observation is compatible with a more general theoretical framework suggesting a cerebellar deficit in dyslexics as being responsible for various difficulties encountered in this patient population with reading, writing and spelling (see [8,53,54]). The above observation is also compatible with our prior study comparing postural control in dyslexic and non dyslexic teenagers while doing the Stroop test [6]. Despite their increased difficulty with such a test, basic parameters of posture stability as measured in dyslexics and non dyslexics were entirely comparable with the exception of the cancellation time in the medium frequency band which were again shorter for dyslexics. In response to the mounting evidence provided by these data, we adduce the hypothesis of the mild inefficiency of cerebellar control of posture in dyslexia. However, such a hypothesis emphasizes the efficiency aspect, dyslexics successfully perform the same postural behaviors as non dyslexics but with greater energetic expenditure. It might also be observed that in more demanding conditions such as balance or dynamic conditions dyslexics differ more clearly from non dyslexics (see [53]). The quiet stance test used here is one of the most common postures humans use to interact with their environment; this test implies multisensory integration and successful stabilization of the body's many components. Yet, this test alone is not sufficient to diagnose postural pathologies. In terms of research however, the quiet stance test has been used to evaluate the effects of prolonged treatment with prisms and soles in dyslexia (e.g. [55]).

Clinical implications

Our study highlights some of the negative effects that convergent prisms can have on postural control in dyslexic and non dyslexic teenagers. Prisms and spherical lenses deteriorate stability and strong accommodation requirements require more energy for dyslexics whose postural control is less efficient than for non dyslexics. Clinical practice often times involves precisely the use of such prisms in conjunction with some convergent action combined with proprioceptive soles [5]. As mentioned above, prisms change not only ocular vergence but also the link with accommodation. Although we cannot exclude *de facto* the benefits which might accrue to some adolescents with respect to the use of convergent prisms, especially adolescents exhibiting some kind of postural syndrome, the present study emphasizes the possible negative effects of prisms on posture control as previously reported with a lower prism diopter (e.g. [16,56–58]). Objective and regular measures of vergence, accommodation and posture, all of which accompany such clinical treatment modalities, could help to improve our understanding of the causal mechanisms of action at work in postural control and eventually strengthen the utility of such treatments. A final point to be made includes the distinction between immediate and long-term effects. The present study has dealt with immediate effects as projected over an interval of 51.2 seconds. How does prolonged exposure to vergence accommodation conflicts ultimately become helpful? This question among others will require further study and analysis. Do the initial negative effects of prisms possibly revert to positive effects improving posture and at what precise period during the course of treatment? Studies of the respective role of prisms, soles and of their interaction are also important.

Beyond the issue of immediate versus long-term exposure effects there are still important questions concerning the existence of postural pathologies in dyslexia and the necessity for prism treatment. Rochelle et al. [2] note that apparent deficits in postural control in developmental dyslexia can be mediated by inclusion of children with hyperactivity. Brookes et al. [59] suggest that mixed results on balance difficulties may be attributable to variability in balance tasks, balance measurement, participant age, and inclusion of comorbid disorders such as ADHD.

The quiet stance posture test used here is not a diagnostic or therapeutic tool but rather a research tool; a similar test has been used to evaluate the effects of prism-sole treatments on dyslexia [55]. Given the negative nature of the immediate effects of prisms and lenses on the posture control of dyslexic and non dyslexic teenagers, and given the difficulty for accommodation experienced by dyslexics, we are inclined to suggest caution and regular follow ups when using prisms as a potentially viable treatment modality in dyslexic teenagers.

Acknowledgments

The authors thank Maria Pia Bucci and Mohamed Djamal for participating in data collection, and Gabi Libede and Paul Locher for English improvement.

Author Contributions

Conceived and designed the experiments: ZK. Performed the experiments: EM. Analyzed the data: ZK EM CG. Contributed reagents/materials/analysis tools: ZK EM CG. Wrote the paper: ZK EM CG.

References

1. Kapoula Z, Bucci MP (2007) Postural control in dyslexic and non-dyslexic children. J Neurol 254: 1174–1183.
2. Rochelle KS, Witton C, Talcott JB (2009) Symptoms of hyperactivity and inattention can mediate deficits of postural stability in developmental dyslexia. Exp Brain Res 192: 627–633.
3. Quercia P, Seigneuric A, Chariot S, Vernet P, Pozzo T, et al. (2005) Ocular proprioception and developmental dyslexia. Sixty clinical observations. J Fr Ophtalmol 28: 713–723.
4. Pozzo T, Vernet P, Creuzot-Garcher C, Robichon F, Bron A, et al. (2006) Static postural control in children with developmental dyslexia. Neurosci Lett 403: 211–215.
5. Vieira S, Quercia P, Michel C, Pozzo T, Bonnetblanc F (2009) Cognitive demands impair postural control in developmental dyslexia: a negative effect that can be compensated. Neurosci Lett 462: 125–129.
6. Kapoula Z, Matheron E, Demule E, Fauvel C, Bucci MP (2011) Postural control during the stroop test in dyslexic and non dyslexic teenagers. PLoS ONE 6(4): e19272. Available: http //dx.plos.org/10.1371/journal.pone.0019272.
7. Nicolson RI, Fawcett AJ (1990) Automaticity: a new framework for dyslexia research? Cognition 35 159–182
8. Nicolson RI, Fawcett AJ, Dean P (2001) Developmental dyslexia: the cerebellar deficit hypothesis. Trends Neurosci 24: 508–511.
9. Brookes RL, Nicolson RI, Fawcett AJ (2007) Prisms throw light on developmental disorders. Neuropsychologia 45: 1921–1930.

10. Schwarz C (1992) [Are prism glasses a sensible measure in treatment of dyslexia?]. Klin Monbl Augenheilkd 200: 599–611.
11. Pestalozzi D (1992) [Further observations of dyslexia patients with prism correction]. Klin Monbl Augenheilkd 200: 614–619.
12. Pestalozzi D (1993) Ophthalmologic aspects of dyslexia: the influence of full prismatic correction of heterophoria on dyslexic symptoms. Ann N Y Acad Sci 682: 397–399.
13. Stavis M, Murray M, Jenkins P, Wood R, Brenham B, et al. (2002) Objective improvement from base-in prisms for reading discomfort associated with mini-convergence insufficiency type exophoria in school children. Binocul Vis Strabismus Q 17: 135–142.
14. Quercia P, Seigneuric A, Chariot S, Bron A, Creuzot-Garcher C, et al. (2007) [Proprioception changes induced by prismatic glasses wear in children suffering from developmental dyslexia]. J Fr Ophtalmol 30: 380–389.
15. Kapoula Z, Le TT (2006) Effects of distance and gaze position on postural stability in young and old subjects. Exp Brain Res 173: 438–445.
16. Matheron E, Le TT, Yang Q, Kapoula Z (2007) Effects of a two-diopter vertical prism on posture. Neurosci Lett 423: 236–240.
17. Matheron E, Kapoula Z (2008) Vertical phoria and postural control in upright stance in healthy young subjects. Clin Neurophysiol 119: 2314–2320.
18. Matheron E, Yang Q, Le TT, Kapoula Z (2008) Effects of ocular dominance on the vertical vergence induced by a 2-diopter vertical prism during standing. Neurosci Lett 444: 176–180.
19. Kapoula Z, Bernotas M, Haslwanter T (1999) Listing's plane rotation with convergence: role of disparity, accommodation, and depth perception. Exp Brain Res 126: 175–186.
20. Ciuffreda KJ, Kenyon RV (1983) Accommodative vergence. In: Schor CM, Ciuffreda KJ, editors. Vergence Eye Movements. Boston: Butterworth-Heinemann, MA.
21. Brautaset Rl, Jennings AJ (2006) Effects of orthoptic treatment on the CA/C and AC/A ratios in convergence insufficiency. Invest Ophtalmol Vis Sci 47: 2876–2880.
22. Chevrie-Muller C, Simon AM, Fournier S (1977) Batterie Langage oral écrit. Mémoire. Attention (L2MA). Paris: Editions du Centre de Psychologie Appliquée.
23. Stein JF, Riddell PM, Fowler MS (1987) Fine binocular control in dyslexic children. Eye (Lond) 1: 433–438.
24. Stein JF, Riddell PM, Fowler S (1988) Disordered vergence control in dyslexic children. Br J Ophthalmol 72: 162–166.
25. Riddell PM, Fowler MS, Stein JF (1990) Spatial discrimination in children with poor vergence control. Percept Mot Skills 70: 707–718.
26. von Noorden GK (1996) Binocular vision and ocular motility: theory and management of strabismus. St.Louis: Mosby. 605 p.
27. Mutti DO, Jones LA, Moeschberger ML, Zadnik K (2000) AC/A ratio, age and refractive error in children. Inv Ophthalmol Vis Sci 41: 2469–2478.
28. Takagi A, Fujimura E, Suehiro S (1985) A new method of statokinesigram area measurement. Application of a statistically calculated ellipse. In: Igarashi M, Black O, editors. Vestibular and visual control on posture and locomotion equilibrium. Basel: Karger. pp 74–79.
29. Dumistrescu M, Lacour M (2006) Nouveaux critères quantitatifs d'analyse du contrôle postural. In: Pérennou D, Lacour M, editors. Efficience et déficiences du contrôle postural. Marseille: Solal éditeur. pp 65–75.
30. Bernard-Demanze L, Dumitrescu M, Jimeno P, Borel L, Lacour M (2009) Age related changes in posture control are differentially affected by postural and cognitive task complexity. Curr Aging Sci 2: 139–149.
31. Naschner LM (1979) Organization and programming of motor activity during posture control. Prog Brain Res 50: 177–184.
32. Kohen-Raz R, Himmelfarb M, Tzur S, Kohen-Raz A, Shub Y (1996) An initial evaluation of work fatigue and circadian changes as assessed by multiplate posturography. Percept Mot Skills 82: 547–557.
33. Paillard T, Costes-Salon C, Lafont C, Dupui P (2002) Are there differences in postural regulation according to the level of competition in judoists? Br J Sports Med 36: 304–305.
34. Lacour M, Bernard-Demanze L, Dumitrescu M (2008) Posture control, aging, and attention resources: models and posture-analysis methods. Neurophysiol Clin 38: 411–421.
35. Paulus W, Straube A, Brandt T (1984) Visual stabilization of posture. Physiological stimulus characteristics and clinical aspects. Brain 107: 1143–1163.
36. Brandt T (1999) Vertigo: Its multisensory syndromes. London: Springer. p 503.
37. Han Y, Lennerstrandt G (1998) Efects of neck muscle proprioceptive activation on the dynamics of monocularly driven horizontal vergence movements. Acta Ophthalmol Scand 76: 283–288.
38. Büttner-Ennever JA (2006) Neuroanatomy of the oculomotor system. Prog Brain Res 151: 1–574.
39. Berthoz A (1988) The role of gaze in compensation of vestibular disfunction: the gaze substitution hypothesis. Prog Brain Res 76: 411–420.
40. Jiang B, Ramamirtham R (2005) The adaptive effect of narrowing the interocular separation on the AC/A ratio. Vis Sci 45: 2704–2709.
41. Mallau S, Vaugoyeau M, Assaiante C (2010) Postural strategies and sensory integration: no turning point between childhood and adolescence. PLoS ONE 5(9): e13078. Available: http://dx.plos.org/10.1371/journal.pone.0013078.
42. Viel S, Vaugoyeau M, Assaiante C (2009) Adolescence: a transient period of proprioceptive neglect in sensory integration of postural control. Motor Control 13: 25–42.
43. Ramus F, Pidgeon E, Frith U (2003) The relationship between motor control and phonology in dyslexic children. J Child Psychol Psychiatry 44: 712–722.
44. Rochelle KS, Talcott JB (2006) Impaired balance in developmental dyslexia? A meta-analysis of the contending evidence. J Child Psychol Psychiatry 47: 1159–1166.
45. Nicolson RI, Fawcett AJ, Brookes RL, Needle J (2010) Procedural learning and dyslexia. Dyslexia 16: 194–212.
46. Patel M, Magnusson M, Lush D, Gomez S, Fransson PA (2010) Effects of dyslexia on postural control in adults. Dyslexia 16: 162–174.
47. Barela JA, Dias JL, Godoi D, Viana AR, de Freitas PB (2011) Postural control and automaticity in dyslexic children: the relationship between visual information and body sway. Res Dev Disabil 32: 1814–1821.
48. Ghulyan V, Paolino M, Lopez C, Dumitrescu M, Lacour M (2005) A new translational platform for evaluating aging or pathology-related postural disorders. Acta Otolaryngol 125: 607–617.
49. Collins JJ, De Luca CJ, Burrows A, Lipsitz LA (1995) Age-related changes in open-loop and closed-loop postural control mechanisms. Exp Brain Res 104: 480–492.
50. Williams HG, McClenaghan BA, Dickerson J (1997) [Spectral characteristics of postural control in elderly individuals]. Arch Phys Med Rehabil 78: 737–744.
51. Palomo-Alvarez C, Puell MC (2008) Accommodative function in school children with reading difficulties. Graefes Arch Clin Exp Ophthalmol 246: 1769–1774.
52. Palomo-Alvarez C, Puell MC (2010) Binocular function in school children with reading difficulties. Graefes Arch Clin Exp Ophthalmol 248: 885–892.
53. Nicolson RI, Fawcett AJ (2005) Developmental dyslexia, learning and the cerebellum. J Neural Transm Suppl 69: 19–36.
54. Nicolson RI, Fawcett AJ (2011) Dyslexia, dysgraphia, procedural learning and the cerebellum. Cortex 47: 117–127.
55. Quercia P, Demougeot L, Dos Santos M, Bonnetblanc F (2011) Integration of proprioceptive signals and attentional capacity during postural control are impaired but subject to improvement in dyslexic children. Exp Brain Res 209: 599–608.
56. Zanfirescu F, Weber B, Marucchi C, Gagey PM, Gentaz R (1988) [Maturation du coefficient de Romberg : influence possible de l'équilibre binoculaire]. Agressologie 29: 661–667.
57. Marucchi C, Zamfirescu F, Gagey PM, Gentaz R, Guillaume P, et al. (1988) [Ophthalmologic determinants of prismatic correction of posture. A retrospective analysis of 39 prescriptions]. Agressologie 29: 693–695.
58. Prevost G (1988) [Eyeglasses and prismatic effects]. Agressologie 29: 697–698.
59. Brookes RL, Tinkler S, Nicolson RI, Fawcett AJ (2010) Striking the right balance: motor difficulties in children and adults with dyslexia. Dyslexia 16: 358–373.

Effect of a Dual Task on Postural Control in Dyslexic Children

Agathe Legrand[1]*, Emmanuel Bui-Quoc[2], Karine Doré-Mazars[1,3], Christelle Lemoine[1], Christophe-Loïc Gérard[4], Maria Pia Bucci[1]

1 Laboratoire de Psychologie et Neuropsychologie Cognitives, IUPDP, Université Paris Descartes, Sorbonne Paris Cité. Institut de Psychologie, Boulogne Billancourt, France, **2** Service d'Ophtalmologie, Hôpital Robert Debré, Paris, France, **3** Institut Universitaire de France, Paris, France, **4** Service de Psychopathologie de l'enfant et de l'adolescent, Hôpital Robert Debré, Paris, France

Abstract

Several studies have examined postural control in dyslexic children; however, their results were inconclusive. This study investigated the effect of a dual task on postural stability in dyslexic children. Eighteen dyslexic children (mean age 10.3±1.2 years) were compared with eighteen non-dyslexic children of similar age. Postural stability was recorded with a platform (TechnoConcept®) while the child, in separate sessions, made reflex horizontal and vertical saccades of 10° of amplitude, and read a text silently. We measured the surface and the mean speed of the center of pressure (CoP). Reading performance was assessed by counting the number of words read during postural measures. Both groups of children were more stable while performing saccades than while reading a text. Furthermore, dyslexic children were significantly more unstable than non-dyslexic children, especially during the reading task. Finally, the number of words read by dyslexic children was significantly lower than that of non-dyslexic children and, in contrast to the non-dyslexic children. In line with the U-shaped non-linear interaction model, we suggest that the attention consumed by the reading task could be responsible for the loss of postural control in both groups of children. The postural instability observed in dyslexic children supports the hypothesis that such children have a lack of integration of multiple sensorimotor inputs.

Editor: Tiziana Zalla, Ecole Normale Supérieure, France

Funding: The authors have no support or funding to report.

Competing Interests: The authors have declared that no competing interests exist.

* E-mail: agathe.legrand@etu.parisdescartes.fr

Introduction

Several studies have explored the effect of a dual task on postural control [1–3], and it has been found that cognitive tasks do influence postural stability. Lacour et al. [4] proposed three models for explaining how cognitive tasks affect postural control. In the cross-domain competition model, attention is shared between the postural performance and the cognitive task; consequently, postural control in a dual-task paradigm is impaired compared to in a single postural task. While several studies of normal adults support this idea [5–7], other investigations have reported opposite findings [8–9]. The nature of the cognitive task used is most likely responsible for the different results. In line with this thinking, the U-shaped non-linear interaction model suggests that the cognitive demand of the secondary task can either improve or diminish postural stability. For instance, an easy cognitive task can shift the focus of attention away from postural control, leading to an improved automatic postural performance [10–12]. However, Huxhold et al. [13] reported that increasing the cognitive demand induces an increase in postural instability. Finally, the third model, the task prioritization model, hypothesizes that subjects prioritize postural control over cognitive activity. This strategy is often used by older people [14] and in cases of pathologies [15].

It should be noted that studies dealing with children's postural control while they perform a cognitive task are quite recent. Indeed, Blanchard et al. [16] studied the effects of a cognitive task on balance in children (between 8 and 10 years old) and reported an improvement in postural stability, in terms of smaller sway variability, when children are performing a task such as counting backward or reading a sentence compared to that recorded when they look at an image. However, they observed that the center of pressure (CoP) path was longer, suggesting that children and adults use different strategies. In contrast, Schmid et al. [17], using a similar task (mentally counting backwards task executed silently), showed a strong perturbation of postural stability in 9-year-old children.

Postural instability has been found to increase in 7-year-old children when they were asked to perform a modified Stroop task [18]; the same phenomenon was found in 5-year-old children, both normal and with developmental coordination disorders, while they were naming simple objects that appeared consecutively on a screen [19]. In a recent study, Olivier et al. [20] examined age-related differences in interference with postural control by cognitive tasks, and showed that the mature level of attention is reached at about 11 years old. In line with the U-shaped non-linear model [4], these authors suggested that there are two independent attentional mechanisms, one for controlling postural control and the other responsible for the cognitive task; two such mechanisms could interfere with each other depending on the difficulty of the tested condition.

The present study examines the question of whether a dual task can influence postural stability in 10-year-old dyslexic children. Dyslexia is a neurobiological disorder characterized by a difficulty in reading acquisition despite adequate intelligence, conventional education and motivation [21]. Different theories have been suggested for the etiology of dyslexia. The phonological theory make the hypothesis that dyslexia is a direct consequence of cognitive deficits specific to the representation and processing of speech sounds [22–24]. Some authors considered that the phonology have a secondary place and that dyslexia is most likely a sensori motor deficit related to: auditory [25], visual [26], cerebellar [27] and the magnocellular impairment [28]. In dyslexic population the oculomotor behavior during reading task has been observed in several studies, and some authors [29–31] showed a different oculomotor pattern during reading with respect to non dyslexic population: longer fixation durations, more frequent fixations, shorter saccade amplitudes and more regressive saccades has been found in dyslexic participants.

Nicolson et al. [32], who reported motor coordination and balance deficits in dyslexic children, advanced the hypothesis that dyslexia is characterized by a cerebellar deficiency. Several subsequent studies were done on the issue, producing conflicting results. For instance, several authors [24,33–34] reported impaired postural control in dyslexia but only in some cases, suggesting that the impairment was not strictly correlated with dyslexia but also with other types of developmental disorders [35].

In a dual-task condition, Nicolson and Fawcett [36] reported that postural stability decreased in dyslexic children, suggesting that this population needs to invest more attentional resources than non-dyslexic children to control their balance. Recent studies [37–38] have suggested that dyslexic children have a postural deficiency syndrome constituting an alteration of postural equilibrium accompanied by a deficit affecting proprioceptive and visual information. A cognitive task, such as reading single words, impairs postural stability in dyslexic children [37]. Interestingly, a vibration of the ankle muscles impaired stability more strongly in dyslexic than in non-dyslexic children, independently of the attentional task; in the condition without vibration, the attentional performance of dyslexics was significantly impaired with respect to the non-dyslexic group of children [38]. According to Nicolson and Fawcett [39], this evidence suggests that the cerebellum, which is responsible for the integration of proprioceptive inputs during balance, could be impaired in the dyslexic population.

In the present study, we compared postural capabilities in a group of dyslexic and non-dyslexic children while they were asked to perform two types of saccadic eye movements (visually guided saccades and voluntary saccades while reading a text silently). Recall that attention is strictly linked to the execution of saccadic eye mouvements [40] and that several structures of the central nervous system in the cerebral cortex (frontal, parietal, occipital) and in the brainstem (paramediane pontine reticular formation and the superior colliculus) play an important role in the postural control [41] as well as in the saccadic eye movement control [42]. Based on these findings, one could expect an interference between oculomotor and postural control. Note that several studies have showed the effect of saccadic eye movement on postural control in adults but none explored this issue in children. For instance, an improvement of postural stability with saccadic eye movements was found [43–47]. In contrast others [48–50] found that saccades increased postural instability. The interest for studing oculomotor tasks together with posture in dyslexic population comes from the fact that studies dealing with oculomotor performance in dyslexics showed poor oculomotor control only during oculomotor cognitive task (as reading) but not during simple oculomotor task as is the case for visually guided saccades [51–54].

Our initial hypothesis was that, in accordance with the U-shaped non-linear interaction model [4], the two oculomotor tasks could influence postural control in dyslexic and non-dyslexic 10-year-old children in different ways given that oculomotor performance and postural capabilities are different in the two groups of children.

Materials and Methods

Subjects

Eighteen dyslexic children participated in the study. The dyslexic children were recruited from the pediatric hospital where they were referred for a complete evaluation of their dyslexia with an extensive examination including neurological/psychological and phonological capabilities. For each child, the time required to read a text, text comprehension, and the ability to read words and pseudowords were evaluated with the L2MA battery [55]. This is the standard test developed by the applied psychology centre in Paris, and is used everywhere in France. Inclusion criteria were scores on the L2MA more than 2 standard deviations from the mean and a normal mean intelligence quotient (IQ, evaluated with the WISC-IV), namely between 80 and 115. The mean age of the dyslexic children was 10.3±0.8 years, the mean IQ was 100±7 and the mean reading age was 8±1 years. The dyslexic children had no signs of hyperactivity or developmental coordination disorder (DCD). Diagnostic and Statistical Manual of Mental Disorders Fourth Edition (DSM-IV) was used to exclude hyperactive children [56]. Dyslexic children were also screened for DCD with the movement assessment battery for children (M-ABC) and their score was above the 21th percentile. A carefully selected age-matched control group (mean age: 10.5±1 years) of 18 non-dyslexic children was chosen. These children had to satisfy the following criteria: no known neurological or psychiatric abnormalities, no history of reading difficulty, and no visual stress or difficulties with near vision. IQ and reading measurements were not available for these children, but their scores for French (reading, comprehension, spelling), mathematics and foreign languages were all beyond the mean scores for the class. Recruitment of controls based on school performance alone has been used by other researchers [57–59].

Both non-dyslexic and dyslexic children underwent an ophthalmological examination accompanied by orthoptic evaluation of their visual functions (median values shown in Table 1).

Visual acuity was normal (≥20/20) for all children in both groups. All children had normal binocular vision (60 seconds of arc or better), as evaluated with the TNO random dot test. The near point of convergence was normal for both groups of children tested (≤5 cm). Moreover, an orthoptic evaluation of vergence fusion capability using prisms and Maddox rod was carried out at far and near distances. The phoria (i.e., latent deviation of one eye when the other eye is covered, using the cover-uncover test) was normal for all children tested. At far distance, the divergence amplitudes were similar in both groups of children examined. In contrast, at near distance, the divergence amplitudes were significantly smaller in the dyslexic group than in the non-dyslexic children. An ANOVA showed a significant main effect of group ($F_{(1,34)} = 6.50$, $p<0.01$). Convergence amplitudes at both far and near distance were similar for dyslexic and non-dyslexic children.

In sum, the orthoptic evaluation showed a tendency toward poor divergence fusional capabilities in dyslexic children.

The investigation adhered to the principles of the Declaration of Helsinki and was approved by our Institutional Human Experi-

Table 1. Clinical characteristics of dyslexic and non-dyslexic children.

	TNO	NPC	Phoria Far	Phoria Near	Div. Far	Div. Near	Conv. Far	Conv. Near
Dyslexic children	40	3	ortho	ortho	4	10	17	30
Non-dyslexic children	40	3	ortho	Exo 2	4	16*	20	30

Clinical characteristics of all children tested. Median values for binocular vision (stereoacuity test, TNO measured in seconds of arc); near point of convergence (NPC measured in cm); heterophoria at far and near distance, measured in prism diopters; ortho = orthophoria; exo = exophoria; vergence fusional amplitudes (divergence and convergence) at far and near distance, measured in prism diopters. Asterisks indicate that the value is significantly different for the group of dyslexic children ($p<0.01$).

mentation Committee (CPP Ile de France I, Hôpital Hotel-Dieu). Written consent was obtained from the children's parents after an explanation of the experimental procedure.

Platform

A platform (principle of strain gauge) consisting of two dynamometric clogs (standards by Association Française de Posturologie, produced by TechnoConcept, Céreste, France) was used to measure postural stability. The position of the feet was as follows: heels 4 cm apart and the feet spread out symmetrically at an angle of 30° with respect to the child's sagittal axis. Arms were vertically along the body. The excursions of the center of pressure (CoP) were measured for 25.6 seconds and the surface of the CoP was calculated following the standards proposed by Gagey et al. [60]; the equipment included a 16-bit analog-digital converter. The sampling frequency of the CoP was 40 Hz.

Stimuli

Visual stimuli were presented on a flat screen (1280×768 pixels), placed 40 cm from the children. The elevation of the screen was adjusted as a function of the height of each child so that its center exactly faced the eyes. Two visual tasks were used for stimulation: a visually guided saccade task and silent reading of a text.

Visually guided horizontal and vertical saccades were elicited by using a simultaneous paradigm to induce reflexive saccades. At the start of each trial, a central black square of 1.4° was switched on for a period of 1500 ms; afterwards the square was switched off, and simultaneously a target (little green man, smiley) of 1.4° appeared at the periphery of the screen (eccentricity of the target was 10° to right or left, up or down) and stayed on for 1500 ms. Children were invited to make a horizontal or vertical saccade to the target. A total of 9 saccades were stimulated for the postural recording. It should be noted that eye movements have not been recorded, consequently we were unable to quantify oculomotor responses.

For the reading task, a six-line test was presented to the child. The mean character width was 0.5° and the text was written in black Courier font on a white background. The paragraph was extracted from *Monsieur Petit*, a text produced by ELFE (Cogni-Sciences, www.cognisciences.com), which allows for a rapid evaluation of the reading capabilities of children aged 7 to 12. We did not give any instructions for reading but we simply asked to the child to read silently. Silent reading was chosen for two reasons: firstly to avoid inducing anxiety in the dyslexic group, secondly to avoid any neck, abdomen and chest muscles activity that are well known to affect postural control [61–62].

Reading task induced mainly horizontal saccades even if some oblique saccades are necessary to start the new line, while with the visually guided paradigm used in our task child has to make both horizontal as well as vertical saccades. Note that Rougier & Garin [47] did not find different effect on posture between these two types of saccade direction. However, it will be interesting to explore further this issue.

Finally, in order to evaluate the reading score, after the recording we asked each child what was the last word he/she had read. The total number of words read in the two different paragraphs was counted.

Postural recording procedure

The child stood on the platform, in front of the screen located 40 cm away from him/her. Postural measurements were made while the child engaged in horizontal and vertical saccades and read a text silently. The child was instructed to stay as stable as possible, with the arms along the body and to look at the screen in order to perform the saccades or read the text. Each condition was performed twice; the order of the two conditions varied randomly between the children. Each postural recording test was followed by a rest lasting for a few minutes.

Data analysis

The posture measurement method is similar to that used in a previous study [63]. We analyzed the surface area and mean speed of the CoP excursion. Surface area is a good measure of CoP spatial variability [64] and mean speed represents a good index of the amount of neuromuscular activity required to regulate postural control [65–66].

Statistical analysis comprised two-way ANOVAs with group of children (dyslexics and non-dyslexics) as between-subject factor and condition (saccades and reading) as within-subject factor. The effect of a factor is significant when the p-value is below 0.05.

Results

Figures show the postural parameters (surface area and mean speed of the CoP) that were measured during the two experimental conditions for dyslexic and non-dyslexic children. Concerning the surface of the CoP (Figure 1), the ANOVA showed a significant effect of group ($F_{(1,34)}=8.57$, $p<0.006$); non-dyslexic children were more stable than dyslexic children. The ANOVA also; showed a significant effect of condition on the surface of the CoP, which was systematically smaller when children were making saccades than when they were reading a text ($F_{(1,34)}=5.64$, $p<0.02$). There are no significant interactions between group of children and condition.

Figure 2 shows the data obtained concerning the mean speed of the CoP. The ANOVA showed a significant interaction between group of children and condition ($F_{(1,34)}=4.85$, $p<0.03$): post hoc comparisons showed that the mean speed of the CoP during

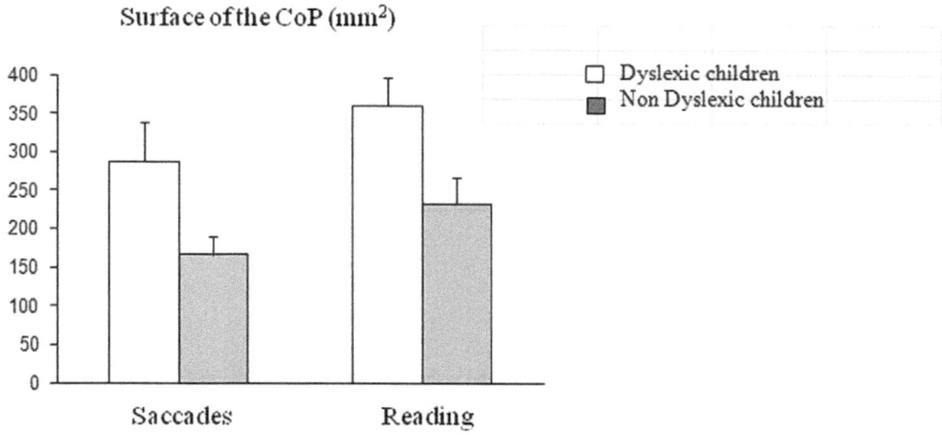

Figure 1. Means and standard deviations for surface area of CoP in the saccade and reading tasks for the two groups of children (dyslexic and non-dyslexic).

reading was significantly greater than during saccades only for the non-dyslexic children ($p<0.01$).

The reading scores for both groups of children were also evaluated by counting the number of words read in the two postural measures. The ANOVA showed a significant difference between the two groups of children ($F_{(1,34)}=9.31$, $p<0.004$); the non-dyslexic children read a larger number of words than the dyslexic children (80±8 and 49±18, respectively).

Discussion

The goal of the study was to compare the effect of a dual task on postural stability in a group of dyslexic and non-dyslexic children. The main findings are as follows: (i) independently of the task, dyslexic children are more unstable than non-dyslexic children; (ii) reading impairs postural stability more than a saccade task in both groups of children. These findings will be discussed individually below.

Poor postural stability in dyslexic children

Several studies have examined postural stability in dyslexic children but the finding that these subjects have balance impairment is still controversial. Indeed, as mentioned in the Introduction, some authors have hypothesized that balance deficits in the dyslexic population are related to other developmental deficits such as attention-deficit/hyperactivity disorder and developmental coordination disorder [35,67]. Note, however, that a recent study [68] reported poor postural control in children and adults with dyslexia even without comorbid attention deficits. Pioneering studies [32,69] suggest that the balance deficits observed in the dyslexic population could be due to an impairment affecting the processing of sensory information by the cerebellum. This hypothesis is based on the finding that dyslexics were impaired in both attentional and balance capabilities when two tasks were performed simultaneously [36]. Subsequent studies have also reported poor postural stability during a dual task in dyslexic children, providing more evidence for the cerebellar hypothesis [28–29]. Studies examining posture in children with cerebellar deficits [70–71] have reported poor postural stability, suggesting a difficulty of these children to integrate multimodal sensory information for balance control and/or a difficulty in properly compensate the deficit of sensory input [41]. Based on our findings, we could assume that dyslexic children are not able to use sensorial inputs in order to assure good postural control particularly when they have to perform a dual task. This hypothesis is in line with the study of Barela et al. [72].

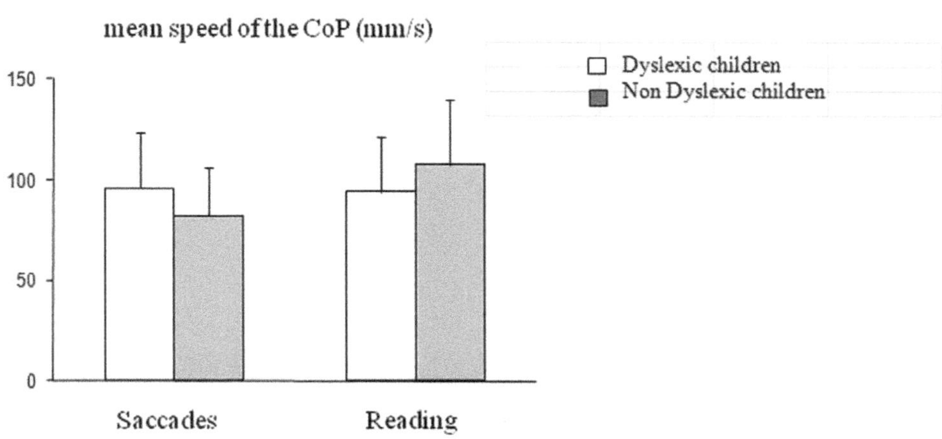

Figure 2. Means and standard deviations for mean speed of CoP in the saccade and reading tasks for the two groups of children (dyslexic and non-dyslexic).

The present data, from dyslexic children without hyperactivity/developmental coordination deficits, are in line with the work of Quercia et al. [64]; indeed, dyslexic children show a significantly larger surface of the CoP during a dual task than non-dyslexic children of comparable age, while the mean speed of the CoP was similar in both groups of children (at least while making saccades). Recall that the mean speed of the CoP, according to Geurts et al. [65] and Maki et al. [66], is believed to reflect the muscular energy used by the body for self-stabilization. Thus, dyslexic children do not seem to use a speed strategy to override their instability more than non-dyslexics do. This finding is new, and needs to be explored further in studies dealing with postural control in different types of dual task in dyslexic and non-dyslexic children in order to better understand whether and how dyslexics are able to use their energy to achieve better balance control.

Reading versus saccading: different effects on postural stability

The second important result of the present study is the different effects of saccadic and reading tasks on postural stability in dyslexic and non-dyslexic children. Indeed, both groups of children showed a greater surface area of the CoP during reading than during the saccade task. Reading is a higher cognitive activity that depends on multiple processes (perception, eye movements, and linguistic/semantic capacities); consequently, during reading, cognition and postural control may require the same mechanisms. Given the difficulty of this task, children might shift their attention towards the reading task, instead of postural stability, leading to poor balance. This occurs for dyslexic and non-dyslexic children, at least for the surface area of the CoP. Interestingly, the results also showed that only non-dyslexic children significantly increased the mean speed of the CoP during reading, suggesting that unlike the dyslexic group, they are able to use their muscular effort to control their equilibrium when they are given a highly cognitively demanding dual task. Dyslexic children did not show this capability, indeed mean speed of CoP did not change in two conditions. Such finding could suggest in dyslexic population a deficit in allocating the muscular energy required for stabilizing the body.

Taken together, all these data are in line with the U-shaped non-linear interaction model [4], which posits that the type of cognitive task can influence postural stability. Thus, we suggest that, in children (both dyslexic and non-dyslexic at about 11 years of age), the more demanding the cognitive task, the worse the postural sway. This has also been reported in previous work [17,20] on non-dyslexic children of similar ages, for whom different cognitive tasks (counting backward or Stroop-type task) led to impaired postural stability. In contrast, these results did not confirm previous findings [16] in which children between 8 and 10 years old changed their postural control strategies by increasing the attentional demand. Note, however, that the results of Blanchard et al.'s [16] study, showing strong interference between cognition and posture, revealed a discordant effect on postural measures depending on the parameter taken into account (sway variability or length of CoP path).

Conclusion

In conclusion, this study, in accordance with previous reports, provided evidence suggesting that dyslexic children have impaired postural stability compared to non-dyslexic children of similar age. Furthermore, a reading task impaired postural control more than a saccadic task; most likely, the attention needed for the reading task leads to poor postural control in both groups of children. The increase in the surface of the CoP in the absence of any increase in the mean speed of the CoP reported in the dyslexic group is in agreement with the hypothesis of sensorimotor theory where the sensory or motor deficit could lead to a multimodal integration difficulties in the cerebellum. These findings could be explored further with eye movement recordings.

Acknowledgments

The authors thank the children who participated in the study. They also thank Zofia Laubitz for revising the English version of the manuscript.

Author Contributions

Conceived and designed the experiments: MPB. Performed the experiments: AL MPB. Analyzed the data: AL MPB. Contributed reagents/materials/analysis tools: CLG EBQ CL. Wrote the paper: AL MPB EQC CLG CL KDM.

References

1. Abernethy B (1988) Dual-task methodology and motor skills research: some applications and methodological constraints. J Hum Mov Stud 14: 101–132.
2. Lajoie Y, Teasdale N, Bard C, Fleury M (1993) Attentional demands for static and dynamic equilibrium. Exp Brain Res 97: 139–144.
3. Huang HJ, Mercer VS (2001) Dual-task methodology: applications in studies of cognitive and motor performance in adults and children. Pediatr Phys Ther 13: 133–140.
4. Lacour M, Bernard-Demanze L, Dumitrescu M (2008) Posture control, aging, and attention resources: models and posture-analysis methods. Neurophysiol Clin 38: 411–421.
5. Shumway-Cook A, Woollacott M (2000) Attentional demands and postural control: the effect of sensory context. J Gerontol Biol Sci 55A: 10–16.
6. Dault MC, Yardley L, Frank J (2003) Does articulation contribute to modifications of postural control during dual-task paradigms? Brain Res Cogn Brain Res 16: 434–440.
7. Pellecchia GL (2003) Postural sway increases with attentional demands of concurrent cognitive task. Gait Posture 18: 29–34.
8. Vuillerme N, Nougier V, Teasdale N (2000) Effects of a reaction time task on postural control in humans. Neurosci Lett 291: 77–80.
9. Andersson G, Hagman J, Talianzadeh R, Svedberg A, Larsen HC (2002) Effect of cognitive load on postural control. Brain Res Bull 58: 135–139.
10. McNevin NH, Wulf G (2002) Attentional focus on supra-postural tasks affects postural control. Hum Mov Sci 21: 187–202.
11. Riley MA, Baker AA, Schmit JM (2003) Inverse relation between postural variability and difficulty of a concurrent short-term memory task. Brain Res Bull 62: 191–195.
12. Wulf G, Mercer J, McNevin N, Guadagnoli MA (2004) Reciprocal influences of attentional focus on postural and suprapostural task performance. J Mot Behav 36: 189–199.
13. Huxhold O, Li SC, Schmiedek F, Lindenberger U (2006) Dual-tasking postural control: aging and the effects of cognitive demand in conjunction with focus of attention. Brain Res Bull 69: 294–305.
14. Shumway-Cook A, Woollacott M, Kerns KA, Baldwin M (1997) The effects of two types of cognitive tasks on postural stability in older adults with and without a history of falls. J Gerontol A Biol Sci Med Sci 52: M232–240.
15. Andersson G, Hagman J, Talianzadeh R, Svedberg A, Larsen HC (2003) Dual-task study of cognitive and postural interference in patients with vestibular disorders. Otol Neurotol 24: 289–293.
16. Blanchard Y, Carey S, Coffey J, Cohen A, Harris T (2005) The influence of concurrent cognitive tasks on postural sway in children. Pediatr Phys Ther 17: 189–193.
17. Schmid M, Conforto S, Lopez L, D'Alessio T (2007) Cognitive load affects postural control in children. Exp Brain Res 179: 375–385.
18. Olivier I, Cuisinier C, Vaugoyeau M, Nougier V, Assaiante C (2007) Dual-task study of cognitive and postural interference in 7-year olds and adults. Neuroreport 18: 817–821.
19. Laufer Y, Ashkenazi T, Josman N (2008) The effects of a concurrent cognitive task on the postural control of young children with and without developmental coordination disorder. Gait Posture 27: 347–351.
20. Olivier I, Cuisinier C, Vaugoyeau M, Nougier V, Assaiante C (2010) Age-related differences in cognitive and postural dual-task performance. Gait Posture 32: 494–499.

21. American Psychiatric Association (1994) Diagnostic and statistical manual of mental disorders (4th ed.). Washington, DC: Author.
22. Liberman I Y (1973) Segmentation of the spoken word and reading acquisition. Bulletin of the Orton Society 23: 65–76.
23. Snowling MJ (2000) Dyslexia (2nd ed.). Oxford, United Kingdom: Blackwell Publishers.
24. Ramus F (2003) Developmental dyslexia: specific phonological deficit or general sensorimotor dysfunction? Curr Opin Neurobiol 13: 212–218.
25. Tallal P (1980) Auditory temporal perception, phonics, and reading disabilities in children. Brain and Language 9: 182–198.
26. Lovegrove WJ, Bowling A, Badcock D, Blackwood M (1980, October 24) Specific reading disability: Differences in contrast sensitivity as a function of spatial frequency. Science 210: 439–440.
27. Fawcett AJ, Nicolson RI (1995) Persistent deficits in motor skill of children with dyslexia. Journal of Motor Behavior 27: 235–240.
28. Stein J (2001) The magnocellular theory of developmental dyslexia. Dyslexia 7: 12–36.
29. Biscaldi M, Gezeck S, Stuhr V (1998) Poor saccadic control correlates with dyslexia. Neuropsychologia 36: 1189–1202.
30. Elterman RD, Daroff RB, Bornstein JL (1980) Eye movement patterns in dyslexic children. Journal of Learning Disabilities 13: 11–16.
31. Hutzler F, Wimmer H (2004) Eye movements of dyslexic children when reading in a regular orthography. Brain and Language 89: 235–242.
32. Nicolson RI, Fawcett AJ, Berry EL, Jenkins IH, Dean P, et al. (1999) Association of abnormal cerebellar activation with motor learning difficulties in dyslexic adults. Lancet 353: 1662–1667.
33. Poblano A, Ishiwara K, de Lourdes Arias M, Garcia-Pedroza F, Marin H, et al. (2002) Motor control alteration in posturography in learning disabled children. Arch Med Res 33: 485–488.
34. Stoodley CJ, Fawcett AJ, Nicolson RI, Stein JF (2005) Impaired balancing ability in dyslexic children. Exp Brain Res 167: 370–380.
35. Rochelle KS, Talcott JB (2006) Impaired balance in developmental dyslexia? A meta-analysis of the contending evidence. J Child Psychol Psychiatry 47: 1159–1166.
36. Nicolson RI, Fawcett AJ (1990) Automaticity: a new framework for dyslexia research? Cognition 35: 159–182.
37. Vieira S, Quercia P, Michel C, Pozzo T, Bonnetblanc F (2009) Cognitive demands impair postural control in developmental dyslexia: a negative effect that can be compensated. Neurosci Lett 462: 125–129.
38. Quercia P, Demougeot L, Dos Santos M, Bonnetblanc F (2011) Integration of proprioceptive signals and attentional capacity during postural control are impaired but subject to improvement in dyslexic children. Exp Brain Res 209: 599–608.
39. Nicolson RI, Fawcett A (2007) Procedural learning difficulties: reuniting the developmental disorders? Trends Neurosci 30: 135–141.
40. Rizzolatti G, Riggio L, Dascola I, Umilta C (1987) Reorienting attention across the horizontal and vertical meridians: evidence in favor of a premotor theory of attention. Neuropsychologia 25: 31–40.
41. Brandt T (2003) Vertigo. Its multisensory syndromes Second Edition Springer.
42. Leigh RJ, Zee DS (2006) The neurology of eye movement. Oxford University Press. New York 4th edn.
43. Uchida T, Hashimoto M, Suzuki N, Takegami T, Iwase I (1979) Effects of periodic saccades on the body sway in human subjects. Neurosci Lett 13: 253–258.
44. Oblak B, Gregoric M, Gyergyek L (1985) Effects of voluntary eye saccades on body sway. 7th Int Symp Int Soc Posturography, Houston, Karger, Basel.
45. Stoffregen TA, Bardy BG, Bonnet CT, Hove P, Oullier O (2007) Postural sway and the frequency of horizontal eye movements. Motor Control 11(1): 86–102.
46. Rougier P, Garin M (2006) Performing saccadic eye movements modifies postural control organisation. Neurophysiol Clin 36(4): 235–243.
47. Rougier P, Garin M (2007) Performing saccadic eye movements or blinking improves postural control. Motor Control 11(3): 213–223.
48. White KD, Post RB, Leibowitz HW (1980) Saccadic eye movements and body sway. Science 208(4444): 621–623.
49. Straube A, Paulus W, Quintern J, Brandt T (1989) Visual ataxia induced by eye movements: posturographic measurements in normals and patients with ocular motor disorders. Clinical Vision science 4(2): 107–113.
50. Glasauer S, Schneider E, Jahn K, Strupp M, Brandt T (2005) How the eyes move the body. Neurology 65(8): 1291–1293.
51. Olson RK, Kliegl R, Davidson BJ (1983) Dyslexic and normal readers eye movements. J. Exp. Psychol. Hum. Percept Perform oct 8; 9(5): 816–825.
52. Bucci MP, Kapoula Z, Brémond-Gignac D (2008) Poor binocular coordination of saccades in dyslexic children. Graefe's Archive for Clinical and Experimental Ophthalmology 246(3): 417–428.
53. Bucci MP, Vernet M, Gerard C, Kapoula Z (2009) Normal speed and accuracy of saccades, vergence and combined saccades vergence movements in dyslexic children. J of Ophthalmology ID 325214. 8 p.
54. Kirkby JA, Blythe HI, Drieghe D, Liversedge SP (2011) Reading Text Increases Binocular Disparity in Dyslexic Children. PLoS ONE 6(11): e27105.
55. Chevrie-Muller C, Simon AM, Fournier S (1997) Batterie Langage oral écrit. Mémoire. Attention (L2MA). Paris: Editions du Centre de Psychologie appliquée.
56. American Psychiatric Association (1996) DSM-IV, Manuel diagnostique et statistique des troubles mentaux. Traduction française. Paris: Masson.
57. Stein JF, Riddell PM, Fowler MS (1987) Fine binocular control in dyslexic children. Eye 1: 433–438.
58. Stein JF, Riddell PM, Fowler S (1988) Disordered vergence control in dyslexic children. Br J Ophthalmol 72: 162–166.
59. Riddell PM, Fowler MS, Stein JF (1990) Spatial discrimination in children with poor vergence control. Percept Mot Skills 70: 707–718.
60. Gagey PM, Bizzo G, Bonnier L, Gentaz R, Guillaume P, et al. (1993) Calcul de la surface du statokinésigramme (SKG). Available: http://pierremarie.gagey.perso.sfr.fr/EllipseConfiance.htm. Accessed 2011 Nov 29.
61. Ivanenko YP, Grasso R, Lacquaniti F (1999) Effect of gaze on postural responses to neck proprioceptive and vestibular stimulation in humans. J Physiol 15(519 Pt 1): 301–314.
62. Bruno E, De Padova A, Napolitano B, Marroni P, Batelli R, Ottaviani F, Alessandrini M (2009) Voice Disorders and Posturography: Variables to Define the Success of Rehabilitative Treatment. Journal of Voice 23(1): 71–75.
63. Legrand A, Bui-Quoc E, Wiener-Vacher S, Ribot J, Lebas N, et al. (2011) Postural control in children with strabismus before and after surgery. Neurosci Lett 501: 96–101.
64. Vuillerme N, Chenu O, Pinsault N, Fleury A, Demongeot J, et al. (2008) Can a plantar pressure-based tongue-placed electrotactile biofeedback improve postural control under altered vestibular and neck proprioceptive conditions? Neuroscience 155: 291–296.
65. Geurts AC, Nienhuis B, Mulder TW (1993) Intrasubject variability of selected force-platform parameters in the quantification of postural control. Arch Phys Med Rehabil 74: 1144–1150.
66. Maki B, Holliday P, Fernie G (1990) Aging and postural control: a comparaison of spontaneous-and induced-way balance tests. J Am Geriatr Soc 38: 1–9.
67. Wimmer H, Mayringer H, Raberger T (1999) Reading and dual-task balancing: evidence against the automatization deficit explanation of developmental dyslexia. J Learn Disabil 32: 473–478.
68. Brookes RL, Tinkler S, Nicolson RI, Fawcett AJ (2010) Striking the right balance: motor difficulties in children and adults with dyslexia. Dyslexia 16: 358–373.
69. Fawcett AJ, Nicolson RI, Dean P (1996) Impaired performance of children with dyslexia on a range of cerebellar tasks. Ann Dyslexia 46: 259–283.
70. Buderath P, Gärtner K, Frings M, Christiansen H, Schoch B, et al. (2009) Postural and gait performance in children with attention deficit/hyperactivity disorder. Gait Posture Feb 29(2): 249–54. Epub 2008 Oct 28.
71. Konczak J, Schoch B, Dimitrova A, Gizewski E, Timmann D (2005) Functional recovery of children and adolescents after cerebellar tumour resection. Brain Jun 128(Pt 6): 1428–1441. Epub 2005 Jan 19.
72. Barela JA, Dias JL, Godoi D, Viana AR, de Freitas PB (2011) Postural control and automaticity in dyslexic children: the relationship between visual information and body sway. Res Dev Disabil 32(5): 1814–1821. Epuib 2011 Apr 16.

Metacognition for Spelling in Higher Education Students with Dyslexia: Is There Evidence for the Dual Burden Hypothesis?

Wim Tops[1,2]*, Maaike Callens[1], Annemie Desoete[1], Michaël Stevens[1], Marc Brysbaert[1]

1 Ghent University, Ghent, Belgium, **2** University of Groningen, Groningen, The Netherlands

Abstract

We examined whether academic and professional bachelor students with dyslexia are able to compensate for their spelling deficits with metacognitive experience. Previous research suggested that students with dyslexia may suffer from a dual burden. Not only do they perform worse on spelling but in addition they are not as fully aware of their difficulties as their peers without dyslexia. According to some authors, this is the result of a worse feeling of confidence, which can be considered as a form of metacognition (metacognitive experience). We tried to isolate this metacognitive experience by asking 100 students with dyslexia and 100 matched control students to rate their feeling of confidence in a word spelling task and a proofreading task. Next, we used Signal Detection Analysis to disentangle the effects of proficiency and criterion setting. We found that students with dyslexia showed lower proficiencies but not suboptimal response biases. They were as good at deciding when they could be confident or not as their peers without dyslexia. They just had more cases in which their spelling was wrong. We conclude that the feeling of confidence in our students with dyslexia is as good as in their peers without dyslexia. These findings go against the Dual Burden theory (Krüger & Dunning, 1999), which assumes that people with a skills problem suffer twice as a result of insufficiently developed metacognitive competence. As a result, there is no gain to be expected from extra training of this metacognitive experience in higher education students with dyslexia.

Editor: Antony Bayer, Cardiff University, United Kingdom

Funding: This study was made possible by an Odysseus Grant, which was awarded to MB by the Flemish Government. The funders however had no role in study design, data collection and analysis, decision to publish, or preparation of the manuscript.

Competing Interests: The authors have declared that no competing interests exist.

* Email: wimtops@gmail.com

Introduction

Getting a degree in higher education depends on three groups of variables: adequate intellectual abilities, will to work (achievement motivation), and knowing how to study. The last component, on which we will focus, is usually referred to as metacognition [1,2,3]. Metacognition was originally defined as cognition about cognition [3,4]. Gradually, it became clear that metacognition involved more aspects. Efklides [2,5,6,7], for instance, distinguished three components of metacognition: metacognitive knowledge, metacognitive skills, and metacognitive experiences.

Metacognitive knowledge refers to beliefs about cognition stored in long term memory. Metacognitive skills deal with the regulation of the cognitive processes needed for good performance. They include (appropriate) effort allocation, time allocation, planning, executing the various steps towards the goal, checking the progress, adapting the modus operandi if necessary, and evaluating the outcome, so that lessons can be learned for future performance. Metacognitive experiences are based on previous involvements with the task at hand (or related learning conditions). They enable the learner to be better aware of the progress made [6] and to make use of alternative metacognitive skills if needed. They include memories of previous experiences with the task, estimates of efforts and time required for successful performance, feeling of difficulty of the task, and feeling of confidence in one's own abilities.

Much research has confirmed the contribution of metacognition to successful learning e.g., [8,9,10]. There is also good evidence that metacognition is involved in the acquisition of adequate reading and writing skills [11,12,13,14,15]. Metacognition therefore may be an important factor in understanding why some people struggle with reading and/or writing [16,17,18,19]. These people are commonly referred to as suffering from dyslexia.

Dyslexia is a specific learning disorder characterized by a persistent problem in learning to read and/or write words or in the automatization of the reading and writing process (Dyslexia Foundation Netherlands; [20]). The level of reading and/or writing is significantly lower than what can be expected on the basis of the educational level and age of the individual. In addition, the impairment is resistant to remedial teaching (defined as meeting the requirements of the "response to instruction" model; [21]), and the reading and writing deficit cannot be attributed to external and/or individual factors such as socio-economic status, cultural background or intelligence.

The term dyslexia is no longer used in the DSM-5 [22], where it is called a specific learning disorder with impairment in reading (word reading fluency and/or accuracy, reading comprehension) and/or written expression (spelling, grammar and punctuation accuracy, organization of written expression). Still, we will continue to use the term throughout the present study, as we have followed the criteria for dyslexia in the selection of participants, as set out by the Dyslexia Foundation Netherlands.

There is evidence for a genetic component in dyslexia (e.g., [23,24]), but the prevalence of the problem also depends on environmental features. For instance, it has been reported that dyslexia is more common in languages with opaque letter-to-sound mappings (such as English) than in languages with simple mappings, such as Italian [25] and Welsh [26]. Beginning readers of languages with inconsistent mappings need more time to reach ceiling performance and, apparently, have higher chances of not getting there. Next to the reading and/or spelling impairment, individuals with dyslexia have been reported to show specific (working) memory problems [27], attentional deficits [28], reduced processing speed [29], problems with fast lexical retrieval and arithmetic [30,31], and less elaborated vocabulary skills [32].

Studies on dyslexia and metacognition come to inconclusive results. Kirby, Silvestri, Allingham, Parrila and Lafave [33] showed that students with dyslexia compensate for their reading difficulties by metacognition. Other studies on metacognition and dyslexia have suggested less sophisticated metacognition in students with dyslexia [16,34]. Job and Klassen [35] found that adolescents with dyslexia were less accurate at predicting their performance. They overestimated their ability on a spelling and ball-throwing task, with a decrease in accurate performance prediction as the difficulty level increased. The authors called this 'optimistic miscalibration'. Mason and Mason [36] reported that adult college students with dyslexia showed deficits in metacognitive skills, resulting in problems with selecting and using effective cognitive strategies.

Kruger and Dunning [37,38] introduced the Dual Burden hypothesis to indicate how people with a skills problem may suffer twice as a result of insufficiently developed metacognitive competence. Not only do these people reach erroneous conclusions and make wrong choices, but their lack of correct metacognitive experiences also hinders them from realising it. Applied to spelling, the knowledge underlying the ability to write without errors is also the knowledge needed to make correct estimates about one's spelling efficiency. Sideridis, Morgan, Botsas, Padeliadu and Fuchs [39] reported some evidence for this possibility, as they observed that knowledge about how to monitor and control one's learning was one of the best predictors of performance in students with dyslexia. Similarly, Trainin and Swanson [40] argued that successful college students with dyslexia have compensated for their cognitive difficulties and processing deficits by relying on metacognition (learning tricks and strategies to cope with the problem, seeking help in time, etc.). Indeed, metacognitive processes (in particular, experiences) make the person aware of the problem and trigger control processes that can serve to help reach the goal that is pursued.

In a recently published Dutch assessment battery for dyslexia in (young) adults [41], three subtests include a measure of metacognition. Two of them are related to spelling. The third applies to morphology and syntax and will not be taken into account in this study because it is not a core deficit in dyslexia. The first spelling test involves a word dictation task, in which participants have to write down spoken words. The second is a proofreading task in which participants have to indicate whether words are correctly written or not. In addition to the primary task, participants also have to indicate how sure they are about their answer (uncertain, almost certain and very certain).

When considering traditional statistical analyses for metacognition in spelling, we saw ourselves confronted with two challenging statistical issues. First, one has to be careful interpreting significant interaction effects in the presence of main effects [42], because a difference between 100 and 120 may be of a similar magnitude as a difference between 10 and 12 (i.e., an increase of 20%). Second, these kinds of analyses often fail to make a clear distinction between performance and metacognition. A proper measure of feeling of confidence or FOC must take into account the difference in skills-levels between the groups. It is easy for people who rarely make spelling errors to feel confident about their performance. Similarly, the best strategy for someone who makes lots of spelling mistakes may be to feel unsure on each trial.

The most elegant way to analyze decision strategies is to make use of signal detection theory, as this nicely separates response criteria from the sensitivity to spelling errors. Figure 1 shows the underlying logic.

Recent advances in statistical methods have made signal detection analysis possible for many more designs than before. DeCarlo [43] showed that the signal detection model can be formulated as a subclass of the generalized linear model. With only one participant and two possible responses, the classical signal detection model can be estimated using a probit regression model with response (e.g., a word is spelled correctly or not) as the dependent variable and type of trial as the predictor (e.g., correct spelling vs. wrong spelling; preferably coded as -0.5 and +0.5). In that case the slope of the regression line corresponds to the distance d' and the intercept agrees with the criterion c.

According to signal detection theory, both correctly and wrongly spelled words trigger a certain amount of evidence for a spelling error. Because of noise in the system, the degree of evidence triggered by correct and wrong spellings is not always exactly the same, but forms two normal distributions (one for correct spellings and one for wrong spellings). In a proficient speller the degree of error provoked by a correctly spelled word is much lower than the degree of error provoked by a wrongly spelled word. So, it will be easy to make a distinction between both distributions. In contrast, for a poor speller, d' will be small and there will be a large overlap between the distributions. So, the distance (d') between the two distributions is an indication of spelling proficiency. This distance is thought to be stable per participant: Individuals cannot manipulate their ability to detect errors.

The second aspect influencing performance is where the response criterion (c) is placed. The total number of judgment errors is minimal when c is placed at the intersection of the two distributions (as shown in Figure 1). This is true for all values of d'. Such optimal performance is called $c = 0$. When c is lower than zero, then the participant has a tendency to judge too many spellings wrong, including a large number of correct spellings. Conversely, when c is set above 0, the participant has a tendency to report too many spellings as correct, including a disproportionately large number of wrong spellings. Within signal detection theory, it is assumed that participants control the position of c as a function of the perceived costs and benefits of the choice alternatives.

In the present study we wanted to investigate whether Kruger and Dunning's [38] dual burden hypothesis applies to the spelling problems experienced by students entering higher education with an assessment of dyslexia. In particular, we wondered whether students with dyslexia would perform less well on spelling because they lack insight into when they are doing well and when not. This metacognitive experience can be measured with Feeling of Confidence (FOC) judgments. If people have no knowledge of their performance, they feel equally confident (or hesitant) on correct and incorrect trials. In contrast, if they have good knowledge, there will be a significant distinction between correct and incorrect trials.

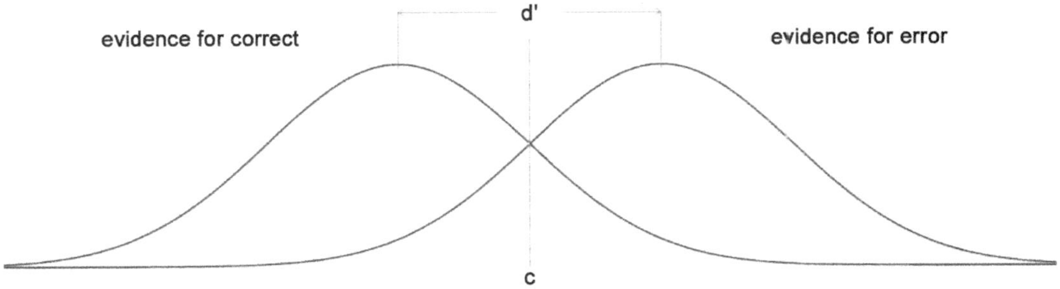

Figure 1. Logic of a signal detection analysis for spelling errors. Both correct spellings and wrong spellings induce a certain degree of evidence for a potential error. This evidence is not fixed but varies from trial to trial as a function of the noise in the system. As a result, there is a normal distribution of evidence when the spelling is correct and a normal distribution of evidence when the spelling is wrong. For someone with good spelling skills, both distributions are far apart, so that there is virtually no overlap between them. This is estimated by the distance d'. We can expect that d' will be considerably larger for controls than for dyslexics. The second variable of interest is c, the place where the decision criterion is placed. When c is at the intersection of the two distributions (as in the figure), it is positioned optimally, because then the smallest number of errors overall is made. In that case, c = 0. When c is lower than 0, the participant makes too many error judgments (i.e., does so for too many words with correct spellings). Conversely, when c is higher than 0, the participant fails to see too many wrong spellings. The degree of deviation in c from 0 is therefore a good indication of the dual burden theory.

It is easy to see how the position of c translates into the Dual Burden theory. Not only would students with dyslexia have a smaller value of d'. In addition, they would position the response criteria at a non-optimal place, so that they either fail to recognize the correct spellings they are capable to discriminate (when c<0) or fail to see the spelling errors that are within their reach (when c>0). Deviations of c from 0 indicate that the person has a suboptimal *Feeling of Confidence* (FOC).

Methods

The study was part of a larger research program in which we also looked at the cognitive profile of the students [29] and their personality profiles [44]. This study was approved by the ethical comity of Ghent University, meaning that the researchers followed the ethical protocol of the university. Students were paid for their participation. All students gave written informed consent and were informed that they could stop at any time if they felt they were treated incorrectly.

Participants

Two hundred first-year undergraduate students of higher education participated in this study. All students had graduated from secondary school and were in their first year of a professional bachelor (in colleges for higher education) leading to a professional bachelor degree (after three years of education) or an academic bachelor (in some colleges for higher education and in university, preparing for a master degree) in the surroundings of Ghent (one of the main cities in the Northern, Dutch-speaking half of Belgium). The group consisted of 100 students diagnosed with dyslexia and a control group of 100 students without dyslexia or other known neurological or functional disorders (ADHD, ASD, …). All had normal or corrected-to-normal vision and were native speakers of Dutch. Dutch is a language with a more transparent letter-sound-mapping than English, but less transparent than Spanish or Italian (e.g., [45]).

All students with dyslexia who applied for special facilities at the local support office (vzw Cursief) in the academic year 2009–2010 were asked to participate in the study until we had a total of one hundred. To find a group of 100 participants with dyslexia who completed the full study, we had to approach an initial cohort of some 120 students. Of these 120 students a small number of students chose not to cooperate once the study was explained to them. A few more students were lost because they failed to show up at appointments. The students with dyslexia had been diagnosed prior to our study by trained diagnosticians in accordance with the definition of SDN (Stichting Dyslexie Nederland [Foundation Dyslexia Netherlands], [20]). They all met the three criteria of the SDN at the moment of their participation. First, their reading and/or writing skills were significantly lower than could be expected given the age and the educational level of the students. Second, all students met the criterion "resistance to instruction" implying that they had attended remedial programs and received individual tutoring in primary or secondary education for a period of minimum 6 months by either a speech-therapist or a remedial teacher. Third, the reading and/or writing impairment could not be attributed to external or individual factors such as cultural background, intelligence or socio-economic status.

To reflect the inflow in the first year of higher education as much as possible and to construct homogenous groups, matching criteria for recruitment of the control students were restricted to field of study, gender and age. To recruit the control students we used different methods. We asked the students with dyslexia for several names of fellow classmates who would be interested in participating. Amongst these names we selected someone at random. If the student with dyslexia failed to give names (which was the case for about half of the participants), we recruited them ourselves by means of electronic platforms or the guidance counselors at the institution in question. There was no difference between the two groups in socio-economical level based on the educational level of the mother, $\chi^2(3) = 4.855$, $p = .183$ or father, $\chi^2(3) = 2.634$, $p = .452$. Educational levels were: lower secondary education, higher secondary education, or post-secondary education either at university or non-university college, as can be seen in Table 1.

Table 1 also shows the results of three literacy tests and one IQ-test we administered to the participants. The verbal tests were word reading (EMT; [46]), pseudoword reading (de Klepel [47];), and word spelling (GL&SCHR; [41]). On all three tests the control group obtained scores within the normal range, whereas the students with dyslexia on average had scores more than 1.5 standard deviations below this level (see the effect sizes in Table 1). The mean fluid IQ measured with the *Kaufman Adolescent and*

Table 1. General Information About the Student Groups With and Without Dyslexia.

		Students without Dyslexia N M (*SD*)	Students with dyslexia N M (*SD*)	Effect size Cohen's *d*
Gender	Male	46	46	
	Female	54	54	
Studies	University	66	66	
	College for higher education	34	34	
Age		19.40 *(1.00)*	19.11 *(0.70)*	NA
Fluid IQ		106.80 *(10.80)*	105.40 *(11.00)*	0.13
Word reading		100.40 *(10.60)*	77.00 *(14.20)*	1.97*
Pseudoword reading		59.70 *(13.10)*	40.90 *(10.50)*	1.59*
Word spelling		24.60 *(2.80)*	17.50 *(4.00)*	2.05*

Note. * p<.01; NA = not applicable; Fluid IQ = Total IQ score on the fluid subtests of the KAIT [48]; Word reading = Dutch word reading, number of words read correctly in 1 minute time (EMT [46]); Pseudoword reading = number of pseudowords read correctly in 1 minute time (de Klepel [47]); word spelling = number of words spelled correctly in a word dictation task (GL&SCHR [41]). Effect sizes calculated according to Cohen's *d* (positive d-values represent better performance of the controls and negative values better performance of the students with dyslexia).

Adult Intelligence Test, Dutch version [48] was 107 ($SD = 10.8$) for the control group and 105 ($SD = 11.0$) for the students with dyslexia. The difference in intelligence was not significant, F (1, 198) = 0.84; $p = .36$.

Test description

For this study two subtests of the *Test for Advanced Reading and Spelling* (Test voor Gevorderd Lezen en Schrijven), also called the GL&SCHR [41] were used. The GL&SCHR is a test battery for the diagnosis of dyslexia in Dutch-speaking (young) adults. The two subtests we analyzed measured word spelling and the ability to detect mistakes in sentences (also known as proofreading). We selected these tests because spelling is one of the major problems in adults with dyslexia [29], is important in (higher) education, and is easy to score unambiguously. Guttman split half correlations of the subtests were .69 and .80.

In the first subtest, *Word spelling*, participants had to write 30 words. Half of the words were rule-based (i.e., their spelling required the correct application of the Dutch phoneme-grapheme and morphosyntactic spelling rules); the other half were memory-based words involving inconsistent sound-letter mappings that must be memorized (mostly because the word is a loan word from another language). The test was computer paced. Each participant was given a blue pen and instructed to put on headphones. Words were presented auditorily with a regular interval of 3 seconds, so that students had to produce an immediate response (as in note taking during lectures). After the first hearing, the headphones were put aside and the participant was given a green pen. The student was allowed to use this to correct any mistakes. In addition, the words the student had missed were read out again by the test administrator and the participant used the green pen to write them down. Besides the word that needed to be written, the response form also contained a three point Likert scale to be completed for each word. For each word the participants were asked how sure they were about their spelling by marking one of these three options (certainly correct, rather certain the spelling is correct, or uncertain). There are three scores for this subtest: one for the number of correct responses, one for the total number of words written during the dictation itself (this variable is beyond the scope of the present paper and is, therefore, not further discussed), and one weighted score in which the certainty per item is taken into account. The last scoring is considered as a measure of metacognitive experience, more precisely the Feeling of Confidence or FOC (for more information, see [2]).

The second subtest, *Spelling rules*, was a proofreading task in which participants had to correct spelling mistakes in 20 words or sentences with a misspelled target word. Participants were asked to correct any misspellings in the words or sentences they noticed (the instructions did not say that each word or sentence contained one spelling error on the target word). As was the case in the previous subtest, students rated how certain they felt about their spelling corrections (certainly correct, rather certain correct, uncertain). There are two scores: one based on the number of well corrected target words (independent of the responses to the other words), and one defined as a weighted score (FOC score). The scores were limited to the target words (i.e., a score of zero was given when participants wrongly corrected a correctly spelled filler word).

For each spelling test, there were two scores: (1) the number of correct responses, and (2) the FOC weighted responses. The latter was implemented by the authors of the GL&SCHR as follows for the spelling test. If the students were very certain and they spelled the word correctly, they received five points. If they were almost certain and the word was spelled correctly they received four points. If they were not certain and the spelling was correct, they were given three points. If they were not certain and the spelling was incorrect, they were given two points. If they were almost certain and the spelling was incorrect, they received one point. And finally, if they were very certain about their spelling but it was incorrect, they received zero points.

A similar FOC weighted coding scheme was used for the proofreading task. If the students corrected the error in the target word well and they were very certain, they received five points. If they corrected the target word well but felt less certain, they obtained four points. If they corrected the target word but felt uncertain, they got three points. If they failed to correct the target word or misspelled it while correcting, they got two points if they felt uncertain, one point if the felt almost certain, and zero points if they felt very certain.

Procedure

The two subtests of the GL&SCHR were part of a larger protocol [29,49]. The complete test battery involved additional tests such as an intelligence test, reading and spelling tests, a study strategies inventory, a personality test and a semi-structured

Table 2. Performances of Students with Dyslexia on Spelling in Comparison With their Non-dyslexic Peers.

	Students with dyslexia		Students without dyslexia		Cohen's *d*			*p*
	M	(SD)	M	(SD)	*d*	lower CI	upper CI	
Word Spelling								
Weighted score (FOC)	91.59	(15.87)	121.40	(12.84)	2.06	1.64	2.48	**
Number correct words	17.49	(4.02)	24.60	(2.81)	2.05	1.63	2.47	**
Proofreading								
Weighted score (FOC)	50.83	(11.74)	62.45	(13.59)	0.92	0.49	1.33	**
Number correct words	10.05	(4.87)	13.81	(8.15)	0.56	0.14	0.98	**

Traditional analysis of the FOC weighted scores.
Note. $p<.05$; $^{**}p<.01$; GL&SCHR = Dutch reading and writing test battery for (young) adults [41].

interview about the socio-emotional and school functioning of the student. The test protocol was split in two counterbalanced parts of about 3 hours each. The order of the tests in part one and part two was determined in such a way that two similar tests were never administered in the same part. There was a break halfway in each session. If necessary, students could take additional breaks. The students with dyslexia started with part one or two according to an AB-design. Their matched control student always started with the same part. The GL&SCHR was taken as a whole in part 2. All tests were administered individually by one of three test administrators (the two first authors and a test psychologist) according to the manual guidelines. After going through the manual guidelines, they observed each other during the first ten test sessions. Afterwards, there was always a brief discussion to key the test administrations as far as possible to one another. Students were tested in a quiet room with the test administrator seated in front of them.

Signal Detection Theory Analysis

Our data fit within the framework of SDT as described in the introduction, but we need to extend it a little bit. First, we do not have a binary decision, but a three-level rating response (certainly correct, rather certain, uncertain). This can be accommodated by using an ordinal probit regression model instead of the binary probit regression model [43]. In that case we still have one estimate for d′ (the slope), but two intercepts: One that corresponds to the first response criterion c1 (between certainly correct and rather certain correct), and one that corresponds to the second criterion c2 (between rather certain correct and uncertain).

Second, we have 200 participants instead of just one participant. This violates the independence assumption of the linear model, so that we have to use a linear mixed effects model, with additional random intercepts and slopes per participant.

Finally, we want to compare students with dyslexia and control subjects. This can be done by adding an extra predictor (Group) to the model. A main effect of Group then indicates that the two groups used different response criteria. An interaction of Group with Type of trial (the word is spelled correctly or not) points to a difference in the ability to discriminate between trials with and without errors.

The analyses were based on the clmm function from the R package Ordinal [50] (see the Supplemental materials). The formula of the model was as follows:

$$\text{Rating} \sim \text{Trial Type} * \text{Group} + (\text{Trial Type} \mid \text{Subject})$$

The rating had three levels (certainly correct, rather certain correct, uncertain), so we had an intercept for the transition between certainly correct and rather certain correct, and a second intercept for the transition between rather certain correct and uncertain. Trial Type was contrast coded: the variable was set to −0.5 for 'correct' trials and +0.5 for 'wrong' trials. By doing this, the intercepts (response criteria) are counted relative to the point where the 'correct' and 'wrong' distributions cross (i.e., where $c = 0$).

Results

First, we analyzed the scores as recommended by the authors of the test. For each test, we had two scores: (1) the number of correct responses, and (2) the FOC weighted responses. Assuming that students with dyslexia are poorer in metacognition than their peers, we expected the difference between both groups to be larger

Table 3. Results of the Signal Detection Theory Analysis for the Word Dictation and Proofreading tasks.

		d′	c1	c2
Word spelling	Control	1.03 (z = 13.31, p<.001)	0.12 (z = 3.27, p<.001)	1.13 (z = 29.15, p<.001)
	Dyslexia	0.71 (z = 10.54, p<.001)	−0.08 (z = −2.73, p<.001)	0.93 (z = 27.8, p<.001)
	Difference	0.32 (z = 3.13, p<.001)	−0.20 (z = −4.37, p<.001)	
Proofreading	Control	1.02 (z = 10.35, p<.001)	−0.32 (z = −8.15, p<.001)	0.94 (z = 22.39, p<.001)
	Dyslexia	0.84 (z = 8.70, p<.001)	−0.42 (z = −10.76, p<.001)	0.85 (z = 20.74, p<.001)
	Difference	0.17 (z = 1.29, p = .197)	−0.09 (z = −1.78, p = .074)	

Note. d′ refers to the distance between the two normal distributions (Figure 1), c1 = the criterion between.
Certainly correct and rather certainly correct, c2 = the criterion between rather certainly correct and uncertain.
The proportional odds assumption claims that the difference for c1 and c2 is identical.

for the FOC weighted scores. As can be seen in Table 2, there was some mixed evidence that the recommended FOC weighted scores resulted in a larger effect size than the percentages of correct responses. There was a difference in the expected direction for the proofreading task but not for the dictation task.

For the reasons outlined in the introduction, we had serious doubts about the usefulness of analyses of variance based on weighted scores. Table 3 shows the outcome of a more promising technique, the SDT analysis, separately for the word dictation task and the proofreading task. The effect of trial type is an estimate of d′ (the distance between the correct and error distribution), the first intercept is an estimate of c1 (response criterion between certainly correct and rather certainly correct), the second intercept is an estimate of c2 (response criterion between rather certainly correct and uncertain).

As expected, d′ was larger for the controls than for the students with dyslexia. This simply refers to their (stable) differences in spelling proficiency. In line with Table 2, the disadvantage of the dyslexic students was larger for the word dictation task than for the proofreading task. More importantly for testing the dual burden theory, both students with dyslexia and control students had their c1 values close to 0 (i.e., the optimal performance level) in the dictation task. This is the criterion between being certain that the spelling is correct and being rather certain that the spelling is correct. The control group tended to be more confident (missing some of the errors they made) than the dyslexic group (thinking some of the correct spellings they made were almost certainly wrong). However, it is not the case that the dyslexic group performed less well than the control group (i.e., the absolute deviation of c1 from 0 was not larger for the dyslexics than for the controls).

A possible objection against the above interpretation is that, although as a group the students with dyslexia did not perform worse, there were very large individual differences with some individuals with dyslexia having very negative c1-values and others having very positive c1-values. This would be reflected in the random intercepts (i.e., the subject-specific deviations of the response criteria). Figure 2 shows a boxplot of the random intercepts in both groups. The variability is not substantially larger in the group of students with dyslexia; it is even slightly smaller.

Table 2 further shows that the values of c2 in the dictation task were rather high (i.e., students needed quite high evidence for a spelling error before they said they were uncertain about their response). Again, however, the similarity between the students with dyslexia and the control students is larger than the difference between the groups.

Very much the same conclusions apply to the Proofreading task, although here both groups tended to be a bit too fast in their transition from certainly correct to rather certain correct (i.e., they put c1 at a level lower than warranted by their spelling proficiency). More importantly, however, there again was no obvious difference between the control group and the dyslexic group, as would be predicted by the Dual Burden theory.

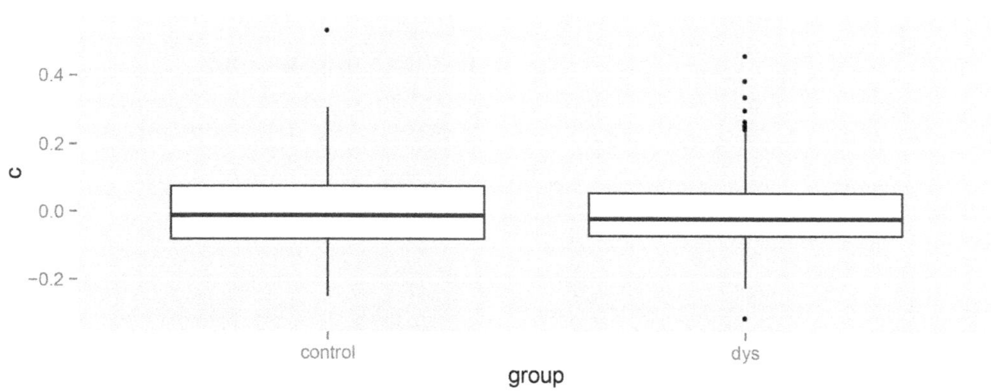

Figure 2. Boxplots of the subject-specific deviations of the response criteria, showing that there was no more variability in c1 scores of the students with dyslexia than in those of the age matched controls.

Discussion

The present study assessed whether undergraduate students in higher education suffer from bad metacognitive skills, as suggested by the dual burden theory [37,38]. According to this theory, spelling errors in students with dyslexia are not only due to low proficiency levels (which cannot easily be changed in an individual), but also to the fact that students with dyslexia fail to realize when they have made a mistake (and hence cannot learn from their errors).

To examine the issue, we ran two tests with Feeling of Confidence (FOC) judgments. According to the dual burden theory, one would expect the difference between students with dyslexia and controls to be larger for scores that take FOC into account than for scores without FOC. However, we searched for an alternative way of analysis, which would give us much more information about the underlying processes. Signal detection is known to be the best framework to model decisions under uncertainty. Such an analysis allows researchers to distinguish criterion setting (which FOC is) from spelling proficiency. Due to recent statistical developments Signal Detection Analyses have become possible for many more designs than the psychophysical experiments on the basis of which they were originally developed.

The signal detection analysis of our data clearly confirmed the difference in proficiency between both groups (d′) and at the same time told us at which positions participants decided to say they were almost certain of their response or not certain at all anymore. As it turned out, the differences in criterion setting were not that much different between students with dyslexia and controls and most certainly not indicative of less rational strategies in students with dyslexia than in other students. Both groups of students seemed to be very smart in their criterion setting. As a result, we feel not justified to say that students with dyslexia in higher education suffer from a double burden (the situation may be different in primary school; this remains to be examined).

At the same time, the signal detection analysis allows us to evaluate the quality of the tests we used and to suggest improvements. For a start, it does not seem that the two-criterion response (certain, almost certain, uncertain) adds much to a single criterion response (certain: yes/no). In the present study, participants clearly put their most important criterion between certain and almost certain; c1). Only when it was clear that their spelling (or spelling correction) did not make sense, did they use the uncertain alternative.

Second, the dictation task also gave clearer data than the proofreading task. One reason for this may be the fact that participants could zoom in on non-target words in the sentence, thinking these were wrong (although they were not). It might be better in the future to alert the participants to the target words (e.g., by printing them in bold) and ask whether this part of the sentences is correctly spelled: yes or no (and how sure the participants are about their correction: sure vs. not sure). These designs will also be more straightforward to analyze. It would, however, require the addition of sentences in which the target words were spelled correctly.

All in all, we conclude that when signal detection theory analysis is used, there is no evidence for a dual burden in students with dyslexia in higher education. Their metacognitive skills are as good as they can be, given the fact that these students are making more mistakes because of their lower proficiency level. Remediation programs focusing on the metacognitive skill of FOC, therefore, are bound to fail. They may even do more bad than good, if the criterion setting is based on implicit learning rather than explicit, declarative knowledge [51].

Finally, because of the added value of the signal detection analysis and because this analysis may be rather daunting for someone starting with it (it took us quite a bit of time too), we include our data and the R program used to analyze them in the supplementary materials. In that way, everyone can first check whether they know how to do the analyses (by comparing their output with our data to Table 3), before they start to analyze other data.

We are convinced that these new types of analysis, although a little bit more complicated to apply, give a better picture of the true metacognitive qualities of people with more limited cognitive skills. After we finished data collection, we discovered another study of Maniscalco and Lau [52] that takes the same approach. These authors employed a new method derived from classical SDT to isolate metacognitive evaluation from task performance on the basis of correct and incorrect decisions. They argue for the use of a relative sensitivity measure instead of an absolute sensitivity measure. Relative sensitivity makes it possible to separate the quality of the information being metacognitively evaluated from the quality of the metacognitive evaluation itself. This (new) type of sensitivity, called *meta-d′*, is another interesting measure to reveal the efficacy of a person's metacognitive experiences.

Supporting Information

File S1 This is a text file with the raw data. For each participant and each trial of the dictation and the proofreading task, it says how certain the participant felt and whether the answer was correct or not.

File S2 This is a file to run the statistical analyses in R. Once you are in the R programming environment, it should run on the data file (if the latter has been placed in your working directory). You must make sure that the package Ordinal is loaded as well. The output of the analyses can directly be compared to the summary in Table 3.

Author Contributions

Conceived and designed the experiments: MC WT MB. Performed the experiments: MC WT. Analyzed the data: WT MC AD MS MB. Contributed reagents/materials/analysis tools: WT MC AD MS MB. Wrote the paper: WT MC AD MS MB.

References

1. Brown A (1987) Metacognition, executive control, self-control, and other mysterious mechanisms. In F Weinert & R Kluwe (Eds.). Metacognition, Motivation, and Understanding. Hillsdale, NJ: Erlbaum, 65–116.
2. Efklides A (2008) Metacognition: Defining its facets and levels of functioning in relation to self-regulation and co-regulation. European Psychologist 13: 277–287.
3. Flavell JH (1976) Metacognitive aspects of problem solving. In LB Resnick (Ed.). The nature of intelligence. Hillsdale, NJ: Erlbaum, 231–235.
4. Flavell JH (1979) Metacognition and cognitive monitoring: A new area of cognitive-developmental inquiry. American Psychologist 34: 906–911.
5. Efklides A (2002) The systemic nature of metacognitive experiences: Feelings, judgments, and their interrelations. In M Izaute, P Chambres, P-J Marescaux (Eds.). Metacognition: Process, function, and use. Dordrecht, The Netherlands: Kluwer, 19–34.
6. Efklides A (2009) The role of metacognitive experiences in the learning process. Psicothema 21: 76–82.

7. Efklides A (2011) Interactions of metacognition with motivation and affect in self-regulated learning: The MASRL model. Educational Psychologist 46: 6–25.
8. Chi MTH, Bassok M, Lewis MW, Reimann P, Glaser R (1989) Self-explanations: How students study and use examples in learning to solve problems. Cognitive Science 13: 145–182.
9. Son LK, Simon DA (2012) Distributed learning: Data, metacognition, and educational implications. Educational Psychology Review 24: 379–399.
10. Winne PH, Hadwin AF (1998) Studying as self-regulated learning. In DJ Hacker, J Dunlosky, AC Graesser (Eds.). Metacognition in educational theory and practice. Mahway, NJ: Erlbaum, 277–304.
11. Hacker DJ, Keener MC, Kircher JC (2009) Writing is applied metacognition. In DJ Hacker, J Dunlosky, AC Graesser (Eds.). Handbook of metacognition in education. New York, NY: Routledge, 154–172.
12. Pressley M, Gaskins IW (2006) Metacognitively competent reading comprehension is constructively responsive reading: how can such reading be developed in students? Metacognition and Learning 1: 99–113.
13. Vanderswalmen R, Vrijders J, Desoete A (2010) Metacognition and spelling performance in college students. In A Efklides, P Misailidi (Eds.). Trends and prospects in metacognition research. New York, NY: Springer, 367–394.
14. Williams JP, Atkins JG (2009) The role of metacognition in teaching reading comprehension to primary students. In DJ Hacker, J Dunlosky, AC Graesser (Eds.). Handbook of metacognition in education. New York, NY: Routledge, 26–43.
15. Zhang LJ (2001) Awareness in reading: EFL students' metacognitive knowledge of reading strategies in an acquisition-poor environment. Language Awareness 10: 268–288.
16. Wong BYL (1996) The ADC's of learning disabilities (1st ed.). San Diego, CA: Academic Press.
17. Butler DL (1998) Metacognition and learning disabilities. In BYL Wong (Ed.). Learning about learning disabilities. USA: Academic Press, 277–307.
18. Perfect TJ, Schwartz BL (2002) (Eds.). Applied Metacognition. UK: Cambridge University Press.
19. Schneider W (2008) The development of metacognitive knowledge in children and adolescents: Major trends and implications for education. Mind, Brain and Education 2: 114–121.
20. Kleijnen R, Bosman A, De Jong P, Henneman K, Pasman J, et al. (2008) Diagnose en behandeling van dyslexie. Brochure van de Stichting Dyslexie Nederland. Geheel herziene versie Diagnosis and treatment of dyslexia. Brochure of the Dutch Dyslexia Foundation. Revision. Bilthoven, The Netherlands: Stichting Dyslexie Nederland.
21. Vaughn S, Fuchs LS (2003) Redefining learning disabilities as inadequate response to instruction: The promise and potential problems. Learning Disabilities Research & Practice 18: 137–146.
22. American Psychiatric Association (2013) Diagnostic and statistical manual of mental disorders (5th ed.). Arlington, VA: American Psychiatric Publishing.
23. Badian N (1999) Reading disability defined as a discrepancy between listening and reading comprehension: A longitudinal study of stability, gender differences, and prevalence. Journal of learning disabilities 32: 138–148.
24. Cope N, Harold D, Hill G, Moskvina V, Stevenson J, et al. (2005) Strong evidence that KIAA0319 on chromosome 6p is a susceptibility gene for developmental dyslexia. American Journal of Human Genetics 76: 581–591.
25. Lindgren SD, De Renzi E, Richman LC (1985) Cross-national comparisons of developmental dyslexia in Italy and the United-States. Child Development 56: 1404–1417.
26. Hanley JR, Masterson J, Spencer L, Evans D (2004) How long do the advantages of learning to read a transparent orthography last? An investigation of the reading skills and reading impairment of Welsh children at 10-years of age. The Quarterly Journal of Experimental Psychology 57: 1393–1410.
27. Szmalec A, Loncke M, Page MPA, Duyck W (2011) Order or Disorder? Impaired Hebb Learning in Dyslexia. Journal of Experimental Psychology, Learning, Memory and Cognition 37: 1270–1279.
28. Hatcher J, Snowling MJ, Griffiths YM (2002) Cognitive assessment of dyslexic students in higher education. British Journal of Educational Psychology 72: 119–133.
29. Callens M, Tops W, Brysbaert M (2012) Cognitive profile of students who enter higher education with an indication of dyslexia. Plos One 7: e38081.
30. De Smedt B, Boets B (2010) Phonological processing and arithmetic fact retrieval: evidence from developmental dyslexia. Neuropsychologia 48: 3973–3981.
31. Göbel SM, Snowling MJ (2010) Number-processing skills in adults with dyslexia. Quarterly Journal of Experimental Psychology 63: 1361–1373.
32. Rose LT, Rouhani P (2012) Influence of verbal memory depends on vocabulary: Oral reading fluency in adolescents with dyslexia. Mind, Brain, and Education 6: 1–9.
33. Kirby JR, Silvestri R, Allingham BH, Parrila R, Lafave CB (2008) Learning strategies and study approaches of postsecondary students with dyslexia. Journal of Learning Disabilities 41: 85–96.
34. Mortimore T, Crozier WR (2006) Dyslexia and difficulties with study skills in higher education. Studies in Higher Education 31: 235–251.
35. Job JM, Klassen RM (2012) Predicting performance on academic and non-academic tasks: A comparison of adolescents with and without learning disabilities. Contemporary Educational Psychology 37: 162–169.
36. Mason A, Mason M (2005) Understanding College Students with Learning Disabilities. Pediatric Clinics of North America 52: 61–70.
37. Krüger J, Dunning D (1999) Unskilled and unaware of it: How difficulties in recognizing one's own incompetence lead to inflated self-assessments. Journal of Personality and Social Psychology 77: 1121–1134.
38. Krüger J, Dunning D (2002) Unskilled and unaware – but why? A reply to Krüger and Müller. Journal of Personality and Social psychology 82: 189–192.
39. Sideridis GD, Morgan PL, Botsas G, Padeliadu S, Fuchs D (2006) Predicting LD on the basis of motivation, metacognition, and psychopathology: A ROC analysis. Journal of Learning Disabilities 39: 215–229.
40. Trainin G, Swanson HL (2005) Cognition, metacognition, and achievement of college students with learning disabilities. Learning Disability Quarterly 28: 261–272.
41. De Pessemier P, Andries C (2009) Test voor Gevorderd Lezen en Schrijven. Test for enhanced reading and writing. Antwerpen, Belgium: Garant Uitgeverij.
42. Loftus GR (1978) On interpretation of interactions. Memory & Cognition 6: 312–319.
43. Decarlo LT (1998) Signal Detection Theory and Generalized Linear Models. Psychological methods 3: 186–205.
44. Tops W, Verguts E, Callens M, Brysbaert M (2013) Do students with dyslexia have a different personality profile as measured with the Big Five? PloS One e64484.
45. Borgwaldt S, Hellwig F (2004) Onset entropy matters: Cross-linguistic sound-spelling analyses and empirical validation. Australian Journal of Psychology 56: 106–107.
46. Brus B, Voeten M (1991) Eén-minuut-test vorm A en B, schoolvorderingstest voor de technische leesvaardigheid bestemd voor groep 4 tot en met 8 van het basisonderwijs. Verantwoording en handleiding Manual of the Dutch version of the One Minute Test. Lisse, The Netherlands: Swets & Zeitlinger.
47. van den Bos K, Spelberg H, Scheepsma A, de Vries J (1999) De klepel vorm A en B, een test voor leesvaardigheid van pseudowoorden. Verantwoording, handleiding, diagnostiek en behandeling Test for pseudoword reading: Manual. Lisse, The Netherlands: Swets & Zeitlinger.
48. Dekker R, Dekker PH, Mulder JL (2004) Kaufman Adolescent and Adult Intelligence Test – Nederlandstalige Versie: Handleiding Manual Dutch version. Leiden, The Netherlands: PITS.
49. Tops W, Callens M, Lammertyn J, Van Hees V, Brysbaert M (2012) Identifying students with dyslexia in higher education. Annals of Dyslexia 62: 186–203.
50. Christensen RHB (2013) Ordinal---Regression Models for Ordinal Data R package version 2013.9–30 http://www.cran.r-project.org/package=ordinal/.
51. Dijkstra KA, Pligt J, Kleef GA (2013) Deliberation versus intuition: Decomposing the role of expertise in judgment and decision making. Journal of Behavioral Decision Making 26: 285–294.
52. Maniscalco B, Lau H (2012) A signal detection theory approach for estimating metacognitive sensitivity form confidence ratings. Consciousness and cognition 21: 422–430.

13

The Submerged Dyslexia Iceberg: How Many School Children Are Not Diagnosed? Results from an Italian Study

Chiara Barbiero[1,2], Isabella Lonciari[2], Marcella Montico[1], Lorenzo Monasta[1], Roberta Penge[3], Claudio Vio[4], Patrizio Emanuele Tressoldi[5], Valentina Ferluga[1], Anna Bigoni[1], Alessia Tullio[1], Marco Carrozzi[2], Luca Ronfani[1]*, for the CENDi (National Committee on the Epidemiology of Dyslexia) working group and for the Epidemiology of Dyslexia of Friuli Venezia Giulia working group (FVGwg)¶

1 Epidemiology and Biostatistics Unit, Institute for Maternal and Child Health - IRCCS "Burlo Garofolo", Trieste, Italy, **2** Child Neurology and Psychiatry Ward, Institute for Maternal and Child Health - IRCCS "Burlo Garofolo", Trieste, Italy, **3** Child Neuropsychiatry Department, UOC NPI B La Sapienza University, Rome, Italy, **4** Child Neuropsychiatry Unit, Hospital of San Donà di Piave, San Donà di Piave, Italy, **5** Psychology Department, University of Padua, Padua, Italy

Abstract

Background: Although dyslexia is one of the most common neurobehavioral disorders affecting children, prevalence is uncertain and available data are scanty and dated. The objective of this study is to evaluate the prevalence of dyslexia in an unselected school population using clearly defined and rigorous diagnostic criteria and methods.

Methods: Cross sectional study. We selected a random cluster sample of 94 fourth grade elementary school classes of Friuli Venezia Giulia, a Region of North Eastern Italy. We carried out three consecutive levels of screening: the first two at school and the last at the Neuropsychiatry Unit of a third level Mother and Child Hospital. The main outcome measure was the prevalence of dyslexia, defined as the number of children positive to the third level of screening divided by the total number of children enrolled.

Results: We recruited 1774 children aged 8–10 years, of which 1528 received parents' consent to participate. After applying exclusion criteria, 1357 pupils constituted the final working sample. The prevalence of dyslexia in the enrolled population ranged from 3.1% (95% CI 2.2–4.1%) to 3.2% (95% CI 2.4–4.3%) depending on different criteria adopted. In two out of three children with dyslexia the disorder had not been previously diagnosed.

Conclusions: This study shows that dyslexia is largely underestimated in Italy and underlines the need for reliable information on prevalence, in order to better allocate resources both to Health Services and Schools.

Editor: Kevin Paterson, University of Leicester, United Kingdom

Funding: The study was funded by the Friuli Venezia Giulia Regional Health Service (Agenzia Regionale della Sanità, resolution n° 42, April 4, 2008) through a grant to the Institute for Maternal and Child Health, IRCCS "Burlo Garofolo", Trieste and by internal research funds of the same Institute (Research project 63/07 Epidemiologia dei Disturbi Specifici dell'Apprendimento in una popolazione scolastica non selezionata). The funders had no role in study design, data collection and analysis, decision to publish, or preparation of the manuscript.

Competing Interests: The authors have declared that no competing interests exist.

* E-mail: ronfani@burlo.trieste.it

¶ Membership of the CENDi (National Committee on the Epidemiology of Dyslexia) working group and the Epidemiology of Dyslexia of Friuli Venezia Giulia working group (FVGwg) is provided in the Acknowledgments.

Introduction

Developmental dyslexia, or specific reading disability, is defined as an unexpected, specific, and persistent failure to acquire efficient reading skills despite conventional education, adequate intelligence, and socio-cultural opportunity. [1,2] Furthermore, this disability significantly interferes with scholastic learning or with daily activities that require reading ability.

Although dyslexia is one of the most common neurobehavioral disorders affecting children, prevalence is uncertain and available data are scanty and dated. Studies conducted in English-speaking countries, mainly in the Nineties, show prevalences ranging from 5 to 17.5%.[3–5] This range is due to the different diagnostic methods and definitions used [4,6,7]. For example, in a population based retrospective birth cohort study, the cumulative incidence rates of dyslexia by the age of 19 years varied from 5.5 to 11.8% depending on the formula used for diagnosis. [8] The geographical setting could also have a role. Dyslexia was found to occur in 9.9% of ten-year-old children living in a metropolitan area vs. 3.9% of children living in small towns. [9].

In Italy, a limited number of studies shows lower prevalences but confirms uncertainty (from 1.3% to 8.5%).[10–18] In the Sixties, in children aged 8 to 10 years living in a metropolitan area of Northern Italy, a prevalence of dyslexia of 1.34% was found using a collective reading test and a spelling test. [11] In studies conducted subsequently adopting the same instruments, on larger and more heterogeneous population samples, higher prevalence was reported, ranging from 3% to 6.5%.[12–14] A prevalence of dyslexia of 3.4% has been reported in a sample of children aged 8 to 10 years, that were first screened by teachers and subsequently underwent reading and writing tests [15] and of 5% in a sample of children of the same age that underwent collective tests on word/non word recognition, word/non word dictation, MT battery. [16] The prevalence of dyslexia estimated in a sample of high school children in Central Italy was 6.5%. [17] A longitudinal study conducted on children of elementary and middle schools living in Isola d'Elba (Tuscany) reported a prevalence of learning disabilities ranging from 0.88 to 1.23% in different school years from 1991 to 1999. [18] A cross national comparison of dyslexia prevalence in Italy and in the United States showed that dyslexia has a higher prevalence in the United States than in Italy and confirmed that the use of different methods and diagnostic criteria actually led to different values of dyslexia prevalence (3.6 to 8.5% in Italy vs. 4.5 to 12.0% in the United States). [19].

As described above, the variability in dyslexia prevalence estimates could be due to the different methods and tests adopted for diagnosis, the type of disability evaluated (i.e. dyslexia vs. learning disabilities), the different age ranges considered, the different geographic setting evaluated, as well as the different language spoken by the children. The key element to be taken into account is the definition of dyslexia adopted. [6] In Italy, an attempt to clearly define diagnostic criteria for dyslexia only dates back to 2007. These criteria were defined during the Montecatini Consensus Conference [20] by a panel of experts from Italian associations and institutions involved with children with learning disabilities, and were revised in 2011 (Text S1). [21,22] In 2010 the Italian Government approved a law to guarantee access to equal educational opportunities for students with learning disabilities (Italian Law n° 170, 8 October 2010). [23] Thus, Italian studies conducted before 2007 suffer from the lack of univocal diagnostic criteria that obviously influence reported prevalence data.

The lack of recent and reliable data on dyslexia prevalence leads to negative effects at the cultural (unmeasured phenomena can be ignored, underestimated or overestimated), clinical (insufficient resources for diagnosis and rehabilitation), and pedagogical level (insufficient resources for schools). Moved by these considerations, associations and institutions (listed in Annex) established a National Committee (CENDi) with the aim to define and apply methods and instruments and to conduct regional researches on the prevalence of dyslexia in representative unselected school populations. This paper describes in detail the methodology adopted and the results of the field study conducted in the Region of Friuli Venezia Giulia of Italy.

Materials and Methods

Cross sectional study carried out in Friuli Venezia Giulia (FVG), a region of North Eastern Italy. The study was approved by the Independent Bioethics Committee of the Institute of Maternal and Child Health - IRCCS "Burlo Garofolo", Trieste, Italy.

Sample

Children aged 8–10 years attending the 4th year of Italian primary schools were enrolled. In Italy, primary school includes children from age six to eleven and is organized in five school years. The 8–10 years of age range was chosen, in accordance with the Montecatini Consensus Conference, [20] for the following reasons: 1) by this age most learning delays are spontaneously resolved; [24,25] 2) a narrow age range reduces the number of developmental variables to be controlled; 3) in this age range, reading compensation strategies are not fixed, so the detection of reading difficulties should be easier.

Exclusion criteria were: 1) children with certification of mental retardation formulated by local health authorities according to the Italian Law n° 104/92 (framework law on disabled persons). [26] The exclusion of children with mental retardation was recommended by the Montecatini Consensus Conference, [20] and is in agreement with the definitions given by ICD-10 and DSM-IV. [1,2] 2) non-Italian nationality; 3) absence from school for more than two months since the first grade.

Bilingual children of Italian nationality and those with chronic diseases not related with learning abilities were not excluded. Pupils with previous diagnosis of dyslexia were included and re-evaluated.

To determine the sample size, the total population of children attending grade four in the Region (9687 children) was considered. A sample size of 1500 children was estimated, hypothesizing a prevalence of dyslexia of 4%, ranging from 3% to 5%, with a precision of 5% and a power of 80%. An extra 15% were enrolled to compensate possible drop outs. Based on the average number of children per class, we decided to randomly extract clusters of grade four classes rather than children. 94 classes were thus randomly extracted, comprising 1774 children.

Identification of Children with Dyslexia and Writing Disorders

The field study started in September 2008, at the beginning of the school year, and ended in October 2009, with the third level evaluation. Parents were adequately informed of the aim of the research and signed the informed consent. To identify children with reading disability, three consecutive levels of evaluation were carried out: the first two directly at school by specifically trained psychologists, the last in the Child Neuropsychiatry Unit of a third level hospital (IRCCS "Burlo Garofolo" of Trieste).

First level evaluation. Considering the large number of children to be screened, the first level evaluation was carried out through collective tests and questionnaires. To avoid discriminations, all children in the selected classrooms were tested, and exclusion criteria were applied afterwards. The evaluation was based on the following tools:

- A short anamnestic questionnaire filled in by parents, with questions concerning the child and his/her family (language spoken at home, age, work, parents' qualifications, health status of the child, handicap certification and previous diagnosis of Learning Disability).
- A specific questionnaire, filled in by the classroom teachers for each child of the selected classes, in order to detect Learning Disabilities (LD). This tool was derived from the validated questionnaire "RSR-DSA. Questionario per la rilevazione di difficoltà e disturbi dell'apprendimento". [27] Since this questionnaire includes 52 items investigating all LDs, for the purpose of this study, 34 specific questions pinpointing dyslexia and closely related disorders (difficulties in math, handwriting, spelling, and reading) were extracted, in agreement with the questionnaire's authors. Answers were scored on a 0 to 3 point scale (0 = never; 1 = sometimes; 2 = often; 3 = always). Children were considered having reading difficulties if: 1) the total score ≥85° percentile or 2) the score on two subgroups of questions specifically addressing dyslexia ≥90° percentile. The diagnostic accuracy of these criteria was tested on a sample of 200

children previously enrolled (100 with diagnosis of dyslexia and 100 controls without reading difficulties) (data not published). The results showed a sensitivity of 82% and a specificity of 100%, with 91% of children correctly classified. The diagnostic accuracy was considered good and comparable with that obtained by more complex screening instruments. [28]

- A dictation task for the forth grade, derived from the "BVSCO – Battery for the assessment of writing skills in children from 7 to 13 years old". [29] To avoid bias due to different reading styles and timing during dictation, the task was recorded on CD and played in the classrooms using a laptop with adequate amplification. The use of a dictation test to screen reading difficulties is supported by studies on the comorbidity between reading and spelling difficulties. [30] Children scoring ≥90° percentile were considered as having learning difficulties, as indicated by the normative data of the tests used. [29]

After applying inclusion/exclusion criteria, children who scored positive by the teachers' questionnaire and/or in the dictation task were selected for the second level evaluation. These criteria allowed to correctly identify all 13 children who had already received a formal diagnosis of dyslexia, except one (Figure 1). This child, however, had just completed a rehabilitation programme before the beginning of the school year which explains his good performance in the tests.

To ensure that all children with reading difficulties were identified, teachers were further asked to indicate 1) children who read more slowly than classmates 2) children who made more reading errors than classmates. All children identified by at least one of these two additional criteria were also selected for second level testing. Furthermore, when possible, in classes in which children with reading difficulties were identified, classmates with adequate performance were also randomly selected for second level evaluation, in order to avoid discrimination from peers.

Second level evaluation. The aim of the second level was to identify children with reading difficulties and adequate cognitive ability through individual tests. Evaluations were conducted at school and carried out by the same researchers involved in the first level evaluation (specifically trained psychologists). The following tools were used for individual testing:

- word and non word reading tasks derived from the DDE-2 Battery (Battery for the assessment of Developmental Dyslexia and Dysorthographia-2) [31] were used to assess reading speed and accuracy. These tasks provided a total of 4 scores (2 for accuracy and 2 for speed). Children were considered to perform poorly if: a) they failed in at least one of four scores (cut-offs: z-score ≤−1.8 standard deviations from the mean for speed scores, a score <5th percentile in the accuracy scores), or b) they failed in at least two of the four scores (cut-offs: z-score ≤−1.5 standard deviations from the mean in speed scores, a score <10th percentile in accuracy scores). The cut-offs selected for the criterion *a* were those indicated by the normative data of the DDE-2 Battery; [31] for the criterion *b*, the CENDi chose less selective cut-offs in order to reduce false negatives to the minimum and to also identify children with mild disorders.
- Vocabulary and Block Design subtests of the WISC-III (Wechsler Intelligence Scale for Children) [32,33] to estimate child's cognitive ability. Since the time at school was insufficient to perform the entire WISC-III scale, these two subtests were selected as the more related to the child's IQ score. [32,33] A weighted score ≤7 in both sub-tests identified a poor IQ, in agreement with those reported in the WISC-III manual.

The second level criteria were defined by CENDi according to the Montecatini Consensus Conference. [20] The selected tests

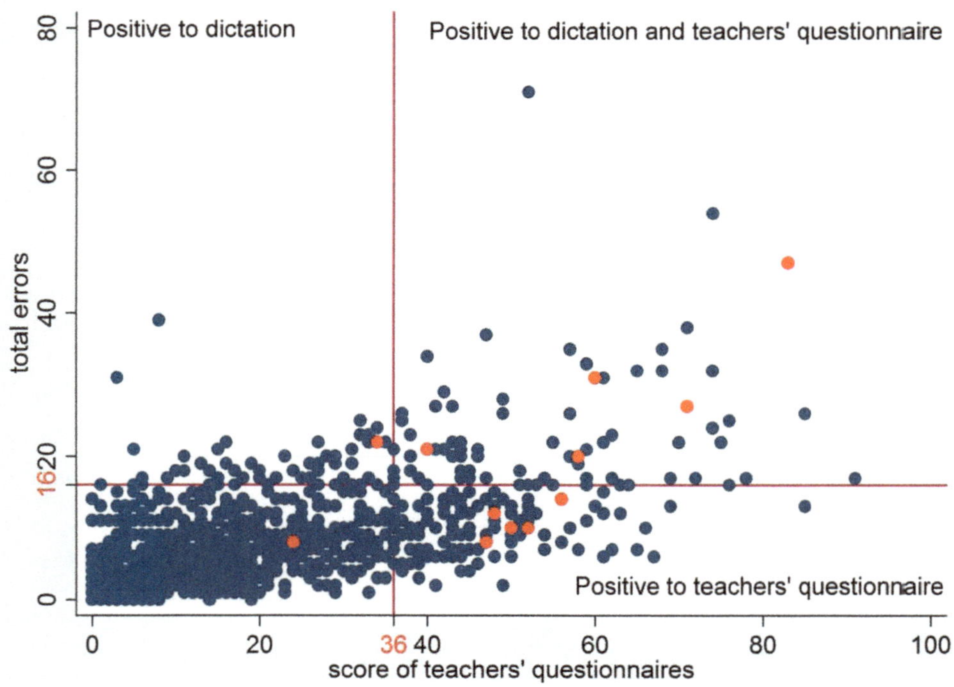

Figure 1. Children positive to the criteria of the first evaluation level. In red children with previously formalised diagnosis of dyslexia.

and cut-offs allowed to correctly identify all children with a prior formal diagnosis of dyslexia, except one. Again, this child had just completed a rehabilitation programme and showed a marked improvement in performance.

Children with adequate WISC-III subtest scores, yet poor performance in reading tasks, were selected for the third level of screening.

Third Level Evaluation

The aim of the third level was to confirm the diagnosis of dyslexia. To avoid bias in the diagnostic process, all children selected at the second level evaluation were referred and evaluated at the Child Neuropsychiatry Unit of the third level hospital IRCCS "Burlo Garofolo". All children were assessed as follows:

a) Detailed questionnaire (see Text S2) filled in by parents and checked during an interview with a psychologist. This standardized protocol allowed to collected anamnestic information about the child's development (speech, gait, autonomy, etc.), kindergarten and primary school attendance (social skills and communication, presence of learning disabilities, etc.), clinically significant events that may have occurred during childhood (i.e. injuries, illnesses) and information regarding formal education of close relatives (school performance, learning difficulties, etc.)
b) Raven's Progressive Matrices PM47 to evaluate in a short time the cognitive performance. [34]
c) MT battery (Prove di lettura MT per la scuola elementare-2) to evaluate speed and accuracy of text reading. [35,36]
d) DDE-2 (Battery for the evaluation of Dyslexia and dysorthography-2) to evaluate speed and accuracy of word and non word reading (tasks 2 and 3) and accuracy of spelling (tasks 6 and 7). [31]
e) Strengths and Difficulties Questionnaire (SDQ) administered to parents to evaluate the mental health status of their child. [37]

To confirm the diagnosis of dyslexia we took into account:

- Six scores (three on accuracy and three on speed) derived from the reading tests (test MT and tasks 2 and 3 from battery DDE-2).
- Parents responses to two questions derived from the detailed questionnaire completed during the third level evaluation: A) presence of early specific reading and/or spelling difficulties B) the child is not independent in performing homework.
- Teachers' positive responses to eight specific questions on decoding skills derived from the questionnaire compiled during the first level evaluation. [27] These items relate to accuracy (skips lines reading, makes more errors in reading than her/his classmates, replaces, omits, adds or reverses letters, makes up words, is fast but incorrect in reading) and speed (the child reads more slowly than her/his peers).

Combining the results of these tests, CENDi experts defined three possible criteria to guide the diagnosis of dyslexia (each criterion requires that all the defined conditions be met):

1. Poor performance (Table 1) on reading tasks in at least three out of six scores.
2. a) Poor performance (Table 1) on reading tasks in at least two scores out of six, in two different reading tests (the poor performance should not refer to two parameters in a single reading test); AND b) parental acknowledgement of the disorder by a positive response to at least one of the two questions A and B of the detailed questionnaire.
3. a) Poor performance (Table 1) on reading tests in at least three out of six scores; AND b) parental recognition of the disorder by a positive answer to both questions A and B of the detailed questionnaire; AND c) teachers' acknowledgement of the disorder by a positive response to at least half of the questions selected by the teachers' questionnaire.

The cut-offs reported in Table 1 were defined by the CENDi experts, according to the normative data and to the recommendations of the Montecatini Consensus Conference. [20] For the third criterion the CENDi decided to choose less selective cut-offs on a higher number of scores, together with the recognition of difficulties by parents and teachers, in order to identify children with a less pronounced form of disability.

An additional fourth criterion was defined to identify children with only phonological difficulties: a) poor performance (Table 1) in at least one score on non word reading tasks; AND b) parental recognition of the disorder by a positive answer to both questions A and B of the detailed questionnaire; AND c) teachers' recognition of the disorder by a positive response to at least half of the questions in the teacher questionnaire. The rationale of this criterion is based on the evidence that children with dyslexia may have difficulties in phonological recoding when measured with non word reading tests. [38].

Children identified by the fourth criterion were considered separately in the prevalence evaluation since CENDi experts considered this criterion weaker than the previous. Any case of discrepancy between the results obtained applying the criteria and the clinician's judgement was also considered separately (i.e. children who were diagnosed dyslexic according to the criteria but not according to the clinician's evaluation and, conversely,

Table 1. Definition of poor performance in reading tasks by diagnostic criteria defined at the third level evaluation.

First and second criteria	
DDE-2*	z-score ≤ -1.8 (speed)
	OR
	percentile <5° (accuracy)
MT§	z-score ≤ -2 (speed)
	OR
	percentile $\leq$5° (accuracy)
Third criterion	
DDE-2*	z-score between -1.8 and -1.5 (speed)
	OR
	percentile between 5° and 10° (accuracy)
MT§	z-score between -2 and -1.5 (speed)
	OR
	between 5° and 10°
Fourth criterion	
DDE-2 non word*	z-score ≤ -1.8 (speed)
	OR
	percentile $\leq$5° (accuracy)

*DDE-2: Battery for the evaluation of Developmental Dyslexia and Dysorthography-2.
§MT: MT battery (Prove di lettura MT per la scuola elementare-2).

children who were diagnosed according to clinician assessment but not according to the criteria). The clinical history of these children and the third level evaluation tests were reviewed by the CENDi experts to confirm or deny the diagnosis.

Children identified by the criteria as dyslexic were subjected to further evaluations: a) Completion of the scale WISC-III; [32,33] b) Math tasks (numerical facts, count backwards, numbers dictation) from the ABCA test; [39] c) the Italian adaptation of the Multidimensional Self-Concept Scale (MSCS); [40] d) Questionnaire "A chi assomiglio", [41] the Italian adaptation of the "Self-Perception Profile for Children"; [42] e) neurological objective examination. The results of the tests applied at points *b*, *c*, *d* were not used for the purpose of this paper and consequently are not presented in this manuscript.

Based on the results of these additional evaluations and on data reported in detailed parents questionnaire, children were considered as non-dyslexic if they had: a) a cognitive delay defined by the results of the WISC-III scale (scores on Verbal IQ and Performance IQ <85); b) diseases or sensory and neurological abnormalities; c) severe psychopathology; d) conditions of environmental, social or cultural disadvantage; e) poor teaching.

Children with suspected neuropsychiatric problems were referred to the Neuropsychiatry Unit for further investigations.

Figure 2 summarizes the procedure for the third level of screening.

Statistical Analysis

Continuous data were presented as means and standard deviations, categorical data as absolute frequencies and percentages.

Prevalence of dyslexia was defined as the number of children positive to the third level of screening (numerator) divided by the total number of children analysed at the first level.

Two values of prevalence were calculated, the first including only cases with diagnosis of dyslexia according to the first three criteria defined by CENDi, and the second also including cases with uncertain diagnosis (defined by the 4th criterion or by discrepancy in diagnosis between criteria and clinical judgment).

To predict the diagnosis of dyslexia in children lost to the third level follow up, a multinomial logistic regression analysis was carried out. The estimation process included the results of the tests conducted at the second level (speed and accuracy in word and non word reading tests) as predictors and the diagnosis of dyslexia as the dependent variable. A step-down procedure was applied to the saturated model retaining only variables with a p-value <0.05. The final logistic model was used to predict the probability of being dyslexic, and ROC (Receiver-Operating-Characteristic) analysis was used to identify the cut-off correctly classifying the highest rate of subjects. Based on this cut-off, subjects lost to the third level follow up were classified as with or without dyslexia and included in the calculation of the total prevalence.

Results

A total of 94 grade four classes were selected using random cluster sampling. Overall, 1774 pupils were contacted, and for 1528 of them parents gave their consent to participate.

First Level Evaluation

Thirty-two children were absent from school on days when the assessments were carried out. The remaining 1496 children participated in the first level evaluation. After application of exclusion criteria, 1365 children were included in the sample and their performance was analysed (Figure 3 and Figure S1). Characteristics of these children are presented in Table 2. Thirteen out of the 1365 children (1%) had already received a formal diagnosis of dyslexia.

Two hundred eighty-three children scored positive in at least one of the two tests of the first level (dictation or teachers' questionnaire) and 62 were identified by the additional questions addressed to the teachers.

Second Level Evaluation

Overall, 396 children were selected for the second level assessment (345 selected at the first level of screening and 51 randomly selected from children with adequate performance). One hundred twenty-one scored positive in the tests and were selected for the third level of screening.

Third Level Evaluation

Ninety-three of 121 children underwent further testing to confirm diagnosis. Parents of 28 children refused to continue in the study. Five children of 93 were excluded since they met the third level exclusion criteria (4 with cognitive delay and 1 with social disadvantage). Of the remaining 88 children, 51 were classified without dyslexia, 35 were diagnosed with dyslexia, 1 was positive only according to the 4th criterion and 1 was positive on the basis of the defined criteria but the clinician did not confirm the diagnosis.

The logistic model built for predicting dyslexia in children lost to the third level follow up retained as significant predictors the speed z-score of the word reading test (adjusted OR 0.13, 95% CI 0.02–0.87 and adjusted OR 0.07, 95% CI 0.01–0.61 respectively) and the speed z-score of the non word reading test (adjusted OR 1.29, 95% CI 1.11–1.51).

The ROC (Receiver-Operating-Characteristic) curve was generated with the predicted probability of the logistic model. The resulting area under the curve was 0.93. The cut-off with the highest percentage of correctly classified (86.2%), gave us a sensitivity of 70.3% and a specificity of 98.0%. Using this cut-off, 7 out of 28 children were considered to be dyslexics.

The prevalence of dyslexia including children who fell in the three diagnostic criteria (n = 35) and children estimated with the logistic model (n = 7) was 3.1% (42/1365) (95% CI 2.2–4.1); adding the child positive to the fourth criterion and that with uncertain diagnosis the prevalence rose to 3.2% (95% CI 2.4–4.3).

Discussion

This study accurately estimated the prevalence of dyslexia in a representative and unselected grade four school population. Prior to the study, out of 1365 children screened, 13 (1%) had a formal diagnosis of dyslexia and 27 (2%) of Learning Disabilities (including dyslexia, dysgraphia, dyscalculia and dysorthography). These findings are similar to those available for other areas in Italy. [43]

The prevalence of dyslexia at the end of the study rose to 3.1–3.2%. Therefore, according to our study, dyslexia is not recognized in two out of three children aged 8–10 years, when the disorder should be clearly expressed and identified. This discrepancy calls for justifications, especially in a Region like FVG which is generally considered quite sensitive to this issue and where attention to the disorder has been recently shown both by Schools and Health Services through workshops, conferences, meeting, circulation of guidelines, and interventions in schools. Since dyslexia has been identified as a specific risk factor for increased internalizing, anxiety and depressive behaviours, [44,45] suicidal ideation, and school failure and drop out, [46] especially

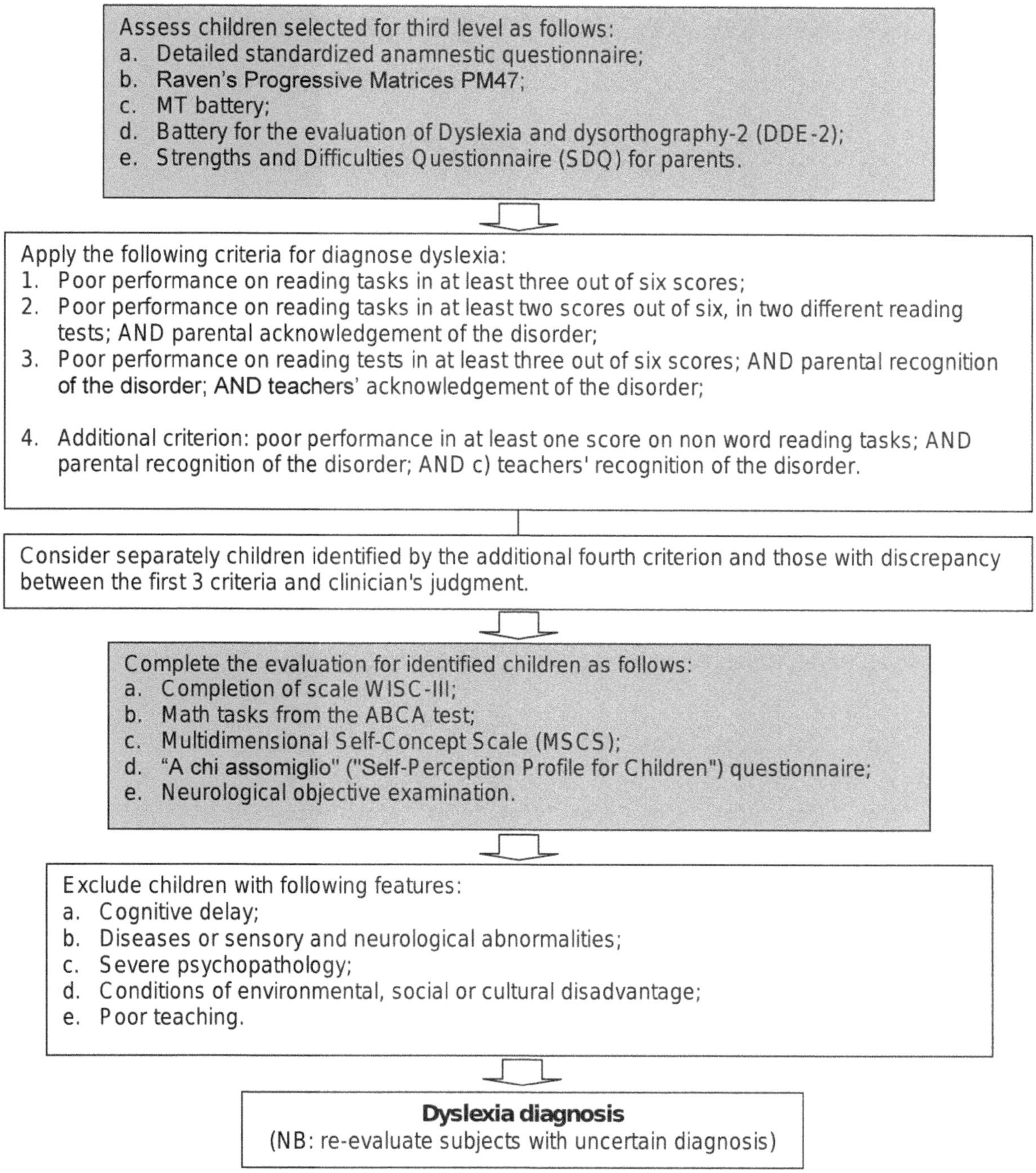

Figure 2. Steps for third level evaluation.

during adolescence, early diagnosis and intervention appear to be crucial for the affected children.

Given the differences in methods, definitions and diagnostic criteria adopted, it is difficult to compare the prevalence data obtained in this study with those previously reported in Italy.[10–18] However, our results are in line with the expected for Italy. The comparison with studies conducted in English-speaking countries is even more complex, as the frequency of dyslexia differs between languages. As addressed in a recent literature review, the neural basis of dyslexia is similar across different languages. However, cross-cultural specificities were evident in the manifestations of dyslexia, as clinically significant difficulties are less common in transparent languages with consistent orthographies (i.e. Italian), if compared to languages with inconsistent orthographies (i.e. English). [6] Poor readers in English, French and Italian showed similar patterns of aberrant neural activation, but Italian subjects present a higher reading accuracy. [47] A cross national comparison of dyslexia prevalence in Italy and in the United States confirmed that dyslexia is more prevalent in the United States than in Italy. Furthermore, in this cross national study, different diagnostic criteria for dyslexia were applied to the enrolled children, thus achieving different values of dyslexia prevalence (3.6 to 8.5% in Italy vs. 4.5 to 12.0% in the United States). [19]

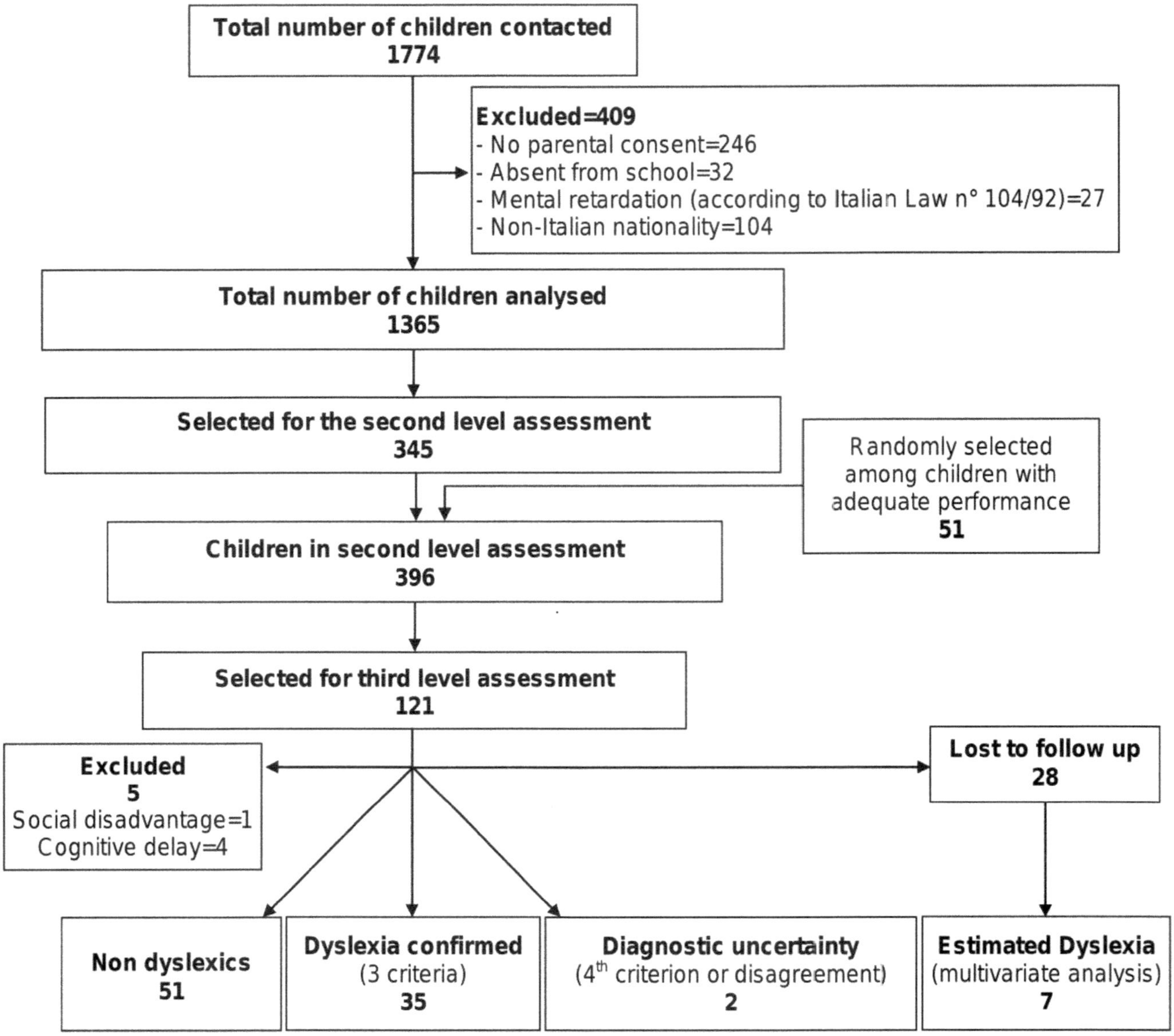

Figure 3. Study flow chart.

Consequently, our estimate of prevalence cannot be extended to different contexts, in particular to populations speaking less phonetically regular languages, like English. However, research on dyslexia has historically focused mainly on the English language, and reliable data on other languages are required to better understand cross-cultural differences and similarities. [6,48] Furthermore, given the important consequences it might have on dyslexic children and on allocation of resources, it would be interesting to understand whether the problem of underestimation of dyslexia prevalence is common to population speaking other languages. The available scientific literature does not allow us to answer this question and ad hoc studies, designed and conducted following clearly defined rigorous methods would be required, in order to guarantee their reproducibility and a clear comprehension of what is being assessed. In our study, to confirm the diagnosis of dyslexia, a detailed and unequivocal diagnostic algorithm, combining the different tests and the cut-offs indicated by the Montecatini Consensus Conference (see Text S1) [20] was developed by the CENDi, thus contributing to a more precise definition of the diagnostic criteria of dyslexia in Italy. The study presents several other strengths: the use of a cluster sampling procedure to enrol a representative sample of regional school pupils aged 8–10 years; the large sample size (about 15% of children attending grade four in Friuli Venezia Giulia); the rigorous application of screening tools by a specifically trained staff; the third level assessment (confirmation of diagnosis) performed in a single third level Neuropsychiatry Unit to avoid bias in the diagnostic process; the involvement in this process of both child neuropsychiatrists and psychologists.

The study has some limitations: given the large sample size, it was not possible to administer individual reading tests to all children at the first level evaluation. Consequently, the CENDi decided to adopt two different tools: a shortened version of a validated questionnaire to be filled in by teachers for each child in the selected classrooms; [27] a dictation test collectively administered to children in a standardized manner. [29] The use of a

Table 2. Main characteristics of the selected population.

Variable		Children (n = 1365)
Sex	Female	663 (48.6%)
	Male	702 (51.4%)
Language spoken at home	Italian	1256 (92.0%)
	Dialect	105 (7.7%)
	Other	4 (0.3%)
Age of the mother, mean (standard deviation)		40.1 (4.71)
Age of the father, mean (standard deviation)		43.2 (5.44)
Mother's formal education level	None/elementary	20 (1.4%)
	Lower secondary	413 (30.4%)
	Upper secondary	729 (53.6%)
	Degree	198 (14.6%)
Father's formal education level	Elementary	22 (1.6%)
	Lower secondary	511 (38.0%)
	Upper secondary	634 (47.2%)
	Degree	177 (13.2%)
Mother with job		1053 (77.4%)
Father with job		1319 (98.2%)
Children with previously formalised dyslexia diagnosis		13 (1.0%)
Children with previously formalised Learning Disabilities diagnosis (dyslexia, dysgraphia, dysorthography, dyscalculia)		27 (2.0%)

dictation test to screen reading difficulties is supported by studies on comorbidity between reading and spelling difficulties. [30] Since these tools have never been used before in screening studies for dyslexia, their use could have resulted in a loss of children with reading difficulties at the first level screening (false negatives). Nevertheless, we believe we have kept this risk to the minimum, considering that: a) children were selected for second level if scores were positive even in one of the two tools; b) a low cut-off (85th percentile) for the teachers' questionnaire was selected to include a large number of children; c) the criteria adopted allowed to correctly identify all 13 children who had already received a formal diagnosis of dyslexia, except one. However, the non-selected child completed a rehabilitation treatment just before the beginning of the study and this should explain the improvement in test performance; d) in addition to the questionnaire, teachers were asked to further point out children with reading difficulties through two simple and standardized questions; children identified by at least one of these two additional criteria were selected for second level analysis, despite results of teachers' questionnaire and dictation tests.

Conclusions

This study shows that the tools and the methodology defined by the CENDi are applicable and allow to estimate the prevalence of dyslexia in an unselected grade four school population in Italy. In our setting the prevalence ranged from 3.1 to 3.2%, in line with expectations. Therefore, it is interesting to notice that in two out of three children with dyslexia the disorder had not been previously diagnosed. These data confirm the need for reliable information on dyslexia prevalence in order to better allocate resources both to Health Services and Schools. Finally, this study provides original and up-to-date information, useful in the debate on trans-cultural features of dyslexia.

Supporting Information

Figure S1 Details on children included and excluded at first and second level evaluation.

Text S1 General criteria for dyslexia diagnosis defined by the Montecatini Consensus Conference (2007) and by the subsequent national Consensus Conferences (2011).

Text S2 Standardized questionnaire filled in by parents.

Acknowledgments

We thank Laura Bravar for the editing of the paper.

The members of the CENDi (National Committee on the Epidemiology of Dyslexia) working group and the Epidemiology of Dyslexia of Friuli Venezia Giulia working group (FVGwg) are: Chiara Barbiero, Marco Carrozzi, Isabella Lonciari, Luca Ronfani, Giorgio Tamburlini, Institute for Maternal and Child Health - IRCCS "Burlo Garofolo"; Marinella Caruso, ANUPI-*Associazione Nazionale Unitaria Psicomotricisti e Terapisti della Neuro e Psicomotricità dell'Età Evolutiva Italiani* (Childhood Neuro and Psycomotricity Therapists Association); Serenella Corbo, ACP-*Associazione Culturale Pediatri* (Cultural Association of Paediatricians); Anna Giulia De Cagno, FLI-*Federazione Logopedisti Italiani* (Italian Federation of Speech and Language Therapists);

Isabella Lonciari, AID-*Associazione Italiana Dislessia* (Italian Dyslexia Association); Massimiliano Parmini, FEDEROTTICA-*Associazione Federativa Nazionale Ottici Optometristi* (National Federation of opticians and optometrists); Roberta Penge, SINPIA-*Società Italiana di Neuro Psichiatria dell'Infanzia e dell'Adolescenza* (Italian Society of Child and Adolescents Neurology and Psychiatry); Alessandra Pinton, SSLI-*Società Scientifica Logopedisti Italiani* (Italian Scientific Society of Speech and Language Therapists); Giovanna Rossini, AITNE-*Associazione Italiana Terapisti della*

Neuropsicomotricità dell'Età Evolutiva (Italian Association of Neurodevelopmental Disorders' Therapists); Claudio Vio, AIRIPA-*Associazione Italiana Ricerca Psicopatologia dell'Apprendimento* (Italian Association for the Research and Clinical Intervention on Learning Psychopathology); Loris Zanier, *Direzione Centrale Salute Integrazione Sociosanitaria e Politiche Sociali, Friuli Venezia Giulia* (Friuli Venezia Giulia Regional Health Service); Edda Colcergnan, Enzo Burchiellaro, *Ufficio Scolastico Regionale del Friuli Venezia Giulia* (Friuli Venezia Giulia Regional School Office).

Author Contributions

Conceived and designed the experiments: CB IL RP CV PET MC LR CENDi FVGwg. Performed the experiments: CB VF AT AB. Analyzed the data: MM LM LR. Contributed reagents/materials/analysis tools: CB IL RP MC MM LM LR. Wrote the paper: CB MM LM LR. Discussed the study findings and participated in decisions concerning ways of reporting findings: CB IL RP CV PET MC LR. Contributed to the final version of the paper and approved it: CB IL MM LM RP CV PET VF AB AT MC LR.

References

1. American Psychiatric Association (1994) Diagnostic and statistical manual of mental disorders, 4th edn. APA.
2. World Health Organization (1993): The international classification of disease, vol.10: classification of mental and behavioural disorders. WHO.
3. Interagency Committee on Learning Disabilities (1987) Learning disabilities: a report to the U.S. Congress. Government Printing Office.
4. Shaywitz SE, Fletcher JM, Shaywitz BA (1994) Issues in the definition and classification of attention deficit disorder. Top Lang Disord 14: 1–25.
5. Demonet JF, Taylor MJ, Chaix Y (2004) Developmental dyslexia. Lancet 363: 1451–60.
6. Peterson RL, Pennington BF (2012) Developmental dyslexia. Lancet 379: 1997–2007.
7. Whitaker S (2004) Inner learning disability. Brit J Learn Disabil 32: 139–143.
8. Katusic SK, Colligan RC, Barbaresi WJ, Schaid DJ, Jacobsen SJ (2001) Incidence of reading disability in a population-based birth cohort, 1976–1982, Rochester, Minn. Mayo Clin Pro 76: 1081–92.
9. Berger M, Yule W, Rutter M (1975) Attainment and adjustment in two geographical areas. II-The prevalence of specific reading retardation. Br J Psychiatry 126: 510–9.
10. Baldini G, Brasca E (1958) L'apprendimento della lettura e della scrittura: aspetti psicopatologici e considerazioni psicopedagogiche. Infanzia Anormale 26: 167–191.
11. Faglioni P, Gatti B, Paganoni AM, Robutti A (1967) La valutazione psicometrica della Dislessia. Infanzia Anormale 81: 628–661.
12. Bisiacchi P, Brotini D, Fornari D (1978) Indagine sull'incidenza della dislessia in un campione di bambini padovani. Formazione e cambiamento;1: 3–16.
13. Sava D, Buffardini C (1981) Dislessia evolutiva: aspetti socio-ambientali e neuropsicologici. Giornale Italiano di Psicologia 8: 405–419.
14. Cassini A, Ciampalini L, Lis A (1984) La dislessia in Italia. Strumenti di rilevazione ed incidenza in alcune regioni. Età Evolutiva 18: 66–73.
15. Levi G, Piredda ML (1982) Strategie semantiche e strategie fonologiche nella costruzione di anangrammi in bambini dislessici. Neuropsichiatria Infantile 250/251: 439–450.
16. Masala C, Petretto DR, Stella G (1998) Studio epidemiologico sui DSA in una popolazione sarda. Psichiatria dell'Infanzia e dell'Adolescenza 65: 648–653.
17. Moreno R, Pianta F, Stella G (2005) L'incidenza dei Disturbi Specifici di Lettura nella Scuola Media Superiore: uno studio comparativo. Dislessia 2: 135–146.
18. Coscarella C (2001) Epidemiologia dei Deficit Specifici di Apprendimento nel territorio dell'Isola d'Elba. Psichiatria dell'Infanzia e dell'Adolescenza 68: 7–15.
19. Lindgren SD, De Renzi E, Richman LC (1985) Cross-national comparisons of developmental dyslexia in Italy and the United States. Child Dev 56: 1404.
20. Consensus Conference (2007) Disturbi evolutivi specifici di apprendimento. Available: www.lineeguidadsa.it/download_documentiDSA/RACCOMANDAZIONI_PRATICA_CLINICA_DSA2007.zip. Accessed 1 September 2012.
21. PARCC (2011) DSA Documento d'intesa. Available: www.lineeguidadsa.it/download_documentiDSA/Raccomandazioni_clinica_DSA11.zip. Accessed 1 September 2012.
22. Istituto Superiore di Sanità (2011) Consensus Conference Disturbi Specifici dell'Apprendimento. Sistema nazionale per le linee guida Ministero della salute. Available: www.lineeguidadsa.it/download_documentiDSA/Raccomandazioni_CC_DSA.zip. Accessed 1 September 2012.
23. Nuove norme in materia di disturbi specifici di apprendimento in ambito scolastico, Public Law N.170 (October 8, 2010). Gazzetta Ufficiale della Repubblica Italiana 2010; 244.
24. Seymour PH, Aro M, Erskine JM (2003) Foundation literacy acquisition in European orthographies. Br J Psychol 94: 143–74.
25. Orsolini M, Fanari R, Tosi V, De Nigris B, Carrieri R (2006) From phonological recoding to lexical reading: A longitudinal study on reading development in Italian Lang Cognitive Proc 21: 576–607.
26. Legge-quadro per l'assistenza, l'integrazione sociale e i diritti delle persone handicappate, Public Law n.104 (February 4, 1992). Gazzetta Ufficiale della Repubblica Italiana 1992;39 (Suppl.Ordinario n.30).
27. Cappa C, Albanesi E, Muzio C, Guglielmino P, Ferraris V, et al. (2012) Uno strumento per la rilevazione di indicatori di rischio di DSA: il questionario RSR-DSA. Dislessia 1.
28. Le Jan G, Le Bouquin Jeannès R, Costet N, Faucon G (2007) Discriminatory validity of dyslexia screening tasks in French school age children. Conf Proc IEEE Eng Med Biol Soc 1: 3781–5.
29. Tressoldi PE, Cornoldi C (2000) Batteria per la valutazione della scrittura e della competenza ortografica nella scuola dell'obbligo (BVSCO, Battery for the assessment of writing skills of children from 7 to 13 years old). Firenze: Giunti OS.
30. Angelelli P, Notarnicola A, Judica A, Zoccolotti P, Luzzatti C (2010) Spelling impairments in Italian dyslexic children: phenomenological changes in primary school. Cortex 46: 1299–1311.
31. Sartori G, Job R, Tressoldi PE (2007) DDE-2. Batteria per la valutazione della dislessia e della disortografia evolutiva (Battery for the assessment of developmental dyslexia and dysorthographia). Firenze: Giunti OS.
32. Wechsler D (2006) WISC-III Wechsler Intelligence Scale for Children – third ed. Firenze: Giunti OS.
33. Orsini A, Picone L (2006). WISC-III Contributo alla taratura italiana. Firenze: Giunti OS.
34. Raven JC (2006) CPM Coloured Progressive Matrices. Firenze: Giunti OS.
35. Cornoldi C, Colpo G (2004). Prove di lettura MT per la scuola elementare –2. Firenze: Giunti OS.
36. Cornoldi C, Tressoldi PE, Perini N (2010) Valutare la rapidità e la correttezza della lettura di brani. Nuove norme e alcune chiarificazioni per l'uso delle prove MT. Dislessia 7: 89–100.
37. Goodman R, Ford T, Simmons H, Gatward R, Meltzer H (2003) Using the Strengths and Difficulties Questionnaire (SDQ) to screen for child psychiatric disorders in a community sample. Int Rev Psychiatry 15: 166–72.
38. Herrmann JA, Matyas T, Pratt C (2006) Meta-analysis of the non word reading deficit in specific reading disorder. Dyslexia 12: 195–221.
39. Lucangeli D, Tressoldi PE, Fiore C (2006) ABCA Test delle abilità di calcolo. Trento: Erickson.
40. Bracken BA (2003) TMA Test di valutazione multidimensionale dell'autostima. Trento: Erickson.
41. Tressoldi PE, Vio C (1996) Diagnosi dei disturbi dell'apprendimento scolastico: dalla segnalazione alla diagnosi funzionale. Trento: Erickson.
42. Harter S (1985) The Self-Perception Profile for Children. University of Denver; Denver, CO.
43. Gruppo di lavoro regionale sui D.S.A. (2011) Alunni con Disturbi Specifici di Apprendimento in Veneto-Monitoraggio Anno Scolastico 2010–11. Available: http://disabilita.istruzioneveneto.it/wp/wp-content/uploads/2011/05/MonitoRegDSA201011.pdf; Accessed 1 September 2012.
44. Mugnaini D, Lassi S, La Malfa G, Albertini G (2009) Internalizing correlates of dyslexia. World J Pediatr 5: 255–64.
45. Willcutt EG, Pennington BF (2000) Psychiatric comorbidity in children and adolescents with reading disability. J Child Psychol Psychiatry 41: 1039–48.
46. Daniel SS, Walsh AK, Goldston DB, Arnold EM, Reboussin BA, et al. (2006) Suicidality, school dropout, and reading problems among adolescents. J Learn Disabil 39: 507–14.
47. Paulesu E, Démonet JF, Fazio F, McCrory E, Chanoine V, et al. (2001) Dyslexia: cultural diversity and biological unity. Science 291: 2165–67.
48. Share DL (2008) On the anglocentricities of current reading research and practice: the perils of overreliance on an "outlier" orthography. Psychol Bull 134: 584–615.

The Genetics of Reading Disability in an Often Excluded Sample: Novel Loci Suggested for Reading Disability in Rolandic Epilepsy

Lisa J. Strug[1,2], Laura Addis[3], Theodore Chiang[1], Zeynep Baskurt[1], Weili Li[1], Tara Clarke[4], Huntley Hardison[5], Steven L. Kugler[6], David E. Mandelbaum[7], Edward J. Novotny[8], Steven M. Wolf[9], Deb K. Pal[3,10]*

1 Child Health Evaluative Sciences, The Hospital for Sick Children, Toronto, Canada, **2** Dalla Lana School of Public Health, University of Toronto, Toronto, Canada, **3** Department of Clinical Neurosciences, Institute of Psychiatry, King's College London, London, United Kingdom, **4** Department of Epidemiology, Mailman School of Public Health, Columbia University Medical Center, New York, New York, United States of America, **5** St. Christopher's Hospital for Children, Philadelphia, Pennsylvania, United States of America, **6** Children's Hospital of Philadelphia and University of Pennsylvania School of Medicine, Philadelphia, Pennsylvania, United States of America, **7** Hasbro Children's Hospital and The Warren Alpert Medical School of Brown University, Providence, Rhode Island, United States of America, **8** Yale University Medical Center, New Haven, Connecticut, United States of America, **9** Beth Israel Medical Center, New York, New York, United States of America, **10** Department of Psychiatry, Columbia University Medical Center, New York, New York, United States of America

Abstract

Background: Reading disability (RD) is a common neurodevelopmental disorder with genetic basis established in families segregating "pure" dyslexia. RD commonly occurs in neurodevelopmental disorders including Rolandic Epilepsy (RE), a complex genetic disorder. We performed genomewide linkage analysis of RD in RE families, testing the hypotheses that RD in RE families is genetically heterogenous to pure dyslexia, and shares genetic influences with other sub-phenotypes of RE.

Methods: We initially performed genome-wide linkage analysis using 1000 STR markers in 38 US families ascertained through a RE proband; most of these families were multiplex for RD. We analyzed the data by two-point and multipoint parametric LOD score methods. We then confirmed the linkage evidence in a second US dataset of 20 RE families. We also resequenced the *SEMA3C* gene at the 7q21 linkage locus in members of one multiplex RE/RD pedigree and the *DISC1* gene in affected pedigrees at the 1q42 locus.

Results: In the discovery dataset there was suggestive evidence of linkage for RD to chromosome 7q21 (two-point LOD score 3.05, multipoint LOD 3.08) and at 1q42 (two-point LOD 2.87, multipoint LOD 3.03). Much of the linkage evidence at 7q21 derived from families of French-Canadian origin, whereas the linkage evidence at 1q42 was well distributed across all the families. There was little evidence for linkage at known dyslexia loci. Combining the discovery and confirmation datasets increased the evidence at 1q42 (two-point LOD = 3.49, multipoint HLOD = 4.70), but decreased evidence at 7q21 (two-point LOD = 2.28, multipoint HLOD = 1.81), possibly because the replication sample did not have French Canadian representation.

Discussion: Reading disability in rolandic epilepsy has a genetic basis and may be influenced by loci at 1q42 and, in some populations, at 7q21; there is little evidence of a role for known DYX loci discovered in "pure" dyslexia pedigrees. 1q42 and 7q21 are candidate novel dyslexia loci.

Editor: Zongli Xu, National Institute of Environmental Health Sciences, United States of America

Funding: This study was supported by the Partnership for Pediatric Epilepsy Research, which includes the American Epilepsy Society, the Epilepsy Foundation, Anna and Jim Fantaci, Fight Against Childhood Epilepsy and Seizures (f.a.c.e.s), Neurotherapy Ventures Charitable Research Fund, and Parents Against Childhood Epilepsy (P.A.C.E.) (DKP); the Epilepsy Foundation through the generous support of the Charles L. Shor Foundation for Epilepsy Research, Inc (DKP); National Institutes of Health grants NS27941 (DAG), NS047530 (DKP); and HG004314 (LJS) from the Human Genome Research Institute (LJS); Natural Sciences and Engineering Research Council of Canada and the Ontario Ministry of Research and Innovation Early Researcher Award program (LJS); European Union Marie Curie Reintegration Award (DKP); Waterloo Foundation (DKP); Charles Sykes Epilepsy Research Trust (DKP); National Institute of Health Research (NIHR) Specialist Biomedical Research Centre for Mental Health of South London and Maudsley National Health Service (NHS) Foundation Trust (DKP). The funders had no role in study design, data collection and analysis, decision to publish, or preparation of the manuscript.

Competing Interests: The authors have declared that no competing interests exist.

* E-mail: deb.pal@kcl.ac.uk

Introduction

Reading disability (RD) is one of the most common developmental conditions in childhood with a prevalence ranging from 5–12% [1]. RD is defined as difficulty in reading and writing not attributable to general intellectual or sensory impairment or to a lack of exposure to an appropriate educational environment (ICD-10). RD may arise from a combination of environmental and genetic components, and there is evidence that the genetic susceptibility to RD is complex [2,3,4,5,6,7,8,9,10,11], with over nine susceptibility loci (*DYX1-DYX9*) mapped [12]. Most genetic studies of RD are based on subjects in whom neurological comorbidities, like epilepsy, have been stringently excluded. Thus we do not know whether the genetic architecture of RD is the same in neurologically comorbid populations.

Epilepsy is often associated with neurodevelopmental disorders [13], and there is strong evidence that the association has a genetic basis in some instances. One common form of childhood epilepsy, Rolandic Epilepsy (RE), is a complex genetic disorder [14] whose electro-encephalographic signature (CentroTemporal Spikes, CTS) has been mapped to the *ELP4* gene at 11p13 [15]. RE is associated with language and academic impairments [16], including speech sound disorder (SSD) (odds ratio 2.5), and RD (OR 5.8). The odds of SSD in relatives of RE probands is 5.4 times that in the general population, and the odds of RD is 2.8 times the general population odds [17]. The strong proband and familial associations with RD and SSD, and the similarity in neurocognitive profiles between probands and siblings [18], suggest that these neurodevelopmental traits in RE are also genetically influenced. We subsequently tested the hypothesis of shared genetic influences for SSD and CTS, and have shown that the 11p13 locus is pleiotropic for SSD and CTS [19]. Other investigators have shown pleiotropic effects across neurodevelopmental phenotypes, for example between RD and SSD [2,3]; RD and ADHD [20]; and RD and specific language impairment (SLI) [21].

The aim of this study was to map loci for RD in RE families and determine whether there is overlap with "pure" RD loci identified in non-comorbid samples. We asked two questions: (i) does reading disability in RE map to loci different from those so far reported in genetic studies of dyslexia in neurologically normal samples [2,3,4], and (ii) does reading disability share inheritance with CTS or SSD in RE families.

Methods

Ethics Statement

The IRBs of New York State Psychiatric Institute and all collaborating centers approved the study. All subjects gave written informed consent.

Design

We employed a two-stage linkage design, the first stage was a genome-wide screen of 38 RE families; the second stage was a follow-up of linkage peaks and reported dyslexia loci in 20 later ascertained RE families. Where an obvious candidate existed, a gene under the linkage peak was resequenced.

Ascertainment

Rolandic Epilepsy probands and their families were recruited from pediatric neurology centers in the US for a genetic linkage study in 2005–2007. Ascertainment was through the proband, with no requirement for other family members to be affected with epilepsy.

Eligibility Criteria

Cases were enrolled if they met stringent eligibility criteria for RE, consisting of typical orofacial seizures, age of onset between 3–12 years, no previous epilepsy type, normal global developmental milestones, normal neurological examination, EEG with centrotemporal sharp waves and normal background, and neuroimaging that excluded an alternative structural, inflammatory or metabolic cause for the seizures. Board-certified experts in epileptology, neurophysiology, and neuroimaging centrally reviewed all of the probands' charts, EEGs, and neuroimaging for eligibility prior to recruitment (see Acknowledgements). Questionable cases were discussed with an independent expert child neurologist specializing in epilepsy. Cases were not required to be comorbid with any neuropsychiatric disorder, and proband RD and SSD affectedness was unknown at time of ascertainment.

Subjects

The first stage genome-wide linkage screen included 38 two or three generation RE families. In the second stage, we included an additional 20 two or three generation RE families. The number of genotyped individuals with RE, RD or both are listed for each family in Table S1.

Phenotyping

A pediatric-trained physician (TC or DKP) interviewed the case families. Both parents were interviewed, either together or separately, and the proband and siblings were also interviewed when age appropriate. The investigator administered a 125-item questionnaire covering perinatal, developmental, medical, educational details, family history and detailed seizure semiology and treatment history. A pediatric neurologist, pediatric neuropsychologist, adult neuropsychologist, and pediatric speech pathologist jointly developed the questionnaire. Questions that were answered positively were followed up in detail by clinical interview to establish ICD-10 diagnoses and to distinguish from global learning disability. The questionnaire included 13 items addressing speech articulation disorder F80.0. A similar batch of questions was used in a high-risk study of phonological disorder (Tunick and Pennington, 2002). The questionnaire also contained nine items addressing the ICD-10 definitions of reading disorder F81.0. RD was thus identified by significant impairment in the development of reading skills not solely accounted for by mental age, sensory problems, mother tongue, or inadequate schooling. Operationally, we asked about difficulties in learning to read in the first year or two of elementary school, reading remediation, and repeating a grade. We also excluded, by clinical interview, hearing impairment, social and educational deprivation, and other factors that were inconsistent with the ICD-10 diagnosis of RD. We checked available school and psychologist's reports for confirmation, and all were consistent with our findings.

A subset of 11 probands and 10 siblings underwent comprehensive neuropsychological evaluation, the details of which are reported elsewhere [18]. In brief, the results of detailed evaluation strongly supported the validity of our ICD-10 estimation of RD. As part of our battery, we used standard instruments to assess general intelligence: *Wechsler Abbreviated Scale of Intelligence*; academic achievement including spelling: *Woodcock-Johnson III* [22]; reading: *Gray Oral Reading Tests 4* [23], *Test of Word Reading Efficiency* [24]; receptive and expressive language: *Clinical Evaluation of Language Fundamentals, 4th Edition* [25], *Boston Naming Test, 2nd Edition* [26]. All tested subjects had a full scale IQ within or above the normal range. Using a definition of impairment as a standard score one standard deviation below normative means in at least two subtests, we found that ICD-10 classifications had a 100% positive predictive value and 90% negative predictive value for reading impairment. At worst, our operational definitions slightly underestimated the actual prevalence of RD.

Genotyping

Blood or saliva samples (Oragene, DNA Genotek, Canada) for DNA extraction were collected from probands and all potentially

Table 1. Genome-wide LOD scores exceeding 2.0 in two-point MMLS linkage analysis for Reading Disability (RD) in original dataset; LOD scores for broader phenotypes (RD or Speech Sound Disorder (SSD) and RD or CentroTemporal Spikes (CTS)) at these loci also listed.

Chromosome	Marker (Flanking)	Max LOD RD	Max LOD RD or SSD	Max LOD RD or CTS
1q42-43	D1S1540 (D1S2709,D1S2850)	2.87 (1.90, −5.06)	1.46 (1.55 −1.62)	1.55 (0.76, −1.56)
2q14.2	D2S2254 (D2S363,D2S347)	2.10 (−0.98, −1.83)	1.24 (0.29, 0.31)	0.45 (0.74, 0.01)
2q14.2	D2S2116 (D2S286, D2S1777)	2.23 (0.12, 1.19)	2.20 (0.60, 1.93)	1.62 (0.77, 0.78)
6q25.2	D6S441 (D6S1687,D6S419)	2.11 (−0.42,1.06)	1.37 (0.04, 0.95)	0.48 (−0.29, 0.35)
7q21.11	D7S660 (D7S2443,D7S1528)	3.05 (2.73, −0.95)	1.75 (1.82, −1.14)	1.13 (1.46, 1.68)

informative available family members. DNA was extracted using standard protocols (15). Individuals were classified as affected or not affected for Reading Disability according to clinical evaluation using operational ICD-10 definitions of reading disorder (F81.0) (who.int/classifications/en). In the first stage, a total of 194 individuals were genotyped at deCODE Genetics, Iceland using the deCODE 1000 marker single tandem repeat (STR) set, which has an average genome-wide resolution of 4 cM. In the second stage, a total of 145 individuals were typed for markers in the same STR set on chromosomes 1–3, 5–7, 11, 12 and 15–17. Twenty additional new markers were typed only in the replication sample. Amplified fragments were typed using ABI 3700 and ABI 3730 DNA analyzers with CEPH family DNA used as standards. Alleles were called automatically and checked for Mendelian consistency and Hardy-Weinberg equilibrium.

Linkage Analysis

We analyzed the data by two-point and multipoint LOD score calculations using the Maximized Maximum LOD Score (MMLS) approach [27], an approximation to the MOD score method [28] which performs maximization over the full unknown trait model. The MMLS procedure specifies that one performs analysis twice, once under dominant and once under recessive disease locus assumptions [29], while keeping other unknown trait model parameters fixed. The consequent increase in type I error is equivalent to half a degree of freedom under a chi-squared distribution [27], and can be conservatively compensated for by increasing the LOD score critical value for significance by 0.3 LOD score units, ie to 3.3. We calculated two-point LOD scores under both dominant and recessive modes of inheritance [27,30,31], with a dominant gene frequency of 0.006, a recessive gene frequency at 0.1, a sporadic rate at 0.002, and penetrance of 0.50 [28,32]. In regions providing significant evidence for linkage with RD, we then maximized over penetrance [27]. Marker allele frequencies were calculated from the dataset. We then followed up two-point results that provided LOD scores greater than 2.0 with multipoint analysis using Genehunter [33], again using the MMLS approach followed by penetrance maximization and computation of heterogeneity LOD scores. We also used multipoint analysis to follow up two-point LOD scores over 2.0 for different affectedness definitions to determine evidence for shared genetic factors, combining the traits: RD *or* CTS; and RD *or* SSD.

Sequencing

We used bi-directional Sanger sequencing for mutation screening of the *SEMA3C* gene in a large 17-member pedigree, 10 affected with RD, of French-Canadian origin included in the original linkage analysis. Genomic DNA from 13 individuals was available for screening. Sanger sequencing was also used to screen the *DISC1* gene in 20 affected families with RE and RD. We designed primers to amplify all of the exons and alternatively spliced exons, as well as the splice sites, promoter and 5′ and 3′ UTRs. We sequenced DNA amplified by PCR using the ABI 3130 DNA Analyzer and interpreted sequence using the Invitrogen Vector NTI Advance Suite. See Table S2 for PCR primer Sequences.

Results

Genome-wide Linkage Analysis of Reading Disability

In two-point analysis of RD in the initial set of families, we observed a LOD score of 3.05 at marker D7S660 in chromosomal band 7q21. The LOD score maximized under a dominant mode of inheritance, with 60% penetrance, at a recombination fraction of 0.01. We also observed LOD scores above 2.0 on chromosomes 1, 2 and 6 (Table 1).

The two-point LOD scores at all these markers decreased when the affectedness definition was extended to RD *or* SSD, and also for the affectedness definition RD *or* CTS (Table 1). Similarly, when we broadened the affectedness definition to RD *or* SSD *or* CTS at the 11p13 locus for CTS/SSD, the two-point LOD score at that locus decreased to -8.90, indicating no evidence of pleiotropy for RD with CTS/SSD at the 11p13 locus. We found little evidence for linkage to known dyslexia loci *DYX1-DYX8* in this dataset (Table 2).

We followed up our two-point results using multipoint analysis for the RD phenotype. Figure 1 shows the maximum multipoint LOD scores for RD on chromosome 7 under a dominant model

Table 2. Maximum LOD scores at DYX loci in the original dataset 'r' indicates maximization of lod score under recessive model, 'd' under dominant model.

Locus	Chromosomal band	Closest marker	Max LOD	Model
DYX1	15q21	D15S659	0.008	30% r
DYX2	6p22.3-p21.3	D6S289	0.83	99% d
DYX3	2p16-p15	D2S337	0.54	30% d
DYX4	6q11.2-q12	D6S1557	0.35	30% d
DYX5	3p12-q13	D3S1276	0.55	85% d
DYX6	18p11.2	D18S453 (SPC/RDG)	0.64	99% r
DYX7	11p15.5	D11S4046	0.09	30% d
DYX8	1p36-p34	D1S2870	0.29	85% d

with 50% penetrance. The largest multipoint LOD score was a HLOD of 3.08 at marker D7S660, the same marker where the maximum two-point score was found. The largest multipoint LOD score on chromosome 1 was a HLOD of 3.03 at marker D1S2833, maximizing under a dominant model with 60% penetrance (Figure 2). The LOD scores at chromosomes 2 and 6 were substantially smaller in multipoint compared to two-point analysis.

We repeated linkage analysis to RD in a second dataset of 20 RE families. In this replication set, we again found evidence of linkage to the 1q42 locus (LOD 1.28 at D1S2833, under a dominant 99% penetrance model). In a combined analysis of both datasets, the evidence for linkage of RD at 1q42 increased to LOD 3.55 at the same marker as in the original dataset, D1S1540, maximizing under a dominant, 70% penetrance trait model. In multipoint linkage analysis the maximum HLOD rose to 4.70 at D1S2833. However, at chromosome 7, the maximum LOD score in the second dataset was at D7S2409 (LOD 0.913, dominant, 99% penetrance), which was 10 cM distant from the linkage peak observed at D7S660 in the original dataset. In combined analysis, the evidence for linkage at D7S660 dropped to 2.28 (Table 3).

Exploring the linkage data by family, sixteen families provided positive LOD scores at the 7q21 region, with the majority of the linkage evidence coming from eight French-Canadian families and three Hispanic families. Interestingly, there were no French-Canadian families in our replication dataset. One particular French-Canadian pedigree, (Figure 3) with 17 individuals (14 genotyped), 10 of which are RD affected, provided a multipoint LOD score of 2.10 at the same marker D7S660 under a dominant mode of inheritance with 99% penetrance. In fact, in a genome-wide analysis of this pedigree alone, D7S660 provided the maximum genome-wide multipoint LOD score. We therefore decided to conduct some resequencing of this pedigree at this locus.

Resequencing SEMA3C

D7S660 sits in a gene-sparse region, except for the *SEMA3C* gene, which resides only 50,000 bp from the start of the microsatellite. Not only is this the closest gene to our linkage peak, but *SEMA3C* is an attractive candidate for further investigation. Semaphorins act as axonal growth cone guidance molecules, especially important in the developing fetal brain, and thus fit well with the theme emerging in the genetics of dyslexia and other neurodevelopmental disorders [34]. We sequenced the exons and alternatively spliced exons, exon-intron junctions, promoter, and 3′ and 5′ UTR of *SEMA3C* from all 13 individuals in the pedigree of French-Canadian origin (Figure 3) for whom we had DNA, (see Table S1 for primers).

No mutations or novel SNPs were found in *SEMA3C* in this pedigree. Eight known SNPs are present here although none segregated with affectedness status for RD. We did not find any evidence for microdeletions or microduplications in this gene. Therefore it is unlikely that *SEMA3C* coding or promoter mutations account for RD in this pedigree, and either intronic regions or other genes and ESTs under the linkage peak at 7q21 need to be investigated.

Resequencing DISC1

The 1q42 locus contains approximately 25 genes in the 1-LOD interval around the linkage peak, and deletions at this locus have previously been associated with rolandic seizures and abnormal EEG [35]. The locus harbors an interesting candidate gene, *Disrupted in Schizophrenia 1* (*DISC1*) which is associated with many psychiatric and neurodevelopmental conditions [36,37,38]. We sequenced the coding, alternatively spliced and regulatory regions of *DISC1* in affected members of 20 families that were linked to the 1q42 locus.

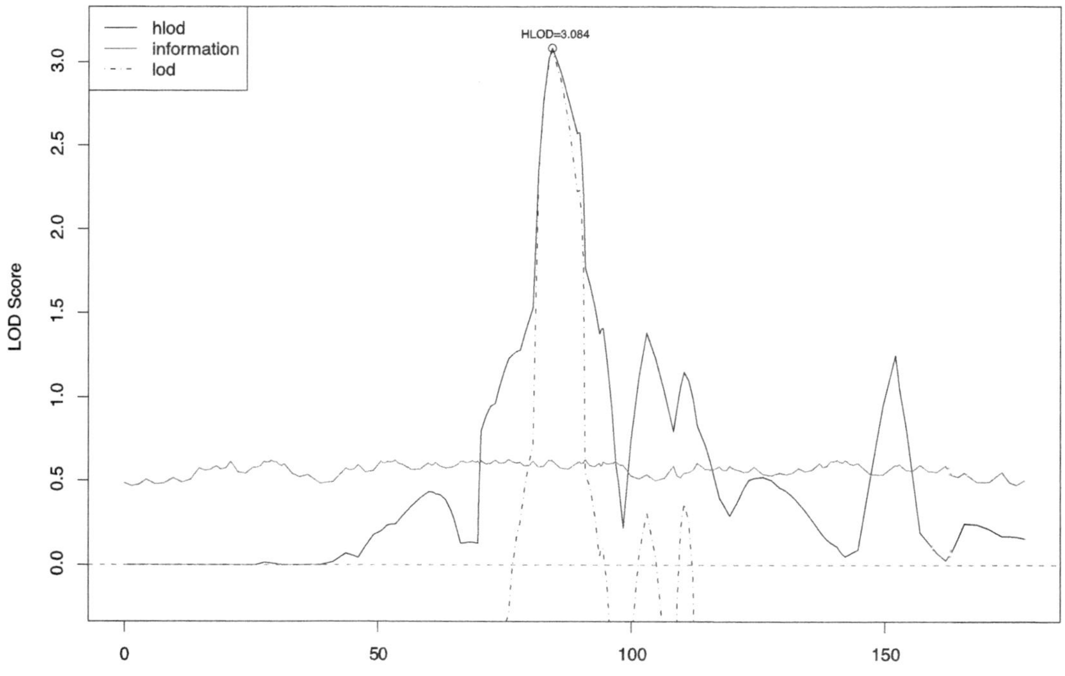

Figure 1. Multipoint analysis of Reading Disability on chromosome 7 in original dataset: maximum HLOD = 3.08 at D7S660 under a dominant mode of inheritance with 50% penetrance. Black line shows the multipoint linkage evidence using a heterogeneity LOD score (HLOD); dotted black line shows the LOD score; and blue line the information content.

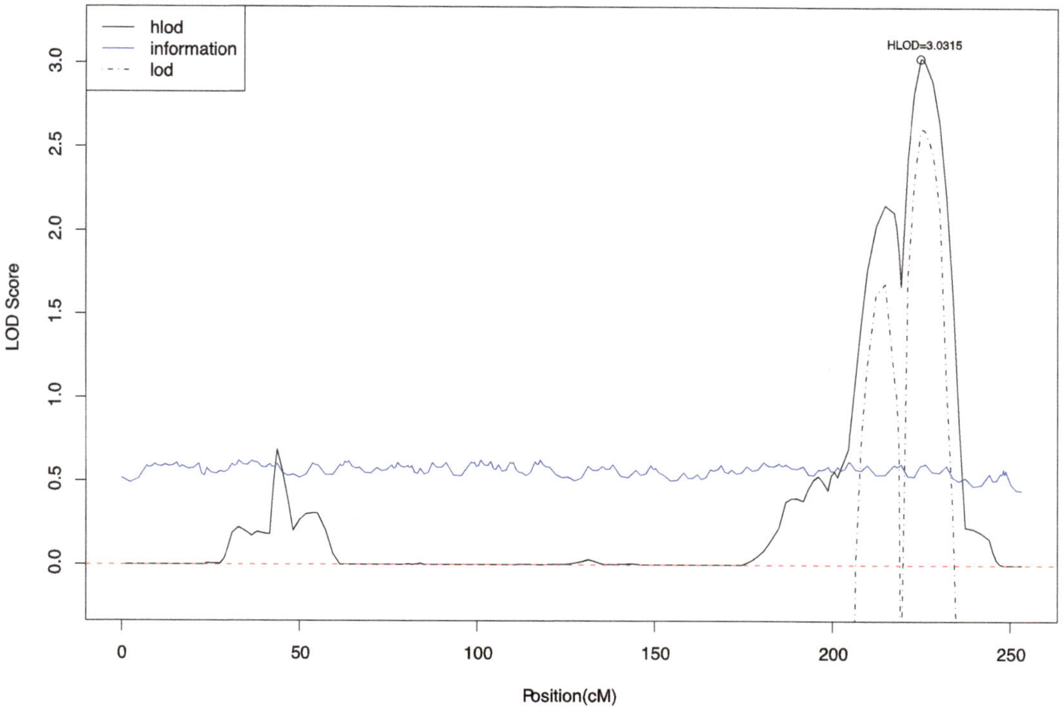

Figure 2. Multipoint analysis of Reading Disability on chromosome 1 in original dataset: maximum HLOD = 3.03 at D1S2833 under a dominant mode of inheritance with 60% penetrance. Black line shows the multipoint linkage evidence using a heterogeneity LOD score (HLOD); dotted black line shows the LOD score; and the blue line the information content.

We found 6 coding SNPs in the sequenced regions; however, none of them were novel, and all occurred at a frequency expected in a Caucasian population, indicating it is unlikely that *DISC1* coding mutations, microdeletions or microduplications, are causative for RD in RE families.

Discussion

We have discovered evidence for possible novel dyslexia loci at 7q21 and 1q42 in families of subjects with rolandic epilepsy, a common type of epilepsy in which speech and language impairments strongly co-aggregate [17,19]. The 7q21 and 1q42 loci have not previously been reported in the dyslexia genetics literature, suggesting that *DYX* loci discovered in relatively "pure" dyslexia samples may not be representative of genetic influences on RD found in samples comorbid for epilepsy. This provides further evidence for the genetic basis of comorbidity in common forms of epilepsy, following our report of pleiotropy between speech sound disorder and centrotemporal EEG spikes [19]. However, in contrast to findings of pleiotropy in non-comorbid RD pedigrees [2,3,20], we found no evidence for shared influences of these two loci for other neurodevelopmental traits associated with RE.

Approximately 55% of RE patients are co-morbid with RD [17], and many are affected by multiple neurodevelopmental comorbidities including SSD, attention deficit hyperactivity disorder (ADHD) and migraine [17,18,39]. The familial aggregation of these cognitive traits in relatives who may or may not have epilepsy or the subclinical EEG of CentroTemporal Spikes [17,18,39] enabled us to perform linkage analysis in pedigrees ascertained through rolandic epilepsy probands. This is in contrast to most published dyslexia genetic studies, which specifically exclude epilepsy and comorbid neurological conditions including SLI and ADHD. The two loci linked to RD in our RE sample have not been reported before, and we did not find confirmatory evidence of linkage at any of the DYX1-DYX8 loci. Our results suggest that the current list of dyslexia loci is not exhaustive, and

Table 3. Maximum LOD scores in the original, replication and combined datasets at chromosomes 1 and 7.

		Maximum two-point LOD			Max multipoint HLOD		
Chr	**Marker**	**Original**	**Replication**	**Combined**	**Original**	**Replication**	**Combined**
1q42-43	D1S2833	2.75	1.28	3.49	3.03	1.87	4.70
1q42-43	D1S1540	2.87	0.69	3.55	2.20	0.84	3.32
7q21.11	D7S2409	1.32	0.91	1.07	1.38	0.004	0.94
7q21.11	D7S2431	1.42	0.10	1.13	0.60	0.01	0.63
7q21.11	D7S660	3.05	0.134	2.28	3.08	0.00	1.81

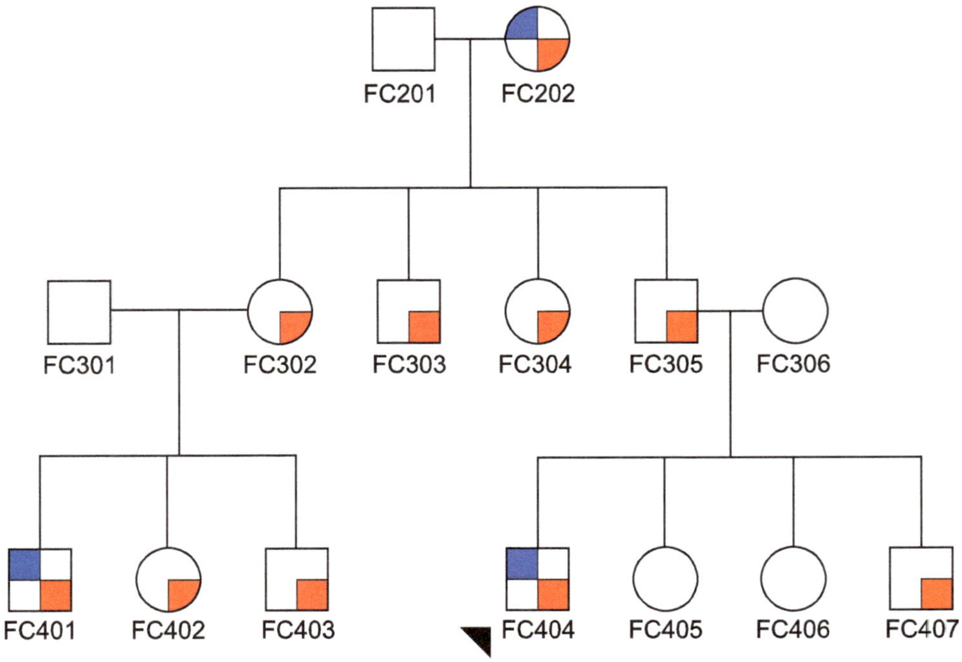

Figure 3. Pedigree of French-Canadian origin multiplex for RE (blue) and reading disability (red); arrow indicates proband.

that considering comorbid samples may increase the understanding of gene pathways, particularly the molecular basis for the observed overlap between conventionally distinct phenotypes such as epilepsy, ADHD, RD and SSD.

The most interesting candidate gene at the 1q42 locus is *DISC1*. *DISC1* has been linked and associated with schizophrenia and bipolar disorder in the general population [36,37], and associated with autism and Asperger's syndrome [38]. More specifically, *DISC1* mutations have been associated with deficits in sustained attention and memory in schizophrenia patients [40,41], an observation that may be pertinent to the deficits in attention and working memory found in rolandic epilepsy [18,42]. However, we did not identify any coding, splicing or regulatory mutations in *DISC1* from sequencing affected family members in this study, suggesting an alternative susceptibility gene, an intronic mutation, or other structural variations.

Our linkage results pointed to the possibility of a second, genetically heterogeneous RD locus enriched in French-Canadian pedigrees at 7q21. A chromosomal deletion at this locus (7q11.23q21.2) has previously been associated with microcephaly, ADHD, and epilepsy with bilateral centrotemporal EEG spikes [43]. The absence of coding and regulatory mutations in *SEMA3C* in one large multiplex French-Canadian pedigree suggests the need to consider other variation in or around this locus.

The genetic basis of dyslexia and speech sound disorder is firmly established in the neurodevelopmental genetics field, yet the occurrence of these common comorbidities among children with epilepsy has not previously been attributed to a genetic etiology. We recently showed pleiotropy at the 11p13 locus for both centrotemporal EEG spikes and speech dyspraxia [19] and this was the first evidence for genetic comorbidity in epilepsy. Here, we show that RD in RE also has a genetic basis and conclude that RD therefore does not result from either abnormal EEG or recurrent seizures. Since rolandic and most other common forms of epilepsy have a complex genetic basis and are often comorbid with RD, SSD, SLI, ADHD and/or migraine, it is reasonable to suggest that the etiological basis for some of these comorbidities in common epilepsies may also be genetic.

Pleiotropy has been demonstrated between SSD and RD in SSD families [2,3], between RD and ADHD in RD families [20], and RD loci may be associated in comorbid individuals [21]. However, despite co-occurrence of RD and SSD in RE individuals and aggregation of both traits in RE families, neither familial aggregation nor linkage analysis suggests pleiotropy between RD and SSD in RE families [17]. These results suggest alternative genetic pathways may be involved in the etiology of these conditions in RE families compared to those in pure dyslexia families. We and others [21] propose that future genetic studies of RD, SSD, SLI and ADHD include collections of comorbid populations, because these traits in comorbid individuals may have genetic bases that are shared with or distinct from "pure" phenotypes. Moreover, the population prevalence and impact of comorbid individuals is likely highly significant. Delineation of genetic heterogeneity will improve statistical power to detect genetic influences. Studies including comorbid populations will contribute to a more comprehensive understanding of the genetic basis of common neurodevelopmental phenotypes.

Supporting Information

Table S1 Breakdown by pedigree of number affected with Rolandic Epilepsy, RE, Reading Disability, RD, or both, in original group 1:n and replication group 2:n.

Table S2 Forward and reverse primer sequences used in the PCR and subsequent Sanger sequencing of a. *SEMA3C* and b. DISC1; nomenclature from Ensembl.

Acknowledgments

Our thanks to members of the IRELAND Study consortium who also referred patients to the study: Linda Leary MD, Frances Rhoads, Maria

Younes MD. Thanks also to Lewis Kull, Cigdem Akman MD, Jeff Rogg MD and Jerry Boxerman MD PhD for reviewing subjects' charts and investigations for eligibility, and to Professor David Greenberg for comments on the manuscript.

Author Contributions

Conceived and designed the experiments: LJS DKP. Performed the experiments: LJS LA. Analyzed the data: LJS LA T. Chiang ZB WL T. Clarke DKP. Contributed reagents/materials/analysis tools: HH SLK DEM EJN SMW. Wrote the paper: LJS LA DKP.

References

1. Shaywitz SE, Shaywitz BA, Fletcher JM, Escobar MD (1990) Prevalence of reading disability in boys and girls. Results of the Connecticut Longitudinal Study. JAMA 264: 998–1002.
2. Stein CM, Schick JH, Gerry Taylor H, Shriberg LD, Millard C, et al. (2004) Pleiotropic effects of a chromosome 3 locus on speech-sound disorder and reading. Am J Hum Genet 74: 283–297.
3. Smith SD, Pennington BF, Boada R, Shriberg LD (2005) Linkage of speech sound disorder to reading disability loci. J Child Psychol Psychiatry 46: 1057–1066.
4. Stein CM, Millard C, Kluge A, Miscimarra LE, Cartier KC, et al. (2006) Speech sound disorder influenced by a locus in 15q14 region. Behav Genet 36: 858–868.
5. Hinshelwood J (1907) Four cases of congenital word-blindness occurring in the same family. Br Med J 1: 608–609.
6. Yale W, Rutter M (1975) The concept of specific reading retardation. J Child Psychol Psychiatry 16: 181–197.
7. Hallgren B (1950) Specific dyslexia (congenital word-blindness); a clinical and genetic study. Acta Psychiatr Neurol Suppl 65: 1–287.
8. Vogler GP, DeFries JC, Decker SN (1985) Family history as an indicator of risk for reading disability. J Learning Disabil 18: 419–421.
9. Pennington BF (1990) The genetics of dyslexia. J Child Psychol Psychiatry 31: 193–203.
10. DeFries JC, Fulker DW, Labuda MC (1987) Evidence for a genetic etiology in reading disability of twins. Nature 329: 537–539.
11. Stevenson J, Graham P, Fredman G, McLoughlin V (1987) A twin study of genetic influences on reading and spelling ability and disability. J Child Psychol Psychiatry 28: 229–247.
12. Scerri TS, Schulte-Korne G (2010) Genetics of developmental dyslexia. Eur Child Adolesc Psychiatry 19: 179–197.
13. Pal DK (2011) Epilepsy and neurodevelopmental disorders of language. Curr Op Neurol 24: 126–131.
14. Bali B, Kugler SL, Pal DK (2005) Genetic influence on Rolandic epilepsy. Ann Neurol 57: 464–465.
15. Strug LJ, Clarke T, Chiang T, Chien M, Baskurt Z, et al. (2009) Centrotemporal sharp wave EEG trait in rolandic epilepsy maps to Elongator Protein Complex 4 (ELP4). Eur J Hum Genet 17: 1171–1181.
16. Staden U, Isaacs E, Boyd SG, Brandl U, Neville BG (1998) Language dysfunction in children with Rolandic epilepsy. Neuropediatrics 29: 242–248.
17. Clarke T, Strug LJ, Murphy PL, Bali B, Carvalho J, et al. (2007) High risk of reading disability and speech sound disorder in rolandic epilepsy families: case-control study. Epilepsia 48: 2258–2265.
18. Smith A, Kavros PM, Clarke T, Dorta N, Tremont G, et al. (2011) Neurocognitive Endophenotype Associated with Rolandic Epilepsy. Epilepsia doi: 10.1111/j.1528-1167.2011.03371.x.
19. Pal DK, Li W, Clarke T, Lieberman P, Strug LJ (2010) Pleiotropic effects of the 11p13 locus on developmental verbal dyspraxia and EEG centrotemporal sharp waves. Genes Brain Behav 9: 1004–1012.
20. Gayan J, Willcutt EG, Fisher SE, Francks C, Cardon LR, et al. (2005) Bivariate linkage scan for reading disability and attention-deficit/hyperactivity disorder localizes pleiotropic loci. J Child Psychol Psychiatry 46: 1045–1056.
21. Scerri TS, Morris AP, Buckingham LL, Newbury DF, Miller LL, et al. (2011) DCDC2, KIAA0319 and CMIP Are Associated with Reading-Related Traits. Biol Psychiatry 70: 237–245.
22. Woodcock R (2001) Woodcock-Johnson Third Edition Tests of Achievment Technical Manual. Chicago, IL: Riverside Publishing.
23. Wiederholt JL, Bryant BR (2001) Gray Oral Reading Tests 4th Edition. Austin, TX: Pro-Ed.
24. Torgesen JK, Wagner RK, Rashotte CA (1999) Test of Word Reading Efficiency. Austin, TX: Pro-Ed.
25. Semel E, Wiig EH, Secord WA (2003) Clinical Evaluation of Language Fundamentals, 4th Edition. San Antonio, TX: Harcourt Assessment.
26. Kaplan E, Goodglass H, Weintraub S (2001) Boston Naming Test, 2nd Edition. Philadelphia, PA: Lippincott, Williams & Wilkins.
27. Hodge SE, Abreu P, Greenberg DA (1997) Magnitude of type I error when single-locus linkage analysis is maximized over models: a simulation study. American Journal of Human Genetics 60: 217–227.
28. Clerget-Darpoux F, Bonaiti-Pellie C, Hochez J (1986) Effects of misspecifying genetic parameters in LOD score analysis. Biometrics 42: 393–399.
29. Greenberg DA, Abreu P, Hodge SE (1998) The power to detect linkage in complex disease by means of simple LOD-score analyses. American Journal of Human Genetics 63: 870–879.
30. Durner M, Greenberg DA (1992) Effect of heterogeneity and assumed mode of inheritance on lod scores. American Journal of Human Genetics 42: 271–275.
31. Abreu PC, Hodge SE, Greenberg DA (2002) Quantification of type I error probabilities for heterogeneity LOD scores. Genet Epidemiol 22: 156–169.
32. Pal DK, Durner M, Greenberg DA (2001) Effect of misspecification of gene frequency on the two-point lod score. European Journal of Human Genetics 9: 855–859.
33. Kruglyak L, Daly MJ, Reeve-Daly MP, Lander ES (1996) Parametric and nonparametric linkage analysis: a unified multipoint approach. American Journal of Human Genetics 58: 1347–1363.
34. Paracchini S, Scerri T, Monaco AP (2007) The genetic lexicon of dyslexia. Annu Rev Genomics Hum Genet 8: 57–79.
35. Vaughn BV, Greenwood RS, Aylsworth AS, Tennison MB (1996) Similarities of EEG and seizures in del(1q) and benign rolandic epilepsy. Pediatr Neurol 15: 261–264.
36. Roberts RC (2007) Schizophrenia in translation: disrupted in schizophrenia (DISC1): integrating clinical and basic findings. Schizophr Bull 33: 11–15.
37. Hashimoto R, Numakawa T, Ohnishi T, Kumamaru E, Yagasaki Y, et al. (2006) Impact of the DISC1 Ser704Cys polymorphism on risk for major depression, brain morphology and ERK signaling. Hum Mol Genet 15: 3024–3033.
38. Kilpinen H, Ylisaukko-Oja T, Hennah W, Palo OM, Varilo T, et al. (2007) Association of DISC1 with autism and Asperger syndrome. Mol Psychiatry.
39. Clarke T, Baskurt Z, Strug LJ, Pal DK (2009) Evidence of shared genetic risk factors for migraine and rolandic epilepsy. Epilepsia 50: 2428–2433.
40. Burdick KE, Hodgkinson CA, Szeszko PR, Lencz T, Ekholm JM, et al. (2005) DISC1 and neurocognitive function in schizophrenia. Neuroreport 16: 1399–1402.
41. Cannon TD, Hennah W, van Erp TG, Thompson PM, Lonnqvist J, et al. (2005) Association of DISC1/TRAX haplotypes with schizophrenia, reduced prefrontal gray matter, and impaired short- and long-term memory. Arch Gen Psychiatry 62: 1205–1213.
42. Kavros PM, Clarke T, Strug LJ, Halperin JM, Dorta NJ, et al. (2008) Attention impairment in rolandic epilepsy: Systematic review. Epilepsia 49: 1570–1580.
43. Burke MS, Carroll JE, Burket RC (1997) Benign rolandic epilepsy and chromosome 7q deletion. J Child Neurol 12: 148–149.

15

Enhanced Recognition Memory after Incidental Encoding in Children with Developmental Dyslexia

Martina Hedenius[1], Michael T. Ullman[2]❡, Per Alm[1], Margareta Jennische[1]❡, Jonas Persson[3]*

1 Department of Neuroscience, Uppsala University, Uppsala, Sweden, 2 Brain and Language Lab, Department of Neuroscience, Georgetown University, Washington, D.C., United States of America, 3 Aging Research Center, Karolinska Institute and Stockholm University, Stockholm, Sweden

Abstract

Developmental dyslexia (DD) has previously been associated with a number of cognitive deficits. Little attention has been directed to cognitive functions that remain intact in the disorder, though the investigation and identification of such strengths might be useful for developing new, and improving current, therapeutical interventions. In this study, an old/new recognition memory paradigm was used to examine previously untested aspects of declarative memory in children with DD and typically developing control children. The DD group was not only not impaired at the task, but actually showed superior recognition memory, as compared to the control children. These findings complement previous reports of enhanced cognition in other domains (e.g., visuo-spatial processing) in DD. Possible underlying mechanisms for the observed DD advantage in declarative memory, and the possibility of compensation by this system for reading deficits in dyslexia, are discussed.

Editor: Linda Chao, University of California, San Francisco, United States of America

Funding: Financial support for this study was provided by the Sven Jerring Foundation and the Foundation Sunnerdahls Disability Fund to MH, MJ and PA, by NIH R01 HD049347 (MTU) and the Mable H. Flory Charitable Trust to MTU, and by a Swedish Research Council grant 2007-1895 to JP. The funders had no role in study design, data collection and analysis, decision to publish, or preparation of the manuscript.

Competing Interests: The authors have declared that no competing interests exist.

* E-mail: martina.hedenius@neuro.uu.se

❡ These authors contributed equally to this work.

Introduction

Developmental dyslexia (DD) is characterized by unexpected difficulties with reading, in the context of typical educational opportunities and intact intellectual and sensory abilities [1]. The disorder, which has a strong genetic component [2], has been estimated to affect about 5–10% of children [3]. Children with DD have difficulties with written word recognition and phonological decoding (using letter-sound mapping knowledge to decode novel words), which may result from underlying phonological impairments [4,5]. In addition, DD has been associated with a number of other deficits [6,7], including of working memory [8,9], executive functions [10], motor function [11], implicit sequence learning [12,13,14], and artificial grammar learning [15] as well as problems with other aspects of language that appear to be primary in nature (i.e. not only a consequence of impaired reading) [16,17,18].

Although much attention has been given to cognitive deficits associated with DD, it is evidently not the case that all cognitive functions are impaired in the disorder. Knowledge about what is well-functioning may be as important for increasing our understanding of the disorder as knowledge about what is impaired. The investigation and identification of cognitive strengths associated with DD could be used for developing new, and improving current, therapeutical interventions. In this study, we examine a previously untested aspect of declarative memory in children with DD, namely recognition memory after incidental encoding.

Declarative memory encompasses memory for factual knowledge (semantic memory) and personally experienced events (episodic memory) [19,20]. It relies on a network of brain structures in which the medial temporal lobe, including the hippocampus and the nearby cortices, plays a critical role [21,22]. Other brain structures of importance in this system include portions of frontal cortex, which play a crucial role in encoding and recall in declarative memory [23,24]. Depending on the specific paradigm used to assess declarative memory, the relative demand on executive functions underlying encoding strategies and recall of information may be increased or decreased. For example, increased demands on working memory and executive functions have been associated with intentional as compared to incidental encoding, and with free recall as compared to recognition [25].

Few studies have directly tested declarative memory functions in DD, and those that have done so have yielded inconsistent findings. Whereas some studies have reported that declarative memory is normal in the disorder [26,27] others have found a deficit [28,29,30]. Consistent with the well-documented phonological impairments associated with DD, some of the contradictory findings appear to be explained by whether verbal or non-verbal material is used to test declarative memory. For example, learning and retention of non-verbal information has been shown to be intact in the paired-associate learning task [31,32], which is a classic declarative (episodic) memory paradigm. The same studies reported impairments at learning when verbal stimuli were used [31]. However, these group differences disappeared when phonological impairments were controlled for, suggesting that the impairment might not be related to declarative memory per se but to underlying phonological problems. Accordingly, in a third study, paired-associate learning with verbal stimuli was found to be intact in DD when short, high-frequency words (which minimizes the effect of phonological processing problems), were used [33].

Another factor that appears to affect the performance of dyslexic participants in tasks probing declarative memory is the extent to which test performance depends on the use of intentional encoding strategies. In line with previous evidence suggesting problems with executive functions in DD [10], one study found that the declarative memory impairment in the DD group appeared to be explained by an inability to develop efficient strategies for encoding [29]. In addition, free recall of previously presented material may be particularly challenging for individuals with DD [9,34].

Declarative memory is a complex phenomenon that depends on the integrity of several underlying functions. Accordingly, a research program aimed at elucidating the status of declarative memory in DD may benefit from a systematic investigation of these underlying functions. One aspect of declarative memory that still remains untested in DD is recognition memory after incidental encoding. Crucially, in this paradigm, subjects are unaware of the subsequent memory test, and incidental encoding is promoted by, for example, a semantic categorization task. Thus, potential group differences in intentional encoding strategies should not be a confounding factor in this task. Moreover, this paradigm does not rely on free recall of information but rather on the identification of a specific item as "old/seen before" or "new/not seen before". These characteristics may make this paradigm particularly suitable for revealing aspects of declarative memory that might function well in DD. Despite these advantages, this paradigm has not yet been used in DD. The present study was designed to fill this gap in the literature.

Methods

Ethics Statement

The study was approved by the ethical review board in the city of Uppsala. All parents or guardians provided informed written consent; children provided informed written assent and received a cinema ticket for their participation.

Participants

Twelve children with developmental dyslexia (DD) and 17 typically developing (TD) control children participated in the study. The two groups did not differ in sex, age and handedness (see Table 1 for participant characteristics of the final set of participants included in statistical analyses).

Children with DD were recruited via speech-language pathology clinics in the cities of Stockholm, Uppsala, Gävle and Västerås, in Sweden. All children with DD had been independently tested and diagnosed with dyslexia by a certified speech-language pathologist within 1.5 years prior to participation in the study. The TD group consisted of a subset of children who were recruited from schools in and around the cities of Stockholm and Uppsala as part of a larger study on memory and language in typically developing children. All children in the study were reported by their parents to be monolingual Swedish-speaking, to have normal (or corrected to normal) vision and hearing, and to have no known cognitive or motor impairment, apart from reading problems in the DD group.

In order to confirm reading problems in the DD group, and the lack thereof in the TD group, two reading tests, assessing phonological decoding and orthographic reading, respectively, were administered on the same day as the declarative memory task. These tests were paper and pencil Swedish adaptations [35]

Table 1. Participant demographics and cognitive characteristics.

Demographics	DD	TD	*t*	*p*
N	11	17	–	–
Age in years	11.0 (0.71)	11.0 (0.49)	0.28	.78
Sex (f/m)	5/6	5/12	$\chi^2 = 0.75$	.39
Handedness	85.1 (16.4)	92.2 (10.2)	1.4	.17
Cognitive scores				
PIQ	87.3 (12.5)	97.1 (15.0)	1.8	.085
Phonological decoding	1.82 (0.87)	5.24 (1.15)	8.4	<.0001
Orthographic reading	2.0 (1.18)	5.76 (1.15)	8.4	<.0001
Nonword repetition	106 (5.3)	111 (5.4)	2.4	.026
TROG	17.9 (1.20)	18.9 (0.70)	2.7	.012
PPVT	150 (15.9)	160 (13.5)	1.8	.089

DD = Children with developmental dyslexia, TD = Typically developing control children, PIQ = Performance IQ; TROG = Test for reception of grammar; PPVT = Peabody picture vocabulary test. Standard deviations are shown in parentheses.

of the computerized phonological decoding and orthographic reading tasks used by Olson, Forsberg, Wise, & Rack [36]. In the phonological decoding test, the task was to decide, and underline with a pencil, which one of three or four pseudo-words was a pseudo-homophone of a real word. (i.e. "sounds" like a real word). The score was the number of correctly identified pseudohomophones within two minutes, with a maximum score of 80. In the orthographic reading test, participants were asked to underline the true word in true word-pseudohomophone pairs. Because the phonological codes for the pairs were identical, the word and its pseudohomophone would be pronounced the same in Swedish. Thus, in order to make a correct response subjects had to use word-specific orthographic knowledge. The score was the number of correctly chosen words in two minutes, with a maximum score of 120.

All TD children had stanine scores ≥4 out of 9 on both reading tests (corresponding to performance at or above −0.75 *SD*). All children in the DD group had stanine scores of ≤3 on both tests, except for one child who had a stanine score of 5 on the orthographic reading test. Because previous evidence suggests that the phonological decoding problems characteristic of DD can sometimes occur together with intact or even superior orthographic skills [37], this child was still included in the DD group.

In addition to these reading tests, all children were also tested on nonword repetition [38], understanding of grammatical structures [39,40], and receptive vocabulary [41] (see Table 1). The DD group performed significantly worse than the TD group on both the nonword repetition test and the grammar test. Receptive vocabulary, by contrast, did not differ significantly between groups (Table 1).

Performance IQ (PIQ), which was assessed by Raven's Standard Progressive Matrices Plus [42], was included for descriptive rather than exclusionary purposes in this study, since we wanted our DD sample to reflect the population of children who are clinically identified and diagnosed with DD in Sweden. In line with evidence suggesting that there is only a weak, if any, relationship between PIQ and the reading problems characteristic of dyslexia [43,44], PIQ is not used as an exclusionary factor for a clinical diagnosis of DD in Sweden. The PIQ range in the DD group was

70–115 and the TD range was 80–140. Because the group difference in PIQ approached significance ($p = .085$; Table 1), PIQ was controlled for in all statistical analyses.

One child in the DD group was excluded from statistical analyses because he was an outlier on the recognition memory test, with a mean d' score of 0.19, which was equal to − 3 *SD* from the mean of all children. All other children fell within 2 *SDs* of the mean. Thus, the final set of participants on which analyses were performed consisted of 11 children in the DD group and 17 children in the TD group.

Stimuli and Procedure

Declarative memory was tested with an object recognition memory task developed by the Brain and Language Lab at Georgetown University. Similar tasks have previously been shown to engage the network of brain structures underlying declarative memory, including medial temporal lobe and frontal structures, for both non-verbal and verbal stimuli [45,46].

The object recognition task consists of three phases; i) incidental encoding, ii) recognition 10 minutes after encoding and iii) recognition 24 hours after encoding. The stimuli were black-and-white line drawings of real objects and made-up objects (Figure 1). The images used for both the real and made-up objects were taken from a variety of sources. For the real objects, items were drawn from, and modified as necessary, various clipart galleries (including free websites and purchased collections), and from a previous study by Snodgrass et al. [47]. For the made-up objects, items were selected and modified from previous studies by Eals and Silverman [48], Laine et al. [49] and Williams and Tarr [50]. The images of made-up objects were selected based on their nameability (that is, low nameability) determined through previous pilot work. All images were resized, touched up, rotated, and/or converted to black-and-white to create the final set of stimuli. The items were presented in a pseudo-randomized order, with no more than 3 consecutive real or made-up objects.

There were three different sets of objects used in this task: i) those presented in the encoding phase (as well as in subsequent phases), ii) those used as foils in the 10 minute recognition phase and iii) those used as foils in the 24 hour recognition phase. Each of these three sets of objects consisted of 32 real objects and 32 made-up objects.

Testing took place in a quiet room under normal classroom lighting conditions. The stimuli were presented on an LCD screen of a portable PC computer running Windows, using E-Prime version 1.2. (Psychology Software Tools). The physical size of the images was 13.7×10.3 centimeters, and the viewing distance was approximately 50 centimeters. Participants were instructed to place their left and right index fingers on the designated buttons on a serial response box (E-prime SRBox) that was placed in front of them, and to make a response by pressing one of these buttons. Preceding each stimulus, a crosshair appeared in the center of the screen for 1000 milliseconds (ms), followed by the item for 500 ms, also in the center of the screen. In cases where the participant responded before 500 ms, the item remained onscreen until the 500 ms finished, to equalize presentation duration across stimuli and subjects. After the item presentation, the crosshair reappeared on the screen until the subject responded, or up to 4500 ms. As soon as the subject made a response through the SRBox, a 200 ms advance tone sounded, followed by 800 ms of fixation. If instead the subject made no response within the 4500 ms response period, a 400 ms time-out tone sounded, followed by 600 ms of fixation. After this the 200 ms advance tone sounded followed by 800 ms of fixation. The next item then began with 1000 ms of fixation.

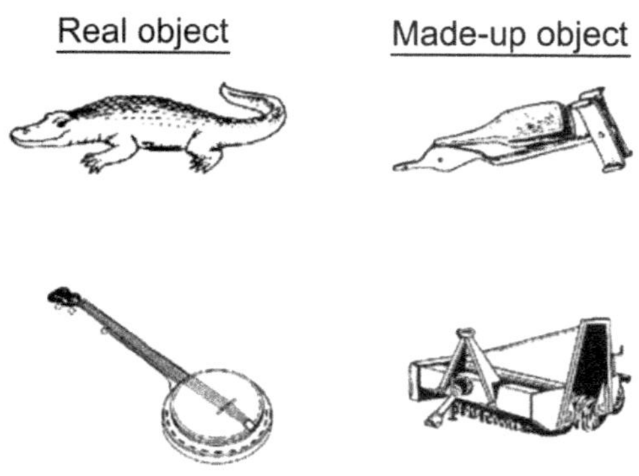

Figure 1. Examples of the real and made-up objects used as stimulus materials.

In the incidental *encoding* phase, participants were told they were going to be presented with pictures of "real" and "made-up" objects on the screen. They were asked to indicate, through a button press, whether the object was real (existed in reality) or made-up (did not exist in reality). Similar categorization tasks have previously been used to promote incidental word encoding [51]. The instructions included 2 sample items to ensure that all participants understood the task and correctly mapped the response buttons. The instructions and sample items were followed by 3 practice items with the same timing parameters as the test items. All instructions were visible on the screen and were simultaneously read aloud to the participants. A reminder appeared at the bottom of the screen throughout the task indicating the mapping of the SRBox buttons (i.e. "real"/ "made-up").

The incidental encoding phase was followed by a 10 minute break during which subjects were encouraged to stretch their legs or have a snack. Just before the subsequent *10 minute recognition* phase, subjects were told they were going to see pictures of real and made-up objects again, some of which they saw previously and some of which they did not. They were asked to indicate, through a button press, whether or not they had seen the object earlier. As in the encoding phase, the instructions included sample items, which were followed by practice items. Presentation and timing was the same as in the encoding phase, but the reminder "real"/"made-up" was changed to "yes"/"no". Additionally, the question "seen before?" was always displayed on the screen, above the "yes" and "no" options. Finally, after a 24 hour interval (+/ −1 hour) subjects were given the *24 hour recognition* phase of the task. Instructions, presentation and timing were the same as in the 10 minute recognition phase.

Responses were captured using E-prime version 1.2. Two versions (A and B) of the task, for which the response buttons for "real"/"made-up" and "yes"/"no" were reversed, were assigned to consecutive participants in each group. Testing took place in a quiet room in the child's school or home over the two consecutive days. Each test session took about 70–90 minutes, including the administration of reading, language and performance IQ tests.

Reaction times (RTs) were calculated for correct responses only, and filtered by excluding responses faster than 300 milliseconds (ms) or greater than 4500 ms. Median RTs were used in order to avoid undue influence from outlier RTs. D-prime (d' = z hits − z false alarms), which takes response bias into account, was used to assess recognition memory accuracy. We report unadjusted *means* and *SDs* unless otherwise indicated. Partial eta-squared (η_p^2) is used as the measure of effect size where appropriate.

Results

Categorization Accuracy and RT during the Incidental Encoding Task

Potential group differences (DD vs. TD) in the incidental encoding task were tested with one-way ANCOVAs (with PIQ as a covariate), with either categorization accuracy (percent correct) for real vs. made-up, or reaction times of correct responses (RTs), as the dependent variable. The DD and TD groups did not differ significantly in accuracy, though the DD group showed somewhat better performance, a pattern that approached significance (DD *mean* = 86.4%, *SD* = 13.9%; TD *mean* = 73.9%, *SD* = 20.3%, $F(1,25) = 3.442$, $p = .075$, $\eta_p^2 = .121$). The two groups did not differ in their reaction times (DD *mean* = 958 ms, *SD* = 150 ms; TD *mean* = 862 ms, *SD* = 241 ms, $F < 1$). Speed-accuracy tradeoff effects during encoding were examined with a partial correlation analysis across subjects (controlling for PIQ) of RT against accuracy. This analysis revealed no association between response speed and accuracy, either across all children ($r(25) = -.163$; $p = .417$) or within any of the two groups (DD group: $r(8) = -.274$, $p = .444$; TD group: $r(14) = -.233$, $p = .384$).

Recognition Memory Accuracy and RT

Potential group differences in recognition memory accuracy across the two recognition sessions (10 minutes and 24 hours) were examined with a 2 (group: DD vs TD)×2 (session: 10 minutes vs 24 hours) ANCOVA with d' scores as the dependent variable. Because the DD group's trend of better performance at distinguishing real and made-up objects in the incidental encoding task could potentially confound performance at recognition, semantic categorization performance during encoding was included along with PIQ as a covariate.

Analyses revealed that the DD group had better recognition memory, as compared to the TD group, across both recognition sessions (Figure 2): the 2×2 ANCOVA produced a significant main effect of group ($F(1,24) = 4.45$, $p = .045$, $\eta_p^2 = .156$), with no main effect of session ($F < 1$), and no group by session interaction ($F < 1$).

Reaction times, by contrast, did not differ significantly between the two groups (mean RTs across both recognition sessions: DD *mean* = 1004 ms, *SD* = 124 ms; TD *mean* = 923 ms, *SD* = 168 ms). The 2 (group: DD vs TD)×2 (session: 10 minutes vs 24 hours) ANCOVA with RT as dependent variable (controlling for PIQ and encoding accuracy) produced no significant effects (main effect of group: $F(1,24) = 1.41$, $p = .248$, $\eta_p^2 = .055$; main effect of session: $F < 1$; group×session interaction: $F < 1$).

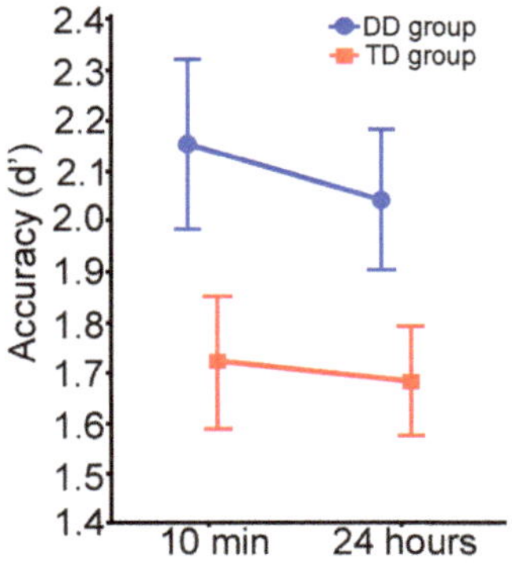

Figure 2. Adjusted means and standard errors for children with developmental dyslexia (DD) and typically developing control children (TD).

Control Analyses

In order to rule out alternative explanations to the observed DD recognition memory advantage, a set of control analyses was performed, with the aim of investigating potentially confounding factors.

First, we asked if group differences in speed-accuracy tradeoff during the recognition memory task could explain the present findings. This question was addressed by partial correlation analyses (controlling for PIQ and encoding accuracy) of RT against d' scores within each recognition session separately. These analyses revealed no evidence of speed-accuracy tradeoffs in either of the two sessions, across all children or within either of the two groups (10 minute recognition session: all children: $r(24) = .017$, $p = .923$; DD group: $r(7) = -.358$, $p = .309$; TD group: $r(13) = .005$, $p = .984$; 24 hour recognition session all: $r(24) = -.170$; $p = .395$; DD group: $r(7) = -.396$, $p = .257$; TD group: $r(13) = -.200$, $p = .457$).

Second, because the two groups were somewhat unbalanced with respect to sex (Table 1), it is possible that the group difference in recognition memory was an artifact produced by the greater number of boys in the TD group. We therefore added sex as a covariate to the model. This 2×2 ANCOVA with three covariates (semantic categorization accuracy, PIQ, and sex) yielded the same pattern as that reported above: a main effect of group, with the DD group showing better recognition memory than the TD group ($F(1,23) = 4.30$, $p = .049$, $\eta_p^2 = .158$). No other main effects or interactions were significant (main effect of sex: $F(1,23) = 1.68$, $p = .207$, $\eta_p^2 = .068$, main effect of session: $F < 1$, group by session interaction: $F < 1$).

Third, the effects of PIQ were more carefully examined. First, we performed a correlation analysis between PIQ and semantic categorization performance (which was the second covariate in the main ANCOVA). This analysis revealed that there was no correlation between PIQ and semantic categorization, across groups or within groups (all *ps* >.6). Next, the relationship between PIQ and the dependent variable (recognition memory) was investigated. There was no correlation between recognition memory mean d' scores and PIQ, either across all children or within the TD group (*ps* >.6). However, there was a marginally significant association between PIQ and recognition memory performance in the DD group ($r = .594$, $p = .054$), confirming the desirability to control for PIQ in the group comparison of recognition memory.

Finally, we followed up on these analyses by creating new DD and TD groups that were matched one-to-one on PIQ. These groups were created by including all DD children for which there was a TD child with an identical PIQ standard score. If there were more than one TD option for a particular DD child (this was the case for one DD child in our data set), we selected the one that would also balance the groups with respect to sex. There were 5 children (3 boys and 2 girls) in each group. All DD children had mean stanine reading scores ≤2 and all TD children had mean stanine reading scores ≥4. The PIQ range was 85–115. These groups were then compared with Mann-Whitney U tests on recognition memory d' scores and reaction times. The results confirmed the pattern observed in the main analysis with a significant DD advantage at recognition memory accuracy (main effect of group across both sessions: $p = .022$) and no group difference in RT (main effect of group across both sessions: $p = .676$).

Correlations between Reading Performance and Recognition Memory

Next, the relationships between reading performance and recognition memory within the two groups were examined. We performed partial correlation analyses (controlling for PIQ and encoding accuracy) between the mean d' score across both sessions and the combined standardized raw scores from the phonological decoding and orthographic reading tests. These analyses revealed a marginally significant association between recognition memory and reading performance in the DD group ($r(7) = .644$, $p = .061$), whereas there was no such association in the TD group ($r(13) = -.081$, $p = .774$). The difference between the correlations between recognition memory and reading in the two groups approached significance ($p = .056$).

Analyses of Object-type Effects

Finally, to examine whether the two groups differed with respect to potential effects of object-type, we performed 2 (object-type: real vs made-up)×2 (group: DD vs TD) ANCOVAs (controlling for PIQ and encoding accuracy) for each of the two recognition sessions. The ANCOVA for the 10 minute session produced a marginally significant main effect of group ($F(1,24) = 4.10$, $p = .054$, $\eta_p^2 = .146$), with better performance for the DD group compared to the TD group (real objects: DD d' *mean* = 3.18, *SD* = 0.72; TD d' *mean* = 2.71, *SD* = 0.81; made-up objects: DD d' *mean* = 1.48, *SD* = 0.60; TD d' *mean* = 1.15, *SD* = 0.62), a significant main effect of object-type ($F(1,24) = 6.39$, $p = .018$, $\eta_p^2 = .210$), with superior memory for real compared to made-up objects, and no object-type×group interaction ($F < 1$). Thus, in the 10 minute session, the DD group showed somewhat better performance for both object types, and both groups showed better performance for real compared to made-up objects.

In the 24 hour session, there was again a marginally significant main effect of group ($F(1,24) = 4.0$, $p = .057$, $\eta_p^2 = .143$), with better DD compared to TD performance (real objects : DD d' *mean* = 2.06, *SD* = 0.31; TD d' *mean* = 2.02, *SD* = 0.26; made-up objects: DD *mean* = 1.95, *SD* = 0.85; TD *mean* = 1.67, *SD* = 1.49), but no effect of object-type ($F(1,24) = 1.33$, $p = .261$, $\eta_p^2 = .052$). The object-type×group interaction was marginally significant ($F(1,24) = 3.99$, $p = .057$, $\eta_p^2 = .142$). Although the lack of significance for this interaction does not support follow-up analyses, the *mean* values suggest that the DD compared to TD advantage in the 24 hour session may be larger for the made-up objects than the real objects.

Discussion

The aim of the present study was to investigate a previously untested aspect of declarative memory in children with DD, namely recognition memory after incidental encoding. Based on previous evidence indicating that declarative memory impairments in DD may be related to less efficient encoding strategies [29] and/or problems with free recall [9,34], we predicted that the present paradigm would yield intact performance in the DD group. Recognition memory was found to be not only intact, but even superior, in the DD group as compared to the TD group. These results were not driven by group differences in PIQ, sex or speed-accuracy trade-off effects.

Developmental dyslexia has previously been associated with a number of linguistic and non-linguistic deficits (see introduction). The present findings indicate that this condition may also entail an enhancement of certain cognitive functions. These findings complement previous reports suggesting enhancements in other aspects of cognition in DD, namely visuo-spatial processing [52,53]. Although the mechanisms underlying the observed enhanced performance at recognition memory are still unknown, we consider several possible explanations.

One explanation that has been proposed to account for enhanced visuo-spatial processing in DD [52], and that could plausibly play a role in the findings here, is that the superior recognition memory performance of the DD group was an effect of an enhanced ability to create semantic labels or associations for the "non-nameable" made-up objects. According to this account, a frequent use of semantic substitutions to compensate for lexical retrieval deficits may make the DD group more adept at creating semantic labels or associations for objects that are difficult to describe, which in turn might have a positive impact on memory performance. This hypothesis would predict performance in the DD group to be enhanced, compared to the TD group, specifically for the made-up objects. Indeed, the marginally significant group×object-type interaction in the 24 hour recognition session hints at the possibility of a group difference in the consolidation of made-up objects (with somewhat better performance in the DD group). However, this hypothesis seems somewhat inconsistent with the fact that the two groups showed an equally large advantage for real as compared to made-up objects in the 10 minute session. Future studies including larger samples might help clarify the nature of these object-type effects and how they may relate to dyslexia.

Alternatively, it may be the case that the superior performance in the DD group was not a result of an enhancement in this group, but rather the result of relatively impaired performance in the TD group. According to the neuronal recycling hypothesis [54], learning to read entails a tradeoff in which the building up of a sight-word lexicon takes place at the cost of certain other visual skills. Support for this hypothesis comes from the tradeoff between reading and other aspects of visual cognition that has been observed in illiterate adults who learn to read [55] and in dyslexic participants following remediation [56]. This hypothesis would predict that the DD advantage at recognition memory observed in the present study would diminish as the dyslexic children improve their reading ability. Although the design of the present study does not allow us to further investigate this hypothesis, a future follow-up study may be warranted to specifically test this prediction.

A third possible explanation for the present findings is that they reflect intricate interactions between the procedural and declarative memory systems. Converging evidence from human and animal studies suggest that the procedural and declarative memory systems rely on at least partly dissociable neural substrates and support different cognitive functions [57]. However, the two systems do not work in isolation. Rather, the relative involvement of the procedural and declarative systems during cognitive task performance appears to be modulated by the to-be-learned material on the one hand [6,58,59,60], and by complex "competitive" and "cooperative" interactions between the two systems on the other (for reviews see [6,61,62]). Competitive interactions, sometimes referred to as a "seesaw effect" [6], may help explain the enhancement of recognition memory observed here. Of particular relevance, animal lesion studies have revealed that damage to one system can actually *enhance* learning by the other [63,64,65]. Such findings have been taken as evidence for a competitive relationship between the two systems that may interfere with learning and processing under normal conditions. The enhanced performance of the unimpaired system has been proposed to reflect the removal of interference by the damaged system [63]. Neuroimaging studies suggest the existence of similar competitive mechanisms in humans [59,66,67]. Since it has been proposed that procedural memory is impaired in DD [6,11], a prediction that is supported by a number of studies [11,12,14,15,68,69,70,71,72], it is possible that the declarative memory enhancement found in the present study may be partially explained by such competitive interactions.

A possible enhancement of aspects of declarative memory is particularly intriguing since evidence suggests that declarative memory may play an important compensatory role for the reading deficits in dyslexia. This phenomenon may reflect the cooperative aspect of the procedural-declarative relationship [6,61,62,73,74]. For example, previous studies indicate that persistent phonological decoding problems in individuals with DD may be associated with an increased reliance on chunking and whole word memorization for reading [75,76]. In addition, behavioral interventions have been found to lead not only to reading improvements, but also to changes in the hippocampus and other medial temporal lobe structures, in both functional and structural imaging studies [77,78]. Similar compensatory mechanisms have previously been reported for populations afflicted with procedural memory impairments (e.g. Parkinson's disease) in which declarative memory has been shown to take over certain cognitive functions that are normally performed by the procedural memory system [73,74,79,80,81].

If declarative memory indeed plays a compensatory role for reading in the present study, we would expect to find a correlation between performance at the recognition memory test and reading scores in the DD group, but not in the TD group. This prediction did not seem to be strictly supported, as the correlation between recognition memory d' scores (across both sessions) and the combined standardized raw scores from the two reading tests did not reach significance. However, the lack of such an effect in the DD group may reflect a lack of power due to the small sample size. Indeed, the correlation approached significance in the DD group ($p = .061$) but not in the TD group ($p = .774$). Moreover, the difference between the two correlations was borderline significant ($p = .056$). Thus, the investigation of a potentially compensatory role of declarative memory in DD requires further studies with larger samples.

The present study has various limitations that may be addressed by future studies. First, samples sizes were relatively small. Thus, the present findings need to be replicated with larger samples in order to ensure their generalizability. In addition, the present study tests only one aspect of declarative memory, and leaves many other aspects unexplored. Future studies would benefit from contrasting the recognition memory paradigm used in the present study with paradigms assessing encoding strategies and recall. Such a within-subjects design would allow for a powerful examination of different aspects of declarative memory, and their status in DD.

Keeping these limitations in mind, the results of the present study are encouraging, as they point to possible cognitive strengths associated with an otherwise difficult and persisting condition. Crucially, knowledge about which aspects of cognition are intact, or even enhanced, in DD, should be of theoretical as well as of clinical and pedagogical interest.

Acknowledgments

We gratefully acknowledge the help of the many schools and families who participated in this study. We also wish to thank Åke Olofsson for helpful comments and advice.

Author Contributions

Conceived and designed the experiments: MH MU MJ. Performed the experiments: MH. Analyzed the data: MH JP PA. Wrote the paper: MH JP MU.

References

1. Lyon GR, Shaywitz SE, Shaywitz BA (2003) A definition of dyslexia. Ann Dyslexia 53: 1–14.
2. Hensler BS, Schatschneider C, Taylor J, Wagner RK (2010) Behavioral genetic approach to the study of dyslexia. J Dev Behav Pediatr 31: 525–532.
3. Shaywitz SE, Shaywitz BA, Fletcher JM, Escobar MD (1990) Prevalence of reading disability in boys and girls. Results of the Connecticut Longitudinal Study. JAMA 264: 998–1002.
4. Bishop DV, Snowling MJ (2004) Developmental dyslexia and specific language impairment: same or different? Psychol Bull 130: 858–886.
5. Catts HW, Kamhi AG, editors (2005) Language and reading disabilties: Pearson Education, Inc.
6. Ullman MT (2004) Contributions of memory circuits to language: The declarative/procedural model. Cognition 92: 231–270.
7. Nicolson RI, Fawcett AJ (2011) Dyslexia, dysgraphia, procedural learning and the cerebellum. Cortex 47: 117–127.
8. Smith-Spark JH, Fisk JE (2007) Working memory functioning in developmental dyslexia. Memory 15: 34–56.
9. Swanson HL, Xinhua Z, Jerman O (2009) Working memory, short-term memory, and reading disabilities: a selective meta-analysis of the literature. J Learn Disabil 42: 260–287.
10. Brosnan M, Demetre J, Hamill S, Robson K, Shepherd H, et al. (2002) Executive functioning in adults and children with developmental dyslexia. Neuropsychologia 40: 2144–2155.
11. Nicolson RI, Fawcett AJ, Dean P (2001) Developmental dyslexia: The cerebellar deficit hypothesis. Trends Neurosci 24: 508–511.
12. Jimenez-Fernandez G, Vaquero JM, Jimenez L, Defior S (2011) Dyslexic children show deficits in implicit sequence learning, but not in explicit sequence learning or contextual cueing. Ann Dyslexia 61: 85–110.
13. Howard JH, Howard DV, Japikse KC, Eden GF (2006) Dyslexics are impaired on implicit high-order sequence learning, but not on implicit spatial context learning. Neuropsychologia 44: 1131–1144.
14. Vicari S, Marotta L, Menghiai D, Molinari M, Petrosini L (2003) Implicit learning deficit in children with developmental dyslexia. Neuropsychologia 41: 108–114.
15. Pavlidou EV, Williams JM, Kelly LM (2009) Artificial grammar learning in primary school children with and without developmental dyslexia. Ann Dyslexia 59: 55–77.
16. Wimmer H, Schurz M (2010) Dyslexia in regular orthographies: manifestation and causation. Dyslexia 16: 283–299.
17. Snowling MJ, Gallagher A, Frith U (2003) Family risk of dyslexia is continuous: individual differences in the precursors of reading skill. Child Dev 74: 358–373.
18. Lyytinen H, Ahonen T, Eklund K, Guttorm T, Kulju P, et al. (2004) Early development of children at familial risk for dyslexia - follow up from birth control to school age. Dyslexia 10: 146–178.
19. Tulving E (1972) Episodic and semantic memory. In: Tulving E, Donaldson W, editors. Organization of memory. New York: Academic Press. 381–403.
20. Tulving E (2002) Episodic memory: From mind to brain. Ann Rev Psychol 53: 1–25.
21. Squire LR, Zola-Morgan S (1991) The medial temporal lobe memory system. Science 253: 1380–1386.
22. Eichenbaum H (2000) A cortical-hippocampal system for declarative memory. Nat Rev Neurosci 1: 41–50.
23. Tulving E, Kapur S, Craik FIM, Moscovitch M, Houle S (1994) Hemispheric encoding/retrieval asymmetry in episodic memory: Positron emission tomography findings. Proc Natl Acad Sci 91: 2016–2020.
24. Nyberg L, McIntosh AR, Cabeza R, Habib R, Houle S, et al. (1996) General and specific brain regions involved in encoding and retrieval of events: what, where, and when. Proc Natl Acad Sci USA 93: 11280–11285.
25. Stuss DT, Knight RT, editors (2002) Principles of Frontal Lobe Function. New York: Oxford University Press.
26. Kibby M (2009) Memory functioning in developmental dyslexia: An analysis using two clinical measures. Arch Clin Neuropsychol 24: 245–254.
27. Kibby MY, Cohen MJ (2008) Memory functions in children with reading disabilities and/or attention deficit/hyperactivity disorder: A clinical investigation of their working memory and long-term memory functioning. Child Neuropsychol 14: 525–546.
28. Kaplan BJ, Dewey D, Crawford S, Fisher GC (1998) Deficits in long-term memory are not characteristic of ADHD. J Clin Exp Neuropsychol 20: 518–528.
29. Kramer JH, Knee K, Delis D (2000) Verbal memory impairments in dyslexia. Arch Clin Neuropsychol 15: 83–93.
30. Menghini D, Carlesimo GA, Marotta L, Finzi A, Vicari S (2010) Developmental dyslexia and explicit long-term memory Dyslexia 16: 213–225.
31. Messbauer VCS, de Jong P (2003) Word, non-word, and visual paired associate learning in Dutch dyslexic children. J Exp Child Psychol 84: 77–96.

32. Li H, Shu H, McBride-Chang C, Liu HY, Xue J (2009) Paired associate learning in Chinese children with dyslexia. J Exp Child Psychol 103: 135–151.
33. Mayringer H, Wimmer H (2000) Pseudoname learning by German-speaking children with dyslexia: evidence for a phonological learning deficit. J Exp Child Psychol 75: 116–133.
34. Vellutino FR, Scanlon DM (1985) Free recall of concrete and abstract words in poor and normal readers. Journal of Experimental Child Psychology 39: 363–380.
35. Olofsson Å (2003) The dyslexic reader and the Swedish language. In: Goulandris N, editor. Dyslexia: Cross-linguistic comparisons. London: Whurr. 137–156.
36. Olson RK, Forsberg H, Wise B, Rack J (1994) Measurement of word recognition, orthographic and phonological skills. In: Lyon GR, editor. Frames of reference for the assessment of learning disabilities: New views on measurement issues. Baltimore: Paul H. Brookes. 243–277.
37. Siegel LS, Share D, Geva E (1995) Evidence for superior orthographic skills in dyslexics. Psychol Sci 6: 250–254.
38. Wass M, Ibertsson T, Lyxell B, Sahlén B, Hällgren M, et al. (2008) Cognitive and linguistic skills in Swedish children with cochlear implants – measures of accuracy and latency as indicators of development. Scand J Psychol 49: 559–576.
39. Bishop DV (1982) T.R.O.G Test for reception of grammar: Chapel Press.
40. Holmberg E, Lundälv E (2002) T.R.O.G. svensk manual. Göteborg: Specialpedagogiska institutet Läromedel.
41. Dunn LM, Dunn LM (1997) Peabody Picture Vocabulary Test Third Edition. Circle Pines: American Guidance Service.
42. Raven J (1998) Standard Progressive Matrices – Plus Version and Mill Hill. Vocabulary Scale, Manual. London: Pearson Assessment.
43. Ferrer E, Shaywitz BA, Holahan JM, Marchione K, Shaywitz SE (2010) Uncoupling of reading and IQ over time: empirical evidence for a definition of dyslexia. Psychol Sci 21: 93–101.
44. Rispens J, van Yperen TA, van Duijn GA (1991) The irrelevance of IQ to the definition of learning disabilities: some empirical evidence. J Learn Disabil 24: 434–438.
45. Henson R (2005) A mini-review of fMRI studies of human medial temporal lobe activity associated with recognition memory. Q J Exp Physiol 58(B): 340–360.
46. Kim H, Cabeza R (2009) Common and specific brain regions in high- versus low-confidence recognition memory. Brain Res 1282: 103–113.
47. Snodgrass JG, Vanderwart M (1980) A standardized set of 260 pictures: Norms for name agreement, image agreement, familiarity, and visual complexity. J Exp Psychol 6: 174–215.
48. Eals M, Silverman I (1994) The Hunter-Gatherer theory of spatial sex differences: Proximate factors mediating the female advantage in recall of object arrays. Ethol Sociobiol 15: 95–105.
49. Cornelissen K, Laine M, Renvall K, Saarinen T, Martin N, et al. (2004) Learning new names for new objects: Cortical effects as measured by magnetoencephalography. Brain Lang 89: 617–622.
50. Williams P, Tarr MJ (1997) Structural processing and implicit memory for possible and impossible figures. J Exp Psychol Learn Mem Cogn 23: 1344–1361.
51. Wagner AD, Schacter DL, Rotte M, Koutstaal W, Maril A, et al. (1998) Building memories: Remembering and forgetting of verbal experiences as predicted by brain activity. Science 281: 1188–1191.
52. Schneps MH, Brockmole JR, Sonnert G, Pomplun M (2012) History of reading struggles linked to enhanced learning in low spatial frequency. scenes. PLoS ONE 7: e35724.
53. Karolyi Cv, Winner E, Gray W, Shermand GF (2003) Dyslexia linked to talent: Global visual-spatial ability. Brain Lang 85: 427–431.
54. Dehaene S, Cohen L (2007) Cultural recycling of cortical maps. Neuron 56: 384–398.
55. Dehaene S, Pegado F, Braga LW, Ventura P, Nunes Filho G, et al. (2010) How learning to read changes the cortical networks for vision and language. Science 330: 1359–1364.
56. Lorusso ML, Facoetti A, Toraldo A, Molteni M (2005) Tachistoscopic treatment of dyslexia changes the distribution of visual-spatial attention. Brain Cogn 57: 135–142.
57. Squire LR, Zola SM (1996) Structure and function of declarative and nondeclarative memory systems. Proc Natl Acad Sci USA 93: 13515–13522.
58. Foerde K, Knowlton BJ, Poldrack RA (2006) Modulation of competing memory systems by distraction. Proc Natl Acad Sci 103: 11778–11783.
59. Poldrack RA, Clark J, Pare-Blagoev EJ, Shohamy D, Moyano JC, et al. (2001) Interactive memory systems in the human brain. Nature 414: 546–550.
60. Shohamy D, Myers C, Grossman S, Sage J, Gluck M, et al. (2004) Cortico-striatal contributions to feedback-based learning: converging data from neuroimaging and neuropsychology. Brain 127: 851–859.
61. Poldrack RA, Packard MG (2003) Competition among multiple memory systems: Converging evidence from animal and human brain studies. Neuropsychologia 41: 245–251.
62. Foerde K, Shohamy D (2011) The role of the basal ganglia in learning and memory: insight from Parkinson's disease. Neurobiol Learn Mem 96: 624–636.
63. Chang Q, Gold PE (2003) Intra-hippocampal lidocaine injections impair acquisition of a place task and facilitate acquisition of a response task in rats. Behav Brain Res 144: 19–24.
64. Mitchell JA, Hall G (1988) Caudate-putamen lesions in the rat may impair or potentiate maze learning depending upon availability of stimulus cues and relevance of response cues. Q J Exp Psychol 40: 243–258.
65. Schroeder JP, Wingard JC, Packard MG (2002) Post-training reversible inactivation of the dorsal hippocampus reveals interference between multiple memory systems. Hippocampus 12: 280–284.
66. Lieberman MD, Chang GY, Chiao J, Bookheimer SY, Knowlton BJ (2004) An event-related fMRI study of artificial grammar learning in a balanced chunk strength design. J Cog Neurosci 16: 427–438.
67. Seger CA, Cincotta CM (2005) The roles of the caudate nucleus in human classification learning. J Neurosci 25: 2941–2951.
68. Vicari S, Finzi A, Menghini D, Marotta L, Baldi S, et al. (2005) Do children with developmental dyslexia have an implicit learning deficit? J Neurol Neurosurg Psychiatry: 1–8.
69. Menghini D, Hagberg GE, Caltagirone C, Petrosini L, Vicaria S (2006) Implicit learning deficits in dyslexic adults: An fMRI study. NeuroImage 33: 1218–1226.
70. Menghini D, Hagberg GE, Petrosini L, Bozzali M, Macaluso E, et al. (2008) Structural correlates of implicit learning deficits in subjects with developmental dyslexia. Ann NY Acad Sci 1145: 212–221.
71. Stoodley CJ, Harrison EPD, Stein JF (2006) Implicit motor learning deficits in dyslexic adults. Neuropsychologia 44: 795–798.
72. Howard JHJ, Howard DV, Japikse KC, Eden GF (2006) Dyslexics are impaired on implicit higher-order sequence learning, but not on implicit spatial context learning. Neuropsychologia 44: 1131–1144.
73. Moody TD, Bookheimer SY, Vanek Z, Knowlton BJ (2004) An implicit learning task activates medial temporal lobe in patients with Parkinson's disease. Behav Neurosci 118: 438–442.
74. Rieckmann A, Fischer H, Backman L (2010) Activation in striatum and medial temporal lobe during sequence learning in younger and older adults: relations to performance. Neuroimage 50: 1303–1312.
75. van der Leij A, van Daal, V (1999) Automatization aspects of dyslexia: speed limitations in word identification, sensitivity to increasing task demands, and orthographic compensation. J Learn Dis 32: 28177–28217.
76. Shaywitz SE, Shaywitz BA (2008) Paying attention to reading: The neurobiology of reading and dyslexia. Dev and Psychopathol 20: 1329–1349.
77. Temple E, Deutsch G, Poldrack R, Miller S, Tallal P, et al. (2003) Neural deficits in children with dyslexia ameliorated by behavioral remediation: evidence from functional MRI. Proc Natl Acad Sci 100: 2860–2865.
78. Eden G, Jones K, Cappell K, Gareau L, Wood F, et al. (2004) Neural Changes following Remediation in Adult Developmental Dyslexia. Neuron 44: 411–422.
79. Beauchamp MH, Dagher A, Panisset M, Doyon J (2008) Neural substrates of cognitive skill learning in Parkinson's disease. Brain Cogn 68: 134–143.
80. Rauch SL, Wedig MM, Wright CI, Martis B, McMullin KG, et al. (2007) Functional magnetic resonance imaging study of regional brain activation during implicit sequence learning in obsessive-compulsive disorder. Biol Psychiatry 61: 330–336.
81. Ullman MT, Pierpont EI (2005) Specific language impairment is not specific to language: The procedural deficit hypothesis. Cortex 41: 399–433.

16

Interval Timing in Children: Effects of Auditory and Visual Pacing Stimuli and Relationships with Reading and Attention Variables

Emma E. Birkett, Joel B. Talcott*

Aston Brain Centre, School of Life and Health Sciences, Aston University, Birmingham, United Kingdom

Abstract

Motor timing tasks have been employed in studies of neurodevelopmental disorders such as developmental dyslexia and ADHD, where they provide an index of temporal processing ability. Investigations of these disorders have used different stimulus parameters within the motor timing tasks that are likely to affect performance measures. Here we assessed the effect of auditory and visual pacing stimuli on synchronised motor timing performance and its relationship with cognitive and behavioural predictors that are commonly used in the diagnosis of these highly prevalent developmental disorders. Twenty-one children (mean age 9.6 years) completed a finger tapping task in two stimulus conditions, together with additional psychometric measures. As anticipated, synchronisation to the beat (ISI 329 ms) was less accurate in the visually paced condition. Decomposition of timing variance indicated that this effect resulted from differences in the way that visual and auditory paced tasks are processed by central timekeeping and associated peripheral implementation systems. The ability to utilise an efficient processing strategy on the visual task correlated with both reading and sustained attention skills. Dissociations between these patterns of relationship across task modality suggest that not all timing tasks are equivalent.

Editor: Aditya Bhushan Pant, Indian Institute of Toxicology Reserach, India

Funding: This work was supported by the Economic and Social Research Council (grant number ES/G013845/1, www.esrc.ac.uk). The funders had no role in study design, data collection, data analysis, decision to publish, nor preparation of the manuscript.

Competing Interests: The authors have declared that no competing interests exist.

* E-mail: j.b.talcott@aston.ac.uk

Introduction

Motor timing in participants with developmental dyslexia and Attention Deficit Hyperactivity Disorder (ADHD) has been investigated with behavioural tasks that require the production of motor responses in synchrony with external pacing stimuli [1,2]. Dyslexia and ADHD are both associated with subtle performance differences in the accuracy and precision of such responses compared to controls [3]. Convergent streams of evidence for perceptual differences in the detection and discrimination of the temporal parameters of auditory, visual and sensory-motor stimuli [4,2] support the hypothesis that poor neural timing is a candidate neuro-cognitive endophenotype of dyslexia [5] and ADHD [2].

ADHD and dyslexia are developmental disorders that are typically identified in childhood. They co-occur at such a high rate (>25%) [6,7] that they almost certainly share underlying cognitive, neurological and genetic risk factors [8,9]. At a neurophysiological level, a risk factor related to timing functions might explain a wide array of the cognitive and behavioural symptoms, both those that are disorder-specific and those that overlap between disorder phenotypes. Although ADHD and dyslexia are defined by independent sets of behavioural symptoms, recent evidence promotes a dimensional rather than a categorical view of developmental disorders and their associated symptoms [10]. This perspective accounts for the overlap between both the diagnostic prevalence and symptoms of these disorders and highlights evidence that common underlying mechanisms likely mediate general population variability on the constructs upon which clinical diagnoses are made (i.e., reading and attention variables) [9].

One target mechanism of impairment identified for both ADHD and dyslexia is in temporal processing [2,5], a construct that includes the ability to segregate and process incoming sequences of stimuli (i.e., rate of perception) [11–13] and the detection of the temporal structure of individual stimuli (i.e., perception of rate) [14,15]. Temporal processing has been measured using an array of neurophysiological and behavioural tasks to estimate detection or discrimination thresholds for rapidly occurring stimuli or those with properties that change in real time. Here we focus on tasks involving motor timing to a periodic sensory event, paradigms that have been employed previously in clinical investigations within the field of learning disabilities [1,3,16–18] and in other populations [19–21].

Tasks of motor timing assess the ability to synchronise movements (typically finger movements) with external pacing stimuli. Such tasks are particularly well-suited for use with children because they allow behavioural assessment of a processing dimension where the accuracy and precision of the response requires temporal processing but not complex subjective judgements about the nature of the stimuli presented. Differences in the ability to perform motor timing tasks between clinical and control groups have been demonstrated for adults, adolescents and children with a history of developmental dyslexia [1,14,17,22], with greater response variability typically demonstrated in the group with dyslexia. Such motor timing skills appear to be sensitive to individual variation in the symptom dimensions relevant to dyslexia diagnosis, such as in reading accuracy and working memory, for both clinical and control samples [1,23,24]. Differences in motor timing have also been reported for ADHD, where performance of clinically-derived, paediatric samples is characterised by greater response variability at the individual level [3,25–27] and difficulties compared to controls in selecting the appropriate response rate [16,25]. Such studies have also shown that motor timing differences can correlate with continuous measures of ADHD symptoms in both clinical and control samples [25,28].

Using motor responses as behavioural indices of temporal processing has an additional advantage over other measures of this construct because response variability can be decomposed into variance components that reflect putative underlying mechanisms [29,30]. For example, the Wing and Kristofferson [29,31] model proposes that two main sources of variance contribute to individual behavioural responses on motor timing tasks: a timekeeping system that monitors the pacing stimuli and generates signals at appropriate intervals, and the peripheral implementation system that produces the motor response based on input from the timekeeper. The Wing and Kristofferson model has been used to investigate the components of timing difficulties in clinical populations, including those with Parkinson's disease and patients with cerebellar lesions [19,32–34]. As applied here to children with varying abilities in reading and attention, this model may highlight the independent and shared components of timing differences associated with these core symptomatic features of dyslexia and ADHD. If the temporal processing differences found in these developmental disorders have a shared causal mechanism, we expect that the efficiency of the timekeeper mechanism will be associated with both literacy and attention variables, even within a typically developing population sample. In contrast, if the shared behavioural difficulties result from different mechanisms, these variables should not share common associations with these skills within the same participants.

Given the evidence of temporal processing deficits in both ADHD and dyslexia [5,35,36], it is tempting to speculate that such a generic functional property of the nervous system may help to explain the high co-morbidity between dyslexia and ADHD. Such a hypothesis has strong face validity. However, studies of groups with ADHD and dyslexia have differed with respect to the sensory modality through which pacing stimuli are delivered: auditory stimuli have been typically employed in investigations of dyslexia [1,14,23,37] but visual or combined auditory-visual stimuli have been predominantly used in studies of ADHD [3,16,26,27]. Investigations of performance under different task parameters show that the high temporal acuity of the auditory system facilitates precise synchronisation of motor behaviour with acoustically-presented pacing stimuli [38–40]. In contrast, motor synchronisation to visual stimuli typically results in greater response-variability [40–43]. This effect has been interpreted as evidence that limited information is available to timekeeping systems in such tasks and prevents effective monitoring and updating of associated output responses [41]. Recent evidence from behavioural [44] and neuroimaging studies [42] further highlights the importance of stimulus mode as a critical variable in understanding intra- and inter-subject differences in motor synchronisation tasks.

To evaluate the potential clinical relevance of motor synchronisation tasks in the context of these important methodological considerations, we examined the behavioural effects of altering task parameters on the timing performance of children. Performance was analysed using the variance model described by Wing and Kristofferson [31]. In addition to comparisons between tasks, we assessed statistical relationships between timing variables and measures of literacy and attention which tap the key cognitive dimensions that form the core deficits in developmental dyslexia and ADHD respectively Both of these analyses allow the validity of the task parameters to be assessed, and are important prerequisites to the application of these methods to clinical samples, including children with developmental disorders.

Methods

Participants

We recruited a group of 25 children from a single primary school classroom. Participants provided informed consent under a protocol approved by the Aston University Institutional Review Board. The research was conducted according to the Declaration of Helsinki. The head teacher at the school provided written informed consent for the study to be carried out in the school and parents were sent letters with an opt-out form to be returned if they did not consent to their child taking part. Following this, the purpose of the study was explained to each child and throughout the study they were continually assessed for their willingness to participate.

Four data sets met the exclusionary criteria for the study: one child had an existing diagnosis of an emotional-behavioural disorder; one had English as a second language and two failed to complete the experimental protocol. The remaining group of 21 children comprised 10 boys and 11 girls (age range 98–127 months; three left-handed). All 21 children had received musical instruction through either home- or school-based music lessons and all had received weekly classroom-based Samba drumming lessons throughout the previous academic year.

Psychometric Measures

The psychometric measures employed in this study assessed cognitive dimensions that are used in deriving diagnoses of developmental dyslexia and ADHD. As applied to population samples, these measures were used to determine the statistical relationships between motor timing performance and reading and attention variables across the normal range.

Verbal and non-verbal reasoning. The Similarities (verbal) and Matrices (non-verbal) subscales from the Wechsler Abbreviated Scale of Intelligence (WASI) [45] were administered to all participants. Age-referenced, standard scores were derived for each child using published norms.

Literacy. The Reading and Spelling subtests from the Wechsler Individual Achievement Test-II UK (WIAT) [46] were completed by all participants. These untimed measures assess accuracy for items graded in difficulty, from which standard scores were obtained for each child.

Attention measures. We obtained teacher ratings of ADHD symptoms using the ADHD Behaviour Rating Scale-Teacher Form [47], a questionnaire with separate sets of items for the assessment of inattention (ADHD-IA) and hyperactivity-impulsivity (ADHD-HI). Both subscales capture the behavioural dimensions associated with ADHD established by the Diagnostic and Statistical Manual of Mental Disorders-IV [48].

The age-standardised Same World, Opposite World task from the Test of Everyday Attention for Children (TEA-Ch) was used to assess attentional control [49]. In each task, two practice trials were followed by two test trials. The time taken to complete the Same World and Opposite World trials was recorded. The score used in statistical analyses was the percentage increase in completion time between the two tasks.

The Score! Subscale from the TEA-Ch battery [49], was also administered to the children. Performance data for each child on this measure of sustained attention was converted to a standard score using age- appropriate norms.

Motor Timing Measures

Simple reaction time. All participants completed a measure of simple reaction time in response to the same individual stimuli as those used in the two modes (auditory and visual) of the finger tapping paradigm (see below). This control measure assessed the speed of simple motor responses. Participants were instructed to respond as quickly as possible to the presentation of a single stimulus with a finger-press. These responses were registered using a flat switch plate, designed to minimise vertical travel when depressed. The plate was contained within a box to prevent participants from viewing their hand whilst making responses, reducing the visual feedback available to participants. Participants responded to 10 reaction time trials in each stimulus modality and the mean reaction time and standard deviation (SD) were calculated for each condition.

Synchronised finger tapping. The primary experimental measure in the study was a synchronisation task in which participants were instructed to tap their index finger of their dominant hand 'in time' with the repeated onsets of externally delivered pacing stimuli. The trials were presented in separate blocks, distinguished only by the different modes of stimulus presentation (auditory or visual). Within each block, participants completed three separate trial sequences, each consisting of 40 isochronous pacing stimuli with onsets timed to achieve an inter-stimulus interval (ISI) of 329 ms (see Figure 1). This tapping rate is comparable to that used previously in studies of motor timing [16,28,33,34]. Responses were registered with the same switch plate described above.

In the auditory condition the stimuli were 47 ms auditory tones presented through computer speakers. The visual stimuli comprised a 2 cm diameter red diamond, presented in the centre of a CRT computer monitor (Dell Trinitron P1130) with a refresh rate of 85 Hz (11.8 frames/sec). Stimuli were presented via E-Prime presentation software [50]. Each constituent stimulus slide was timed to ensure that its offset was synchronised with the end of the fourth refresh cycle (i.e., 47 ms after stimulus presentation). At the end of this frame, the stimulus slide was replaced with a blank screen of 282 ms duration (24 frames). The timing of the stimulus and blank slide ensured that the interval between the onset of two successive stimuli was fixed at 376 ms (32 frames). Although the decay characteristics of monitor phosphors made it likely that the duration of the visual stimuli were notionally less than the 47 ms stimulus duration [51,52], our method for timing stimuli ensured the reliability of the crucial component of the timing task, namely the consistency of the onset to onset interval.

Two further blocks of filler sequences were interspersed between trial runs to reduce potential effects related to entrainment of the stimulus presentation rate. Auditory and visual distracter blocks were comprised of three synchronisation trials each, with 20 pacing stimuli presented at an ISI of 517 ms. The order of the 4 blocks (2 speeds×2 modalities) was randomised for each child.

The tasks in the test battery were presented in a fixed order, and divided across two or three testing sessions, each of which lasted approximately 20 minutes.

Data Analysis

The first five finger tap responses from every trial run were removed from analyses to account for stabilisation of responses. An inter-response interval (IRI) was calculated for each of the 30 remaining responses in each trial. IRIs that that were outside the range of 50% of the target interval (i.e., greater than 495 ms or less than 165 ms against the 329 ms target interval) were removed from the analysis as invalid responses on the basis that they likely resulted from response errors (for e.g., doubled responses). Data were not analysed for a given trial if more than 10 responses were deemed invalid (9.5% of total trials in the dataset). Mean and standard deviation (SD) of IRIs were calculated for each trial. The

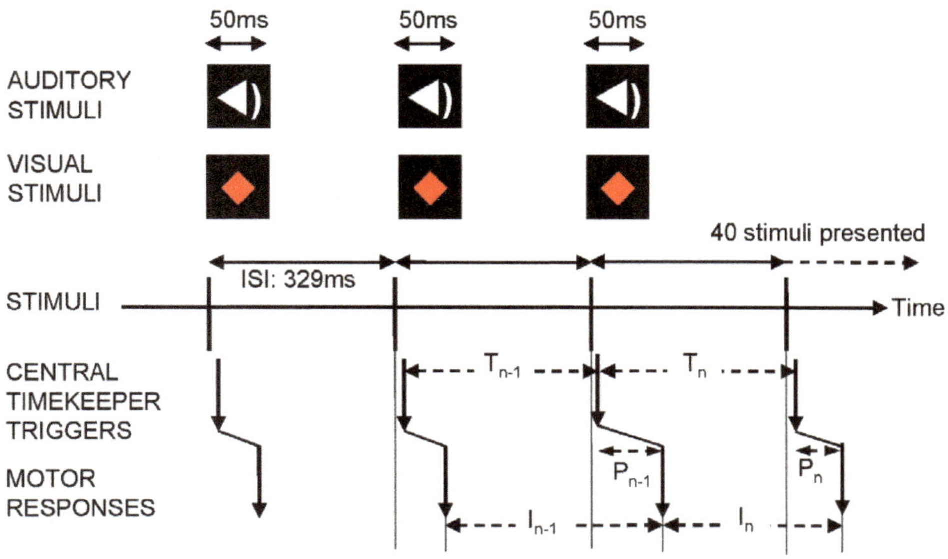

Figure 1. Representation of finger tapping stimuli, response synchrony and variance components. Stimulus intervals of 329 ms are represented by the lines with bidirectional arrows. A central timekeeping mechanism generates response triggers with intervals T_n which are subject to peripheral implementation delays (P_n) and result in the recorded inter-response intervals of motor responses (I_n). The mean difference from the absolute interval is calculated as inter-stimulus interval (ISI) minus I_n.

mean difference from the absolute interval was also obtained and defined as the difference between the target ISI and the IRI achieved by the participant, averaged within a trial.

From the raw data collected for each trial, estimates of the different components of timing variance were calculated using a method consistent with that described by Wing and Kristofferson [31]. This approach to the analysis of timing data assumes that for any stimulus interval, the corresponding inter-response interval (IRI) is the sum of the interval generated by a timekeeper mechanism (T_n) and any delays in implementation of the response from the periphery (P_n), including both those delays resulting from the motor responses at the beginning (P_{n-1}) or end of that interval (P_n). These two components are assumed to be independent, random variables, so the duration of any response interval (I_n) can be represented by Equation 1.This is also illustrated in Figure 1.

Equation 1: $I_n = T_n - P_{n-1} + P_n$

Equation 2: $\mathrm{var}(I_n) = \sigma_T^2 + 2\sigma_P^2$

Equation 3: $\mathrm{cov}(I_{n-1}, I_n) = -\sigma_P^2$

Equation 4: $\sigma_T^2 = \mathrm{var}(I_n) + 2\mathrm{cov}(I_{n-1}, I_n)$

Equation 5: $\sigma_P^2 = -\mathrm{cov}(I_{n-1}, I_n)$

Equation 6: $ACF = \dfrac{-\hat{\sigma}_P^2}{\hat{\sigma}_T^2 + 2\hat{\sigma}_P^2}$

The components described in the model cannot be observed directly from the participant's IRIs. However, the statistical dependences within human motor timing performance, detailed by Wing & Kristofferson [29,31], provide quantifiable parameters of the system and allow estimation of the variance in these components. Variance in motor timing performance is more heavily influenced by variance in the implementation system (σ_P^2) than that in the timekeeper system (σ_T^2), denoted by Equation 2. Each implementation delay has a differential effect on two adjacent intervals (I_n and I_{n-1}), resulting in statistical dependence between these intervals and a negative correlation between them (Equation 3). The model only accounts for dependencies between adjacent intervals, and therefore assumes that non-adjacent IRIs are independent. Rearrangement of these equations allows estimation of the variance attributable to the timekeeper and implementation systems from the observed data. Timekeeper variance is estimated as the sum of the variance of the intervals plus twice the covariance of successive intervals (Equation 4). Implementation variance is estimated as the negative covariance across successive intervals (Equation 5).

Consistent with the method introduced by Kooistra et al [20], we implemented additional terms in the model. First, a drift parameter was added to the terms in Equation 1 to account for any linear trends over successive intervals. In addition, the implementation and timekeeper components were calculated based on the actual number of taps, to account for the fact that variance estimates result from a limited set of possible population samples rather than an unbiased independent sample, as assumed by Equations 2 and 3. Finally, any estimates of timekeeper or implementation variance with negative values were corrected to zero. Negative estimates of variance are theoretically impossible. Statistically, however, they are not unexpected because the tail of the sampling distribution of variance estimates can fall below zero, despite predictions of positive variance by the model [20,53]. Such negative variance estimates do not necessarily signify a poor fit of the variance model to the data. The strategy of zero truncation has been shown to be an adequate method to account for such estimates [20,53]. The resulting corrected estimates of timekeeper ($\hat{\sigma}_T^2$) and implementation variance ($\hat{\sigma}_P^2 o$) were used in subsequent analyses. The full derivation of these adjusted parameters are explained detail in Kooistra et al [20].

We also obtained the lag one auto-correlation function (ACF) from the data. This is defined as the covariance of successive intervals divided by the variance of intervals as shown in Equation 6. The ACF provides a ratio of the two variance components, in the absence of individual differences in variance magnitude, where larger values indicate a greater proportion of timekeeper variance relative to implementation variance.

Results

Psychometric, Literacy and Attention Measures

Descriptive statistics obtained for the psychometric measures and reaction time task are provided in Table 1.

Motor Timing Measures

Stimulus modality in simple reaction time. A paired samples t-test showed that there was no significant difference in simple reaction time to auditory stimuli compared to visual stimuli ($t_{(20)} = 1.12$, n.s.).

Stimulus modality in synchronised finger tapping. Mixed-factors analyses of variance were conducted to assess motor timing performance across the within-subjects factors of mode (auditory, visual) and trial number (one, two and three). Trial number was included to assess the influence of practice effects that may arise in motor timing tasks [41].

Performance measures across the stimulus modes are shown in Figure 2. The effect of modality on mean IRI was marginally significant with slightly larger intervals produced in the auditory condition (mean 325 ms, S.E. 0.69) compared to the visual condition (mean 303 ms, S.E. 5.50; $F_{(1,12)} = 3.56$, $p = 0.08$, $\eta^2 = 0.23$). In addition, there was a mean effect of trial ($F_{(2,24)} = 3.69$, $p < 0.05$, $\eta^2 = 0.22$). Average IRIs were smaller in the third trial (mean 309 ms), compared to 317 ms and 315 ms in trials 1 and 2, but the means of these conditions were not significant in pairwise post hoc tests.

IRI variability did not significantly differ across the stimulus modalities and there was no effect of trial. Additional interaction effects were not statistically significant. For the mean differences from the absolute interval, the main effect of stimulus modality was significant ($F_{(1,12)} = 21.05$, $p < 0.01$, $\eta^2 = 0.64$), with greater asynchrony between IRI and ISI demonstrated under visual conditions (mean = 49 ms, S.E. 3.03) compared to that in auditory conditions

Table 1. Descriptive statistics for the group of 21 children.

Measure	Mean	SD
Age (months)	115.0	9.2
Verbal Reasoning (SS)	119.4	9.4
Non-verbal Reasoning (SS)	104.9	10.5
Reading (SS)	106.9	10.2
Spelling (SS)	104.9	12.3
ADHD-IA Rating	4.8	5.4
ADHD-HI Rating	2.9	4.1
Attentional Control % increase in time	32.4	18.5
Sustained Attention (SS)	96.9	15.5
Auditory Reaction Time (ms)	335.5	81.7
Visual Reaction Time (ms)	320.2	44.7

SS: standard score (mean = 100, SD = 15), ADHD-IA: Inattention subscale score, ADHD-HI: Hyperactivity-Impulsivity subscale score.

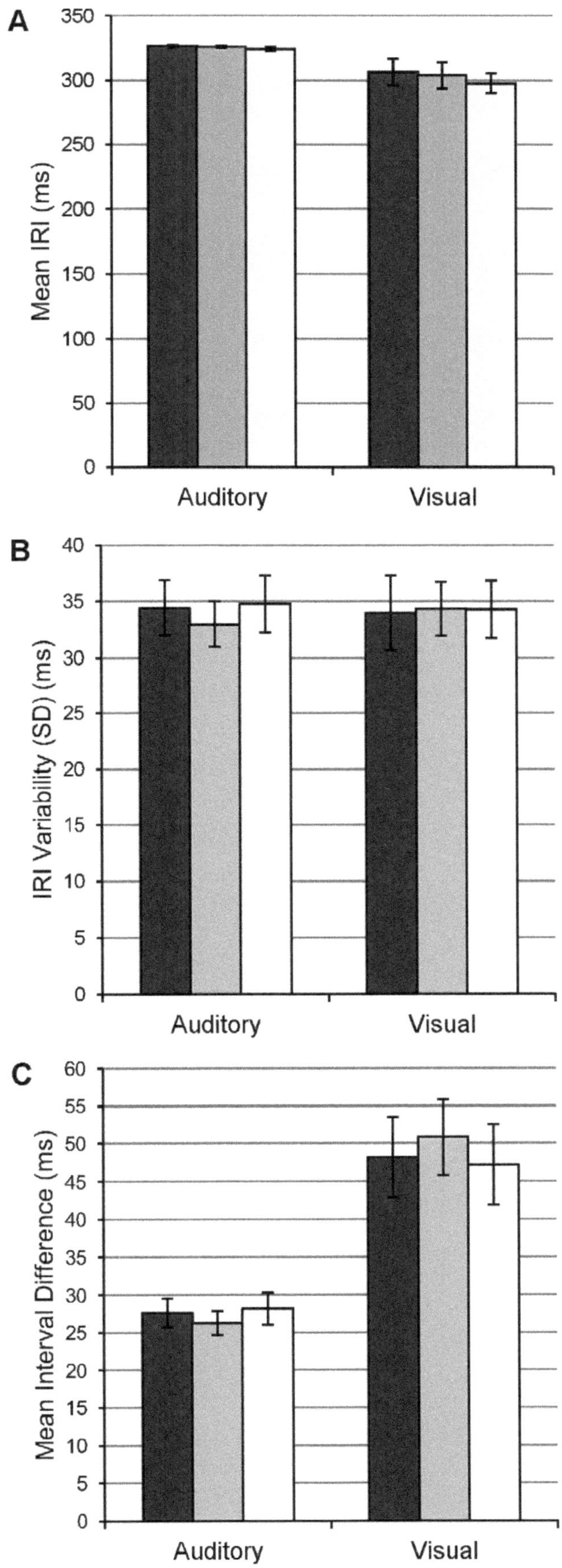

Figure 2. Effect of stimulus modality on finger tapping accuracy. Behavioural data across the three trials (bars: trial 1 - dark grey, trial 2 - light grey, trial 3 - mid grey)) within the two stimulus modalities. Data presented are (A) mean IRI, (B) IRI variability and (C) mean interval difference. Error bars show SEM.

(mean = 27 ms, S.E. 1.06). Trial number did not have a significant effect on the absolute interval difference nor were there any significant interaction effects.

Stimulus modality and decomposed timing variance. The variance in responses on the tapping tasks for each group and task modality was decomposed into timekeeper ($\hat{\sigma}_T^2$) and implementation ($\hat{\sigma}_P^2$) variance, as shown in Figure 3. Stimulus modality had a significant effect on timekeeper variance ($F_{(1,12)} = 5.33$, $p<0.05$, $\eta^2 = 0.31$) with larger estimates obtained when tapping to visual stimuli (mean 907 ms^2, S.E. 126.5) than to auditory stimuli (mean 611 ms^2, S.E. 83.3). The effect of modality on implementation variance was not significant ($F_{(1,12)} = 3.82$, $p = 0.07$, $\eta^2 = 0.22$), although the means (as illustrated in Figure 3) suggest that implementation variance was greater under auditory conditions (351 ms^2, S.E. 55.8) compared to visual conditions (172 ms^2, S.E. 26.7). A post hoc analysis collapsed across trials showed that this difference was significant statistically ($t_{(52)} = 3.02$, $p<0.01$). Neither timekeeper nor implementation variance was significantly affected by trial number nor were there significant interaction effects involving these variance components.

An assessment of the effect of modality on the ratio of timekeeper to implementation variance yielded a significant main effect ($F_{(1,12)} = 5.32$, $p<0.05$, $\eta^2 = 0.28$). ACF was significantly lower in the auditory condition (mean = −0.28, S.E. 0.02) compared to the visual condition (mean = −0.16, S.E. 0.03) indicating that timekeeper variance is lower relative to implementation variance under auditory stimulation. The effect of trial and additional interaction effects were not significant statistically.

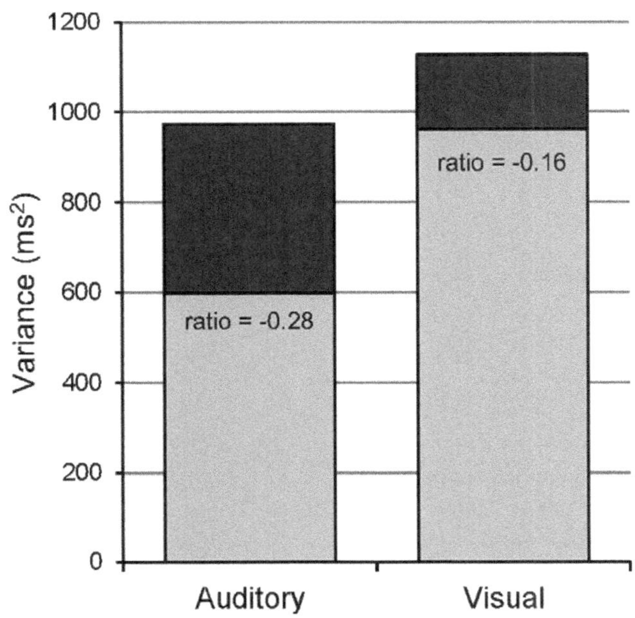

Figure 3. Effect of stimulus modality on decomposed performance variance. Cumulative mean estimates of variance. Timekeeper (light grey) and implementation variance (dark grey) are shown across the two stimulus conditions. Ratio values indicate the ACF which represents the relative amounts of variance from each source.

Relationships between Motor Timing and Cognitive/ Behavioural Measures

Predictive relationships between the timekeeper and implementation variance components and performance on psychometric measures of cognition and behaviour can help illuminate the relevance of timing deficits for developmental disorders such as dyslexia and ADHD on which measures of literacy and attention tap core symptoms. To evaluate these relationships, we calculated Pearson's product moment correlations, using component measures of motor skill and psychometric performance to reduce the risk of Type 1 error associated with the large number of multiple comparisons that would arise from conducting pair-wise correlations between all of the measures in our task set. Summary measures of timing performance were created by averaging each of the timing variables (timekeeper variance, implementation variance and ACF) across the three trials within each modality. These composite values were considered appropriate because none of the variance components were influenced by trial number. When appropriate, variables were transformed to adhere to normality assumptions. The effects of outliers were also evaluated to ensure the validity of the correlation coefficients obtained [54]. The results of these analyses are shown in Table 2.

Associations with auditory timing. Auditory implementation variance was positively correlated with performance on the measure of sustained attention, with poorer attention associated with decreased implementation variance.

Associations with visual timing. Reading scores correlated positively with timekeeper variance and negatively with implementation variance. Sustained attention performance in the children was negatively associated with visual implementation variance, and positively with the visual ACF ratio measure. Thus, poorer sustained attention was associated with increased implementation variance overall, as well as relative to timekeeper variance.

A series of multiple regressions were performed to evaluate the importance of different timing variables as predictors of the cognitive/behavioural measures of interest. In the first analysis, reading ability was entered as the dependent variable, with the independent variables visual timekeeper variance and visual implementation variance entered in a fixed order, two-step model. This showed that visual implementation variance was a significant predictor ($\beta = -0.53$, $t_{(19)} = -2.69$, $p<0.05$) and alone accounted for 24% of the variance in reading accuracy scores ($r^2 = 0.28$, $F_{(1,19)} = 7.23$, $p<0.05$). In contrast, timekeeper variance was not a significant predictor when entered alone at Step 1 ($\beta = 0.43$, $t_{(19)} = 2.08$, n.s.) or in the presence of implementation variance ($\beta = 0.20$, $t_{(18)} = 0.83$, n.s.). With both variables included at step 2, the equation remained significant but did not explain more variance in Reading performance beyond that contributed by implementation variance ($\Delta r^2 = 0.03$, $F_{(1,19)} = 3.9$, $p<0.05$).

A second regression analysis evaluated the proportion of variance in sustained attention predicted by visual ACF, auditory implementation variance and visual implementation variance. Because implementation variance contributes to the ACF, only visual ACF was entered into the regression. The two predictors were entered step-wise into the equation in order of their strength of association with the dependent variable. The ACF in the visual modality was a significant predictor of sustained attention ($\beta = 0.65$, $t_{(19)} = 3.76$, $p<0.01$), accounting for 40% unique variance in this variable($r^2 = 0.43$, $F_{(1,19)} = 14.16$, $p<0.01$). The model remained significant with the inclusion of auditory implementation variance as a predictor ($F_{(2,18)} = 10.78$, $p<0.01$) and accounted for a further 9% of the variance in sustained attention ($\Delta r^2 = 0.12$, $\beta = 0.36$, $t_{(18)} = 2.16$, $p<0.05$).

A final regression examined whether the dependent variable of visual implementation variance was more strongly related to reading performance or sustained attention, which were entered simultaneously as predictors. The model was significant ($r^2 = 0.43$, $F_{(2,18)} = 5.80$, $p<0.05$) accounting for over 30% of the variance in visual implementation variance. Only reading performance was a significant unique predictor ($\beta = -0.42$, $t_{(18)} = -2.17$, $p<0.05$), in contrast to sustained attention ($\beta = -0.36$, $t_{(18)} = -1.86$, n.s.). These analyses suggest that reading ability is closely associated with implementation variance, whereas sustained attention is related more to the relative proportions of implementation variance and timekeeper variance.

Table 2. Pearson's product moment correlations and partial correlations.

	1.	2.	3.	4.	5.	6.	7.	8.	9.	10.	11.	12.
1. Reading	–	0.82**	−0.20	−0.14	−0.06	0.30	−0.04	0.43	−0.04	−0.53**	0.32	0.39
2. Spelling	.66**	–	−0.32	−0.14	0.12	0.02	−0.03	0.32	−0.05	−0.34	0.34	0.27
3. ADHD-IA	−.32	−.46*	–	0.80**	−0.07	−0.03	−0.07	−0.07	0.15	−0.04	−0.15	−0.03
4. ADHD-HI	−.38	−.38	.83**	–	0.23	0.08	−0.05	0.20	0.33	−0.09	−0.14	0.18
5. Attention Control	−.27	−.02	−.08	.18	–	−0.40	0.20	0.39	0.08	0.04	0.04	0.12
6. Sustained Attention	.28	−.10	−.03	.08	−.44	–	−0.05	0.29	0.50*	−0.48*	−0.21	0.65**
7. Auditory TK variance	−.09	−.08	−.07	−.10	.18	−.04	–	0.21	0.05	0.10	0.62**	0.08
8. Visual TK variance	.22	.05	−.09	.10	.33	.28	.18	–	0.09	−0.56**	0.20	0.74**
9. Auditory IMP variance	−.10	−.13	.16	.28	.04	.56*	−.01	.02	–	−0.14	−0.55**	0.25
10. Visual IMP variance	−.49*	−.24	−.03	−.07	.09	−.46*	.11	−.55*	−.17	–	0.03	−0.79**
11. Auditory ACF ratio	.16	.20	−.18	−.19	−.01	−.28	.66**	.10	−.59**	.13	–	0.04
12. Visual ACF ratio	.20	.05	−.05	.16	.06	.65**	.09	.75**	.32	−.77**	−.10	–

*$p<0.05$;
**$p<0.01$.
Pearson's product moment correlations (top right) between psychometric variables of interest and motor timing performance, with partial correlations controlling for verbal and non-verbal reasoning (bottom left). TK = Timekeeper, IMP = Implementation, ACF = Autocorrelation function.

Discussion

Motor timing tasks provide clinically useful measures of temporal processing, which may help understand the mechanisms involved in developmental disorders such as ADHD and dyslexia for which deficits in implicit and explicit timing functions are a common feature [2,5,35,36]. The increased recognition that risk factors for developmental disorders are expressed continuously in the population [8] underpins the need to establish the extent of overlap between disorder phenotypes on dimensions such as temporal processing. Previous studies of motor timing have presented stimuli via different stimulus modalities, however, with interval timing in ADHD assessed primarily using visual pacing stimuli and in developmental dyslexia with auditory stimuli. Here we provided a comprehensive assessment of such stimulus modality effects on paced motor timing performance in children, within the context of relationships with measures of literacy and attention variables. The addition of a variance decomposition method enabled us to evaluate sources of variability in finger tapping performance in children and to assess the contribution of these different underlying mechanisms to literacy ability and attention skills. The Wing and Kristofferson model [31] enabled separation of components that reflect the variability of both the ongoing timekeeping and the motor implementation of timing signals.

Modality Dependent Effects

The data confirmed our hypothesis that finger tapping performance is strongly modulated by the modality of the pacing stimuli. Average IRIs in the auditory condition corresponded more closely with the target interval, compared to the visual condition where the intervals produced were significantly shorter and more asynchronous (Figure 2). In visual conditions, synchronisation of outputs with stimuli may be more difficult due to the lack of accurate temporal information available to a timekeeping mechanism [55], resulting in poorer precision of the clocking output for implementation [41]. Previous research has suggested that under such conditions participants may select and implement a response strategy irrespective of available information, for example asynchronies between stimuli and responses or feedback from internal timekeeping mechanisms [41,42]. This response strategy hypothesis is supported by converging evidence from behavioural and brain imaging experiments. Errors in timing performance are typically neither noticed nor corrected under visually paced conditions, yet such errors are corrected sufficiently when performance is paced with auditory stimuli [41,56]. Furthermore, neural areas engaged in updating of motor responses and recalibrating sensory-motor coupling are particularly active in auditory timing tasks but less so when timing is visually paced [42,57].

Adopting stereotyped motor responses [41] would be expected to reduce implementation variance relative to timekeeper variance. Consistent with this explanation, we found that typically developing children had reduced implementation variance and increased timekeeper variance when pacing stimuli were presented visually. This pattern of result poses questions for the validity of using visually paced timing tasks alone in motor timing studies; the premise that timed motor outputs are always generated in concert with external pacing stimuli cannot be assumed. In sum, visually paced tasks may fail to adequately assess the internal timekeeping capacities that are of most interest when focusing on temporal processing and the putative difficulties thereof in relevant clinical populations.

In contrast to the results obtained with visual stimulation, participant responses in auditory conditions were characterised by lower estimates of timekeeper variance, coupled with higher estimates of implementation variance. This confirms that children, like adults [38,40,41], have relatively invariant output from timekeeper mechanisms when synchronising motor responses with auditory stimuli. This result reinforces evidence for the increased temporal precision of the auditory system compared to the visual system [38,40] and highlights the important effects of task parameters in research of this kind. Studies employing visual, or bimodal auditory-visual stimuli [3,16,27] may underestimate the true capacities of central timing processes. Therefore, when considering questions of temporal processing in developmental populations, our results suggest that more confidence can be placed in results from auditory stimulated motor timing tasks than for similar visual paradigms [1,14,18,24,28].

Relationships between Timing and Cognitive Variables

Timing tasks may explain unique variance in the underlying neuro-cognitive mechanisms of impairment in developmental disorders [2,17,18]. We therefore assessed the relationships between interval timing variables and the reading and attention variables that tap core behavioural symptoms upon which developmental dyslexia and ADHD are diagnosed. These two disorder phenotypes have been repeatedly studied with measures of interval timing, with visual tasks often used in investigations of ADHD [3,16,27,58] and auditory tasks most frequent in studies of dyslexia [14,23,59].

The statistical associations between timing performance and indices of cognition and behaviour provide further support for the importance of the differences between timing assessed with visual and auditory pacing stimuli. Both sustained attention and reading ability were statistically associated with the relative contribution of implementation variance in finger tapping performance, and particularly for data derived from the visually paced task. Participants with low scores on these cognitive dimensions had relatively larger estimates of implementation variance on the visually paced task. Under visually paced conditions, timing mechanisms may lack precision, effects that are hypothesised to result from a combination of the inefficiency of the visual control mechanisms for generating internal rhythms [42,60] and the poorer functional coupling of these mechanisms with the motor system [42,57]. A stereotyped, motor-focused strategy has been suggested to be the most efficient approach to such tasks [41,42] and would be predicted to result in reduced implementation variance. Our data suggest however, that children with lower scores on reading and attention measures do not consistently implement such a strategy on a visually paced task. Alternatively, it appears as if these children do not adequately account for imperfect timing signals. The specific demands of the visual timing task may elicit reallocation of cognitive resources to facilitate task completion [61], resulting in correlations between timing performance and reading and sustained attention variables similar to those that might be predicted for a measure of processing speed [62].

As applied in this study, the introduction of time series analysis to data obtained from motor timing tasks has helped to illuminate the potential links between individual variability in timing performance and in the cognitive dimensions that underlie highly prevalent developmental disorders. The Wing & Kristofferson model [31] has been applied previously to data obtained from other clinical populations with varying results [63–65], demonstrating the limitations of this approach for the analysis of data with very large IRIs, linear trends or negative variance estimates.

Such parameters would not be unexpected in data derived from clinical groups, compared to that obtained from highly practiced individuals. The proportion of trials where the resulting data did not satisfy the assumptions of the model was comparatively modest in our sample compared to that reported in clinical groups [61,62]. However, this proportion would be expected to increase in studies of children with developmental disorders. Rather than posing intractable problems for interpretation, however, such atypical data sets may provide additional information (for e.g., individual trends within time series [65–67]) useful for understanding the nature and extent of timing deficits in clinical or developmental populations [64,68].

Conclusions

Previous investigations of motor timing have reported associations between auditory paced timing tasks and measures of literacy, even in control populations [1,24]. Our results do not provide strong evidence for this association. In contrast, they highlight the variable nature in the way auditory and visual tasks are processed behaviourally, as well as differences in the way that performance on temporal processing tasks correlates with cognitive constructs associated with highly prevalent disability phenotypes. They also highlight the methodological importance of assessing the construct of attention in temporal processing tasks [18,61], particularly in clinical populations where attention difficulties often co-occur with the primary diagnostic symptoms [6,7]. While the use of visual timing tasks may ultimately be useful for demonstrating the quality of processing difficulties experienced by children with attention deficits or reading difficulties, such measures may not adequately assess the timekeeping capability of central neural mechanisms. Our evidence suggests that central timekeeping mechanism(s) may be more accurately assessed with auditory paced tasks.

Author Contributions

Conceived and designed the experiments: EEB JBT. Performed the experiments: EEB. Analyzed the data: EEB. Contributed reagents/materials/analysis tools: EEB JBT. Wrote the paper: EEB JBT.

References

1. Thomson JM, Goswami U (2008) Rhythmic processing in children with developmental dyslexia: Auditory and motor rhythms link to reading and spelling. Journal of Physiology - Paris 102: 120–129. doi:10.1016/j.jphysparis.2008.03.007.
2. Rubia K, Halari R, Christakou A, Taylor E (2009) Impulsiveness as a timing disturbance: neurocognitive abnormalities in attention-deficit hyperactivity disorder during temporal processes and normalization with methylphenidate. Philosophical Transactions of the Royal Society B 364: 1919–1931. doi:10.1098/rstb.2009.0014.
3. Rubia K, Noorloos J, Smith A, Gunning B, Sergeant J (2003) Motor timing deficits in community and clinical boys with hyperactive behavior: The effect of methylphenidate on motor timing. Journal of Abnormal Child Psychology 31: 301–313.
4. Hulslander J, Talcott J, Witton C, Defries J, Pennington BF, et al. (2004) Sensory processing, reading, IQ, and attention. Journal of Experimental Child Psychology 88: 274–295. doi:10.1016/j.jecp.2004.03.006.
5. Farmer ME, Klein RM (1995) The evidence for a temporal processing deficit linked to dyslexia: A review. Psychonomic Bulletin & Review 2: 460–493.
6. Willcutt EG, Pennington BF (2000) Comorbidity of reading disability and attention-deficit/hyperactivity disorder: Differences by gender and subtype. Journal of Learning Disabilities 33: 179–191. doi:10.1177/002221940003300206.
7. Pauc R (2005) Comorbidity of dyslexia, dyspraxia, attention deficit disorder (ADD), attention deficit hyperactive disorder (ADHD), obsessive compulsive disorder (OCD) and Tourette's syndrome in children: A prospective epidemiological study. Clinical Chiropractic 8: 189–198. doi:10.1016/j.clch.2005.09.007.
8. Pennington BF (2006) From single to multiple deficit models of developmental disorders. Cognition 101: 385–413. doi:10.1016/j.cognition.2006.04.008.
9. Plomin R, Kovas Y (2005) Generalist genes and learning disabilities. Psychological Bulletin 131: 592–617. doi:10.1037/0033-2909.131.4.592.
10. Cramer AOJ, Waldorp LJ, van der Maas HLJ, Borsboom D (2010) Comorbidity: A network perspective. Behavioral and Brain Sciences 33: 137–193. doi:10.1017/S0140525X09991567.
11. Klein RM (2002) Observations on the temporal correlates of reading failure. Reading and Writing: An Interdisciplinary Journal 15: 207–232.
12. Share DL, Jorm AF, Maclean ROD, Matthews R (2002) Temporal processing and reading disability. Perception: 151–178.
13. Tallal P, Miller S, Fitch R (1993) Neurobiological basis of speech: A case for the preeminence of temporal processing. Annals of the New York Academy of Sciences 682: 27–47.
14. Wolff PH, Michel GF, Ovrut M, Drake C (1990) Rate and timing precision of motor coordination in developmental dyslexia. Developmental Psychology 26: 349–359.
15. Witton C, Talcott J, Hansen P, Richardson A, Griffiths T, et al. (1998) Sensitivity to dynamic auditory and visual stimuli predicts nonword reading ability in both dyslexic and normal readers. Current Biology 8: 791–797.
16. Ben-Pazi H, Gross-Tsur V, Bergman H, Shalev RS (2003) Abnormal rhythmic motor response in children with attention-deficit-hyperactivity disorder. Developmental Medicine and Child Neurology 45: 743–745.
17. Wolff PH (2002) Timing precision and rhythm in developmental dyslexia. Reading and Writing: An Interdisciplinary Journal 15: 179–206.
18. Zelaznik HN, Vaughn AJ, Green JT, Smith AL, Hoza B, et al. (2012) Motor timing deficits in children with Attention-Deficit/Hyperactivity disorder. Human Movement Science 31: 255–265. doi:10.1016/j.humov.2011.05.003.
19. Ivry RB, Keele SW (1989) Timing functions of the cerebellum. Journal of Cognitive Neuroscience 1: 136–152.
20. Kooistra L, Snijders TAB, Schellekens JMH, Kalverboer AF, Geuze RH (1997) Timing variability in children with early-treated congenital hypothyroidism. Acta Psychologica 96: 61–73.
21. Madison G (2011) Intelligence and temporal accuracy of behaviour: unique and shared associations with reaction time and motor timing. Nature Reviews Neuroscience: 175–183. doi:10.1007/s00221-011-2817-6.
22. Thomson JM, Fryer B, Maltby J (2006) Auditory and motor rhythm awareness in adults with dyslexia. Literacy 29: 334–348. doi:10.1111/j.1467-9817.2006.00312.x.
23. Thomson JM, Fryer B, Maltby J, Goswami U (2006) Auditory and motor rhythm awareness in adults with dyslexia. Journal of Research in Reading 29: 334–348. doi:10.1111/j.1467-9817.2006.00312.x.
24. Waber DP, Weiler MD, Bellinger DC, Marcus DJ, Forbes PW, et al. (2000) Diminished motor timing control in children referred for diagnosis of learning problems. Developmental Neuropsychology 17: 181–197. doi:10.1207/S15326942DN1702.
25. Ben-Pazi H, Shalev RS, Gross-Tsur V, Bergman H (2006) Age and medication effects on rhythmic responses in ADHD: possible oscillatory mechanisms? Neuropsychologia 44: 412–416. doi:10.1016/j.neuropsychologia.2005.05.022.
26. Rubia K, Taylor E, Smith AB, Oksannen H, Overmeyer S, et al. (2001) Neuropsychological analyses of impulsiveness in childhood hyperactivity. British Journal of Psychiatry 179: 138–143.
27. Toplak ME, Tannock R (2005) Tapping and anticipation performance in attention deficit hyperactivity disorder. Perceptual and Motor Skills 100: 659–675.
28. Pitcher TM, Piek JP, Barrett NC (2002) Timing and force control in boys with attention deficit hyperactivity disorder: Subtype differences and the effect of comorbid developmental coordination disorder. Human Movement Science 21: 919–945. doi:10.1016/S0167-9457(02)00167-7.
29. Wing AM, Kristofferson AB (1973) The timing of interresponse intervals. Perception & Psychophysics 13: 455–460.
30. Vorberg D, Wing AM (1996) Modelling variability and dependence in timing. In: Heuer H, Keele SW, editors. Handbook of perception and action: Vol. 3. Motor skills. London: Academic Press. 181–261.
31. Wing AM, Kristofferson AB (1973) Response delays and the timing of discrete motor responses. Perception & Psychophysics 14: 5–12.
32. O'Boyle DJ, Freeman JS, Cody FWJ (1996) The accuracy and precision of timing of self-paced, repetitive movements in subjects with Parkinson's disease. Brain 119: 51–70.
33. Freeman JS, Cody FWJ, O'Boyle DJ, Craufurd D, Neary D, et al. (1996) Abnormalities of motor timing in Huntington' s disease. Parkinsonism & Related Disorders 2: 81–93.
34. Harrington DL, Haaland KY, Hermanowicz N (1998) Temporal processing in the basal ganglia. Neuropsychology 12: 3–12.
35. Toplak ME, Dockstader C, Tannock R (2006) Temporal information processing in ADHD: Findings to date and new methods. Journal of Neuroscience Methods 151: 15–29. doi:10.1016/j.jneumeth.2005.09.018.
36. Goswami U (2011) A temporal sampling framework for developmental dyslexia. Trends in Cognitive Sciences 15: 3–10. doi:10.1016/j.tics.2010.10.001.
37. Overy K, Nicolson RI, Fawcett AJ, Clarke EF (2003) Dyslexia and music: Measuring musical timing skills. Dyslexia 9: 18–36. doi:10.1002/dys.233.

38. Fendrich R, Corballis PM (2001) The temporal cross-capture of audition and vision. Perception & Psychophysics 63: 719–725.
39. Patel AD, Iversen JR, Chen Y, Repp BH (2005) The influence of metricality and modality on synchronization with a beat. Experimental Brain Research 163: 226–238. doi:10.1007/s00221-004-2159-8.
40. McAuley JD, Henry MJ (2010) Modality effects in rhythm processing: Auditory encoding of visual rhythms is neither obligatory nor automatic. Attention, Perception, & Psychophysics 72: 1377–1389. doi:10.3758/APP.
41. Kolers PA, Brewster JM (1985) Rhythms and responses. Journal of Experimental Psychology: Human Perception and Performance 11: 150–167.
42. Jancke L, Loose R, Lutz K, Specht K, Shah NJ (2000) Cortical activations during paced finger-tapping applying visual and auditory pacing stimuli. Cognitive Brain Research 10: 51–66.
43. Elliott MT, Wing AM, Welchman AE (2010) Multisensory cues improve sensorimotor synchronisation. European Journal of Neuroscience 31: 1828–1835. doi:10.1111/j.1460-9568.2010.07205.x.
44. Loras H, Sigmundsson H, Talcott J, Ohberg F, Stensdotter A (2012) Timing continuous or discontinuous movements across effectors specified by different pacing modalities and intervals. Experimental Brain Research 220: 335–447. doi:10.1007/s00221-012-3142-4.
45. Wechsler D (1999) Wechsler abbreviated scale of intelligence. San Antonio: Psychological Corporation.
46. Wechsler D (2005) Wechsler individual achievement test Second UK Edition. London: Harcourt Assessment.
47. Barkley RA, Murphy KR (1998) Attention-deficit hyperactivity disorder: A Clinical Workbook. New York: Guilford Press.
48. American Psychiatric Association (2000) Diagnostic and statistical manual of mental disorders. 4th ed. Washington DC: American Psychiatric Association.
49. Manly T, Robertson IH, Anderson V, Nimmo-Smith I (1999) The test of everyday attention for children (TEA-CH). Bury St Edmunds: Thames Valley Test Company. p.
50. Schneider W, Eschman A, Zuccolotto A (2002) E-Prime. Pittsburgh,PA: Psychology Software Tools Inc.
51. Bridgeman B (1998) Durations of stimuli displayed on video display terminals: (n - 1)/f + persistence. Psychological Science 9: 232–233. doi:10.1111/1467-9280.00045.
52. Elze T (2010) Misspecifications of stimulus presentation durations in experimental psychology: A systematic review of the psychophysics literature. PLoS ONE 5: e12792. doi:10.1371/journal.pone.0012792.
53. Collier GL, Ogden RT (2004) Adding drift to the decomposition of simple isochronous tapping: An extension of the Wing – Kristofferson model. Journal of Experimental Psychology: Human Perception and Performance 30: 853–872. doi:10.1037/0096-1523.30.5.853.
54. Tabachnick B, Fidell L (2001) Using multivariate statistics. 4th ed. Boston: Allyn and Bacon.
55. Repp BH, Penel A (2002) Auditory dominance in temporal processing: New evidence from synchronization with simultaneous visual and auditory sequences. Perception 28: 1085–1099. doi:10.1037//0096-1523.28.5.1085.
56. Kato M, Konishi Y (2006) Auditory dominance in the error correction process: A synchronized tapping study. Brain Research 1084: 115–122. doi:10.1016/j.brainres.2006.02.019.
57. Jantzen K, Steinberg F, Kelso J (2005) Functional MRI reveals the existence of modality and coordination-dependent timing networks. NeuroImage 25: 1031–1042. doi:10.1016/j.neuroimage.2004.12.029.
58. Rubia K, Overmeyer S, Taylor E, Brammer M, Williams SCR, et al. (1999) Hypofrontality in attention deficit hyperactivity disorder during higher-order motor control: A study with functional MRI. American Journal of Psychiatry 156: 891–896.
59. Wolff PH, Cohen C, Drake C (1984) Impaired motor timing control in specific reading retardation. Neuropsychologia 22: 587–600.
60. Grahn J a (2012) See what I hear? Beat perception in auditory and visual rhythms. Experimental Brain Research 220: 51–61. doi:10.1007/s00221-012-3114-8.
61. Heron J, Roach NW, Whitaker D, Hanson JVM (2010) Attention regulates the plasticity of multisensory timing. European Journal of Neuroscience 31: 1755–1762. doi:10.1111/j.1460-9568.2010.07194.x.
62. McGrath LM, Pennington BF, Shanahan M a, Santerre-Lemmon LE, Barnard HD, et al. (2011) A multiple deficit model of reading disability and attention-deficit/hyperactivity disorder: searching for shared cognitive deficits. Journal of Child Psychology and Psychiatry 52: 547–557. doi:10.1111/j.1469-7610.2010.02346.x.
63. O'Boyle DJ, Freeman JS, Cody FWJ (1996) The accuracy and precision of timing of self-paced, repetitive movements in subjects with Parkinson's disease. Brain 119: 51–70. doi:10.1093/brain/119.1.51.
64. Pastor M, Jahanshahi M, Artieda J, Obeso J (1992) Performance of repetitive wrist movements in Parkinson's disease. Brain 115: 875–891.
65. Duchek JM, Balota DA, Ferraro FR (1994) Component analysis of a rhythmic finger tapping task in individuals with senile dementia of the Alzheimer type and in individuals with Parkinson's disease. Neuropsychology 8: 218–226.
66. Madison G, Forsman L, Blom Ö, Karabanov A, Ullén F (2009) Correlations between intelligence and components of serial timing variability. Intelligence 37: 68–75. doi:10.1016/j.intell.2008.07.006.
67. Forsman LJ, Madison G, Ullén F (2009) Neuroticism is correlated with drift in serial time interval production. Personality and Individual Differences 47: 229–232. doi:10.1016/j.paid.2009.02.020.
68. Madison G (2001) Variability in isochronous tapping: Higher order dependencies as a function of intertap interval. Journal of Experimental Psychology: Human Perception and Performance 27: 411–422. doi:10.1037//0096-1523.27.2.411.

Reading Performance Is Enhanced by Visual Texture Discrimination Training in Chinese-Speaking Children with Developmental Dyslexia

Xiangzhi Meng[1,5], Ou Lin[1], Fang Wang[2,4], Yuzheng Jiang[3], Yan Song[2,4]*

1 Department of Psychology, Peking University, Beijing, China, 2 State Key Laboratory of Cognitive Neuroscience and Learning & IDG/McGovern Institute for Brain Research, Beijing Normal University, Beijing, China, 3 School of languages and communication, Beijing Jiaotong University, Beijing, China, 4 Center for Collaboration and Innovation in Brain and Learning Sciences, Beijing Normal University, Beijing, China, 5 The Joint PekingU-PolyU Center for Child Development and Learning, Peking University, Beijing, China

Abstract

Background: High order cognitive processing and learning, such as reading, interact with lower-level sensory processing and learning. Previous studies have reported that visual perceptual training enlarges visual span and, consequently, improves reading speed in young and old people with amblyopia. Recently, a visual perceptual training study in Chinese-speaking children with dyslexia found that the visual texture discrimination thresholds of these children in visual perceptual training significantly correlated with their performance in Chinese character recognition, suggesting that deficits in visual perceptual processing/learning might partly underpin the difficulty in reading Chinese.

Methodology/Principal Findings: To further clarify whether visual perceptual training improves the measures of reading performance, eighteen children with dyslexia and eighteen typically developed readers that were age- and IQ-matched completed a series of reading measures before and after visual texture discrimination task (TDT) training. Prior to the TDT training, each group of children was split into two equivalent training and non-training groups in terms of all reading measures, IQ, and TDT. The results revealed that the discrimination threshold SOAs of TDT were significantly higher for the children with dyslexia than for the control children before training. Interestingly, training significantly decreased the discrimination threshold SOAs of TDT for both the typically developed readers and the children with dyslexia. More importantly, the training group with dyslexia exhibited significant enhancement in reading fluency, while the non-training group with dyslexia did not show this improvement. Additional follow-up tests showed that the improvement in reading fluency is a long-lasting effect and could be maintained for up to two months in the training group with dyslexia.

Conclusion/Significance: These results suggest that basic visual perceptual processing/learning and reading ability in Chinese might at least partially rely on overlapping mechanisms.

Editor: Hengyi Rao, University of Pennsylvania, United States of America

Funding: This study was supported by a grant from the Natural Science Foundation of China (81371206) to XM, National Key Basic Research Program of China (2014CB846103) to YS, and NSFC (81171016, 31271203) to XZ and YS. The funders had no role in study design, data collection and analysis, decision to publish, or preparation of the manuscript.

Competing Interests: The authors have declared that no competing interests exist.

* Email: songyan@bnu.edu.cn

Introduction

Developmental dyslexia is a disorder characterized by difficulty in learning to read without lack of motivation, educational opportunities or intellectual insufficiency [1]. The root cause of dyslexia remains controversial. In past decades, two major frameworks were established to explain the origin, mechanisms and symptoms of developmental dyslexia. The first framework, from a linguistic point of view, hypothesizes a core deficit in accessing and/or manipulating phonemic information in children and adults with developmental dyslexia [2], [3]. The second, from a nonlinguistic perspective, posits that the phonological deficit occurring on the linguistic level may stem from more fundamental deficits in information processing within the sensory domain, such as acoustic-auditory information processing, auditory temporal processing [4–7], and/or visual processing [8], [9].

Accordingly, the remediation of dyslexia has also followed these two lines: the linguistic/phonological and the nonlinguistic orientated treatments. Aside from a large number of studies showing the remedial effect of linguistic programs, mostly targeted at improving phonological skills [10–12] and reading skills in developmental dyslexia, an increasing number of studies have reported that nonlinguistic intervention programs also substantially improve reading performance in individuals with dyslexia. These nonlinguistic training methods include auditory temporal training/musical training [5], [13–16], visual programs aimed at improving the function of the magnocellular system [17] or alleviating the crowding phenomenon by increasing letter spacing [18], and action video games that significantly improve reading speed in individuals with dyslexia by efficiently improving attention abilities [19]. The effects of these nonlinguistic intervention protocols suggest that training the perceptual and cognitive skills underpinning poor phonological development and/or poor reading would be beneficial to reading and phonological development [15].

Indeed, studies directly involving visual perceptual learning did reveal a positive effect on reading speed. Perceptual learning is evidenced by an improvement of perceptual performance as a function of training [20], which has been shown to enlarge visual span size and produce corresponding improvement in reading speed in young children [21] and older adults [22]. The texture discrimination task (TDT) is one of the most intensively studied PL tasks. In this task, a texture stimulus is first presented for a short time, followed by a blank interval (stimulus-to-mask onset asynchrony, SOA), and then by the mask. The subjects need to decide whether the fixation letter was "T" or "L", and then indicate the texture target orientation (horizontal or vertical). Behavioral performance on both tasks was measured as the proportion of correct responses for different SOAs. Our recent behavioral study reported that Chinese-speaking children with dyslexia exhibited visual perceptual learning deficits [23]. In this study, when all of the participants were asked to perform the classical TDT with the SOA at 300 ms, the SOA for reaching 80% accuracy did not show improvement over 5 days of training in the children with dyslexia while this SOA steadily decreased over the training sessions in the control group. When an adaptive procedure was used to determine the SOA for each participant during training, both the children with dyslexia and the control group attained perceptual learning; more importantly, over individual participants, the SOA was negatively correlated with their performance in Chinese character recognition. These findings suggest that deficits in visual perceptual processing and learning might, in part, underpin the reading difficulty in Chinese.

In the current study, we further examined whether visual perceptual learning has a positive effect in improving the performance of reading. Before and after 10 sessions of TDT training, a series of reading measures were performed in two groups of children (dyslexia children and typically developed control children). This study can provide a more detailed picture of the relationship between visual perceptual learning and developmental dyslexia. Of particular empirical importance, if visual perceptual training can benefit the development of reading skills in children with dyslexia, this finding will have significant implications for the prevention and diagnosis and the design of educational curricula for developmental dyslexia.

Materials and Methods

Ethics Statement

All experimental procedures were approved by the Ethics Committee of the Department of Psychology, Peking University. The research was conducted according to the principles expressed in the Declaration of Helsinki. Written consent was obtained from all of the children as well as their parents. All experiments were performed at the joint PekingU-PolyU center for Child Development and Learning of Peking University.

Participants

Thirty-six Chinese-speaking children, eighteen with dyslexia, eighteen with typical readers, in grades four, five, and six, were recruited to participate in this study according to the procedures described below. None of the participants had a history of neurological diseases or psychiatric disorders. In particular, the DSM-IV Attention-Deficit/Hyperactivity Disorder (ADHD) Scale [24] was used to exclude children with ADHD. All of the participants were right-handed and had normal or corrected-to-normal vision. Informed consent was obtained from each participant and their parents.

The children were placed in the dyslexia group if their scores on the character recognition test were at least 1.5 grades below the norm (below), and if their reading fluency test scores were lower than the mean scores for their grades (below). Additionally, they had typically developed IQ scores, as assessed by *Raven's Standard Progressive Matrices* [25]. The chronological age- and IQ -matched control children were selected from among their peers (Table 1). Similar procedures for recruiting children with dyslexia or with reading impairment were implemented by previous studies [26].

Prior to the TDT training, each group of children was split into two equivalent training and non-training groups on the performance of all of the reading measures, IQ, and TDT (Table 2).

Linguistic tests

Two reading measures, character recognition accuracy and reading fluency, were utilized to assess the participants' reading abilities, and to investigate the relationship between visual perceptual processing/learning and the accuracy and fluency of reading skills. The reason for using two reading measures was that a review of the literature revealed that both accuracy and fluency are important for reading development and that both are impaired in children with dyslexia [27], [28]. Additionally, only a few studies have directly addressed the association between reading measures and visual perceptual processing/learning [21–23]. Therefore, we also used two reading measures to classify which specific reading skills (recognition accuracy or the speed) are associated with the visual perceptual processing/learning ability and which are enhanced by visual perceptual training. This study will probably permit us to infer what psychological processes are involved in visual perceptual learning.

The Standardized Chinese Character Recognition Test [29] consists of 210 characters, and is divided into ten groups based on the reading-difficulty level. The participants were asked to write down a compound word based on a constituent morpheme provided on the sheet. Their performance was measured by the total number of correct characters (morphemes) that they could utilize in word compositions. The participants had to know morpheme combination rules to form a compound word. The scores from this test formed the index of the participants' Chinese character recognition performance.

In this standardized Chinese character recognition test [29], the medium difficulty characters with a high degree of differentiation were stratified, sampling from the character corpus of primary school textbooks for each grade. Then, 5102 children from grades 1–5 were tested with the tests for their own grades. The mean and standard deviation of the performance of character recognition were calculated for each grade. The standard Z scores for each grade were then obtained with $(X_{raw\ score} - Mean_{certain\ grade})/$ standard $deviation_{certain\ grade}$ as the norm. The total number of correct characters each participant completed corresponds to a specific reading grade through the norm. For example, if a child was in fifth grade when tested and the total number of characters

Table 1. Characteristics of the participants, with standard deviation in parenthesis.

	Group with dyslexia	Control group	t	P
N	18	18		
Gender/Boys	15	11		
Age (years)	10.34 (0.78)	10.41 (0.74)	0.294	NS
Raven (Percentile)	69 (17.17)	75 (18.11)	1.039	NS
Reading fluency (Mean)	28.06 (5.87)	49.56 (9.01)	8.479	<.001
Vocabulary (Mean)	2446.8 (254.57)	3054.1 (182.61)	8.224	<.001

For age, the numbers are mean years for the dyslexia and control groups. For the Raven, the numbers are mean percentiles for the dyslexia and control groups. For reading fluency, the numbers represent means of items that the dyslexia and control groups answered correctly. For Chinese character recognition, the numbers are the numbers of characters children could use correctly in word composition.

completed correctly corresponded to third grade on the norm, he/she would be identified as a participant with dyslexia.

The Reading Fluency Test was composed of 95 sentences [30]. Each sentence was paired with five multiple-choice pictures. The participants were asked to read each sentence and select, from five pictures, the one that best illustrated the meaning of the sentence. For instance, for the sentence "She is playing with a ball in front of the house", if a participant circles the picture of a girl playing a ball in front of a house, the answer is correct. If the participant circles pictures in which three or two children are playing ball in the yard or in the house, the answers are incorrect. The children were encouraged to complete as many paragraphs as possible within a ten-minute time period. The total number of sentences that the participants could understand determined the performance score. This task required the rapid retrieval and retention of lexical information and construction of sentential representation. All of the sentences in this test are composed of high frequency characters and words; therefore, it is very easy for participants to grasp the meaning of each sentence. We used this test to evaluate children's reading speed by the total number of sentences they can accomplish. Because participants in this study were recruited from grades four, five, and six, each participant's reading fluency score was compared to the mean score of the grade he/she belonged to. The mean score was calculated from the total number of correct answers the grade children completed, divided by the total number of children participating from that grade.

Additionally, *Raven's Standard Progressive Matrices* were used to measure the children's nonverbal Intelligence Quotient (IQ). The scoring procedures were based on the Chinese norm [25].

Visual perceptual learning test and training

Stimuli. A texture discrimination task (TDT) was employed that has been used in a number of visual perceptual learning studies [31–33]. The stimuli, white (54 cd/m^2) on a uniform black background, were displayed on a 21-inch gamma linearized CRT monitor (1024×768 pixels at 85 Hz) at a 110 cm viewing distance. All of the stimuli were generated by a MATLAB program. All of the experiments were performed using E-prime (1.0) software.

The visual stimulus was a texture display made of 19×19 high-contrast horizontal line segments positioned in the central visual field, covering an area of a 14°×14° visual angle (Figure 1). The lines were .46°×.04° in size and spaced .76° apart. The position of each line segment was jittered randomly by 0°~.1°. A randomly rotated letter "T" or "L" was presented at the bottom of the texture stimulus for subjects to fixate. A target was generated by tilting three adjacent bars in the texture stimuli from horizontal to 135°, forming either a horizontal (Figure 1) or a vertical configuration. The target array was embedded either in the upper left or upper right quadrant of the visual field at a location of 2.5°~5° away from the fixation. A mask of the same size as the stimulus was made of 19×19 randomly oriented V-shaped patterns except at the fixation, where a superimposed "T" and

Table 2. Characteristics of training and non-training groups of participants, with standard deviation in parenthesis.

	Group with Dyslexia			Control group		
	Training group	Non-training group	p	Training group	Non-training group	p
N	9	9	n.s.	9	9	n.s.
Age (years)	10.5 (0.7)	10.2 (0.9)	n.s.	10.4 (0.8)	10.4 (0.7)	n.s.
Raven (Percentile)	68.9 (15.6)	69.4 (19.6)	n.s.	75 (20.3)	75.6 (16.8)	n.s.
TDT threshold SOAs of Pre-test (ms)	555 (297)	615 (289)	n.s.	377 (197)	451 (215)	n.s.
Reading fluency	26.3 (4.2)	29.8 (6.9)	n.s.	51.4 (10.5)	47.6 (7.4)	n.s.
Vocabulary	2454.7 (306)	2438.8 (209)	n.s.	3065.4 (135)	3042.7 (228)	n.s.

For age, the numbers are mean years for training and non-training groups with dyslexia and control. For the Raven, the numbers are mean percentiles for each group of participants. For reading fluency, the numbers represent means of items that each group of participants answered correctly. For Chinese character recognition, the numbers are the numbers of characters children could use correctly in word composition.

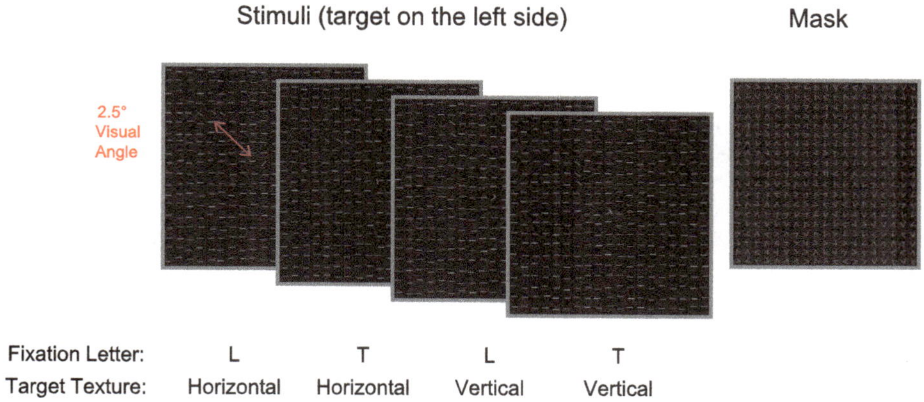

Figure 1. Experimental stimuli displays. The texture stimulus (left) was composed of three adjacent diagonal bars (vertically or horizontally aligned) embedded within a background of horizontal bars, with a letter "T" or "L" as the fixation. The mask (right) was made of randomly oriented "V", with superimposed "T" and "L" at the fixation position.

"L" were used to mask the "T" or "L" in the stimulus pattern (Figure 1).

Procedure. During each test trial, observers first fixated for 500 ms on a small central cross, where the fixation letter ("T" or "L") was displayed (Figure 2). Subsequent to a 300 ms blank, the texture stimulus was presented for 36 ms, followed by a blank interval (stimulus-to-mask onset asynchrony, SOA), and then by the mask for 100 ms. The central cross remained on the CRT until the observers gave their responses, first reporting the fixation letter ("T" or "L") and then indicating the texture target orientation (horizontal or vertical). No feedback was given. The response was deemed correct when judgments on both the letter and the target texture were correct.

The staircase followed a 2-down-1-up rule, which resulted in a 66.7% convergence rate. Each staircase (approximately 60 trials) consisted of four preliminary reversals and six experimental reversals. The geometric mean of the experimental reversals was taken as the threshold for each staircase. There were three staircases in the test sessions (pre- and post-test, approximately 20 minutes) and six staircases in the training sessions (approximately 50 minutes). For all of the participants, the step-size was 36 ms until the fourth reversal and then changed to 24 ms. During the training, the horizontal or vertical target array was always presented at a fixed location (either in the upper-left or upper-right visual-field quadrant, "the trained location"), which was counterbalanced across participants.

To ensure that the children understood how to perform the task, all of the participants practiced the task without mask at the beginning of the experiment. First, the children were told only to do the central letter discrimination task and to ignore the target texture task (40 trials). Then, they were asked to process the central letter and peripheral stimuli simultaneously (40 trials). Finally, they practiced the task with the formal experimental program (with mask for 40 trials).

The participants were assigned to two training groups, one with dyslexia and one control group, and completed ten sessions of TDT training within four weeks with two or three sessions per week. All reading measures and TDT were administered to the participants before and after training. In addition, a follow-up testing with all of these reading measures was conducted to the participants of two training groups two months post TDT training to investigate whether the training effect was long-lasting and maintainable.

The participants in the two non-training groups participated in the same TDT threshold and all of the same linguistic measurements as the training groups in the pre- and post-tests. However, they were not trained with the TDT. The time interval between pre- and post-tests was the same as the training groups.

Data analysis

We first investigated whether there was difference in the TDT thresholds in the pre-test between the dyslexia and control groups.

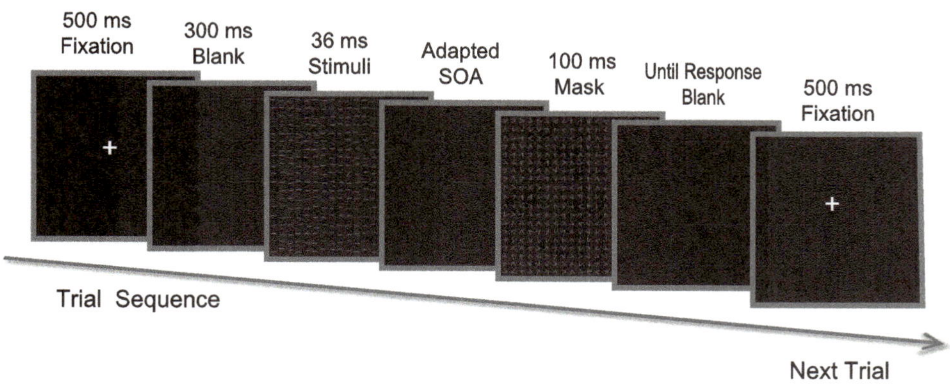

Figure 2. Trial sequences of texture discrimination task.

Next, the TDT learning effect on TDT processing was estimated. Then, we compared the slopes of the learning curves between the two training groups. Finally, ANOVAs were conducted for the TDT thresholds and the two reading measures, reading fluency and vocabulary in the test sessions, to examine whether the TDT training effects were significant and whether the TDT training affects the performance in the vocabulary test and the reading fluency test. The factors were Participant (dyslexia vs. control; between-subjects factor), Training Group (training vs. non-training, between-subjects factor) and Testing Time (pre- vs. post-test; within-subjects factor).

All of the ANOVAs were conducted with SPSS software. If any significant interactions related to Training Group were found, the subsequent simple effects were analyzed. In all of the analyses, in cases of sphericity violations, the significance levels of the F ratios were adjusted by the Greenhouse-Geisser correction.

Results

The TDT performance in the pre-test

Before training, the TDT threshold in the pre-test for the dyslexia group (584.89±59.75 ms) was significantly higher than that of control group (414.08±59.75 ms, $t_{34} = -2.063$, $p<.048$). Moreover, we compared the performance without mask in the practice. There were no significant differences in the central letter task between children with dyslexia and control children (accuracy: 94.31% vs. 95.83%; $t_{34} = 0.954$, $p>0.351$). However, when they were asked to discriminate both the central letter and peripheral stimuli simultaneously, children with dyslexia exhibited much lower accuracy than control children (75.97% vs. 89.44%; $t_{34} = 3.903$, $p<0.001$).

The "training'" and "non-training" groups had similar pre-test TDT thresholds ($t_{34} = 0.771$, $p>.446$), therefore the observers in the training and non-training groups were homogeneous in the behavioral dimension before the training.

The effect of TDT training on TDT

The TDT threshold SOAs for the two training groups of children in 10 sessions were averaged separately. Learning curves depict the learning progress of the two training groups of children (Figure 3).

A repeated-measures ANOVA of 2 Participants (Controls vs. Dyslexia)×2 Training Group (Training vs. Non-training)×2 Testing Time (Post- vs. Pre-test) was conducted to estimate the training effects of TDT. The main effect of Training Group was significant ($F_{1,32} = 5.09$, $p<.05$), suggesting that the training group had a lower TDT threshold SOA (347.61±44.09 ms) than the non-training group (493.72±45.79 ms). The main effect of Participants was also significant ($F_{1,32} = 6.58$, $p<.05$), suggesting that the dyslexia group (503.72±42.10 ms) had a higher threshold SOA than the control group (337.61±43.32 ms). The main effect of testing time was also significant ($F_{1,32} = 29.99$, $p<.0001$), suggesting that the threshold SOA for post-test (341.84±27.79 ms) was significantly lower than that of pre-test (499.49±42.25 ms).

The interaction between Training Group and Testing Time was significant ($F_{1,32} = 6.78$, $p<.05$). The post-hoc simple effect analyses showed that the threshold SOA of post-test (229.28±39.29 ms) was significantly lower than pre-test (465.93±59.75 ms) in the training group ($p<.0001$, Bonferroni's correction), but not in the non-training group ($p>.05$, Figure 4). In addition, the three-way interaction of Testing time×Participant×Training group was not significant ($F_{1,32} = 0.447$, $p>.507$). All of these results indicate that both the children with dyslexia and the control group could attain perceptual learning.

However, further analysis of the learning curves (Figure 3) show that there is a difference in the learning speed between the two training groups. We fitted the learning curve with a logarithmic function ($y = -a \times \ln(x)+b$) for each child. The "y" is the threshold SOA in each session, the "x" is the session number. The "a" indicates the slope of the learning curve. The results show that the slope of learning curve for the dyslexia group is marginally smaller than that of the control group (62.2±69.6 vs. 7.4±42.8; $t_{16} = 2.012$, $p = 0.061$), indicating that the learning speed for the control group is faster than that of dyslexia group. Secondly, we calculated the averaged vertical distance between the threshold SOA and the logarithmic function across all of the training sessions. The averaged distance of the dyslexia group was significantly larger than that of the control group (73.7±23.4 vs. 45.4±19.2; $t_{16} = -2.798$, $p<0.014$), indicating that the threshold SOA for the group with dyslexia had much more fluctuation than that of control group during the training.

The effect of TDT training on reading measures

The same repeated-measures ANOVA of 2 Participants (Controls vs. Dyslexia)×2 Training Group (Training vs. Non-training)×2 Testing Time (Post- vs. Pre-test) was conducted to estimate the training effects of perceptual training on reading measures. Reading fluency performance was enhanced in the post-

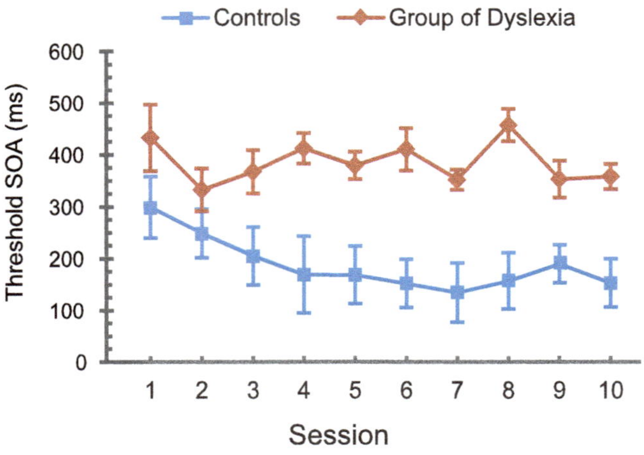

Figure 3. The perceptual learning curves for two training groups of children. The error bars represent standard errors.

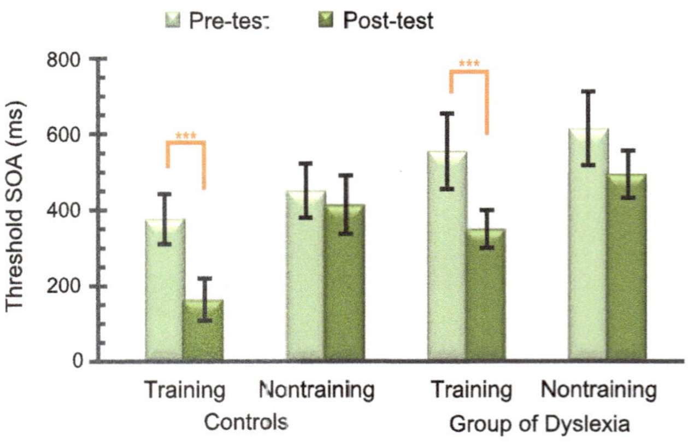

Figure 4. The threshold SOA (mean ± standard error) of TDT performance in the pre- and post- test.

test compared to the pre-test in the dyslexia training group. Specifically, the main effect of Testing Time was significant ($F_{1,32} = 16.3$, $p<.001$). The interaction of Participants and Testing Time was also significant ($F_{1,32} = 4.73$, $p<.05$). Simple effect analyses indicate that the performance of reading fluency was significantly improved in the post-test compared to that in the pre-test for the participants with dyslexia ($p<.001$, Bonferroni's correction), whereas this comparison was not significant in control group ($p>.1$). The interaction of Testing Time, Participants, and Training Group was also significant ($F_{1,32} = 6.77$, $p<.05$). Simple effect analyses revealed that reading fluency performance in the post-test (41.00±2.57) significantly outperformed that of the pre-test (26.33±2.53) for the dyslexia training group ($p<.0001$, Bonferroni's correction). However, this comparison did not reach significance in the non-training group of children with dyslexia or in the control groups ($p>.1$, Bonferroni's correction, Figure 5). After 2 months, the performance improvement of reading fluency in the training group of dyslexia was still maintained, as revealed by a non-significant paired two-tailed t-test between the post-test and the follow-up test ($t_8 = 1.11$, $p>.1$).

The same repeated-measures ANOVAs of 2 Participants (Controls vs. Dyslexia)×2 Training Group (Training vs. Non-training)×2 Testing Time (Post- vs. Pre-test) was also conducted to estimate the training effects of perceptual training on vocabulary. However, neither the main effect of Training Group nor its interactions with other factors were significant, suggesting that the TDT training did not affect the performance of vocabulary.

Discussion

The focus of this study was to examine whether visual perceptual training with an individually adaptive visual texture discrimination task could benefit reading performance in developmental dyslexia. Both the children with dyslexia and control children decreased TDT threshold SOAs from TDT training, but the children with dyslexia had higher threshold SOAs and slower learning speed, further confirming that children with dyslexia indeed have deficits in visual perceptual processing and learning. More importantly, reading fluency performance was significantly enhanced only in the dyslexia training group, and this enhancement could be maintained up to two months post TDT training. These results suggest that visual perceptual training might have a positive effect in improving performance of reading fluency.

The enhanced reading fluency performance can be explained in three ways. First, temporal processing is one of the possible causes that underlie the training effect. A major study reported the

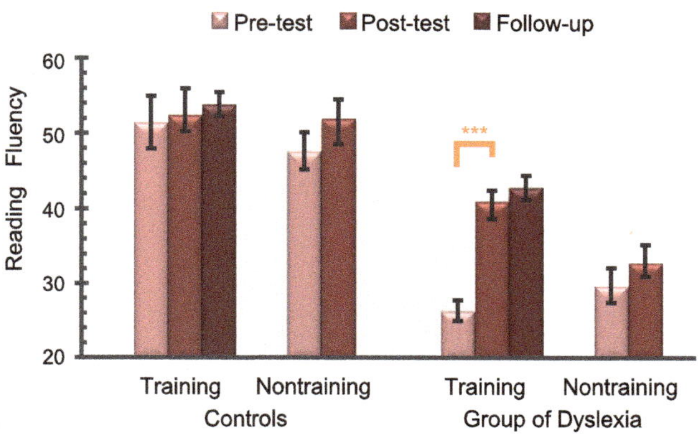

Figure 5. The reading fluency performance (mean ± standard error) in the pre-, post- and follow-up test.

temporal processing deficit in people with dyslexia [34]. In the present TDT task, the participants had to make judgments about the orientation of the central letter and the peripheral target bars in the short time span of SOA between stimuli and mask. Previous research has shown that TDT learning involves temporal processing to disentangle target stimuli from mask [35], [36]. Similarly, a recent study found that TDT learning was mostly temporal learning, which is the temporal learning of target–mask separation [37]. Additionally, TDT training improved participants' temporal processing speed and probably enabled them to separate the target and the mask rapidly within a very brief threshold SOA [38], [39]. In the current study, reading fluency is a speeded comprehension task which requires participants to analyze the visual stimuli accurately and quickly, retrieve the phonological information, and access the meaning of reading materials immediately. Therefore, TDT might enhance reading fluency performance of individuals with dyslexia by strengthening their temporal processing ability. Compared to normal readers, children with dyslexia had a deficiency in temporal processing which resulted in low efficiency in separating target and mask prior to training; they might be more sensitive to the adaptive and intensive TDT training than normal counterparts and exhibited training effects.

Second, visual perceptual training possibly enlarged and strengthened the readers' visual span and improved their reading speed through training their peripheral visual field. This interpretation is compatible with the findings from studies in people with amblyopia [21], in normally sighted young adults [40–42], and even in people with central vision loss [43]. In our study, even without the mask, children with dyslexia exhibited more difficulty than control children when they were asked to process central letter and peripheral stimuli simultaneously [44]. This result suggests that, at least, part of their deficit in TDT learning is not related to temporal processing. The peripheral field in individuals with dyslexia is possibly weak and therefore had difficulty in processing the visual attributes and forming representations of stimuli presented in the peripheral field [45], and visual perceptual training might be a potential effective treatment for these individuals with dyslexia.

The third explanation for these results involves spatial attention. Previous reports have suggested that the developmental dyslexia had attention deficit [46–48], and there may be a causal link between visual spatial attention and reading acquisition [49], and reading speed was improved through strengthening attention abilities [19]. Meanwhile, our recent ERP studies found that visual perceptual learning also involved spatial attention regulation [50], [51], and TDT training might also improve reading fluency performance by enhancing their spatial attention ability. Further study will be necessary to clarify the underlying mechanisms.

TDT training improves reading fluency in the children with dyslexia, but not the performance of vocabulary. Previous findings have suggested that visual processing in the peripheral visual field, temporal processing, and visual spatial attention might be the potential processes involved in perceptual learning [37], [43], [50]. Meanwhile, as stated earlier, reading fluency mainly targeted reading speed which demanded a certain amount of ability in temporal processing and spatial attention. Additionally, visual processing in the peripheral visual field was critically important in continuous text reading [39]. In contrast, vocabulary test, as a character recognition task, was mostly involved separate character recognition and word composition, which put less demands on temporal processing, peripheral field visual processing, and spatial attention than did reading speed task, reading fluency test. That's plausible the reason why TDT training enhanced performance in reading fluency instead of vocabulary in the children of dyslexia. In addition, it might be the ceiling effect that resulted in the unchanged reading fluency performance in normal control group.

These findings are of two-fold practical significance: first, it has implications for the early prevention or diagnosis of potential dyslexia. Commonly, dyslexia cannot be identified until the child has failed in learning to read and write, and studies show that these children rarely catch up [52]. However, because dyslexia is a constitutional impairment, if we know more about early risk signs of dyslexia, early prevention starting before they learn to read should be possible and effective. If visual perceptual processing/learning is associated with and possibly shares common mechanisms with the development of reading skills, adaptive visual perceptual learning programs/games with very basic visual stimuli prior to school years would be beneficial for preventing at-risk readers from developing into dyslexia.

Second, effective training program should be individualized and adaptive. From the findings of the current study and the previous study [23], the perceptual learning curves and learning speed have great individual differences; in order to obtain gains for each individual, the procedural arrangement and learning pace for individuals with dyslexia should be determined in accordance with their individual basic processing and learning abilities.

Conclusions

Our results demonstrate that visual perceptual learning can significantly enhance the performance of reading fluency in Chinese-speaking children with developmental dyslexia, further suggesting that that basic visual perceptual processing/learning and reading ability in Chinese might at least partially rely on overlapping mechanisms.

Acknowledgments

We are grateful to all of the children, teachers, and schools that participated in this study.

Author Contributions

Conceived and designed the experiments: YS XM. Performed the experiments: OL FW YJ. Analyzed the data: XM OL FW. Contributed reagents/materials/analysis tools: XM YS. Contributed to the writing of the manuscript: XM YS. Supervised the work and provided conceptual and technical insights: YS.

References

1. Shaywitz SE, Shaywitz BA (2005) Dyslexia (specific reading disability). Biol Psychiatry 57: 1301–1309.
2. Ramus F (2003) Developmental dyslexia: specific phonological deficit or general sensorimotor dysfunction? Curr Opin Neurobiol 13: 212–218.
3. Wagner RK, Torgesen JK (1987) The nature of phonological processing and its causal role in the acquisition of reading skills. Psychological Bulletin 101: 192–212.
4. Tallal P (1980) Auditory temporal perception, phonics, and reading disabilities in children. Brain Lang 9: 182–198.
5. Tallal P, Miller SL, Bedi G, Byma G, Wang X, et al. (1996) Language comprehension in language-learning impaired children improved with acoustically modified speech. Science 271: 81–84.
6. Witton C, Talcott JB, Hansen PC, Richardson AJ, Griffiths TD, et al. (1998) Sensitivity to dynamic auditory and visual stimuli predicts nonword reading ability in both dyslexic and normal readers. Curr Biol 8: 791–797.
7. Ahissar M, Protopapas A, Reid M, Merzenich MM (2000) Auditory processing parallels reading abilities in adults. Proc Natl Acad Sci U S A 97: 6832–6837.
8. Stein JF (1994) Developmental dyslexia, neural timing and hemispheric lateralisation. Int J Psychophysiol 18: 241–249.
9. Stein J, Walsh V (1997) To see but not to read; the magnocellular theory of dyslexia. Trends Neurosci 20: 147–152.
10. Bradley L, Bryant PE (1978) Difficulties in auditory organisation as a possible cause of reading backwardness. Nature 271: 746–747.
11. Shaywitz BA, Shaywitz SE, Blachman BA, Pugh KR, Fulbright RK, et al. (2004) Development of left occipitotemporal systems for skilled reading in children after a phonologically- based intervention. Biol Psychiatry 55: 926–933.
12. Lovio R, Halttunen A, Lyytinen H, Näätänen R, Kujala T (2012) Reading skill and neural processing accuracy improvement after a 3-hour intervention in preschoolers with diffic processing deficits of language-learning impaired children ameliorated by training. Science 271: 77–81.
13. Merzenich MM, Jenkins WM, Johnston P, Schreiner C, Miller SL, et al. (1996) Temporal processing deficits of language-learning impaired children ameliorated by training. Science 271: 77–81.
14. Temple E, Deutsch GK, Poldrack RA, Miller SL, Tallal P, et al. (2003) Neural deficits in children with dyslexia ameliorated by behavioral remediation: evidence from functional MRI. Proc Natl Acad Sci U S A 100: 2860–2865.
15. Bhide A, Power A, Goswami U (2013) A rhythmic musical intervention for poor readers: a comparison of efficacy with a letter-base intervention. Mind, Brain and Education 7(2): 113–123.
16. Moritz C, Yampolsky S, Papadelis G, Thomson J, Wolf M (2013) Links between early rhythm skills, musical training, and phonological awareness. Read Writ 26: 739–769.
17. Chouake T, Levy T, Javitt DC, Lavidor M (2012) Magnocellular training improves visual word recognition. Front Hum Neurosci 6: 14.
18. Zorzi M, Barbiero C, Facoetti A, Lonciari I, Carrozzi M, et al. (2012) Extra-large letter spacing improves reading in dyslexia. Proc Natl Acad Sci U S A 109: 11455–11459.
19. Franceschini S, Gori S, Ruffino M, Viola S, Molteni M, et al. (2013) Action video games make dyslexic children read better. Curr Biol 23: 462–466.
20. Gibson EJ (1969) Principles of perceptual learning. New York: Appleton-Century-Crofts.
21. Chung ST, Legge GE, Cheung SH (2004) Letter-recognition and reading speed in peripheral vision benefit from perceptual learning. Vision Res 44: 695–709.
22. Yu D, Cheung SH, Legge GE, Chung ST (2010) Reading speed in the peripheral visual field of older adults: Does it benefit from perceptual learning? Vision Res 50: 860–869.
23. Wang Z, Cheng-Lai A, Song Y, Cutting L, Jiang Y, et al. (2014) A perceptual learning deficit in Chinese developmental dyslexia as revealed by visual texture discrimination training. Dyslexia in press. DOI:10.1002/dys.1475.
24. American Psychiatric Association (1994) Diagnostic and statistical manual of mental disorders (4th ed.). Washington, DC: American Psychiatric Association Press.
25. Zhang HC, Wang XP (1985) Raven standard progressive matrices: Chinese city revision. Beijing: The National Revision Collaborative Group.
26. Siok WT, Perfetti CA, Jin Z, Tan LH (2004) Biological abnormality of impaired reading isconstrained by culture. Nature 43: 71–76.
27. Xue J, Shu H, Li H, Li W, Tian X (2013) The Stability of Literacy-Related Cognitive Contributions to Chinese Character Naming and Reading Fluency. J Psycholinguist Res. 42: 433–450.
28. Norton ES, Wolf M (2012) Rapid Automatized Naming (RAN) and Reading Fluency: Implications for Understanding and Treatment of Reading Disabilities. Annu Rev Psychol. 63: 427–452.
29. Wang XL, Tao BP (1996) Chinese character recognition test battery and assessment scale forprimary school children. Shanghai: Shanghai Education Press.
30. You H, Gaab N, Wei N, Cheng-Lai A, Wang Z, et al. (2011) Neural deficits in second language reading: fMRI evidence from Chinese-speaking children with English reading impairment. NeuroImage 57: 760–770.
31. Karni A, Sagi D (1991) Where practice makes perfect in texture discrimination: Evidence for primary visual cortex plasticity. Proc Natl Acad Sci U S A 88: 4966–4970.
32. Schwartz S, Maquet P, Frith C (2002) Neural correlates of perceptual learning: A functional MRIstudy of visual texture discrimination. Proc Natl Acad Sci U S A 99: 17137–17142.
33. Yotsumoto Y, Watanabe T, Sasaki Y (2008) Different dynamics of performance and brainactivation in the time course of perceptual learning. Neuron 57: 827–833.
34. Farmer ME, Klein RM (1995) The evidence for a temporal processing deficit linked to dyslexia: A review. Psychon Bull Rev 2: 460–493.
35. Schubö A, Schlaghecken F, Meinecke C (2001) Learning to ignore the mask in texture segmentation tasks. J Exp Psychol Hum Percept Perform 27: 919–931.
36. Censor N, Bonneh Y, Arieli A, Sagi D (2009) Early-vision brain responses which predict human visual segmentation and learning. J Vis 9: 12.1–9.
37. Wang R, Cong LJ, Yu C (2013) The classical TDT perceptual learning is mostly temporal learning. J Vis 13: 9.1–9.
38. Polat U (2009) Making perceptual learning practical to improve visual functions. Vision Res 49: 2566–2573.
39. Sterkin A, Yehezkel O, Bonneh YS, Norcia A, Polat U (2009) Backward masking suppresses collinear facilitation in the visual cortex. Vision Res 49: 1784–1794.
40. Yu D, Legge GE, Park H, Gage E, Chung ST (2013) Development of a training protocol to improve reading performance in peripheral vision. Vision Res 50: 36–45.

41. Chung ST, Truong SR (2013) Learning to identify crowded letters: does the learning depend on the frequency of training? Vision Res 77: 41–50.
42. Bernard JB, Arunkumar A, Chung ST (2012) Can reading-specific training stimuli improve the effect of perceptual learning on peripheral reading speed? Vision Res 66: 17–25.
43. Chung ST (2011) Improving reading speed for people with central vision loss through perceptual learning. Invest Ophthalmol Vis Sci 52: 1164–1170.
44. Lin O (2013) Texture discrimination training and reading development in Chinese-speaking school children. Peking University thesis, Beijing, June.
45. Martelli M, Di Filippo G, Spinelli D, Zoccolotti P (2009) Crowding, reading, and developmental dyslexia. J Vis 9: 14.1–18.
46. Facoetti A, Paganoni P, Turatto M, Marzola V, Mascetti GG (2000) Visual-spatial attention in developmental dyslexia. Cortex 36: 109–123.
47. Facoetti A, Lorusso ML, Paganoni P, Umiltà C, Mascetti GG (2003) The role of visuospatial attention in developmental dyslexia: evidence from a rehabilitation study. Brain Res Cogn Brain Res 15: 154–164.
48. Roach NW, Hogben JH (2008) Spatial cueing deficits in dyslexia reflect generalised difficulties with attentional selection. Vision Res 48: 193–207.
49. Franceschini S, Gori S, Ruffino M, Pedrolli K, Facoetti A (2012) A causal link between visual spatial attention and reading acquisition. Curr Biol 22: 814–819.
50. An A, Sun M, Wang Y, Wang F, Ding Y, et al. (2012) The N2pc is increased by perceptual learning but is unnecessary for the transfer of learning. PLoS One 7: e34826.
51. Wang F, Zhong X, Huang J, Ding Y, Song Y (2013) Comparison of perceptual learning of real and virtual line orientations: an event-related potential study. Vision Res 93: 1–9.
52. Shaywitz BA, Shaywitz S, Pugh KR, Fulbright RK, Mencl WE, et al. (2001) The neurobiology of dyslexia. Clin Neurosci Res 1: 291–299.

18

Attentional Modulation of Auditory Steady-State Responses

Yatin Mahajan*, Chris Davis, Jeesun Kim

The MARCS Institute, University of Western Sydney, Penrith, New South Wales, Australia

Abstract

Auditory selective attention enables task-relevant auditory events to be enhanced and irrelevant ones suppressed. In the present study we used a frequency tagging paradigm to investigate the effects of attention on auditory steady state responses (ASSR). The ASSR was elicited by simultaneously presenting two different streams of white noise, amplitude modulated at either 16 and 23.5 Hz or 32.5 and 40 Hz. The two different frequencies were presented to each ear and participants were instructed to selectively attend to one ear or the other (confirmed by behavioral evidence). The results revealed that modulation of ASSR by selective attention depended on the modulation frequencies used and whether the activation was contralateral or ipsilateral. Attention enhanced the ASSR for contralateral activation from either ear for 16 Hz and suppressed the ASSR for ipsilateral activation for 16 Hz and 23.5 Hz. For modulation frequencies of 32.5 or 40 Hz attention did not affect the ASSR. We propose that the pattern of enhancement and inhibition may be due to binaural suppressive effects on ipsilateral stimulation and the dominance of contralateral hemisphere during dichotic listening. In addition to the influence of cortical processing asymmetries, these results may also reflect a bias towards inhibitory ipsilateral and excitatory contralateral activation present at the level of inferior colliculus. That the effect of attention was clearest for the lower modulation frequencies suggests that such effects are likely mediated by cortical brain structures or by those in close proximity to cortex.

Editor: Manuel S. Malmierca, University of Salamanca- Institute for Neuroscience of Castille and Leon and Medical School, Spain

Funding: The study was supported by MARCS Institute research fund. The funders had no role in study design, data collection and analysis, decision to publish, or preparation of the manuscript.

Competing Interests: The authors have declared that no competing interests exist.

* Email: y.mahajan@uws.edu.au

Introduction

A listener in a typical everyday situation receives multiple auditory inputs some of which may be relevant and others not. As such, the listener has to selectively attend to particular inputs and sustain this attention over time. It is through sustained selective attention that a listener is able to enhance task-relevant processing and suppress irrelevant processing [1,2].

The neurophysiological mechanisms underlying selective auditory attention and its neural correlates have been studied using various electrophysiological methods (EEG, MEG and electrocorticography). Early research on the attentional modulation of cortical responses typically examined event-related potentials (ERPs) and paralleled the early behavioral work on aural discrimination by using simple transient stimuli, such as tone bursts and tone pips. Use of these stimuli provided a high degree of control over stimulus properties and presentation times. Results showed larger auditory P1, N1 and T-complex responses to attended stimuli [3,4] and reduced activity to unattended stimuli [1,5].

Recently, another neurophysiological measure, the auditory steady state response (ASSR) has been used to examine the effect of attention on neurophysiological responses underlying selective auditory attention. The ASSR consists of evoked responses from central auditory pathway and auditory cortex when presented with rapid periodic/rhythmic auditory stimuli that lead to synchronization of cortical oscillations to its frequency and phase [6]. The ASSR can be generated by modulating an auditory input (carrier signal: white noise or pure tones) either in an amplitude (AM) or frequency (FM) domain or both [7].

One benefit of using ASSR is that the modulating frequency of the auditory stream will be represented in the neural response, and multiple modulation frequencies can be used in a single stimulus paradigm to record ASSR simultaneously. Since the modulation frequencies used to record ASSR are predefined, precise frequency analyses can be performed at those frequencies. When the modulating auditory streams are attended, the attention typically influences the activity of neurons that match the temporal structure of the input and so neural responses will be tied to the timing of the attended events. These properties of ASSR enable the researchers to study the neural correlates of auditory selective attention such that the cortical responses (ASSR) are 'tagged' to the multiple modulation frequencies used that may be attended or unattended in a stimulus paradigm called 'frequency tagging'.

Frequency tagging for ASSR was first introduced in a binaural interaction experiment to study the contribution of ipsilateral and contralateral pathways at the level of human auditory cortex [8]. Frequency tagging when used to evaluate auditory selective attention typically involves presentation of different auditory input in each ear with each ear modulated by a particular modulation frequency. The listener attends to sounds in one ear while ignoring the stimulus from the other ear. The ASSR is tagged for both the attended and unattended modulation frequencies from each ear. The effects of selective attention can be investigated from the resultant power of the ASSR. Furthermore, the effect of attention at different levels of auditory system can be probed with the frequency tagging paradigm by using a number of modulation frequencies. That is, the effects of attention can be assessed at different loci along central auditory pathway because such are activated by differing modulation frequencies, e.g., primary and secondary auditory cortices responsive to 4–16 Hz, the medial geniculate body of upper brainstem to 16–32 Hz and lower brainstem and other brainstem regions to 32–256 Hz AM frequency [9–11].

There have been only a handful of studies investigating the effect of selective attention on ASSR that have used frequency tagging. A summary of the findings and methods used in these studies is presented in Table 1. With the exception of [8,12], all the studies shown in Table 1 employed an active attention task in which either a change in modulation frequency or carrier frequency was to be detected while paying attention to a particular ear and simultaneously ignoring the auditory stream from the other. Three general results can be drawn from these studies. First, the power of the ASSR was modulated by the deployment of attention. That is, apart from two studies [13,14], the power of the ASSR was increased for the stream of rhythmic auditory stimuli that was attended compared to the stream that was unattended or ignored.

Second, it appears that the enhancement of ASSR by attention is clearest in the hemisphere contralateral to the stimulated ear. Müller et al. [15] reported that attention enhanced the power of contralateral ASSR tagged to 20 Hz and suppressed ipsilateral 20 Hz ASSR. Bharadwaj et al. [16] found significantly increased ASSR in the hemisphere contralateral to attended sound source and only a trend of enhancement in the ipsilateral one. Ross et al. [17] also reported increased 40 Hz ASSR amplitude on attention in the contralateral hemisphere during monaural stimulation. The other studies did not report results as a function of contralateral and ipsilateral activations per se, but rather in terms of attention effects in the left or right hemisphere. Of these studies all but one [14] reported an effect of attention in left hemisphere; Lazzouni et al. [14] reported modulation of ASSR in the right hemisphere. A reason why attention might have a more potent effect contralaterally than ipsilaterally is there are more neurons and connections from subcortical structures to contralateral cortical ones [18]. It should be noted, however, that although the suppression of ipsilateral responses compared to contralateral responses is reported in a number of frequency tagging paradigms [8,12,14], these studies either had no attention related task or did not alternate the modulation frequencies across the ears. Alternating the frequencies and attentional load across the ears allows for the ipsilateral and contralateral auditory pathways to potentially contribute equally for each frequency providing a fairer

Table 1. A summary of research on attentional modulation of ASSR using the frequency tagging paradigm.

Study	Number of participants/ Carrier Signal	Modulation frequencies	Effect of Attention on ASSR	Hemispheric lateralization	Task (Listening)
Linden et al., 1987	10 (5 females)/500 Hz	37 and 41 Hz	No effect	NR	Active (Change in carrier) frequency)
Fujiki et al., 2002	12 (5 females)/1000 Hz	26.1 and 20.1 Hz	NR	Left hemisphere laterality; suppression of ipsilateral responses in right hemisphere	Active (No task)
Kaneko et al., 2003	10 (4 females)/1000 Hz	39.1 and 41.1 Hz	NR	Binaural suppression of ipsilateral responses; contralateral hemisphere dominance	Active (No task)
Bidet-Caulet et al., 2007	12 (8 females)/659–784 Hz	21 and 29 Hz	Increased responses when attending; decreased when unattended	Left hemisphere laterality	Active (Target detection and localization)
Müller et al., 2009	15 (6 females)/500 Hz	20 and 45 Hz	Contralateral responses enhanced and ipsilateral responses suppressed only for 20 Hz	Left hemisphere laterality	Active (Target detection, change in modulation frequency)
Xiang et al., 2010	28 (15 females)/250–500 Hz	4 and 7 Hz	Responses enhanced by attention for each frequency tested	NR	Active (Deviant tone detection)
Lazzouni et al., 2010	15 (8 females)/1000 Hz	39 and 41 Hz	No effect of attention on ASSR power but increased ASSR amplitude (time-domain)	Right Hemisphere laterality; Binaural suppression of ipsilateral responses	Active (Target detection, change in carrier)
Bhardwaj et al., 2014	10 (2 females)/Vowels	35 and 45 Hz	Increased responses for attended frequencies	Larger responses in contralateral hemisphere	Active (Target detection)
Current Study	23 (10 females)/White noise	16, 23.5, 32.5 and 40 Hz	Contralateral responses enhanced for 16 and 23.5; ipsilateral responses suppressed for 16 Hz	No hemispheric laterality	Active (Target detection, change in modulation frequency)

Note: NR = Not Relevant.

assessment of hemispheric dominance related to attention. Indeed, in this regard, only one study [15] has employed a suitable design to properly assess the effect of attention on ASSR as a function of ipsilateral and contralateral responses in a frequency tagging paradigm.

Third, the Table 1 suggests that the modulation of ASSR by attention may depend on the modulation frequencies used; however the results are inconsistent. Müller et al. found significant attentional modulation only for 20 Hz and not for 45 Hz ASSR. Other studies have found significant attentional modulation of ASSR when tagged to 35–45 Hz modulation frequencies [14,16]. Moreover, using an active listening oddball paradigm with 20 Hz and 40 Hz AM frequencies, Skosnik et al. [19] found increased ASSR amplitude for attended 40 Hz targets compared to 20 Hz ones. Although the existing data suggests that attentional modulation of ASSR might depend on the modulation frequencies being used in the paradigm, such a conclusion may not be appropriate as it relies on cross experiment comparisons that often involve the change of many factors. In our view then, to resolve the apparent inconsistencies in the existing research an experiment is required that systematically examines multiple modulation frequencies. Furthermore, examining multiple modulation frequencies in a single experiment is worthwhile, since no previous study has ever used more than two modulation frequencies to evaluate the effect of attention on ASSR.

In sum, attention has been found to modulate the ASSR, with the strength (direction) of this activation influenced by the stimuli input, i.e., activation in the hemisphere contralateral to the attended ear produces increased amplitude and reduced amplitude in the ipsilateral hemisphere. Further, the left hemisphere is reported to be more sensitive to attentional modulation than right. The findings are inconsistent on how different modulation frequencies may interact with the attention effect.

The purpose of the present research was to build on the above research that has used a frequency tagging paradigm with the aim of determining how selective sustained attention modulates cortical responses (ASSR) as a function of contralateral/ipsilateral activations across different modulation frequencies. The results will contribute to the growing body of literature evaluating the neural correlates of selective auditory attention by frequency tagging.

Materials and Methods

Ethics Statement

The methods of the present research were approved by the human research ethics committee at the University of Western Sydney. Written informed consent was obtained from each participant before the experiment.

Participants

Twenty three participants (10 females), aged 22–35 years were recruited using notice board advertisements around the university campus. All the participants were right handed as assessed by Edinburgh handedness inventory and reported no significant neurological and psychological history. All the participants had normal hearing bilaterally with hearing thresholds of $\leq$15 dB HL at 500 Hz, 1000 Hz and 2000 Hz determined by screening audiometry.

Experimental stimuli

The experimental stimuli consisted of four 'standard' 30 second long white noise stimuli amplitude modulated at 16 Hz, 23.5 Hz, 32.5 Hz and 40 Hz with 100% modulation depth sampled at the rate of 44,100 Hz. The stimuli were ramped with 20 ms rise time at the onset and 20 ms fall time at the offset to avoid clicks. The white noise was used as a carrier signal in order to evoke reliable and robust ASSR. The broadband signal when used to elicit ASSR, produces larger magnitude of ASSR as compared to pure tone and band-limited noise as carrier signals [20]. The stimuli were created using the signal processing toolbox of MATLAB and were presented at a comfortable level around 70–75 dB SPL for all the participants. The experiment was completed in two sessions. In one session, the participants were presented with 16 Hz and 23.5 Hz AM stimuli and in the other session the 32.5 Hz and 40 Hz AM stimuli. The two sessions of recording were counterbalanced between the participants.

During each session the participants were presented each of the two stimuli in each of their two ears dichotically such that the one ear was stimulated by 16 Hz or 32.5 Hz and other ear by 23.5 Hz or 40 Hz modulated white noise. The ear of stimulation was counterbalanced equally between the two sets of stimuli such that a particular amplitude modulated stimulus was presented equally to both left and right ears and at the same time the opposite ear was stimulated with a different stimulus.

The experiment also consisted of 'target' stimuli, in which the modulation frequency changed multiple times during 30 seconds of stimulation (based on paradigm used by Müller et al.). The stimuli with 16 Hz and 23.5 Hz amplitude modulation changed to 40 Hz modulation for 2 seconds, either two, three or four times within 30 seconds of stimulation for target stimuli before returning to original modulation rate. The target stimuli with 32.5 Hz and 40 Hz amplitude modulation changed to 12.5 Hz modulation frequency. The target stimuli were also counterbalanced equally between ears in two sessions of recording. The two frequencies using as stimulus pairs were selected so that there was a relatively small difference between them; this was done to minimize involuntary switching of attention to one of the frequencies. That is, as part of a pilot study conducted to determine the best combination of modulation frequencies, we found that when the difference in frequencies was large (e.g., 16 and 40 Hz) then participants' attention involuntarily switched to higher modulation frequency (i.e. the 40 Hz). Further, even if the stimulus intensity was equalized across all the modulation frequencies, the perceived loudness of the higher modulation rate stimulus was greater than the lower one and this plausibly would induce an involuntary attention switch towards the high modulation frequency. To minimize this possible effect, we selected modulation frequencies pairs that were closer together (i.e., 16 and 23.5 Hz, 32.5 and 40 Hz) and this combination did not produce any involuntary attention switches.

Experimental procedure

An attention switch paradigm was used to direct attention to the stimulus presented in the designated ear for the dichotic stimuli, (see Fig. 1). The trial started with a fixation cross presented at the center of the screen for 500 ms. Then, a cue in the form of the words 'RIGHT' or 'LEFT' appeared on the screen indicating the participants which ear to attend to and after 1 second the set of paired stimuli (16 or 23.5 Hz; 32.5 or 40 Hz) were presented for 30 seconds. The cue remained on the screen for the duration of the stimuli. The participants were instructed to attend to the ear cued and press the response button as fast as they can whenever they heard a change in modulation frequency of the stimuli ('target'). A total of 72 trials were presented in one experimental session. Out of these 72 trials, 48 were standard trials that contained no targets and 24 trials had targets in them. In 12 target trials, the location of the targets and attention cue were same, i.e., if the cue was 'RIGHT', the target also appeared during right ear stimulation; these trials represent the 'congruent' condition. The 'incongruent' condition consisted of the remaining 12 target trials in which the cue and the stimulation ear were at opposite locations. The reaction times for detecting the targets were recorded and slower reaction times were expected in the incongruent condition compared to the congruent one (assuming that attention manipulation had been successful).

Electrophysiological recording

The participants were seated on a comfortable chair while the electrode cap was fitted. Prior to the fitting of the electrode cap, the scalp of each participant was combed to reduce the time taken to achieve the optimal scalp electrode impedance [21]. The raw electroencephalograph (EEG) was recorded with a BioSemi Active-Two amplifier system (BioSemi, Amsterdam, Netherlands). The 64 Ag-AgCl electrodes were mounted on a nylon electrode cap according to the international standard 10-10 system [22]. There were two electrodes on the electrode cap (CMS & DRL) which served as online references. Six additional electrodes were also placed on the participants. Four of them were bipolar electrodes placed above and below the left eye and outer canthi of both the eyes to monitor vertical and horizontal eye movements (EOG channels) respectively and two electrodes were placed on two mastoids. The raw EEG recording was sampled at 512 Hz with online band-pass filtering of.05–200 Hz. This raw EEG data was stored for every participant for later offline analysis.

EEG data analysis

The pre-processing and analysis of the stored raw EEG data was carried out using EEGLAB version 10 [23] and custom written functions in MATLAB (The Mathworks, Natick, MA). Initially, any obvious artifact was removed after visually inspecting the data. Then the EEG data was re-referenced to the average of both the mastoids. The resultant EEG activity was band-pass filtered (1 Hz high pass and 70 Hz low pass; 12 dB per octave roll-off). The filtered data then was epoched into a pre-stimulus period of 200 ms and post stimulus period of 30 seconds. Only the standard trials were included in the EEG analysis. The epoched data then was subjected to *runica*, an ICA (Independent component analysis) algorithm incorporated in EEGLAB to detect and remove eye blinks, horizontal eye movements and other artifacts (muscle, line noise artifacts). The ICA algorithm resulted in 64 components and based on the scalp topography, activity power spectrum and activity over trials, the artifactual components were identified and removed from the EEG data. To remove the effect of onset and offset ERP responses, the epochs were averaged from 1 s to 29.5 s in the ICA corrected epochs to form ASSR responses. The averaged ASSR responses were calculated for each modulation frequency in four conditions namely, 'right attended', 'right unattended', 'left attended' and 'left unattended'.

These time domain ASSR responses were then subjected to a Fourier transformation using a custom written MATLAB script to convert them into frequency domain (FFTs). The FFTs were used to calculate the absolute ASSR power for each condition for every modulation frequency at the two most lateral electrodes (T7 and T8) on the scalp depicting left and right hemispheric activity respectively. These two electrodes were selected as the greater distance between the locations of T7 and T8 makes them the best electrodes to compare neural activity between the two hemispheres, as opposed to using two fronto-central electrodes. To determine if the ASSR at the modulation frequencies of interest evoked at T7 and T8 was significant across participants, the mean absolute power at the two neighboring frequencies on the either side of the modulation frequency were computed and compared with the power at the modulation frequency of interest using a t-test in the resultant FFTs. Results revealed that across all the conditions the power of the ASSR at the frequency of interest was a significant response.

Data analysis

To determine how attention modulates the ASSR as a function of modulation frequency and hemisphere by ear of stimulation (ipsilateral and contralateral), the data on the absolute power of the ASSR obtained through FFT was subjected to a 4 ('modulation frequency'; 16 Hz, 23.5 Hz, 32.5 Hz & 40 Hz)×2 ('stimulation ear'; left vs. right)×2 ('attention'; attended vs. unattended)×2 ('hemisphere by stimulation' (ipsilateral vs. contralateral)) within participant factorial ANOVA. The reaction times obtained in the target detection task were also analyzed with a 4×2×2 repeated measures ANOVA, with 'Frequency' (four modulation frequencies), 'congruency' (congruent vs. incongruent) and 'stimulation ear' (left vs. right) as within participant factors. This analysis provided an index of the differential attention paid to the experimental stimuli. For both above mentioned ANOVA analyses, wherever the assumption of sphericity was violated the Greenhouse-Geisser correction was applied. The significant results obtained are reported in the section below.

Results

Reaction times

Table 2 shows the reaction times obtained for four modulation frequencies across congruent and incongruent conditions. The ANOVA results indicated that congruency significantly altered the reaction times ($F(1,17) = 24.77$, $p<.001$, $\eta_p^2 = .56$) and the modulation frequencies and the ear of stimulation had no significant main effect on reaction times. As evident from Table 2, reaction times were slower when participants attended to targets in the incongruent conditions across the different modulation frequencies. Similar reaction times between right and left ears and slower response times to targets in incongruent conditions across modulation frequencies when considered together, suggest that participants paid and sustained attention to the appropriate ear as instructed at the beginning of each trial.

ASSR

Fig. 2 and Fig. 3 show the grand mean FFTs of the ipsilateral and contralateral activation patterns for the 16 Hz/23.5 Hz and 32.5 Hz/40 Hz modulation frequencies respectively as a function

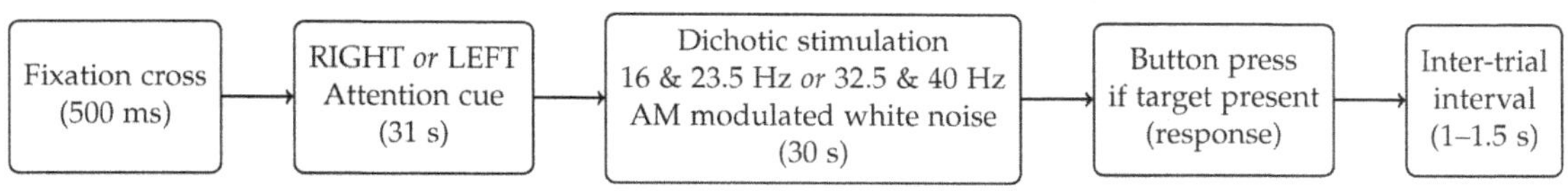

Figure 1. A depiction of the trial sequence.

Table 2. Mean reaction times for targets across modulation frequencies for the congruent and incongruent condition. Standard deviations are given in parentheses.

Frequency	Congruent		Incongruent	
	Left	Right	Left	Right
16 Hz	493 (134.27)	489 (116.85)	531 (138.71)	574 (168.75)
23.5 Hz	492 (122.04)	535 (144.49)	559 (139.36)	584 (152.18)
32.5 Hz	532 (152.54)	532 (133.57)	572 (127.33)	596 (117.65)
40 Hz	510 (153.30)	501 (149.97)	587 (141.44)	545 (142.54)

of attention (i.e., presented to the attended and unattended ear). The presence of clear and robust peaks in the FFTs indicates that the multiple frequencies presented had the desired effect of driving auditory responses at those frequencies. The results of repeated measures ANOVA revealed that there was a significant three-way interaction between frequency, attention and activation pattern, $F(3,66) = 5.76$, $p = .005$, $\eta_p^2 = .20$ (there was no significant main effect of modulation frequency, attention, ear of stimulation or hemisphere by stimulation). To understand this complex three way interaction, first the ipsilateral and contralateral activations were combined from the two ears for each attended and unattended condition across the four modulation frequencies. Then, a follow up two-way ANOVA was computed with factors 'attention' (attended & unattended) and 'hemisphere by stimulation' (ipsilateral & contralateral) for each modulation frequency (16 Hz, 23.5 Hz, 32.5 Hz & 40 Hz).

The results of this ANOVA revealed that there was no significant main effect of attention and hemisphere by stimulation across all the modulation frequencies. There was a significant interaction between these factors for the 16 Hz ($F(1,22) = 14.40$, $p = .001$, $\eta_p^2 = .39$) and 23.5 Hz ($F(1,22) = 10.47$, $p = .004$, $\eta_p^2 = .32$) modulation frequencies. To investigate this interaction, subsequent one-way ANOVAs were conducted on each 16 Hz and 23.5 Hz modulation frequency. For the 16 Hz modulation, the power of the ASSR for attended compared to the unattended stimuli was significantly suppressed for ipsilateral activation ($F(1,22) = 9.17$, $p = .005$) and significantly enhanced for contralateral activation ($F(1,22) = 9.93$, $p = .006$). A similar significant suppression on attended ipsilateral stimulation was found for 23.5 Hz, ($F(1,22) = 8.46$, $p = .008$), but attention did not affect contralateral stimulation ($F(1,22) = .21$, $p = .64$). For 32.5 Hz and 40 Hz AM frequencies, attention did not alter the power of the ASSR, although the change in power was in the enhancement direction for 32.5 Hz and suppression for 40 Hz for both ipsilateral and contralateral stimulation, respectively. These results are illustrated in Fig. 4. The complete statistical analysis has been summarized in supplementary Table S1.

Discussion

The aim of the present research was to determine the extent to which auditory sustained selective attention modulates the strength of ASSR for ipsilateral and contralateral stimulation across different modulation frequencies. The results from the behavioral task demonstrated an effect of selective attention: responses were slower to incongruent (target presented on the unattended side) versus congruent targets depicting successful manipulation of attention. Below we consider the effects of this allocation of attention on the ASSR as a function of the various experimental manipulations.

Attentional modulation of ASSR

To our knowledge, this is the first study that has used a frequency tagging paradigm with more than two modulation frequencies to test the effect of attention on ASSR. This design allows for the direct comparison of the effect of attention on ASSR by multiple modulation frequencies. Our results indicated that attention significantly modulated the power of ASSR and, except for two studies [13,14] listed in Table 1, our results are in general agreement with other studies. The inconsistencies with the results of the studies in Table 1 may be explained by the differences in the experimental tasks used to manipulate the attention. The participants in the current study (and in [15,24]) attended to a change in the modulation frequency or the temporal envelope of stimuli which revealed modulation of ASSR. In the two studies that failed to show any significant modulation of ASSR power [13,14], the participants' task was to attend to changes in carrier frequency (or to spectral change). This difference in task raises the possibility that the attentional modulation of the ASSR requires that attention be directed to modulation frequency change rather than a change in the carrier frequency. In other words, it appears that attending to the stimulus parameter that drive the ASSR (modulation frequency) is essential for its modulation whereas attending to any other stimulus change (carrier frequency) is not. Further, we found that the attentional modulation of ASSR depended on the modulation frequencies and pattern of activation, which are discussed below.

Attentional modulation of ASSR across modulation frequencies and hemispheric dominance

The results indicated that selective attention influenced the power of ASSR for the 16 and 23.5 Hz modulation frequencies whereas this was not the case for the two other modulation frequencies used. These results are in general agreement with two studies (see Table 1), that also reported significant modulation by attention for 20–29 Hz ASSR [15,24]. It has been reported that white noise when amplitude modulated using a range of modulation frequencies (4–256 Hz) tends to preferentially stimulate different parts of central auditory pathway [9]. That is, the primary auditory cortex and the neural structures closer to the cortex like the medial geniculate body and a portion of lower brainstem appear to be more sensitive to 16–32 Hz AM frequencies, whereas the lower brainstem structures are more responsive to >40 Hz AM frequencies. Based on this selective responsiveness of neural structures within the auditory system, we suggest that assemblies more proximal to the cortex are likely to be more susceptible to attentional effects than those more distal from the cortex. Such a differential sensitivity would result in lower modulation frequencies being the ones most likely to show an attention effect. This claim that the activity of neural structures

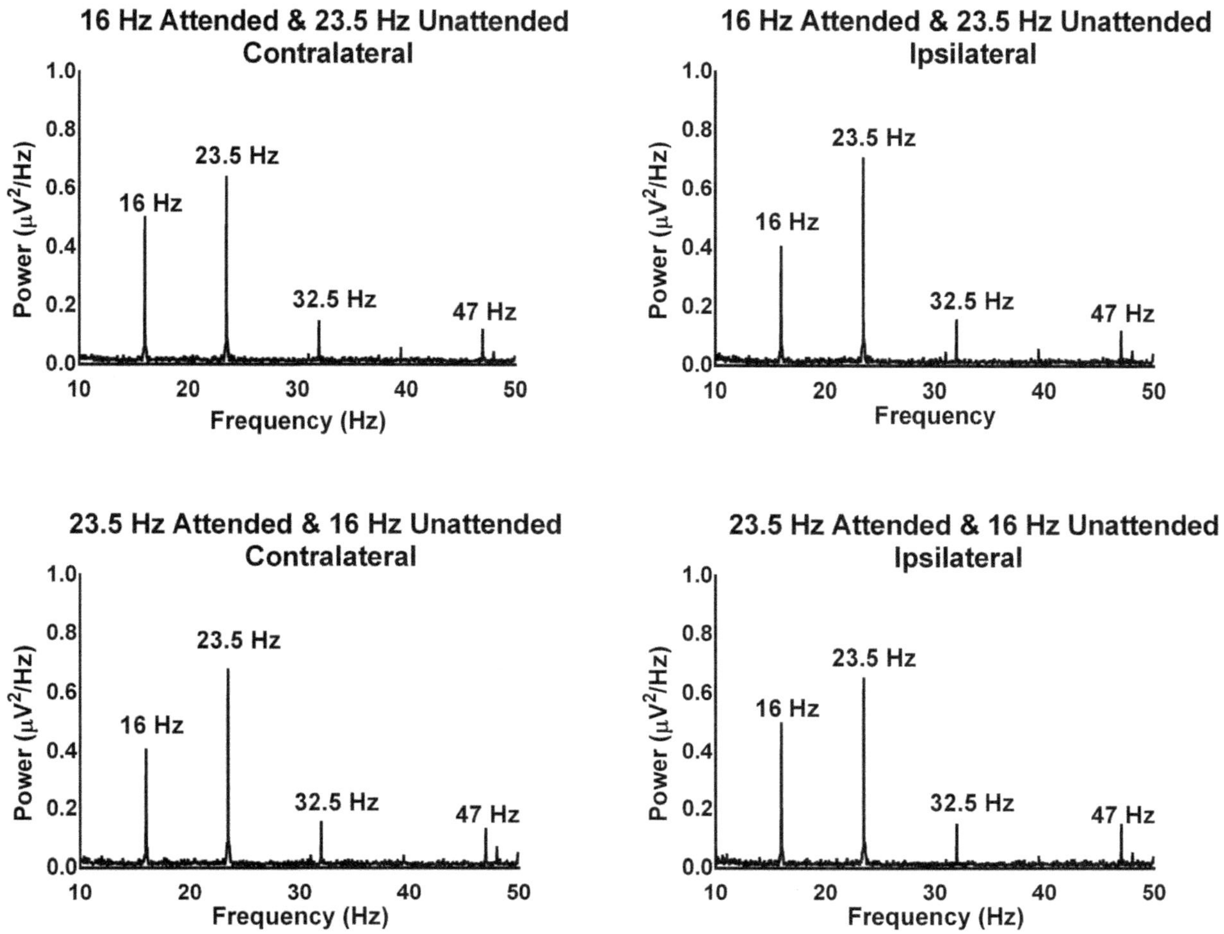

Figure 2. The grand mean FFTs for 16 and 23.5 Hz modulation frequencies during attended and unattended conditions across ipsilateral and contralateral activations combined from the two electrodes (T7 & T8). The power in the FFTs is an absolute value expressed in terms of squared microvolts per every 1 Hz of frequency (μV^2/Hz). The first harmonics for both 16 and 23.5 Hz are also shown.

higher in auditory system will be more open to attention modulation than those located down the auditory hierarchy is supported by a series of studies that have reported no effects of attention on auditory brainstem responses [1].

The results of the present study are inconsistent with the results of a number of previous studies that have found significant modulation of ASSR by attention for modulation rates between 35–45 Hz [16,17,19]. In line with the explanation proposed by Müller et al to clarify the lack of attentional modulation of 45 Hz ASSR in their study, this discrepancy might have stemmed from methodological differences between the studies. For example, Skosnik et al. found attention effects only for 45 Hz ASSR and not 20 Hz ASSR (they also used binaural stimulation of these frequencies with clicks as carrier signals in an oddball paradigm). Ross et al. used only monaural stimulation in their target detection task for 40 Hz ASSR (change in modulation frequency) and used a concurrent visual control task for unattended condition, thus involving two modalities in contrast to the present study that investigated effect of attention with in a single modality. Lastly, in a MEG study, Bharadwaj et al used rapid presentation of vowels (A, E, I, O and U) at 35 and 45 Hz spatially to the participants two ears based on his/her head related transfer functions. The task was to attend to one spatial stream and count a particular vowel in that stream and like Ross et al a visual control task was used as an unattended condition.

In the current study, there was no separate unattended control condition as we considered the modulation frequency presented opposite to the attended ear to be unattended. Furthermore, we suggest that in examining the effects of auditory selective attention on ASSR, it is important that the unattended or control condition should only involve the auditory modality. That is, a visual attention control task in an auditory selective paradigm may stimulate additional cortical areas and pathways apart from auditory ones; hence the results will not be specific to auditory stimulation alone. The differences in the stimulation pattern (binaural vs. monaural vs. dichotic), unattended conditions (visual control vs. attention switch) between previous studies [16,17,19] and the present study might indicate that the current results are specific to the experimental manipulations we used and as such do not conflict with previous results per se. In support of the idea that modulation effects might be influenced by the precise paradigm used, our paradigm was based on Müller et al's paradigm in terms of having an attention switching task between the ears and to detect a change in modulation frequencies. They also reported attention effects only for 20 Hz and not 45 Hz modulation frequencies.

As shown in Table 1, previous research found significant attentional modulation of ASSR either in left hemisphere and right ear [15,17,24] or in the right hemisphere [14]. Since the task in the current study was to detect a change in the modulation

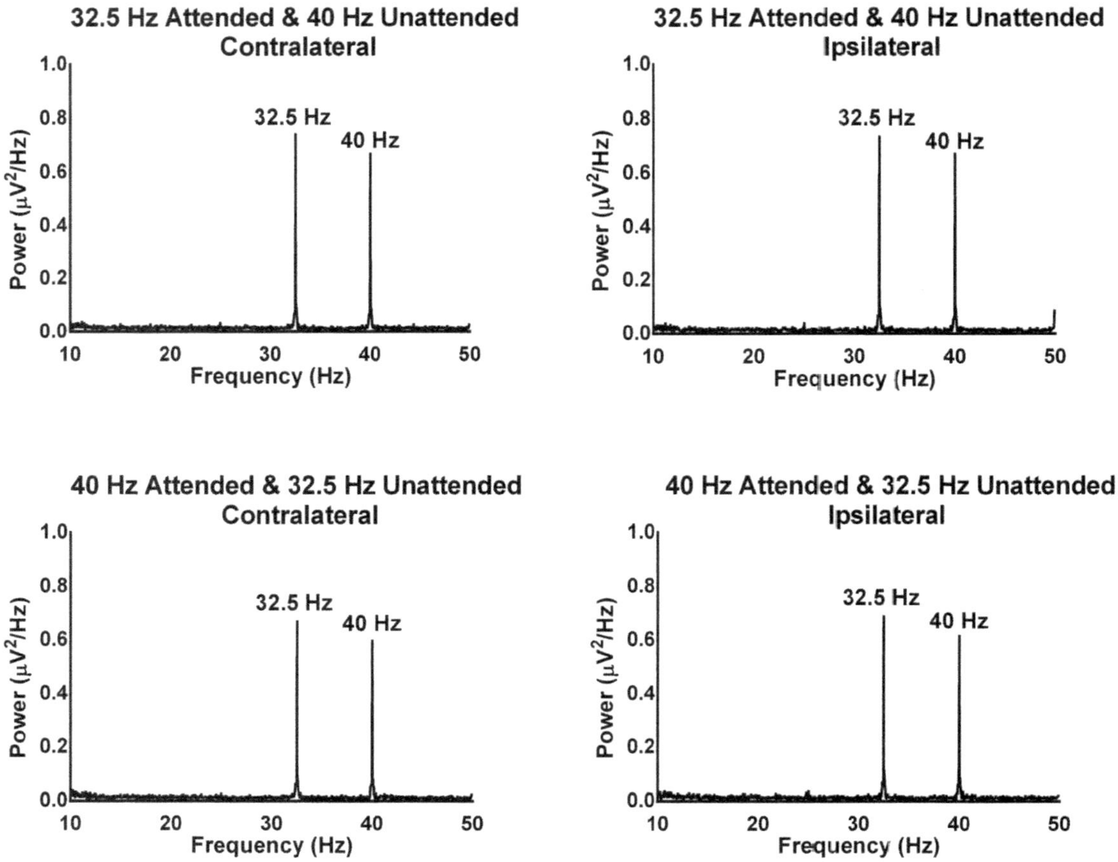

Figure 3. The grand mean FFTs for 32.5 and 40 Hz modulation frequencies during attended and unattended conditions across ipsilateral and contralateral activations combined from the two electrodes (T7 & T8). The power in the FFTs is an absolute value expressed in terms of squared microvolts per every 1 Hz of frequency ($\mu V^2/Hz$).

frequency, i.e., a change in the temporal envelope, left hemisphere laterality was expected for the attentional modulation as opposed to right hemisphere when a change in carrier frequency was to be detected (spectral change; [14]). However, the results revealed neither an ear effect nor any hemispheric laterality effect. The reason for the lack of an influence of hemispheric laterality is not clear. A notable difference between our study and previous ones is that we used white noise as a carrier signal, whereas previous studies used pure tones of different frequencies (see Table 1). We employed white noise as a carrier signal to evoke reliable, robust and larger ASSR responses since the white noise activates a larger region of the basilar membrane, which in turn provides more sensory input to higher cortical structures [25]. Except for one study [16] that used vowels as stimuli to evoke ASSR, other studies used pure tones as carrier signals and have reported attentional modulation of ASSR in either left or right hemisphere. The type of carrier signal (broadband or pure tone) or the band width of the carrier signal (large for white noise and small for pure tone) might determine the laterality of the ASSR when modulated by the attention. In line with the findings of previous studies that have showed hemispheric laterality of ASSR, it is plausible that that narrow band carrier signal when used to evoke ASSR is more likely to elicit clear hemisphere laterality during attentional modulation as compared to a broadband signal as in present study. Support to this proposal comes from a recent experiment [26] on hemispheric laterality of various auditory processing tasks such as gap detection, frequency discrimination and intensity discrimination. The results showed that no hemispheric lateralization was found for psychoacoustic thresholds obtained from these tasks with broad band stimuli whereas clear left hemisphere laterality was found for pure tones.

Additionally, it has been reported that in conventional central masking scenarios, the power of the ASSR reduces in both the hemispheres when evoked monaurally in the presence of contralaterally presented continuous white noise [27]. Applying similar principles to the results of the present study, it is possible that the continuous white noise stimulation from each ear might have reduced the power of ASSR in both hemispheres and in effect eliminated any hemispheric differences that might have been evident during attentional modulation. Though, it must be noted that this account is speculative and further systematic investigations would be needed to confirm this.

Attentional modulation of ASSR across ipsilateral and contralateral activations

It was found that attention differentially affected ASSR power as a function of ipsilateral versus contralateral stimulation. When attended, the ASSR was suppressed for ipsilateral stimulation at modulation frequencies of 16 and 23.5 Hz and enhanced for contralateral stimulation at 16 Hz (the effect for 23.5 Hz was in the enhancement direction but was not significant). In general, these results agree with those of Müller et al who also reported similar suppression and enhancement effects for 20 Hz frequency

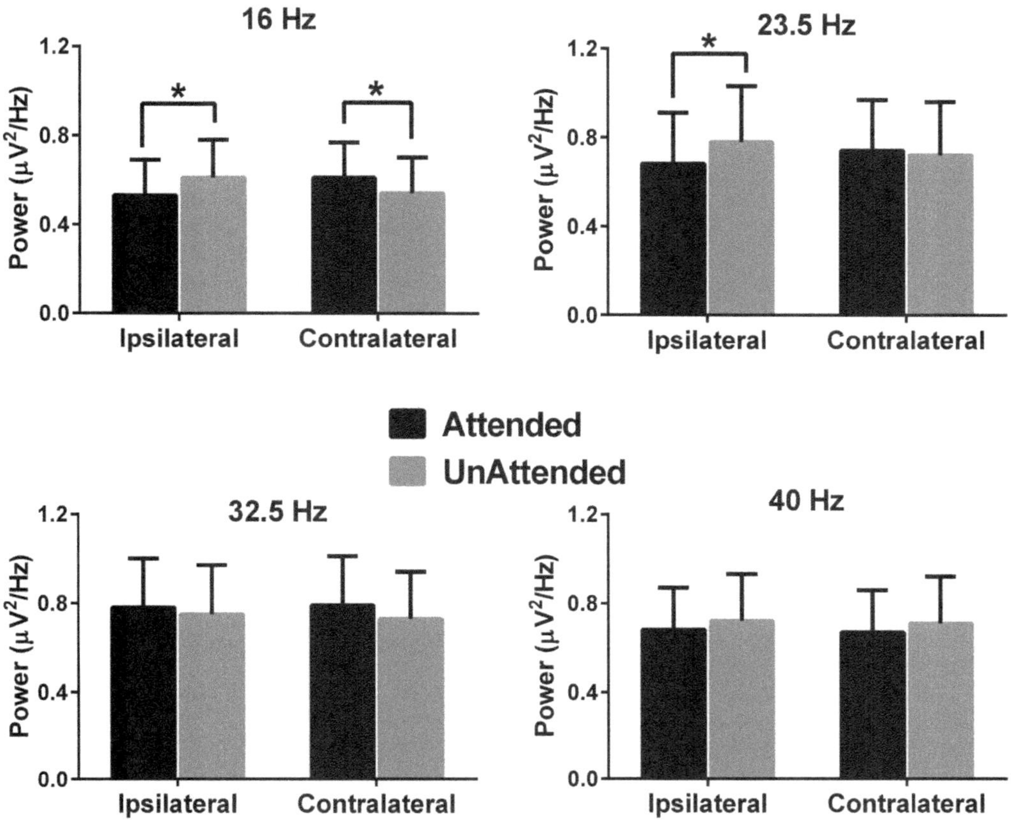

Figure 4. The bar graphs represent the absolute power measured from FFTs, when white noise was modulated with a particular modulation frequency and was attended or unattended. The bars represent neural activity from the ipsilateral and contralateral activations combined from T7 and T8 sites. An asterisk above the bar graphs indicates significant differences at $p<.05$.

for ipsilateral and contralateral stimulation, respectively and did not find any significant effects for the 45 Hz ASSR.

Müller et al. explained these findings based on an experiment by Staines et al. [28] that examined the somatosensory system and where an enhancement for contralateral and suppression for ipsilateral stimulation was found. In the study by Staines et al it was found that task relevant stimulation increased the BOLD response in the somatosensory cortex contralateral to stimulation and decreased it in the ipsilateral one. Staines et al. pointed out that this was unexpected since the suppression in the ipsilateral cortex occurred in response to task-relevant somatosensory stimulation (the task was to detect a change in frequency of vibrotactile stimulation, no matter on what side it occurred). The explanation that was given for this inhibitory effect was that, making the ipsilateral cortex less responsive would mitigate the effects that potentially conflicting inputs would have on a behaviorally relevant task. Müller et al. explained their ASSR modulation assuming that information is likely to be more relevant when processed by the contralateral mechanisms than when processed by ipsilateral ones. That is, relevant contralateral activity gets enhanced by attention whereas ipsilateral activity gets suppressed. A problem with this account is that the basis of the assumption that relevant and irrelevant stimulation map to contralateral and ipsilateral mechanisms has not been made clear. Also, the ipsilateral effect has not been found across stimulation frequencies. For example, Bhardwaj et al. found an enhancement effect for contralateral ASSR for 35 Hz and 45 Hz modulations but no ipsilateral effect for these modulation frequencies.

There are several other approaches for explaining the finding that attention leads to contralateral enhancement and ipsilateral suppression. One approach builds on two proposals that have been made about findings using dichotic listening. First, it has been reported that the dichotic listening leads to a cortical level competition between the two auditory inputs from the two ears [8,12]. This competition may lead to either summation or suppression of neural responses. Fujiki et al. [8] and Kaneko et al. [12] found suppression of ipsilateral activity in both the hemispheres during dichotic listening when compared with monaural stimulation. While there was no task associated with Fujiki et al's and Kaneko et al's frequency tagging paradigms, the listeners were attending to the stimuli. The present study which employed a task-relevant dichotic listening frequency tagging paradigm would have produced similar ipsilateral suppressive effects on ASSR power. The binaural rivalry from the two ears in response to dichotic stimulation led to the suppression of ipsilateral activity during attention. Secondly, it is well-known that during dichotic listening, there is a shift of hemispheric balance towards the hemisphere contralateral to the stimulation owing to the relatively large number of contralateral neural connections [29]. This property might have led to enhanced and larger ASSR on attention for the contralateral side during dichotic stimulation in the present study. It should be pointed out that the suppression and summation of ASSR reported for dichotic listening in Fujiki et a. [8] and Kaneko et al. [12] was with higher modulation frequencies (26, 39 & 41 Hz) than those used in present study. Given this, and the lack of ipsilateral suppression by Bhardawaj et al. [16] and that the differential effects of attention in the present study were present only for two of the four tested modulation frequencies, it would appear that attentional effects on the ASSR are complex and likely depend on the experimental procedures used to manipulate attention. We therefore suggest that our interpretation of attentional effects on ASSR based on dichotic listening should be viewed with some caution.

A slightly different explanation suggests that the pattern of enhancement and inhibition as a function of neural connectivity may be ultimately due to the anatomical arrangement and function of the inferior colliculus (IC). The IC contains EI cells (excitatory-inhibitory cells) that enhance contralateral input and suppresses the ipsilateral input [30,31]. This arrangement may influence processing at cortical regions and result in relative inhibition of ipsilateral activity and enhancement of contralateral activity. It is known that, selective attention enhances the underlying neuronal output and increases the synchronization of the local neuronal output [32]. Accordingly, during selective attention the overall neural firing of the EI cells at the level of ICs will also increase; with EI cells being excitatory and inhibitory in nature, the increased output will be inhibited at ipsilateral cortex and enhanced on the contralateral cortex. Indeed, bilateral activation at the level of ICs in an auditory selective attention task, where the participants had to selectively attend to an increasing or decreasing pitch in one ear and ignore the stimulus in the other, has been reported [33]. Rinne et al. [33] observed increased activations at the level of ICs, while attending the stimuli contralaterally than ipsilaterally. These findings suggests that on attention, the selective auditory processing at cortical level is mediated both by the increased neuronal output at the level of ICs and by the excitatory-inhibitory properties of the EI cells which alter the contralateral and ipsilateral activations at cortical level.

Conclusions

The results of the present study indicate that modulation of ASSR by selective attention: 1) depends upon the modulation frequencies used in the paradigm (with 16 and 23.5 Hz being modulated by attention). 2) Also depends upon the pattern of activation at the cortical level, with contralateral activations from either ear enhanced the ASSR and ipsilateral activations suppressed the ASSR. 3) Can be probed efficiently using a frequency tagging paradigm in which participants monitor a change in the temporal envelope.

The results of the present study contribute to the limited but emerging body of research on auditory selective attention using an ecologically valid frequency tagging scenario and also stress the importance of replication of research. Future studies may usefully look into the attentional modulation of low frequencies (3–8 Hz) to which primary and secondary auditory cortices are highly responsive. Based on current findings we would predict a significant modulation of low frequency ASSR as well. Also an experimental comparison between different carrier stimuli is required to examine the relationship between ipsilateral/contralateral activations and attention.

Supporting Information

Table S1 The ANOVA results. The significant interactions are presented in bold.

Author Contributions

Conceived and designed the experiments: YM CD JK. Performed the experiments: YM CD. Analyzed the data: YM. Contributed reagents/materials/analysis tools: YM. Wrote the paper: YM CD JK.

References

1. Giard M-H, Fort A, Mouchetant-Rostaing Y, Pernier J (2000) Neurophysiological mechanisms of auditory selective attention in humans. Front Biosci 5: d84.
2. Choi I, Rajaram S, Varghese LA, Shin-Cunningham BG (2013) Quantifying attentional modulation of auditory-evoked responses from single trial electroencephalography. Front Hum Neurosci 7: 115.
3. Hillyard SA, Hink RF, Schwent VL, Picton TW (1973) Electrical signs of selective attention in the human brain. Science 182: 177–180.
4. Woldorff MG, Gallen CC, Hampson SA, Hillyard SA, Pantev C, et al. (1993) Modulation of early sensory processing in human auditory cortex during auditory selective attention. Proc Natl Acad Sci 90: 8722–8726.
5. Michie PT, Solowij N, Crawford JM, Glue LC (1993) The effects of between-source discriminability on attended and unattended auditory ERPs. Psychophysiology 30: 205–220.
6. Reagan D (1989) Human brain electrophysiology: Evoked potentials and evoked magenetic fields in science and medicine. New York: Elsevier. 546 p.
7. Picton TW, John MS, Dimitrijevic A, Purcell D (2003) Human auditory steady-state responses. Int J Audiol 42: 177–219.
8. Fujiki N, Jousmaki V, Hari R (2002) Neuromagnetic responses to frequency-tagged sounds: a new method to follow inputs from each ear to the human auditory cortex during binaural hearing. J Neuroscience 22: RC205.
9. Giraud A-L, Lorenzi C, Ashburner J, Wable J, Johnsrude I, et al. (2000) Representation of the temporal envelope of sounds in the human brain. J Neurophysiol 84: 1588–1598.
10. Liégeois-Chauvel C, Lorenzi C, Trébuchon A, Régis J, Chauvel P (2004) Temporal envelope processing in the human left and right auditory cortices. Cereb Cortex 14: 731–740.
11. Miller LM, Escabi MA, Read HL, Schreiner CE (2002) Spectrotemporal receptive fields in the lemniscal auditory thalamus and cortex. J Neurophysiol 87: 516–527.
12. Kaneko K, Fujiki N, Hari R (2003) Binaural interaction in the human auditory cortex revealed by neuromagnetic frequency tagging: no effect of stimulus intensity. Hear Res 183: 1–6.
13. Linden DR, Picton TW, Gilles H, Kenneth BC (1987) Human auditory steady-state evoked potentials during selective attention. Electroenceph Clin Neurophysiol 66: 145–159.
14. Lazzouni L, Ross B, Voss P, Lepore F (2010) Neuromagnetic auditory steady-state responses to amplitude modulated sounds following dichotic or monaural presentation. Clin Neurophysiol 121: 200–207.
15. Müller N, Schlee W, Hartmann T, Lorenz I, Weisz N (2009) Top-down modulation of the auditory steady-state response in a task-switch paradigm. Front Hum Neurosci 3:1
16. Bharadwaj HM, Lee AKC, Shin-Cunningham BG (2014) Measuring auditory selective attention using frequency tagging. Front Integr Neurosci 8: 1.
17. Ross B, Picton T, Herdman A, Pantev C (2004) The effect of attention on the auditory steady-state response. Neurol Clin Neurophysiol 22–22.
18. Evans E (1982) Functions of the auditory system. In: Barlow HB, Mollon, JD, editors. The senses. Cambridge: Cambridge University Press. p.239.
19. Skosnik PD, Krishnan GP, O'Donnell BF (2007) The effect of selective attention on the gamma-band auditory steady-state response. Neuroscie Lett 420: 223–228.
20. John MS, Dimitrijevic A, Picton TW (2003) Efficient stimuloi for evoking auditory steady-state responses. Ear Hear 24: 406–423.
21. Mahajan Y, McArthur G (2010) Does combing the scalp reduce scalp electrode impedances? J Neurosci Meth 188: 287–289.
22. Oostenveld R, Praamstra P (2001) The five percent electrode system for high-resolution EEG and ERP measurements. Clin Neurophysiol 112: 713–719.
23. Delorme A, Makeig S (2004) EEGLAB: an open source toolbox for analysis of single-trial EEG dynamics including independent component analysis. J Neurosci Meth 134: 9–21.
24. Bidet-Caulet A, Fischer C, Besle J, Aguera PE, Giard MH, et al. (2007) Effects of selective attention on the electrophysiological representation of concurrent sounds in the human auditory cortex. J Neurosci 27: 9252–9261.
25. Ross B (2014) Steady-state auditory evoked responses. In: Celesia GG, editor. Handbook of clinical neurophysiology: Disorders of peripheral and central auditory processing. Amsterdam: Elsevier. 10: pp. 137–154.
26. Sininger YS, Bhatara A (2012). Laterality of basic auditory perception. Laterality 17: 129–149.
27. Kawase T, Maki A, Kanno A, Nakasato N, Sato M, et al. (2012) Contralateral white noise attenuates 40-Hz auditory steady-state fields but not N100m in auditory evoked fields. Neuroimage 59: 1037–1042.
28. Staines WR, Graham SJ, Black SE, McIlroy WE (2002) Task-relevant modulation of contralateral and ipsilateral primary somatosensory cortex and the role of a prefrontal-cortical sensory gating system. Neuroimage 15: 190–199.
29. Hugdalh K, Westerhausen R, Alho K, Medvedev S, Laine M, Hämäläinen H (2009) Attention and cognitive control: unfolding the dichotic listening story. Scand J Psychol 50: 11–22.

30. Sanes DH, Malone BJ, Semple MN (1998) Role of synaptic inhibition in processing of dynamic binaural level stimuli. J Neurosci 18: 794–803.
31. Xiong XR, Liang F, Li H, Mesik L, Zhang KK, et al. (2013) Interaural level difference-dependent gain control and synaptic scaling underlying binaural computation. Neuron 79: 738–753.
32. Womelsdorf T, Fries P (2007) The role of neuronal synchronization in selective attention. Curr Opin Neurobiol 17: 154–160.
33. Rinne T, Balk MH, Koistinen S, Autti T, Alho K, Sams M (2008) Auditory selective attention modulates activation of human inferior colliculus. J Neurophysiol 100: 3323–3327.

Reduced Neural Integration of Letters and Speech Sounds in Dyslexic Children Scales with Individual Differences in Reading Fluency

Gojko Žarić[1,2]*, Gorka Fraga González[3,5], Jurgen Tijms[3,4,5], Maurits W. van der Molen[3,5,6], Leo Blomert[1,2]†, Milene Bonte[1,2]

1 Department of Cognitive Neuroscience, Faculty of Psychology and Neuroscience, University of Maastricht, Maastricht, Netherlands, **2** Maastricht Brain Imaging Center (M-BIC), Maastricht, Netherlands, **3** Department of Psychology, University of Amsterdam, Amsterdam, Netherlands, **4** IWAL Institute for Dyslexia, Amsterdam, Netherlands, **5** Rudolf Berlin Center, Amsterdam, Netherlands, **6** Amsterdam Brain and Cognition, University of Amsterdam, Amsterdam, Netherlands

Abstract

The acquisition of letter-speech sound associations is one of the basic requirements for fluent reading acquisition and its failure may contribute to reading difficulties in developmental dyslexia. Here we investigated event-related potential (ERP) measures of letter-speech sound integration in 9-year-old typical and dyslexic readers and specifically test their relation to individual differences in reading fluency. We employed an audiovisual oddball paradigm in typical readers (n = 20), dysfluent (n = 18) and severely dysfluent (n = 18) dyslexic children. In one auditory and two audiovisual conditions the Dutch spoken vowels/a/and/o/were presented as standard and deviant stimuli. In audiovisual blocks, the letter 'a' was presented either simultaneously (AV0), or 200 ms before (AV200) vowel sound onset. Across the three children groups, vowel deviancy in auditory blocks elicited comparable mismatch negativity (MMN) and late negativity (LN) responses. In typical readers, both audiovisual conditions (AV0 and AV200) led to enhanced MMN and LN amplitudes. In both dyslexic groups, the audiovisual LN effects were mildly reduced. Most interestingly, individual differences in reading fluency were correlated with MMN latency in the AV0 condition. A further analysis revealed that this effect was driven by a short-lived MMN effect encompassing only the N1 window in severely dysfluent dyslexics versus a longer MMN effect encompassing both the N1 and P2 windows in the other two groups. Our results confirm and extend previous findings in dyslexic children by demonstrating a deficient pattern of letter-speech sound integration depending on the level of reading dysfluency. These findings underscore the importance of considering individual differences across the entire spectrum of reading skills in addition to group differences between typical and dyslexic readers.

Editor: Sonja Kotz, Max Planck Institute for Human Cognitive and Brain Sciences, Germany

Funding: This project is funded by the Netherlands Initiative Brain and Cognition, a program of the Organization for Scientific Research (NWO), as a part of the "Fluent reading neurocognitively decomposed: The case of dyslexia - HCMI 10-59" research program under grant number 056-14-015. http://www.nwo.nl/en/research-and-results/research-projects/97/2300163097.html. The funders had no role in study design, data collection and analysis, decision to publish, or preparation of the manuscript.

Competing Interests: The authors have declared that no competing interests exist.

* Email: gojko.zaric@maastrichtuniversity.nl

† Deceased.

Introduction

Though many children learn to read without any problems, 5% to 10% of children are affected by developmental dyslexia and never acquire proficient reading skills despite normal cognitive abilities and schooling opportunities [1,2]. A lack of reading fluency has been pinpointed as the most persistent and impaired characteristic of developmental dyslexia [3], although studies also show a large inter-individual variability in the level of reading (dys)fluency [4,5]. A first important step in obtaining reading fluency in alphabetic orthographies, the formation of solid letter-speech sound correspondences, poses an immediate hurdle for beginning dyslexic readers [6–9]. Accordingly, in addition to tackling well-known difficulties in phonological processing, i.e. recognizing and manipulating the sound structure of language [10,11], many dyslexia interventions contain a condition focused on teaching letter-speech sound correspondences [12–14]. In recent years, the neurofunctional basis of the difficulties in building these correspondences has been elucidated by neuroimaging findings showing reduced neural integration of letters and speech sounds in dyslexic children [15–17] and adults [18]. How this reduced neural integration scales with individual differences in the level of reading (dys)fluency remains an interesting and open question.

In largely transparent languages, accurate letter-speech sound identification and discrimination is typically observed after one year of reading instruction [19]. However, evidence from neuroimaging studies shows a dissociation between knowing which letters belong to which speech sounds and the automatic neural integration of these associations, with the latter showing a much more protracted period of incremental learning throughout primary school in typical readers [20,21]. One of the first studies in this domain recorded magnetoencephalography (MEG) in literate Finnish adults and indicated a dynamic process of letter-speech sound integration with audiovisual convergence starting around 225 ms in bilateral temporal cortices [22]. Subsequent functional magnetic resonance imaging (fMRI) evidence revealed the involvement of the superior temporal sulcus, as well as auditory cortex (superior temporal gyrus/planum temporale) [23]. More specifically, results indicated a modulating influence of letters on speech sounds as a consequence of feedback from the superior temporal sulcus to the superior temporal gyrus, but only if the letter and speech sound were presented simultaneously and in a passive listening paradigm [23–25].

Evidence for the protracted developmental time-course of letter-speech sound integration comes from a series of studies measuring electroencephalography (EEG) responses in a passive crossmodal "oddball" paradigm [16,21,26]. In an oddball paradigm, at a latency of 100–200 ms, a mismatch negativity (MMN) response is elicited by a rare sound (deviant, or oddball) that is presented in a sequence of frequent (standard) sounds [27]. The MMN represents an automatic change detection response sensitive to deviation from traces in auditory short-term memory [27,28]. Multiple experiments have shown that the MMN is sensitive to language-specific speech sounds in adults and in children [27,29–37], as well as to audiovisual integration [21,26,38–42]. Furthermore, in school-aged children the speech evoked MMN response may be followed by an additional late negativity (Late MMN or LN) in a broader time window from 300 to 700 ms, the amplitude of which decreases in adulthood [43–45], suggesting fast and automatic discrimination and representation of speech syllables in adults while the developing brain still needs additional processing resources to reach to the same result. In the paradigm of Froyen and colleagues [16,21,26], in an auditory and two audiovisual experimental blocks, the Dutch speech sound/a/was presented as the standard stimulus, and the Dutch speech sound/o/as the deviant stimulus. In the audiovisual blocks, the letter 'a' was presented together with the standard and deviant speech sounds, leading to a double violation: the deviant speech sound/o/violated the expectation built by both the standard speech sound/a/and the letter 'a'. In order to investigate the temporal window of integration the letter 'a' was presented either simultaneously, or 200 ms before speech sound onset. Due to the double violation, literate adults showed a significant enhancement of the MMN response in the audiovisual as compared to auditory blocks, but, reminiscent of the fMRI findings [23–25], only when letters and speech sounds were presented simultaneously, indicating an early and automatic audiovisual integration [26]. Using the same paradigm, 8 year-old typically reading children after one year of reading instruction only showed a significant audiovisual enhancement of a late negativity (LN) evoked around 650 ms after speech sound onset and only when the letter preceded the speech sound, indicating a slow and immature neural integration of letters and speech sounds [21]. A more developed, bit still not adult-like pattern was apparent in 11 year-old typically reading children after four years of reading instruction. That is, these more advanced readers showed a cross-modal enhancement of the earlier MMN when the letter preceded the speech sound, and a cross-modal LN enhancement when the letter and speech sound were presented simultaneously [21]. Although adults did not show these late letter effects in this passive paradigm using simple speech stimuli [26], orthographic influences on spoken language processing around 400–700 ms have been reported in adults when using a more complex metaphonological task [46,47]. Thus, whereas the observed cross-modal MMN enhancement may be a neurophysiological marker of initial and automatic letter-speech sound integration and/or representation [27,28]), the crossmodal LN enhancement may reflect more elaborate, explicit associative processes that, in children but not in adults, are recruited for the integration of simple letter-speech pairs.

The same crossmodal MMN paradigm [16,21,26], was used in 11 year-old dyslexic children after 4 years of reading instruction, and indicated reduced integration of letters and speech sounds, with significant letter effects only in the late LN window [16]. Further evidence for a reduced sensitivity to letter-speech sound associations in dyslexia comes from fMRI studies showing an underactivation of superior temporal cortex during letter-speech sound integration in 9-year-old dyslexic children [15] and adults [18], as well as from the absence of a crossmodal MMN enhancement for spoken-written syllable pairs in dyslexic adults [41]. Similarly, recent studies suggest reduced orthographic-phonological integration in dyslexics on word reading tasks [48–51].

In the current study, we investigate EEG measures of letter-speech sound integration in 9-year-old typical and dyslexic readers and specifically test whether they scale with behavioral measures of reading fluency and reading-related skills. To this end we employ an adapted version of the audiovisual paradigm of Froyen and colleagues [16] in typical readers ($n = 20$) and age-matched dyslexic children ($n = 36$) with variable levels of reading (dys)-fluency. By focusing on 9-year old children, we extend previous ERP findings to a different age group, 2.5 years after reading instruction, intermediate between the previously studied age groups, namely typical readers with 1 or 4 years of reading instruction [21] and dyslexic readers with 4 years of reading instruction [16]. This age range also coincides with the age of participants from a previous fMRI study reporting reduced neural letter-speech sound integration in dyslexics, as well as correlations between these neural measures and behavioral reading scores [15], allowing us to further investigate the same processes with a different technique at the same level of development. As the morphology, amplitude and timing of ERP components are known to be age dependent [52–56], we chose to use a chronologically age matched control group, rather than a reading age matched control group. Finally, including a larger group of dyslexic children with variable levels of reading fluency, allowed us to demonstrate brain-behavior relations not only across typical and dyslexic readers but also to show interindividual differences within the group of dyslexic readers.

Methods

Participants

In total, 61 children (41 dyslexic and 20 typical readers) participated in the EEG experiment. All children were 3rd graders, native Dutch speakers, having received 2.5 years of reading instruction. Data of 56 children were included in the analysis, including 36 dyslexic readers (9.0 years old, range: 8.2–9.9; 16 girls; 6 left-handed, as assessed by an adapted version of Annett's handedness questionnaire [57], and 20 age-matched typical readers (8.8 years old range: 8.3–9.5; 12 girls; 2 left-handed). Data of five children with dyslexia were discarded, 4 children did not complete the EEG measurement and 1 child moved excessively during the EEG measurement.

Dyslexic children were recruited from a specialized institute for dyslexia and reading problems. Prior to the present study, they were diagnosed as dyslexic after an extensive cognitive psycho-diagnostic procedure by the institute. Each of the dyslexic children scored in the lowest 10 percentile of the age appropriate group on standard reading tests (see below). Other behavioral scores such as phonological skills or rapid automatized naming (RAN), were not included as selection criteria. Typical readers had reading score percentile of 25 or higher and were recruited from 3rd grades of primary schools in the same area and had similar social-demographic characteristics. All children had a normal hearing and normal or corrected to normal vision, as reported by parents. Comorbidity with behavioral and/or attention disorders was assessed with the Child Behavior Checklist (CBCL) from the Achenbach system of empirically based assessment (ASEBA) [58] which was completed by the parents, and used as an exclusion criterion. Children with below average IQ were also excluded from the experiment. Written informed consent was obtained from the parents of each child. Each child received a small present after the experiment and travel costs were reimbursed. The approval for the research was obtained from a local ethical committee of the Developmental Psychology department of the University of Amsterdam.

Behavioral tests

Prior to the EEG measurements, each of the children performed standard language tests including the word reading, spelling, letter-speech sound identification, letter-speech sound discrimination, rapid automized naming (RAN) and basic reaction time subtests of the 3DM battery (Dyslexia Differential Diagnosis; 3DM, [19], as well as a one-minute word reading test (EMT) [59], and reading of a short story 'De kat' ('The cat') [60]. In addition, we used a paper and pencil version of the RAVEN Coloured Progressive Matrices to assess non-verbal IQ scores (RAVEN CPM) [61]. We performed a median split of the 36 dyslexic children based on their fluency score to form groups of dysfluent dyslexic readers (n = 18) and severely dysfluent dyslexic readers (n = 18) (for similar approaches see [62–64]). Because our three individual word reading fluency measures were highly correlated ($r > .919$), reading fluency was quantified using a composite score of the 3DM word reading tests, the EMT, and "De Kat". Subject characteristics and the results of the behavioral tests are shown in Table 1. Group differences were tested using one way ANOVAs for each of the pairwise group comparisons and are reported in the Results section.

Stimuli

The stimuli were the same as in Froyen et al. [16,21,26] including auditory stimuli consisting of the Dutch vowels/a/and/o/spoken by a native Dutch female speaker. The vowels were digitally recorded (sampling rate 44.1 kHz, 16 bit quantization), band-pass filtered (180–10.000 Hz), resampled at 22.05 kHz and matched for loudness with Praat software [65]. Phoneme duration was 384 ms for vowel/a/and 348 ms for vowel/o/. Vowels were presented binaurally through headphones at a comfortable listening level of ~65dB as measured with an analog loudness meter. The visual stimulus was a white, lower case letter "a", presented in size 40 "Arial" font in the center of a computer screen with a black background. The stimuli were presented using Presentation 14.4 (Neurobehavioral Systems, Inc., Albany, CA).

Experimental Design

In one auditory and two audiovisual oddball paradigms, we presented the vowel/a/as the standard (83%) and the vowel/o/as the deviant (17%) stimulus. In the auditory condition participants listened to the vowels while watching silent movies. In the two audiovisual conditions, the presentation of the standard or deviant vowel was paired with a white letter "a", presented for 500 ms at the center of a black computer screen. Between the successive letter presentations a white fixation cross appeared in the same location. Both auditory and audiovisual trials had a trial length of 1700 ms. The two audiovisual conditions differed in the stimulus onset asynchrony (SOA) between letter and vowel presentation. In the first audiovisual condition (AV0), the letter and vowel appeared simultaneously, and in the second audiovisual condition (AV200), the letter appeared 200 ms before the vowel. During the audiovisual conditions, participants performed a simple visual target detection task to ensure fixation on the screen. The visual target consisted of a color picture of a wrapped present, which was presented instead of the letter in 3,5% of the trials (10 trials per block) and required a button press. This paradigm was the same as the one used in Froyen et al., [16,21,26] except for the following two changes. First, the trial length was increased from 1250 ms to 1700 ms because the experiment was part of a larger study involving coherence analysis at lower frequencies. Second, in order to obtain sufficient deviant trials within 76 minutes of measurement time, the number of deviants was increased from 10% to 17%, a percentage that was previously shown to lead to reliable mismatch responses [29,66]. Participants performed three blocks of each condition, each block consisting of 288 trials. Per condition a total of 150 deviant and 714 standard trials were presented. Standards and deviants were presented in pseudo-random order: two successive deviants were required to be separated by at least three standards, and deviants could not be one of the first two trials of a block. The blocks of the same condition were presented in consecutive fashion, the order of the conditions was pseudorandomized and counterbalanced, with one of the cross-modal conditions always being presented first.

EEG data recording and analysis

EEG data were recorded at a 1024 Hz sampling rate and a DC-104 Hz recording bandwidth using the Biosemi Active Two system (Biosemi, Amsterdam, Netherlands). EEG was measured from 64 active-channels, placed according to the 10–20 international system (Electro-cap International Inc., with CMS and DRL electrodes at the approximate locations of PO1 and PO2), and the CMS was used as a recording reference. Eye-movements were measured using 4 additional Flat-Type Active electrodes, 2 were placed below and above left eye and 2 at the outer canthi of each eye. In addition 2 electrodes were placed on the right and left mastoids and used for offline re-referencing. The offset range of the electrodes was kept between −20 mV and 20 mV.

For the analysis we discarded the first 2 trials of each block, as well as the first epoch after each deviant and, in the audiovisual conditions, the first 2 epochs after catch trials to account for possible movement artifacts due to button presses [67]. Per participant, we included data of the 150 deviant trials and of 150 standard trials chosen randomly from the pool of 480 standard trials. Data were analyzed using the v11.0.0b EEGLAB toolbox [68](http://www.sccn.ucsd.edu/eeglab) and custom Matlab scripts (MATLAB 2011b, The MathWorks, Natick, MA). EEG data pre-processing included offline rereferencing to the average of the left and right mastoids, applying a bandpass filter of 1–70 Hz and downsampling to 256 Hz. The EEG data was epoched from −500 ms to 1200 ms with respect to the auditory (Auditory and AV0 condition) or visual (AV200) stimulus and baseline corrected with respect to the mean signal in the 500 ms baseline period. Removal of artifacts was performed in two steps. First, the data were visually inspected and epochs containing non-stereotypical artifacts including high amplitude, high-frequency muscle noise,

Table 1. Behavioral reading scores: Descriptive data and statistical group comparisons for typical readers, dysfluent and severely dysfluent dyslexic readers.

	Typical Readers		**Dysfluent Readers**		**Severely Dysfluent Readers**							
N	20		18		18							
Age	8.80±0.38		8.99±0.46		9.01±0.41		F(2,53) = 1.50 p = .233					
Sex ratio (m:f)	8:12		9:9		11:7							
Handedness (L:R)	2:18		3:15		3:15		Typical and Dysfluent		Typical and Severely Dysfluent		Dysfluent and Severely Dysfluent	
	M	**SD**	**M**	**SD**	**M**	**SD**	**F(1,36)***	**p**	**F(1,36)**	**p**	**F(1,34)***	**p**
Word reading - *accuracy [%]* [a]												
3DM High Frequency Words - HF	99.12	1.12	95.84	3.84	90.97	6.60	13.28	**.001**	29.56	**.000**	7.31	**.011**
3DM Low Frequency Words - LF	97.25	3.23	94.58	4.30	76.33	15.31	4.72	**.036**	35.67	**.000**	23.71	**.000**
3DM Pseudowords - PW	87.37	9.65	77.27	15.26	64.80	16.07	6.07	**.019**	28.19	**.000**	5.70	**.023**
3DM Total Word Accuracy *[T]* [b]	49.50	9.06	39.44	9.08	25.67	8.83	11.65	**.002**	67.15	**.000**	21.29	**.000**
Word reading – *fluency*												
3DM HF*[T]*	52.95	7.58	34.44	3.45	26.94	4.28	90.16	**.000**	164.29	**.000**	33.53	**.000**
3DM LF*[T]*	54.65	9.02	35.89	2.54	26.17	4.26	72.56	**.000**	149.32	**.000**	69.15	**.000**
3 DM PW *[T]*	53.00	9.44	33.78	5.43	26.83	4.42	57.41	**.000**	115.23	**.000**	17.70	**.001**
3DM Total Word Fluency *[T]*	53.95	9.34	33.83	2.41	26.17	3.96	78.62	**.000**	136.87	**.000**	39.28	**.000**
One minute test - EMT *[C]* [c]	6.05	1.76	2.61	.61	1.56	.70	61.83	**.000**	102.22	**.000**	23.16	**.000**
Story reading – *fluency*												
'De Kat' *[T]*	54.70	8.04	36.33	2.20	29.39	5.72	87.81	**.000**	122.44	**.000**	23.12	**.000**
Letter –speech sound coupling *[T]*												
3DM Spelling – *accuracy*	50.60	9.14	35.89	5.96	34.22	7.45	33.66	**.000**	36.13	**.000**	.55	.464
3DM Spelling – *RT*	54.55	8.70	39.11	6.99	38.22	8.17	35.83	**.000**	35.35	**.000**	.12	.728
L-SS identification - *accuracy*	46.95	7.70	42.94	11.63	40.11	12.24	1.60	.214	4.34	**.044**	.51	.481
L-SS discrimination - *accuracy*	50.20	9.25	46.06	8.96	41.00	8.39	1.89	.177	10.23	**.003**	2.98	.094
L-SS identification – *RT*	52.80	7.08	45.00	7.39	42.56	8.08	11.03	**.002**	17.35	**.000**	.90	.350
L-SS discrimination - *RT*	51.10	8.01	46.76	9.71	49.28	9.05	2.22	.145	.43	.514	.63	.434
Phoneme deletion – *accuracy [T]*	52.70	7.63	41.94	7.18	36.89	8.04	19.28	**.000**	38.69	**.000**	3.83	.059
Rapid naming (RAN) *[T]*												
Letters	50.05	7.13	41.35	6.53	34.28	7.34	14.77	**.000**	45.12	**.000**	9.04	**.005**
Digits	50.65	10.92	40.94	6.04	35.11	8.89	10.64	**.002**	22.81	**.000**	5.09	**.031**
Pictures	49.95	7.27	40.41	7.68	41.11	12.53	15.01	**.000**	7.26	**.011**	.04	.845
RAN Total	49.85	9.91	38.76	6.86	32.83	9.15	20.36	**.000**	37.82	**.000**	4.67	**.038**
Basic reaction time *[T]*	60.70	9.61	62.29	7.70	66.95	10.69	.302	.586	3.59	.066	2.16	.151
Raven matrices *[C]*	7.04	1.49	6.81	1.68	7.34	1.25	.21	.651	.46	.503	1.19	.282

[a]Raw scores b T scores (M = 50, SD = 10) c C scores (M = 5, SD = 2).
* For RAN, basic reaction time, phoneme deletion and L-SS discrimination degrees of freedom were: F(1,35) and F(1,33) as data for one subject was missing.

swallowing and electrode cable movements, were rejected. Secondly, stereotypical artifacts, including eye movements, eye blinks and heart beat artifacts were corrected with extended INFOMAX ICA [69] as implemented in EEGLAB. ICA was performed on 64 scalp channels resulting in 64 components per condition per participant which were classified as EEG or artificial activity based on scalp topography, time course and power-frequency spectra [70]. Single electrodes containing high amplitude noise were interpolated using spherical interpolation after the data was reconstructed. Component activations representing non-brain artifacts were removed, and EEG data were reconstructed from the remaining component activations representing brain activity. In typical readers, the reconstructed data was based on a mean (SD) number of 41 (4) components per subject in the auditory condition, 47 (4) in the Av0 condition and 44 (5) in the Av200 condition. The number of EEG components in the two subgroups of dyslexic children corresponded to - dysfluent dyslexics: 43 (4) components per subject in the auditory condition, 48 (4) in the Av0 condition and 46 (4) in the Av200 condition; severely dysfluent dyslexics: 42 (8) components per subject in the auditory condition, 45 (7) in the Av0 condition and 44 (7) in the Av200 condition. The reconstructed data was baseline corrected and low pass filtered at 30 Hz.

Event related potentials (ERPs) were obtained by averaging the epochs per stimulus per condition for each participant separately. In typical readers, the mean (SD) number of epochs included in the averages for the standards and deviants corresponded to 149 (1) and 149 (1) in the auditory condition, 148 (2) and 149 (2) in the AV0 condition and 148 (2) and 149 (1) in the AV200 condition. In dysfluent dyslexics these values were 149 (1) and 148 (2) in the auditory condition, 148 (2) and 148 (2) in the AV0 condition and 148 (2) and 148 (2) in the AV200 condition. Lastly, in severely dysfluent these values were 148 (5) and 148 (5) in the auditory condition, 148 (2) and 148 (2) in the AV0 condition and 148 (2) and 147 (3) in the AV200 condition.

We evaluated the presence of the mismatch negativity (MMN) and late negativity (LN) by analyzing ERPs evoked by standard and deviant stimuli in the auditory and both audiovisual conditions, in each of our subject groups. As maximal cross-modal effects were expected across fronto-central electrodes [16,21], analysis was performed on four fronto-central sites (Fz, Cz, FC3, FC4). The timing of the MMN and LN responses was measured by determining individual peak latencies within their respective time windows: (1) 100 to 250 ms for the MMN and (2) 600 ms–750 ms for the LN [16,21]. The amplitude of the MMN and LN responses was measured by determining the mean amplitude in the 50 ms around the individual peak latencies. We first applied mixed model ANOVAs with stimulus (2 levels: standard and deviant), condition (3 levels: Au, Av0, Av200) and electrode (4 levels) as within subjects factors and group (3 levels: typical, dysfluent dyslexic and severely dysfluent dyslexic readers) as between subjects factor. Because MMN and LN responses were detected in all conditions and all subject groups, we subsequently performed our analyses of crossmodal letter effects on the difference waves obtained by subtracting the ERPs evoked by standards from those of deviants. MMN/LN amplitude and latency measures were analyzed using mixed model ANOVAs on pairs of conditions (Au-Av0; Au-Av200) and electrode (4 levels: Fz, Cz, FC3, FC4) as within subject factors. We report Greenhouse-Geisser corrected p-values. In a further analysis, we separately analyzed the N1 and P2 responses to standard and deviant stimuli to investigate the relation between the crossmodal MMN effects and these event-related responses. N1 and P2 amplitudes were statistically assessed using repeated measures ANOVAs with Stimulus (2 levels: standard, deviant) and Electrode (4 levels: Fz, Cz, FC3, FC4) as within subject factors.

We used linear regression to investigate the relation between individual differences in ERP correlates of letter-sound associations and behavioral measures of reading fluency and related skills. ERP measures consisted of (1) MMN latency in the two audiovisual (AV0 and AV200) conditions, and (2) the MMN and LN letter-effect in the two audiovisual conditions (i.e. the MMN/LN amplitude enhancement in the audiovisual as compared to auditory conditions, [16,21,26]). For linear regression, ERP measures were quantified using composite scores across 4 fronto-central electrodes (Fz, Cz, FC3 and FC4). Our selection of behavioral measures of interest was based on (1) our research aim, i.e. to test the relation between reading fluency and cross-modal ERP measures, and (2) results of a large-scale study in Dutch, Hungarian and Portuguese school children in which factor analysis of test scores on 3DM subtests identified verbal working memory, phonemic awareness, RAN, letter-speech sound accuracy and letter-speech sound speed as separate factors [71]. Thus, reading fluency, was quantified using a composite score of the 3DM word reading tests, the EMT, and "De Kat". Furthermore, the other behavioral measures included reading accuracy (3DM), letter-speech sound coupling accuracy (spelling, letter-speech sound identification and discrimination, $r > .406$) and speed (spelling, letter-speech sound identification and discrimination, $r > .391$), phonological awareness (3DM phoneme deletion accuracy) and rapid auditory naming (3DM RAN total score). We employed simple linear regressions with one of the ERP measures as a predictor and one of the behavioral composite scores as a dependent variable to probe relations of each ERP measure specifically to the behavior. As we conducted several linear regressions, i.e. 12 for latencies and 24 for amplitudes, once for all the children and once only for dyslexics, we accounted for multiple comparisons by using FDR corrections [72] and report p values relative to obtained q(FDR) thresholds.

Results

Behavioral tests: Typical readers, Dysfluent and Severely Dysfluent Dyslexic readers

The dyslexic readers were divided into a dysfluent and a severely dysfluent group, using a median split based on their reading fluency scores (see Methods). A comparison of behavioral test scores showed significantly lower scores for severely dysfluent as compared to dysfluent dyslexics on all word reading tests (fluency as well as accuracy), as well as on rapid automatized naming (Table 1). The dyslexic subgroups did not significantly differ on any of the other behavioral tests. Both dyslexic groups scored significantly lower than typical readers on all language tests with the exception of the accuracy of letter-speech sound discrimination and identification (comparable in dysfluent and typical readers) and the speed of letter-speech sound discrimination (comparable in all three groups). Non-verbal IQ and speed of processing (reaction times) were comparable across the three groups.

Auditory MMN and LN effects

Because these measures served as a baseline for assessing cross-modal enhancement effects, we first analyzed the MMN and LN responses evoked in the auditory condition. In each of the three subject groups, the deviant elicited a comparable auditory MMN, with the expected fronto-central topographical distribution (Figures 1 and 2). Comparable MMN responses lead to a main effect of Stimulus ($F(1, 53) = 105.26$, $p = .000$, $\eta^2 = .665$), without

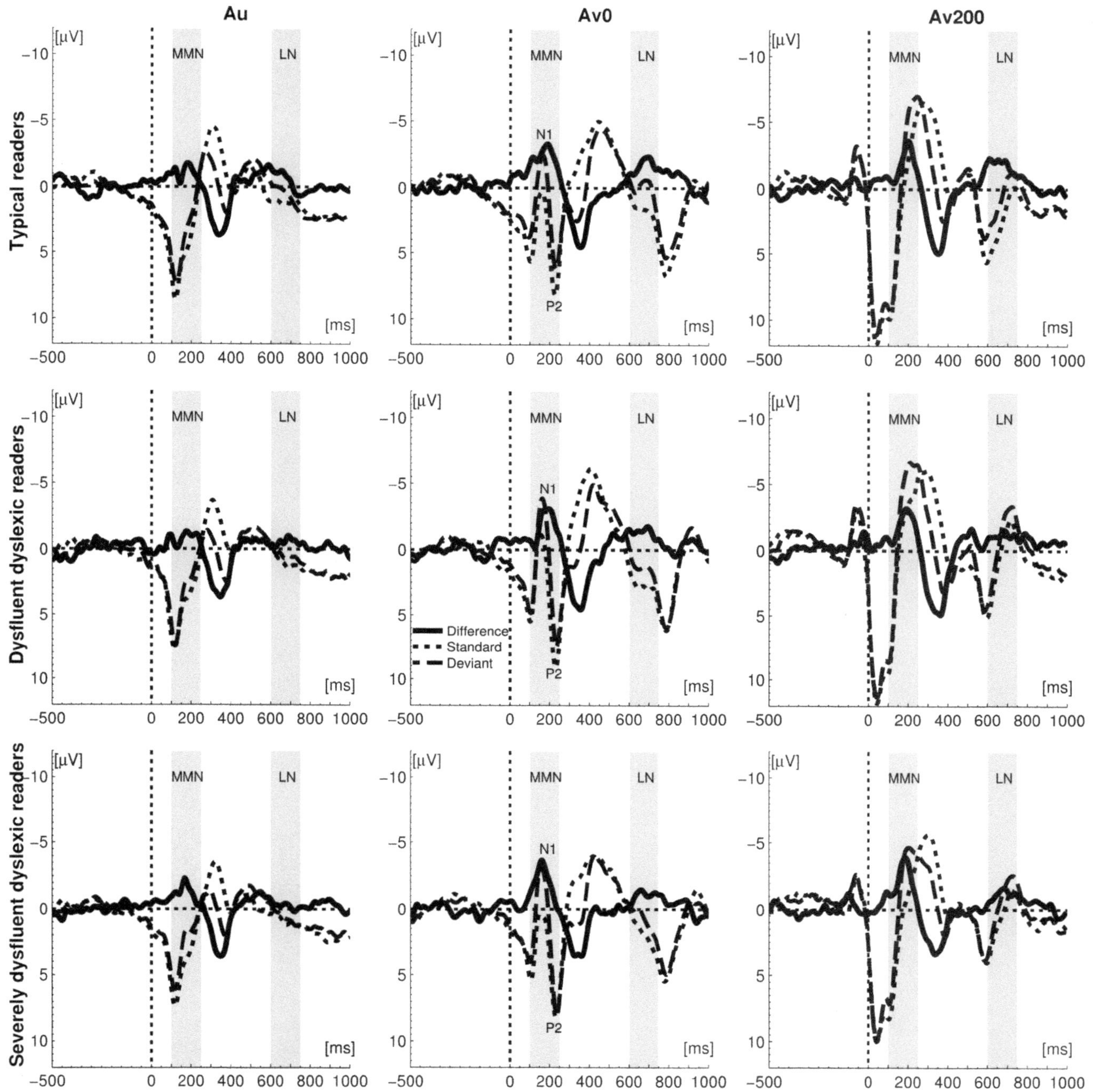

Figure 1. Grand average event-related potentials (ERP) and difference waves. Grand average ERPs averaged over 4 frontocentral electrodes for standard (dotted line), deviant (dashed line) and their difference (solid line) in auditory (Au) and two audiovisual conditions (Av0 and Av200) with time intervals of interest shaded in light grey. N1 and P2 peaks of standard and deviant ERPs are also marked in synchronous audiovisual condition (Av0).

significant group differences. We also did not observe significant group differences in the latency of the auditory MMN.

In each group, the vowel deviant additionally elicited a weaker and more sustained auditory LN response around 670–690 ms after stimulus onset (Figures 1 and 2). Statistical analyses indicated a comparable auditory LN response across groups, with a significant main effect of Stimulus ($F(1, 53) = 64.44$, $p = .000$, $\eta^2 = .549$) and no significant group differences for amplitudes or latencies. In sum, in each of the three groups the deviant vowel sound/o/elicited comparable MMN and LN responses with respect to the standard vowel sound/a/.

Letter-effects: MMN and LN amplitude enhancements

In both cross-modal conditions (Av0 and Av200) the deviant vowel sound/o/elicited MMN and LN responses with respect to the standard vowel sound/a/(Fig. 1 and Fig. 2). In these blocks, the letter "a" was presented together with the standard and deviant vowels, leading to a double violation: the deviant speech sound/o/violated the expectation built by both the standard

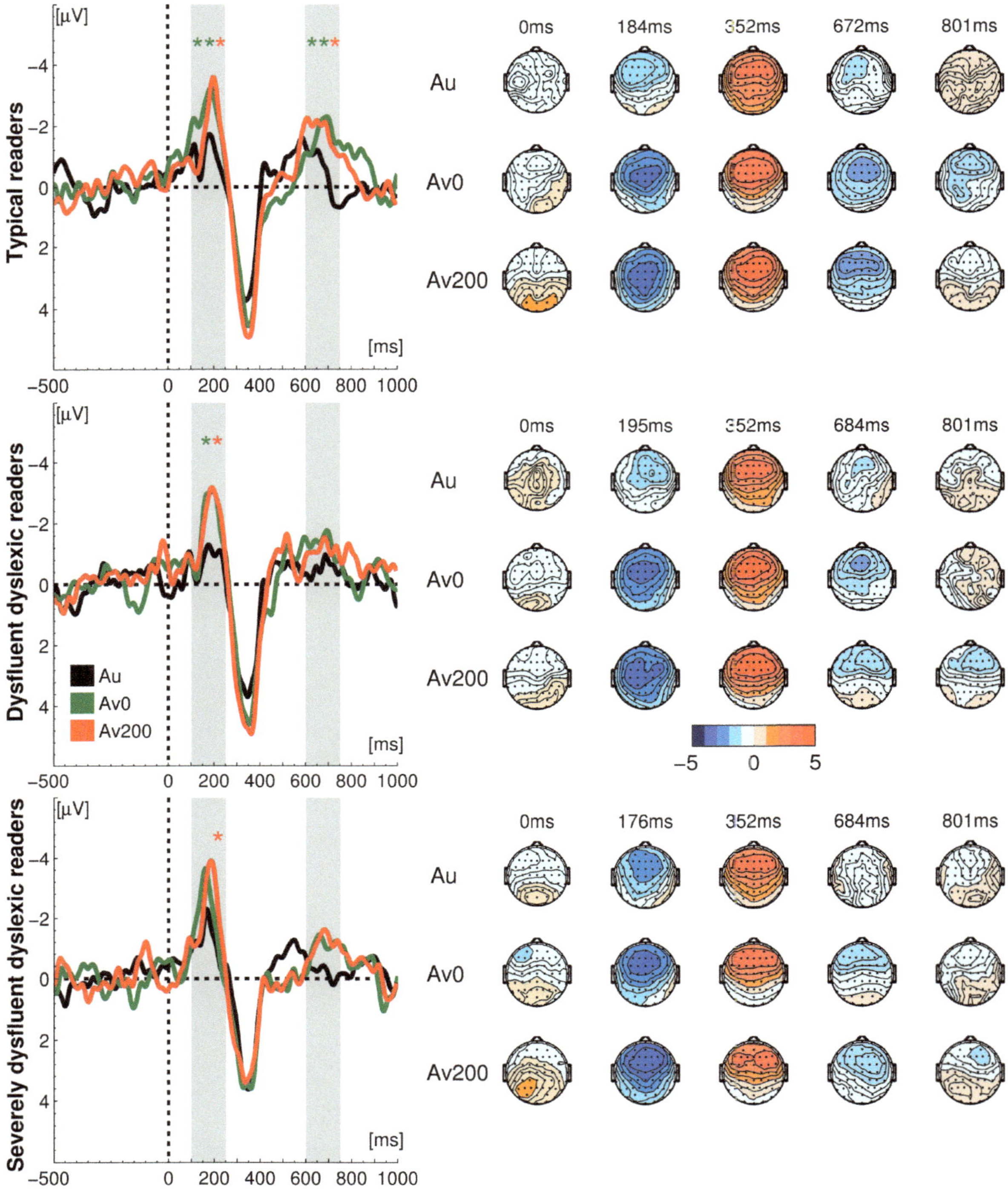

Figure 2. Difference waves and topographical maps. I. Difference waves (averaged over 4 frontocentral electrodes) with time intervals of interest shaded in gray. Significant differences between conditions are marked with asterisks (*p< = .05;**p< = .01): green asterisk – AV0 vs. Au difference, red asterisk – Av200 vs. Au difference. II. Topographical distribution of average amplitudes in difference waves over 64 scalp electrodes.

speech sound/a/and the letter 'a'. To assess the neural integration of letters and speech sounds we tested whether this double violation significantly enhanced the cross-modal as compared to the auditory MMN and LN responses [16,21,26]. To this end, we first performed a mixed model ANOVA with stimulus (standard, deviant), condition (auditory, AV0, AV200) and electrodes (4 fronto-central electrodes) as within-subject factors and subject group as between-subject factor. In the MMN window, this overall analysis indicated stronger responses to deviants as compared to standards (Stimulus $F(1,53) = 294.61$, $p = .000$, $\eta^2 = .848$), and stronger cross-modal as compared to auditory (mismatch) responses (Condition $F(2,99) = 50.61$, $p = .000$, $\eta^2 = .488$; Stimulus*Condition: $F(2,105) = 12.29$, $p = .000$, $\eta^2 = .188$), as well as a tendency for groups to differ in their response amplitudes across conditions (Condition*Group ($F(4,99) = 2.18$, $p = .081$, $\eta^2 = .076$). Pairwise group comparisons showed that this tendency was driven by significant differences between severely dysfluent dyslexics and typical readers (Condition*Group: $F(2,69) = 3.87$, $p = .027$, $\eta^2 = .097$), while there were no differences in other cases.

Also in the later LN window, the overall mixed-model ANOVA indicated stronger responses to deviants as compared to standards (Stimulus $F(1,53) = 267.28$, $p = .000$, $\eta^2 = .835$) and stronger cross-modal as compared to auditory (mismatch) responses (Condition $F(1,73) = 9.47$, $p = .001$, $\eta^2 = .152$; Stimulus*Condition: $F(2,99) = 8.78$, $p = .000$, $\eta^2 = .142$) together with significant group differences in response amplitudes across conditions (Condition*Group: $F(3,73) = 3.87$, $p = .015$, $\eta^2 = .127$). Pairwise group comparisons showed that the significant group difference in response amplitudes across conditions was driven by significant differences between severely dysfluent dyslexics and typical readers (Condition*Group: $F(1,51) = 4.49$, $p = .027$, $\eta^2 = .111$) as well as between dysfluent dyslexics and typical readers (Condition*Group: $F(1,49) = 6.80$, $p = .006$, $\eta^2 = .159$), but not by a difference between the two dyslexic groups ($F(1,46) = 0.48$, $p = .549$, $\eta^2 = .014$).

We further analyzed these condition and group effects by performing mixed model ANOVAs on the MMN difference waves with Condition (AV0 versus Auditory; AV200 versus Auditory) and electrodes (4 fronto-central electrodes) as within subjects factors. In the simultaneous cross-modal condition (AV0), significant MMN amplitude enhancements were observed in typical readers ($F(1,19) = 10.92$, $p = .004$, $\eta^2 = .365$) as well as in dysfluent dyslexics ($F(1,17) = 7.63$, $p = .013$, $\eta^2 = .310$), whereas in severely dysfluent dyslexics this enhancement was not significant ($F(1,17) = 3.43$, $p = .082$, $\eta^2 = .168$). When letter presentation preceded speech sound onset (AV200) significant cross-modal MMN enhancements were found in all three subject groups (typical readers: $F(1,19) = 7.21$, $p = .015$, $\eta^2 = .275$; dysfluent dyslexics: $F(1,17) = 5.93$, $p = .026$, $\eta^2 = .259$; severely dysfluent dyslexics: $F(1,17) = 6.09$, $p = .024$, $\eta^2 = .264$).

As for the LN window, in typical readers the presence of a letter significantly enhanced the LN amplitude in both cross-modal conditions (AV0 vs. Auditory: $F(1,19) = 10.90$, $p = .004$, $\eta^2 = .365$; AV200 vs. Auditory: $F(1,19) = 7.85$, $p = .011$, $\eta^2 = .292$). In contrast, in the dyslexic groups the LN letter effects only resulted in non-significant trends (AV0 vs. Auditory, dysfluent: $F(1,17) = 3.93$, $p = .064$, $\eta^2 = .188$; severely dysfluent: $F(1,17) = 3.98$, $p = .062$, $\eta^2 = .190$; Av200 vs. Auditory, dysfluent: ($F(1,17) = 3.44$, $p = .081$, $\eta^2 = .168$; severely dysfluent: $F(1,17) = 2.41$, $p = .139$, $\eta^2 = .124$).

In summary, in both cross-modal conditions, our results showed early (MMN) and late (LN) letter effects in typical readers. Although the group differences in MMN and LN letter effects were subtle, the dysfluent group resembled typical readers in the presence of an MMN letter effect, whereas they resembled the severely dysfluent group in the lack of a significant LN letter effect. The severely dysfluent group differed most from typical readers in both the lack of a significant LN letter effect and in only showing a significant MMN letter effect in the AV200 condition.

Letter effects: MMN and LN latency

We investigated the timing of the letter effects, by analyzing MMN and LN latencies in both crossmodal conditions. As already indicated by our regression analysis, groups tended to differ in MMN response latency in the simultaneous crossmodal (AV0) condition (Group ($F(2,53) = 5.85$, $p = .062$, $\eta^2 = .181$). In particular, severely dysfluent dyslexics showed a significantly shorter MMN latency than both the typical readers ($F(1,36) = 8.59$, $p = .006$, $\eta^2 = .193$), and the dysfluent dyslexics ($F(1,34) = 7.65$, $p = .009$, $\eta^2 = .184$), whereas the latter groups showed similar latencies ($F(1,36) = 0.07$, $p = .787$, $\eta^2 = .002$). No significant group differences were found for MMN latency in the asynchronous cross-modal condition (AV200), or for LN latency in either of the cross-modal conditions.

ERP - behavior relations

We used linear regression to investigate the relation between individual differences in MMN/LN responses in the crossmodal conditions and behavioral measures of reading fluency and related skills. Results showed that such a relation was present for the latency of the MMN response elicited in the simultaneous crossmodal condition (AV0). First, across both typical and dyslexic readers, MMN latency in the AV0 condition significantly correlated (significance threshold q(FDR) = .010) with individual differences in word reading fluency ($r = .368$; $p = .005$; Table 2, Figure 3), word reading accuracy ($r = .398$; $p = .002$) and phoneme deletion accuracy ($r = .343$; $p = .001$). When restricting the analysis to the dyslexic readers, a significant relation was only shown for reading fluency ($r = .554$; $p = .000$). Remarkably, in both cases, longer MMN peak latencies were found in the more fluent readers, a result that is further investigated in our analysis of the N1-P2 responses underlying the MMN effect. None of the other ERP-behavior regressions reached statistical significance.

Relation between MMN and N1-P2 responses

In a final analysis we aimed to further investigate the origin of the *shorter* MMN latency in severely dysfluent dyslexics as compared to both other groups, as well as the corresponding regression results in the simultaneous cross-modal (AV0) condition (Figure 3) by analyzing the timing of the MMN with respect to the evoked N1 and P2 responses (Figure 1). Results showed that in severely dysfluent dyslexics, letter-speech sound pairs only elicited a deviancy effect in the N1 window (main effect of Stimulus $F(1,17) = 28.32$, $p = .000$, $\eta^2 = .625$), but not in the P2 window ($F(1,17) = .03$, $p = .860$, $\eta^2 = .002$), as can also be seen in Figure 1. In contrast, typical readers as well as dysfluent dyslexics showed a deviancy effect in both the N1 and the P2 windows (main effects of Stimulus typical readers N1: $F(1,19) = 32.27$, $p = .000$, $\eta^2 = .629$; P2: $F(1,19) = 6.49$, $p = .020$, $\eta^2 = .255$); dysfluent dyslexics N1: $F(1,17) = 14.24$, $p = .002$, $\eta^2 = .456$ and P2: $F(1,17) = 10.15$, $p = .005$, $\eta^2 = .374$). The absence of a P2 deviancy effect in the severely dysfluent dyslexics thus most likely explains their shorter MMN latency.

Discussion

The present study investigated ERP measures of letter-speech sound integration in typically reading and dyslexic children after 2,5 years of reading instruction and specifically investigated how these ERP measures relate to individual differences in reading fluency and related skills. For this purpose we employed a passive oddball paradigm and tested cross-modal enhancement of the MMN and LN due to an audiovisual violation (vowel sound/o/vs. vowel sound/a/and letter 'a') as compared to an auditory only violation (vowel sound/o/vs. vowel sound/a/; [21]). Our results show robust neural integration of letters and speech sounds in the typical readers, albeit at a different temporal integration window compared to adults [26]. Furthermore, they confirm and extend previous findings in dyslexic children by demonstrating reduced letter-speech sound integration, with different patterns of integration deficiency depending on the level of reading dysfluency (Table 3).

Table 2. Regression of word reading fluency and accuracy with the MMN latency in Av0 condition: Regression coefficients for behavioral measures and latency of MMN in Av0 condition averaged over 4 electrodes (significant p values for q(FDR) = .010 are denoted in bold).

	Av0 MMN latency [ms]							
	All children				Dyslexic children			
	R^2	β	t(54)	p	R^2	β	t(34)	p
Word reading – *fluency*								
M_{3DM} Total Word Fluency, EMT, 'De Kat'	.136	.368	2.91	**.005**	.307	.554	3.88	**.000**
Word reading - *accuracy [%]*								
3DM Total Word Accuracy	.159	.398	3.19	**.002**	.139	.372	2.34	.025
Letter –speech sound coupling								
M_{3DM} Spelling, L-SS identification, L-SS discrimination – *accuracy [%]*	.073	.271	2.05	.046	.044	.209	1.23	.227
M_{3DM} Spelling, L-SS identification, L-SS discrimination – *RT [sec/item]*	.031	−.176	−1.30	.199	.000	.006	0.03	.975
Phoneme deletion – *accuracy [%]*	.117	.343	2.66	**.010**	.089	.298	1.80	.082
Rapid naming (RAN) *[ms]*	.103	−.321	−2.47	.017	.095	−.308	−1.86	.072

Typical readers: enhanced (and non-selective) neural sensitivity?

Typical readers after 2,5 years of reading instruction showed cross-modal enhancements of the MMN and LN responses independent of the precise timing of letter and speech sound presentation (AV0 and Av200), indicating a broad temporal window of integration. This contrasts with previous results of adults, who only showed a cross-modal enhancement in the MMN window, and only when letters and speech sounds were presented simultaneously [26]. Furthermore, the present results showed a different pattern of cross-modal effects as compared to previous findings in both typical beginning readers after 1-year of reading instruction and advanced typical readers after 4-years of reading instruction [21]. That is, in the younger readers cross-modal enhancement only reached significance in the LN window and only when the letter preceded the speech sound (AV200). In the advanced readers this pattern shifted with significant cross-modal enhancement in the earlier MMN window when the letter preceded the speech sound (AV200) and additionally in the LN window when letters and speech sounds were presented simultaneously (AV0). In comparison to the younger readers, the observed emergence of a cross-modal MMN enhancement may reflect the initial development of an early detection and integration of letter-sound pairs in 9-year-old children [27,28]. In comparison to the more advanced readers, who only showed a cross-modal LN enhancement in the simultaneous AV0 condition, the unspecific cross-modal LN enhancement independent of the timing of letter presentation, may suggest immature and non-selective further processing of letter-sound congruency in 9-year-olds. On a more general level, the pattern of stronger and/or less selective cross-modal effects in our intermediate group of typical readers is consistent with a developing neural system for audiovisual speech and letter-sound processing that undergoes dynamic changes throughout primary school years [6,73,74]. In particular, they may reflect enhanced neural sensitivity for letter-sound congruency after 2.5 years of reading instruction, before developing into a more selectively tuned system with advanced reading practice. Similar nonlinear patterns of an initial sensitivity increase during early school years, followed by reduced and more selective sensitivity in adults, have been observed for print selective visual N1 responses [53] and ERP phonological priming effects during an auditory lexical decision task [52]. On the other hand, also methodological differences between the present study and the previous ERP studies by Froyen and colleagues [16,21,26] may have (at least partly) contributed to the relatively strong cross-modal ERP effects in our typical readers. For example, unlike these previous studies, we used active electrodes for EEG data acquisition and ICA-based EEG preprocessing, which both lead to improvement of ERP signal-to-noise ratio. Another factor that may have increased signal-to-noise ratio is an increase in trial length from 1250 ms to 1700 ms. In addition, we employed a full within-subjects design as compared to a partial within-subjects design [21]. To further understand the development of brain mechanisms for letter-speech sound integration and their relation to reading acquisition, it is important to apply similar cross-modal neuroimaging paradigms in a longitudinal set-up and follow the same children while they are learning to read.

Dyslexic children: crossmodal MMN effect scales with reading dysfluency

ERP data of dyslexic children showed normal auditory MMN and LN responses together with reduced effects of letter-speech sound congruency. Most interestingly results indicated different

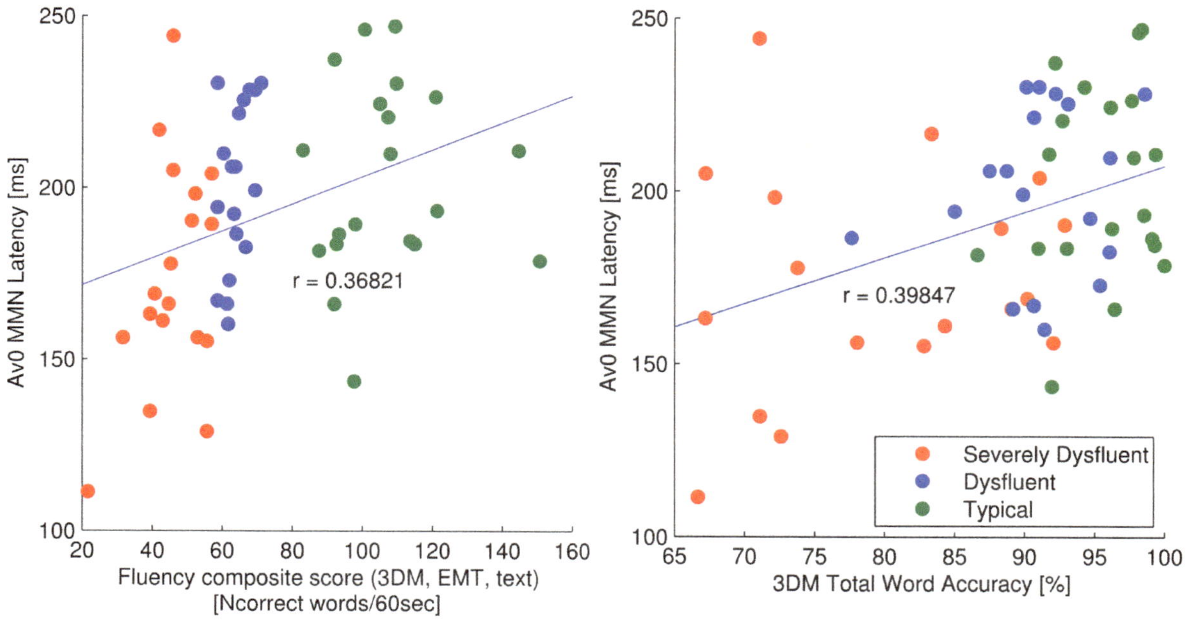

Figure 3. Correlations of word reading fluency and accuracy with the MMN latency in Av0 condition. Relation of composite fluency (3DM word reading fluency, EMT, 'De Kat') and 3DM Accuracy (HFW, LFW, PW) raw scores with MMN latency in Av0 condition with the strength of correlation represented by r.

patterns of integration deficiency depending on the level of reading fluency. In particular, in our regression analysis behavioral measures of reading fluency significantly predicted the latency of the MMN response in the simultaneous cross-modal condition (AV0), not only across typical and dyslexic readers, but also within the group of dyslexic readers. Further analyses indicated that this relation could be explained by a short-lasting, reduced MMN response, encompassing only the N1 window in severely dysfluent dyslexics as compared to a longer lasting MMN response, encompassing both the N1 and P2 windows in dysfluent dyslexic and typical readers. In addition, in the AV0 condition, MMN latency correlated significantly with reading accuracy and phonological awareness (phoneme deletion) across typical readers and dyslexics, but not within the dyslexic group alone.

Although relatively little is known about the functional relevance of the P2, recent evidence suggests that this response is specifically sensitive to the audiovisual integration of orthographic and phonological units [47] as well as of visual articulatory gestures and speech [74–77]. For example, in an elegant study by Baart et al. [75], audiovisual integration of articulatory gestures (lipread speech) and sine-wave speech was compared between participants trained to perceive the sine-wave speech in either a 'speech' or 'nonspeech' mode. Whereas lipread speech modulated the N1 response in both processing modes, the P2 was only modulated in listeners who recognized the sine-wave speech as speech, thus suggesting more general audiovisual convergence in the N1 window followed by speech specific audiovisual integration in the P2 window. This speech specificity of the P2 response would also concur with its putative neural source in the posterior superior temporal sulcus [78], a region involved in the integration of audiovisual speech [79] and of letters and speech sounds [23,80]. Moreover activity in this region has been found to scale with interindividual differences in audiovisual speech perception (McGurk effect) in typically reading children and adults [73,81] and to show reduced letter-speech sound integration in dyslexic children [15]. By analogy, we would speculate that the N1 deviancy effect shown in the simultaneous audiovisual (AV0) condition indicates audiovisual convergence common across the three children groups, followed by a speech specific integration of letters and speech sounds in the P2 window in typical readers and dysfluent dyslexics, which is reduced or absent in severely dysfluent dyslexics. Recently, a diminished speech-specificity of audiovisual integration was also found for spoken-written syllable pairs in Finnish dyslexic adults [41].

A similar pattern of results or relation with behavior (reading fluency) was not observed in the asynchronous crossmodal (AV200) blocks, possibly indicating a diminished recruitment of speech specific integration processes in this condition. This may also explain why typical adult readers, with selectively tuned neural systems for letter-speech sound integration, only show congruency effects when letters and speech sounds are presented simultaneously (AV0 blocks, [23,26]). These findings deserve further study however, especially in relation to the nature of possible audiovisual integration deficits in dyslexics, because in a previous study with 11 year old dyslexic readers, behavioral measures of word reading fluency (MMN), non-word reading fluency and letter-phoneme matching (LN) were found to correlate with MMN/LN letter effects in the AV200 condition [16].

Further evidence for brain-behavior relations with respect to letter-speech sound integration comes mainly from fMRI studies. [15], for example found a positive correlation between letter-speech sound congruency effects measured in the planum temporale/Heschl's sulcus and both reading accuracy and the speed of letter-speech sound matching across 9-year old typical and dyslexic readers. Cross-modal fMRI congruency effects measured in the planum temporale during a rhyme judgment task were also found to positively correlate with literacy skills [82] as well as with phonological awareness [17] in 8–11 year old typical readers. However, in the latter study no correlation was found between cross-modal integration and phonological awareness in dyslexic children, which was suggested to indicate a decoupling of these processes in dyslexia [17]. Although most

Table 3. Summary of results.

	Severely dysfluent dyslexic	Dysfluent dyslexic	Typical
MMN			
Av0 vs. Au	**No**	Yes	Yes
Av200 vs. Au	Yes	Yes	Yes
LN			
Av0 vs. Au	**No**	**No**	Yes
Av200 vs. Au	**No**	**No**	Yes
Av0			
N1 difference	Yes	Yes	Yes
P2 difference	**No**	Yes	Yes

studies thus find a relation between reading and/or phonological skills and ERP/fMRI indices of letter-speech sound integration, the type of relation shows some variability as well as its presence or absence in dyslexic readers. These differences may relate to the dependency of neural effects of letter-speech sound congruency on task demands [25,46] the type of speech/letter units, e.g. consonants, vowels, syllables [38,83] and/or the depth of the orthography [84]. Importantly, the present results show that the severity of reading (dys)fluency may also lead to differences in the observed brain-behavior correlations across studies. It would thus be interesting to further investigate these brain-behavior relationships in a larger-scale cross-national study including children of varying reading (dys)fluency, and deep and shallow orthographies, using the same paradigm with stimuli of grain sizes with different relevance in the different orthographies. Furthermore, the observed relation between reading fluency/accuracy and cross-modal ERP modulations across typical as well as dyslexic readers is compatible with a continuity model of reading dysfunction [80], although our results do not exclude the possibility of dyslexia subtypes.

Given the present focus on letter-speech sound integration, it may seem surprising that behavioral measures of letter-speech sound coupling showed the weakest differences across reading groups and did not correlate with ERP measures of letter-speech sound coupling. However, these findings are in agreement with previous ERP and fMRI evidence revealing a dissociation between children's knowledge of which letters belong to which speech sounds and the automatic neural integration of these associations [19–21]. The present results thus provide additional support for the notion that behavioral measures alone may not to be a sensitive indicator for letter–speech sound integration [6,21].

Normal auditory responses and subtle reduction of LN letter effect in dyslexics

Results showed comparable auditory MMN and LN responses to vowels in all three groups. This absence of group differences was expected because vowels typically elicit normal MMN and/or LN responses in dyslexic children [16,85] whereas deficient change detection responses are typically reported for more subtle speech changes involving e.g. stop consonants (e.g. [85,86]). Correspondingly, we did not find any correlations between auditory MMN and LN responses and behavioral measures of reading or reading-related skills.

Our results also confirm weak neural integration of letters and speech sounds in 9 year old dyslexic children [15], with reduced or absent audiovisual LN effects in both groups and a short-lived MMN effect in the AV0 condition in severely dysfluent dyslexics. The timing of these effects was different than those previously reported in 11 year old dyslexics, for whom MMN letter effects did not, but the LN letter effect in the AV200 condition did, reach significance [16]. These differences could relate to developmental or strategy changes in dyslexic readers after 2.5 versus 4 years of reading instruction, but could also relate to methodological differences between the two studies and/or differences in the severity of reading dysfluency (see above).

Interestingly, an attenuated late negativity to spoken/ba/ deviants as compared to/da/standards has been proposed as a potential endophenotype for dyslexia [36]. That is, this negativity in a broader time window (300–700 ms) overlapping with our crossmodal LN (600–750 ms) was found to be attenuated in both dyslexic children and their siblings without dyslexia [36], and to be associated with rare variants in a candidate gene region for dyslexia [43]. As compared to perceptual aspects of letter-speech sound congruency in the MMN window, the observed LN letter effect may reflect cognitive, explicit associative and/or attentional processes [16,21,36,87], present depending on familiarity and complexity of the stimuli. Whereas in adults these type of late orthographic-phonological interactions may only occur during complex metaphonological tasks [46,47] and pseudoword-word priming tasks [51], in typically reading children they seem to be recruited during the integration of simple letter-vowel pairs (present findings and [21]), letter strings [88], integration of audiovisual words [89] and a visual lexical decision task with phonological distractors [49], with disrupted recruitment in dyslexic children (present findings and [16,49]). If this process is disrupted, as was the case in both dyslexic groups then the automaticity in adulthood may not be reached [18], as it may be prevented by an incapability to access and/or manipulate the representations [15,51,90], and/or reduced attentionally-mediated integration [36,43,50,51]. The additional attenuation of the early MMN in severely dyslexic children may signal a more basic failure in forming a clear letter-speech sound representation [6], and concurs with the suggested timing of sublexical orthographic-phonological integration during online visual word recognition [91]. Similarly, Roeske and colleagues [92] observed an association between specific genetic markers and a speech evoked late negativity across dyslexic children independently of the severity of their reading problems, while a significant association with the earlier speech evoked MMN was present only in the most severe dyslexics. Thus, the crossmodal MMN enhancement would represent a successful representation of an audiovisual stimulus, and the crossmodal LN enhancement would characterize availability of the represented stimulus for further manipulation.

Finally, Blau and colleagues [15] showed that Dutch dyslexic children of the same age as our participants, exhibit reduced neural integration of letters and speech sounds in the planum temporale/Heschl sulcus and the superior temporal sulcus, thus showing both reduced integration in the STS and feedback to the auditory cortex [23]. As the severely dysfluent dyslexics in our study showed both early and late deficiencies, while dysfluent dyslexics showed only a late deficiency, it would be interesting to investigate whether the early MMN deficiency would stem from the reduced integration in the STS while the LN deficiency would be a product of a reduced feedback.

Conclusion

The present ERP study investigated letter-speech sound integration in 9-year-old typically reading and dyslexic children by using a well-studied oddball paradigm with simple vowel sounds and letters and demonstrated that early (speech specific) audiovisual integration processes scale with individual differences in reading (dys)fluency. Results further indicated enhanced neural sensitivity to letter-speech sound associations in 9-year-old typical readers, together with disrupted sensitivity in dyslexic readers. In future studies, this ERP paradigm could be used to investigate whether and how systematic training of phonological skills and/or letter speech-sound coupling changes this disrupted neural integration of letters and speech sounds in dyslexic children. Furthermore, an extension to longitudinal designs using units of different complexity and grain sizes (e.g. vowels, consonants, syllables, words), possibly in the context of more naturalistic online reading tasks, could lead to a more complete understanding of the dynamic neural changes contributing to successful and hampered reading acquisition.

Acknowledgments

We dedicate this paper to our co-author, professor Leo Blomert, who passed away on November 25, 2012. His contributions to the project prior to his passing were significant. This project is part of the research program "Fluent reading acquisition neurocognitively decomposed: the case of dyslexia (HCMI 10–59)" funded by the Netherlands Initiative Brain and Cognition (NIHC), a part of the Netherlands Organization for Scientific Research (NWO) under grant number 056-14-015. We thank Suzanne van Grieken, Marlena van Langevelde, Gert-Jan Munneke, Jitka Annen, Mandy Meijer, Helene Vos and Jorinde Wesseling for their help during data collection and Nienke van Atteveldt for useful comments on the manuscript. Last but not least, a special thanks goes to the children participating in the research and their parents.

Author Contributions

Conceived and designed the experiments: GŽ LB MB. Performed the experiments: GŽ GFG JT. Analyzed the data: GŽ MB. Contributed to the writing of the manuscript: GŽ MB MvdM.

References

1. Blomert L (2005) Dyslexie in Nederland. Amsterdam: Uitgeverij Nieuwezijds. Available: http://www.boomtestuitgevers.nl/upload/Dyslexie_in_Nederland_Leo_Blomert.pdf. Accessed 2014 April 16.
2. Lyon GR, Shaywitz SE, Shaywitz BA (2003) A definition of dyslexia. Ann Dyslexia 53: 1–14. Available: http://link.springer.com/10.1007/s11881-003-0001-9. Accessed 2014 February 14.
3. Shaywitz SE, Morris R, Shaywitz BA (2008) The education of dyslexic children from childhood to young adulthood. Annu Rev Psychol 59: 451–475. Available: http://www.ncbi.nlm.nih.gov/pubmed/18154503. Accessed 2013 February 10.
4. Katzir T, Kim, Wolf M, Morris R, Lovett MW (2008) The Varieties of Pathways to Dysfluent Reading: Comparing Subtypes of Children With Dyslexia at Letter, Word, and Connected Text Levels of Reading. J Learn Disabil 41: 47–66. Available: http://www.ncbi.nlm.nih.gov/pubmed/18274503. Accessed 2013 September 10.
5. Leinonen S, Müller K, Leppänen PHT, Aro M, Ahonen T, et al. (2001) Heterogeneity in adult dyslexic readers: Relating processing skills to the speed and accuracy of oral text reading *. Read Writ 14: 265–296. doi:10.1023/A:1011117620895.
6. Blomert L (2011) The neural signature of orthographic-phonological binding in successful and failing reading development. Neuroimage 57: 695–703. Available: http://www.ncbi.nlm.nih.gov/pubmed/21056673. Accessed 2013 January 29.
7. Ehri LC (2005) Learning to Read Words: Theory, Findings, and Issues. Sci Stud Read 9: 167–188. Available: http://www.tandfonline.com/doi/abs/10.1207/s1532799xssr0902_4.
8. Share DL (1995) Phonological recoding and self-teaching: sine qua non of reading acquisition. Cognition 55: 151–218; discussion 219-26. Available: http://www.ncbi.nlm.nih.gov/pubmed/7789090.
9. Wimmer H, Schurz M (2010) Dyslexia in regular orthographies: manifestation and causation. Dyslexia 16: 283–299. Available: http://www.ncbi.nlm.nih.gov/pubmed/20957684. Accessed 2013 December 9.
10. Snowling M (1998) Dyslexia as a Phonological Deficit: Evidence and Implications. Child Psychol Psychiatry Rev 3: 4–11. Available: http://www.journals.cambridge.org/abstract_S1360641797001366.
11. Ramus F, Szenkovits G (2008) What phonological deficit? Q J Exp Psychol (Hove) 61: 129–141. Available: http://www.ncbi.nlm.nih.gov/pubmed/18038344. Accessed 2013 March 3.
12. Aravena S, Snellings P, Tijms J, van der Molen MW (2013) A lab-controlled simulation of a letter–speech sound binding deficit in dyslexia. J Exp Child Psychol 115: 691–707. Available: http://linkinghub.elsevier.com/retrieve/pii/S0022096513000659. Accessed 2013 May 27.
13. Bus AG, Ijzendoorn MH Van (1999) Phonological Awareness and Early Reading: A Meta-Analysis of Experimental Training Studies. J Educ Psychol 91: 403–414. doi:10.1037/0022-0663.91.3.403.
14. Tijms J, Hoeks J (2005) A computerized treatment of dyslexia: benefits from treating lexico-phonological processing problems. Dyslexia 11: 22–40. Available: http://www.ncbi.nlm.nih.gov/pubmed/15747805. Accessed 2013 March 4.
15. Blau V, Reithler J, van Atteveldt N, Seitz J, Gerretsen P, et al. (2010) Deviant processing of letters and speech sounds as proximate cause of reading failure: a functional magnetic resonance imaging study of dyslexic children. Brain 133: 868–879. Available: http://www.ncbi.nlm.nih.gov/pubmed/20061325. Accessed 2013 May 22.
16. Froyen D, Willems G, Blomert L (2011) Evidence for a specific cross-modal association deficit in dyslexia: an electrophysiological study of letter-speech sound processing. Dev Sci 14: 635–648. Available: http://www.ncbi.nlm.nih.gov/pubmed/21676085. Accessed 2013 February 15.
17. McNorgan C, Randazzo-Wagner M, Booth JR (2013) Cross-modal integration in the brain is related to phonological awareness only in typical readers, not in those with reading difficulty. Front Hum Neurosci 7: 388. Available: http://www.pubmedcentral.nih.gov/articlerender.fcgi?artid=3719029&tool=pmcentrez&rendertype=abstract. Accessed 2013 August 7.
18. Blau V, van Atteveldt N, Ekkebus M, Goebel R, Blomert L (2009) Reduced neural integration of letters and speech sounds links phonological and reading deficits in adult dyslexia. Curr Biol 19: 503–508. Available: http://www.ncbi.nlm.nih.gov/pubmed/19285401. Accessed 2013 August 15.
19. Blomert L, Vaessen AA (2009) 3DM Differential diagnostics for dyslexia: Cognitive analysis of reading and spelling. Amsterdam: Boom Test Publishers.
20. Booth JR, Burman DD, Van Santen FW, Harasaki Y, Gitelman DR, et al. (2001) The development of specialized brain systems in reading and oral-language. Child Neuropsychol 7: 119–141. Available: http://www.tandfonline.com/doi/abs/10.1076/chin.7.3.119.8740. Accessed 2013 September 9.
21. Froyen DJW, Bonte ML, van Atteveldt N, Blomert L (2009) The long road to automation: neurocognitive development of letter-speech sound processing. J Cogn Neurosci 21: 567–580. Available: http://www.ncbi.nlm.nih.gov/pubmed/18593266. Accessed 2014 April 8.
22. Raij T, Uutela K, Hari R (2000) Audiovisual integration of letters in the human brain. Neuron 28: 617–625. Available: http://www.ncbi.nlm.nih.gov/pubmed/11144369.
23. Van Atteveldt N, Formisano E, Goebel R, Blomert L (2004) Integration of letters and speech sounds in the human brain. Neuron 43: 271–282. Available: http://www.ncbi.nlm.nih.gov/pubmed/15260962.
24. Van Atteveldt NM, Formisano E, Blomert L, Goebel R (2007) The effect of temporal asynchrony on the multisensory integration of letters and speech sounds. Cereb Cortex 17: 962–974. Available: http://www.ncbi.nlm.nih.gov/pubmed/16751298. Accessed 2013 August 28.
25. Van Atteveldt NM, Formisano E, Goebel R, Blomert L (2007) Top-down task effects overrule automatic multisensory responses to letter-sound pairs in auditory association cortex. Neuroimage 36: 1345–1360. Available: http://www.ncbi.nlm.nih.gov/pubmed/17513133. Accessed 2013 August 26.

26. Froyen D, Van Atteveldt N, Bonte M, Blomert L (2008) Cross-modal enhancement of the MMN to speech-sounds indicates early and automatic integration of letters and speech-sounds. Neurosci Lett 430: 23–28. Available: http://www.ncbi.nlm.nih.gov/pubmed/18023979. Accessed 2013 October 21.
27. Näätänen R (2001) The perception of speech sounds by the human brain as reflected by the mismatch negativity (MMN) and its magnetic equivalent (MMNm). Psychophysiology 38: 1–21.
28. Näätänen R, Paavilainen P, Rinne T, Alho K (2007) The mismatch negativity (MMN) in basic research of central auditory processing: a review. Clin Neurophysiol 118: 2544–2590. Available: http://www.ncbi.nlm.nih.gov/pubmed/17931964. Accessed 2013 August 6.
29. Bonte ML, Poelmans H, Blomert L (2007) Deviant neurophysiological responses to phonological regularities in speech in dyslexic children. Neuropsychologia 45: 1427–1437. Available: http://www.ncbi.nlm.nih.gov/pubmed/17187830. Accessed 2013 February 2.
30. Cheour-Luhtanen M, Alho K, Kujala T, Sainio K, Reinikainen K, et al. (1995) Mismatch negativity indicates vowel discrimination in newborns. Hear Res 82: 53–58. Available: http://www.sciencedirect.com/science/article/pii/037859559400164L. Accessed 2013 March 18.
31. Cheour M, Shestakova A, Alku P, Ceponiene R, Näätänen R (2002) Mismatch negativity shows that 3–6-year-old children can learn to discriminate non-native speech sounds within two months. Neurosci Lett 325: 187–190.
32. Csépe V (1995) On the origin and development of the mismatch negativity. Ear Hear 16: 91–104. Available: http://scholar.google.com/scholar?hl=en&btnG=Search&q=intitle:On+the+origin+and+development+of+the+mismatch+negativity#0. Accessed 2013 December 3.
33. Eulitz C, Lahiri A (2004) Neurobiological Evidence for Abstract Phonological Representations in the Mental Lexicon during Speech Recognition. J Cogn Neurosci 16: 577–583.
34. Kasai K, Nakagome K, Iwanami A, Fukuda M, Itoh K, et al. (2002) No effect of gender on tonal and phonetic mismatch negativity in normal adults assessed by a high-resolution EEG recording. Brain Res Cogn Brain Res 13: 305–312. Available: http://www.ncbi.nlm.nih.gov/pubmed/11918996.
35. Lohvansuu K, Hämäläinen JA, Tanskanen A, Bartling J, Bruder J, et al. (2013) Separating mismatch negativity (MMN) response from auditory obligatory brain responses in school-aged children. Psychophysiology 50: 640–652. Available: http://www.ncbi.nlm.nih.gov/pubmed/23577828. Accessed 2014 January 23.
36. Neuhoff N, Bruder J, Bartling J, Warnke A, Remschmidt H, et al. (2012) Evidence for the late MMN as a neurophysiological endophenotype for dyslexia. PLoS One 7: e34909. Available: http://www.pubmedcentral.nih.gov/articlerender.fcgi?artid=3351484&tool=pmcentrez&rendertype=abstract. Accessed 2013 May 22.
37. Winkler I, Kujala T, Tiitinen H, Sivonen P, Alku P, et al. (1999) Brain responses reveal the learning of foreign language phonemes. Psychophysiology 36: 638–642. Available: http://www.ncbi.nlm.nih.gov/pubmed/10442032.
38. Andres AJD, Oram Cardy JE, Joanisse MF (2011) Congruency of auditory sounds and visual letters modulates mismatch negativity and P300 event-related potentials. Int J Psychophysiol 79: 137–146. Available: http://www.ncbi.nlm.nih.gov/pubmed/20888870. Accessed 2013 February 21.
39. Colin C, Radeau M, Soquet A, Demolin D, Colin F, et al. (2002) Mismatch negativity evoked by the McGurk-MacDonald effect: a phonetic representation within short-term memory. Clin Neurophysiol 113: 495–506. Available: http://www.ncbi.nlm.nih.gov/pubmed/11955994.
40. Mittag M, Takegata R, Kujala T (2011) The effects of visual material and temporal synchrony on the processing of letters and speech sounds. Exp Brain Res 211: 287–298. Available: http://www.ncbi.nlm.nih.gov/pubmed/21516331. Accessed 2013 October 16.
41. Mittag M, Alho K, Takegata R, Makkonen T, Kujala T (2013) Audiovisual attention boosts letter-speech sound integration. Psychophysiology 50: 1034–1044. Available: http://www.ncbi.nlm.nih.gov/pubmed/23848280. Accessed 2013 October 21.
42. Stekelenburg JJ, Vroomen J, de Gelder B (2004) Illusory sound shifts induced by the ventriloquist illusion evoke the mismatch negativity. Neurosci Lett 357: 163–166. Available: http://www.ncbi.nlm.nih.gov/pubmed/15003275. Accessed 2013 June 6.
43. Czamara D, Bruder J, Becker J, Bartling J, Hoffmann P, et al. (2011) Association of a rare variant with mismatch negativity in a region between KIAA0319 and DCDC2 in dyslexia. Behav Genet 41: 110–119. Available: http://www.ncbi.nlm.nih.gov/pubmed/21104116. Accessed 2013 August 20.
44. Hommet C, Vidal J, Roux S, Blanc R, Barthez MA, et al. (2009) Topography of syllable change-detection electrophysiological indices in children and adults with reading disabilities. Neuropsychologia 47: 761–770. Available: http://www.ncbi.nlm.nih.gov/pubmed/19126410. Accessed 2013 October 25.
45. Cheour M, Korpilahti P, Martynova O, Lang AH (2001) Mismatch negativity and late discriminative negativity in investigating speech perception and learning in children and infants. Audiol Neurootol 6: 2–11. Available: http://www.ncbi.nlm.nih.gov/pubmed/11173771.
46. Lafontaine H, Chetail F, Colin C, Kolinsky R, Pattamadilok C (2012) Role and activation time course of phonological and orthographic information during phoneme judgments. Neuropsychologia 50: 2897–2906. Available: http://www.ncbi.nlm.nih.gov/pubmed/22971812. Accessed 2013 October 31.
47. Pattamadilok C, Perre L, Ziegler JC (2011) Beyond rhyme or reason: ERPs reveal task-specific activation of orthography on spoken language. Brain Lang 116: 116–124. Available: http://www.ncbi.nlm.nih.gov/pubmed/21211833. Accessed 2013 October 31.
48. Hasko S, Bruder J, Bartling J, Schulte-Körne G (2012) N300 indexes deficient integration of orthographic and phonological representations in children with dyslexia. Neuropsychologia 50: 640–654. Available: http://www.ncbi.nlm.nih.gov/pubmed/22245008. Accessed 2014 July 29.
49. Hasko S, Groth K, Bruder J, Bartling J, Schulte-Körne G (2013) The time course of reading processes in children with and without dyslexia: an ERP study. Front Hum Neurosci 7: 570. Available: http://www.pubmedcentral.nih.gov/articlerender.fcgi?artid=3791381&tool=pmcentrez&rendertype=abstract. Accessed 2013 October 17.
50. Savill NJ, Thierry G (2012) Decoding ability makes waves in reading: deficient interactions between attention and phonological analysis in developmental dyslexia. Neuropsychologia 50: 1553–1564. Available: http://www.ncbi.nlm.nih.gov/pubmed/22426204. Accessed 2014 July 9.
51. Savill NJ, Thierry G (2011) Reading for sound with dyslexia: evidence for early orthographic and late phonological integration deficits. Brain Res 1385: 192–205. Available: http://www.ncbi.nlm.nih.gov/pubmed/21316349. Accessed 2014 July 9.
52. Bonte ML, Blomert L (2004) Developmental dyslexia: ERP correlates of anomalous phonological processing during spoken word recognition. Brain Res Cogn Brain Res 21: 360–376. Available: http://www.ncbi.nlm.nih.gov/pubmed/15511652. Accessed 2013 October 24.
53. Maurer U, Brem S, Kranz F, Bucher K, Benz R, et al. (2006) Coarse neural tuning for print peaks when children learn to read. Neuroimage 33: 749–758. Available: http://www.ncbi.nlm.nih.gov/pubmed/16920367. Accessed 2014 February 12.
54. Oades RD, Dmittmann-Balcar A, Zerbin D (1997) Development and topography of auditory event-related potentials (ERPs): Mismatch and processing negativity in individuals 8?22 years of age. Psychophysiology 34: 677–693. Available: http://doi.wiley.com/10.1111/j.1469-8986.1997.tb02143.x. Accessed 2014 July 10.
55. Shafer VL, Morr ML, Kreuzer JA, Kurtzberg D (2000) Maturation of mismatch negativity in school-age children. Ear Hear 21: 242–251. Available: http://cat.inist.fr/?aModele=afficheN&cpsidt=1410810. Accessed 2014 July 10.
56. Ponton CW, Eggermont JJ, Kwong B, Don M (2000) Maturation of human central auditory system activity: evidence from multi-channel evoked potentials. Clin Neurophysiol 111: 220–236. Available: http://www.ncbi.nlm.nih.gov/pubmed/10680557.
57. Annett M (1979) Family handedness in three generations predicted by the right shift theory. Ann Hum Genet 42: 479–491. Available: http://doi.wiley.com/10.1111/j.1469-1809.1979.tb00681.x. Accessed 2014 April 16.
58. Achenbach TM, McConaughy SH (2003) The Achenbach System of Empirically Based Assessment (ASEBA). In: Reynolds CR, Kamphaus RW, editors. Handbook of psychological and educational assessment of children. New York, NY: Guilford Press. pp. 406–430.
59. Brus BT, Voeten MJM (1973) Eén-minuut test, vorm A en B; Verantwoording en Handleiding. Nimegen: Berkenhout Testmateriaal.
60. De Vos T (2007) Schoolvaardigheidstoets Technisch Lezen. Amsterdam: Boom test uitgevers.
61. Raven J, Raven JC, Court JH (1998) Coloured progressive matrices. Oxford, UK: Oxford Psychologists Press.
62. Faulkner HJ, Levy BA (1999) Fluent and nonfluent forms of transfer in reading: words and their message. Psychon Bull Rev 6: 111–116. Available: http://www.ncbi.nlm.nih.gov/pubmed/12199304.
63. Fuchs D, Fuchs LS, Compton DL (2004) Identifying Reading Disabilities by Responsiveness-to-Instruction: Specifying Measures and Criteria. Learn Disabil Q 27: 216–227. Available: http://www.jstor.org/stable/1593674?origin=crossref. Accessed 2014 April 11.
64. Stanovich KE, Feeman DJ, Cunningham AE (1983) The development of the relation between letter-naming speed and reading ability. Bull Psychon Soc 21: 199–202. Available: http://link.springer.com/10.3758/BF03334686. Accessed 2014 April 11.
65. Boersma P, Weenink D (2002) Praat: doing phonetics by computer (Version 4.0.26). Available: http://www.fon.hum.uva.nl/praat.
66. Bonte ML, Mitterer H, Zellagui N, Poelmans H, Blomert L (2005) Auditory cortical tuning to statistical regularities in phonology. Clin Neurophysiol 116: 2765–2774. Available: http://www.ncbi.nlm.nih.gov/pubmed/16256430. Accessed 2013 March 19.
67. Luck SJ (2005) An introduction to the event-related potential technique. Cambridge, MA: The MIT Press.
68. Delorme A, Makeig S (2004) EEGLAB: an open source toolbox for analysis of single-trial EEG dynamics including independent component analysis. J Neurosci Methods 134: 9–21 Available: http://www.sciencedirect.com/science/article/pii/S0165027003003479. Accessed 2013 June 23.
69. Lee TW, Girolami M, Sejnowski TJ (1999) Independent component analysis using an extended infomax algorithm for mixed subgaussian and supergaussian sources. Neural Comput 11: 417–441. Available: http://www.ncbi.nlm.nih.gov/pubmed/9950738.
70. Jung TP, Makeig S, Humphries C, Lee TW, McKeown MJ, et al. (2000) Removing electroencephalographic artifacts by blind source separation. Psychophysiology 37: 163–178. Available: http://www.ncbi.nlm.nih.gov/pubmed/10731767.

71. Vaessen A, Bertrand D, Tóth D, Csépe V, Faísca L, et al. (2010) Cognitive development of fluent word reading does not qualitatively differ between transparent and opaque orthographies. J Educ Psychol 102: 827–842. Available: http://doi.apa.org/getdoi.cfm?doi=10.1037/a0019465. Accessed 2013 July 9.
72. Benjamini Y, Hochberg Y (1995) Controlling the false discovery rate: a practical and powerful approach to multiple testing. J R Stat Soc Ser B 57: 289–300. Available: http://www.jstor.org/stable/10.2307/2346101. Accessed 2013 November 15.
73. Nath AR, Fava EE, Beauchamp MS (2011) Neural correlates of interindividual differences in children's audiovisual speech perception. J Neurosci 31: 13963–13971. Available: http://www.pubmedcentral.nih.gov/articlerender.fcgi?artid=3203203&tool=pmcentrez&rendertype=abstract. Accessed 2014 April 4.
74. Knowland VCP, Mercure E, Karmiloff-Smith A, Dick F, Thomas MSC (2014) Audio-visual speech perception: a developmental ERP investigation. Dev Sci 17: 110–124. Available: http://www.ncbi.nlm.nih.gov/pubmed/24176002. Accessed 2014 February 25.
75. Baart M, Stekelenburg JJ, Vroomen J (2014) Electrophysiological evidence for speech-specific audiovisual integration. Neuropsychologia 53: 115–121. Available: http://www.ncbi.nlm.nih.gov/pubmed/24291340. Accessed 2014 February 24.
76. Pilling M (2009) Auditory event-related potentials (ERPs) in audiovisual speech perception. J Speech Lang Hear Res 52: 1073–1081. Available: http://www.ncbi.nlm.nih.gov/pubmed/19641083. Accessed 2014 March 4.
77. Van Wassenhove V, Grant KW, Poeppel D (2005) Visual speech speeds up the neural processing of auditory speech. Proc Natl Acad Sci U S A 102: 1181–1186. Available: http://www.pubmedcentral.nih.gov/articlerender.fcgi?artid=545853&tool=pmcentrez&rendertype=abstract. Accessed 2013 June 24.
78. Liebenthal E, Desai R, Ellingson MM, Ramachandran B, Desai A, et al. (2010) Specialization along the left superior temporal sulcus for auditory categorization. Cereb Cortex 20: 2958–2970. Available: http://www.pubmedcentral.nih.gov/articlerender.fcgi?artid=2978244&tool=pmcentrez&rendertype=abstract. Accessed 2014 April 3.
79. Beauchamp MS, Lee KE, Argall BD, Martin A (2004) Integration of auditory and visual information about objects in superior temporal sulcus. Neuron 41: 809–823. Available: http://www.ncbi.nlm.nih.gov/pubmed/15003179.
80. Van Atteveldt NM, Blau VC, Blomert L, Goebel R (2010) fMR-adaptation indicates selectivity to audiovisual content congruency in distributed clusters in human superior temporal cortex. BMC Neurosci 11: 11. Available: http://www.pubmedcentral.nih.gov/articlerender.fcgi?artid=2829029&tool=pmcentrez&rendertype=abstract.
81. Nath AR, Beauchamp MS (2012) A neural basis for interindividual differences in the McGurk effect, a multisensory speech illusion. Neuroimage 59: 781–787. Available: http://www.pubmedcentral.nih.gov/articlerender.fcgi?artid=3196040&tool=pmcentrez&rendertype=abstract. Accessed 2014 March 19.
82. McNorgan C, Awati N, Desroches AS, Booth JR (2013) Multimodal Lexical Processing in Auditory Cortex Is Literacy Skill Dependent. Cereb Cortex. Available: http://www.ncbi.nlm.nih.gov/pubmed/23588185. Accessed 2014 March 5.
83. Mittag M, Thesleff P, Laasonen M, Kujala T (2013) The neurophysiological basis of the integration of written and heard syllables in dyslexic adults. Clin Neurophysiol 124: 315–326. Available: http://www.ncbi.nlm.nih.gov/pubmed/22939780. Accessed 2013 February 7.
84. Holloway ID, van Atteveldt N, Blomert L, Ansari D (2013) Orthographic Dependency in the Neural Correlates of Reading: Evidence from Audiovisual Integration in English Readers. Cereb Cortex. Available: http://www.ncbi.nlm.nih.gov/pubmed/24351976. Accessed 2014 March 4.
85. Csépe V (2003) Auditory event-related potentials in studying developmental dyslexia. In: Csépe V, editor. Dyslexia: Different brain, different behavior. New York, NY: Kluwer Academic Publishers – Plenum Publishers. pp. 81–112.
86. Schulte-Körne G, Deimel W, Bartling J, Remschmidt H (1998) Auditory processing and dyslexia: evidence for a specific speech. Neuroreport 9: 337–340.
87. Shestakova A, Huotilainen M, Čeponienė R, Cheour M (2003) Event-related potentials associated with second language learning in children. Clin Neurophysiol 114: 1507–1512. Available: http://linkinghub.elsevier.com/retrieve/pii/S1388245703001342. Accessed 2014 April 4.
88. Maurer U, Brem S, Bucher K, Brandeis D (2005) Emerging neurophysiological specialization for letter strings. J Cogn Neurosci 17: 1532–1552. Available: http://www.ncbi.nlm.nih.gov/pubmed/16269095.
89. Jost LB, Eberhard-Moscicka AK, Frisch C, Dellwo V, Maurer U (2013) Integration of Spoken and Written Words in Beginning Readers: A Topographic ERP Study. Brain Topogr. Available: http://www.ncbi.nlm.nih.gov/pubmed/24271979. Accessed 2013 December 17.
90. Ramus F, Ahissar M (2012) Developmental dyslexia: the difficulties of interpreting poor performance, and the importance of normal performance. Cogn Neuropsychol 29: 104–122. Available: http://www.ncbi.nlm.nih.gov/pubmed/22559749. Accessed 2013 November 1.
91. Grainger J, Holcomb PJ (2009) Watching the Word Go by: On the Time-course of Component Processes in Visual Word Recognition. Lang Linguist Compass 3: 128–156. Available: http://www.pubmedcentral.nih.gov/articlerender.fcgi?artid=2740997&tool=pmcentrez&rendertype=abstract.
92. Roeske D, Ludwig KU, Neuhoff N, Becker J, Bartling J, et al. (2011) First genome-wide association scan on neurophysiological endophenotypes points to trans-regulation effects on SLC2A3 in dyslexic children. Mol Psychiatry 16: 97–107. Available: http://www.ncbi.nlm.nih.gov/pubmed/19786962. Accessed 2014 June 5.

Auditory Conflict Resolution Correlates with Medial–Lateral Frontal Theta/Alpha Phase Synchrony

Samantha Huang[1]*, Stephanie Rossi[1], Matti Hämäläinen[1,2], Jyrki Ahveninen[1]

1 Harvard Medical School, Athinoula A. Martinos Center for Biomedical Imaging, Department of Radiology, Massachusetts General Hospital, Charlestown, Massachusetts, United States of America, **2** Harvard–MIT Division of Health Sciences and Technology, Cambridge, Massachusetts, United States of America

Abstract

When multiple persons speak simultaneously, it may be difficult for the listener to direct attention to correct sound objects among conflicting ones. This could occur, for example, in an emergency situation in which one hears conflicting instructions and the loudest, instead of the wisest, voice prevails. Here, we used cortically-constrained oscillatory MEG/EEG estimates to examine how different brain regions, including caudal anterior cingulate (cACC) and dorsolateral prefrontal cortices (DLPFC), work together to resolve these kinds of auditory conflicts. During an auditory flanker interference task, subjects were presented with sound patterns consisting of three different voices, from three different directions (45° left, straight ahead, 45° right), sounding out either the letters "A" or "O". They were asked to discriminate which sound was presented centrally and ignore the flanking distracters that were phonetically either congruent (50%) or incongruent (50%) with the target. Our cortical MEG/EEG oscillatory estimates demonstrated a direct relationship between performance and brain activity, showing that efficient conflict resolution, as measured with reduced conflict-induced RT lags, is predicted by theta/alpha phase coupling between cACC and right lateral frontal cortex regions intersecting the right frontal eye fields (FEF) and DLPFC, as well as by increased pre-stimulus gamma (60–110 Hz) power in the left inferior fontal cortex. Notably, cACC connectivity patterns that correlated with behavioral conflict-resolution measures were found during both the pre-stimulus and the pre-response periods. Our data provide evidence that, instead of being only transiently activated upon conflict detection, cACC is involved in sustained engagement of attentional resources required for effective sound object selection performance.

Editor: Lawrence M. Ward, University of British Columbia, Canada

Funding: This work was supported by National Institutes of Health Awards R01MH083744, R21DC010060, R21DC014134, R01HD040712, R01NS037462, and 5R01EB009048. This research was carried out at the Athinoula A. Martinos Center for Biomedical Imaging at the Massachusetts General Hospital, using resources provided by the Center for Functional Neuroimaging Technologies, P41EB015896, and a P41 Biotechnology Resource Grant supported by the National Institute of Biomedical Imaging and Bioengineering (NIBIB), National Institutes of Health. The research environment was additionally supported by National Center for Research Resources Shared Instrumentation Grants S10RR014978, S10RR021110, S10RR019307, S10RR014798, and S10RR023401. The funders had no role in study design, data collection and analysis, decision to publish, or preparation of the manuscript.

* Email: samhuang@nmr.mgh.harvard.edu

Introduction

Speech perception in everyday acoustic environments is a considerable computational challenge. When several persons speak at the same time, the spectrotemporal overlap of competing signals may hinder the segregation of the competing sound streams to form distinct perceptual objects (*i.e.*, object formation) [1]. Even if the relevant and irrelevant sounds can be perceptually grouped into distinct objects, similarity of these objects can make it difficult for the listener to direct attention to correct object in the auditory scene (*i.e.*, object selection) [1]. This could happen, for example, when one hears conflicting pieces of advice in an emergency situation, and the inherently most salient instead of most relevant object tends to prevail. While the top-down modulations of auditory neurons supporting perceptual object formation (for a review, see [2]) under the control of higher-order frontoparietal areas (for reviews, see [3,4]) have been documented, a paucity of information exists on how the higher-order brain regions work together to support selection of relevant sound objects amongst competing or conflicting sound objects.

The question about how different brain regions work together to select relevant objects while ignoring conflicting stimuli in a multitalker environment falls within the cognitive realm of conflict processing. In the visual domain, conflict processing has been intensively studied using the classic Flanker task [5], in which flanking distractor letters or arrows interfere with judgments about central target letters or target arrow direction, respectively. Much like in a multitalker setting where more salient voices can be assumed to complicate speech-object selection in the auditory domain [1], the more salient/numerous flankers significantly interfere with the selection of the relevant visual object and the motor responses associated with it. In addition to the Flanker task, other widely used conflict tasks include the Stroop color-word task [6], requiring the subject to identify the color of the letters instead of reading the word, and the Simon spatial compatibility task where a conflict arises when subjects need to respond with the hand opposite to the side of screen where a visual target appears [7]. A large body of evidence from human neuroimaging studies, using different tasks (although mainly visual) typically report activations in anterior cingulate cortex (ACC), lateral prefrontal cortices (PFC) (including dorsolateral PFC, DLPFC, and inferior frontal cortex, IFC), anterior insula (AI), and parietal cortices [8–14]. However, given the methodological limitations, such as the poor temporal resolution of the prevailing neuroimaging technique of fMRI, it is not completely clear how these regions work together as a functional network during conflict processing.

In order to disentangle specific processes and mechanisms that underlie attentional control during conflict resolution, it is necessary to use imaging tools with high temporal resolution, such as magnetoencephalography (MEG) and EEG that provide a direct measure of post-synaptic neuronal processes. Findings from event-related potential (ERP) studies using various conflict tasks suggest that the components N200 (also known as N2) [15] and N450 [16] are related to stimulus-level conflict, while the error-related negativity (ERN) component [15] reflects response-level conflict (for a review, see [17]). A limitation of such conventional ERP analyses are that task-modulated non-phase-locked "induced" dynamics of EEG data are not-present trial-averaged responses, and that they do not allow inferences of interregional dynamics during conflict processing [18]. However, accumulating evidence suggests that functional coupling across distant brain areas during attention and cognitive control can be explicitly quantified based on interregional phase locking of neuronal oscillations [19,20], occurring at distinct frequency ranges. It appears that low-frequency (<30 Hz) oscillations at the theta (4–7 Hz), alpha (7–15 Hz), and beta (15–30 Hz) ranges are particularly relevant for longer-range coupling associated with top-down modulation of neurons [21–23]. Evidence from human studies suggests that such coupling may be enhanced in task-relevant networks during auditory attention [24], as well as visually-delivered working memory [25] and conflict-processing tasks [26,27]. It has been also noninvasively shown that, during auditory orienting, interregional interactions at the gamma band are modulated by the phase of theta in humans [28]. As suggested by extracellular measurements in cats [29] and human MEG studies [30], inter-regional phase locking may also increase at the beta band during attention and/or cognitive control tasks.

Previous auditory fMRI studies suggest that ACC is essential for selective attention to task-relevant sound features [31,32] and auditory feedback monitoring [33]. It is specifically activated when the subject is asked to pay attention selectively to one of two dichotically presented phonemes and ignore a simultaneously presented competing stimulus [34]. However, only a small number of auditory behavioral [35,36] and neuroimaging [32,34] studies on perceptual conflicts have been conducted in the auditory domain, especially at the early stage of object identification and selection, that is, the stimulus conflict. Here, we therefore tested the hypothesis that ACC may also support selective listening in complex auditory settings such as multitalker environments. To achieve this goal, we used non-invasive estimates of neuronal oscillations [24,37,38] to investigate the ACC and DLPFC oscillatory phase locking patterns predicting fast and efficient conflict processing using a modified auditory flanker interference task, in which participants were required to identify a spoken "A" or "O" from acoustically similar or distinct flankers. Source localization of neuronal oscillations was facilitated by using anatomical MRI constraints to limit the potential solutions to the cortical gray matter [39,40], where non-invasively measurable MEG and EEG activities are generated [41], and by combining the complementary information provided by simultaneously measured MEG and EEG [42]. A priori regions of interest (ROIs) including the caudal ACC (cACC) and DLPFC in each hemisphere were first defined based on the Desikan-Killiany atlas [43]. The cACC seed roughly corresponded to the anterior mid-cingulate cortex area that has also been termed "dorsal ACC" in previous conflict processing studies [44]. Seed-based oscillatory phase locking estimates between these ROIs and all cortical locations were then calculated using the debiased weighted phase lag index (wPLI), to test the specific hypothesis that conflict processing is associated with increased cortico-cortical low-frequency phase locking between ACC and lateral prefrontal regions.

Materials and Methods

Participants

The study protocol was approved by the Partners Human Research Committee, the Institutional Review Board (IRB) of the Massachusetts General Hospital. Potential subjects were first screened with a phone interview to ensure that they had normal hearing and had not been exposed regularly to environments with excessively loud noise. Twelve right-handed college-level educated adults with normal hearing and no neurological disorders, psychiatric conditions, or learning disabilities, gave written informed consent prior to testing.

Task and stimuli

During MEG/EEG acquisitions, subjects ($N = 12$, age 20–33 years, 6 females) were presented with an auditory spatial-phonetic flanker interference task modified based on previous psychoacoustic studies [35] (**Figure 1**). Each sound trial, presented at a randomly varying inter-trial onset interval of 2.95–3.05 s, included two 400 ms "flankers" simulated horizontally from 45° to the right and left using generic head-related transfer functions [45], and a 400 ms target sound coming from straight ahead that started 300 ms after the flankers. The delay was introduced to the target, as very few subjects were able to discriminate the target from simultaneous flankers. The setting was thus analogous to certain previous visuospatial flanker studies [46,47], with the additional delay being also justified because of the serial nature of phonetic sound-object processing [48]. The flankers and targets consisted of a voice sounding out the American English letters "A" or "O", obtained from the Psychology Experiment Building Language (PEBL) Sound Archive version 0.1. The pitch of the flankers was digitally manipulated to be 3.1 semitones lower or higher than the target, such that the listener always heard three sounds coming from three different directions at three different pitches. Equiprobably, the subject heard either a congruent set of voices ("A_{Left}-A_{Middle}-$A_{\mathbf{Right}}$" or "O_{Left}-O_{Middle}-O_{Right}") or an incongruent/conflicting set of voices ("A_{Left}-O_{Middle}-A_{Right}" or "O_{Left}-A_{Middle}-O_{Right}"). In all trials, subjects were instructed to ignore the flanking distractors and pay attention only to the middle target by pressing a button with the index finger of one hand if the target was "A" and with the index finger of the opposite hand if the target was "O". The hand/target letter order was switched after each of two 16-minute runs (324 trials per run), in an counterbalanced order across the subjects. Subjects' responses were recorded together with the MEG/EEG raw data and reaction time (RT) was measured from the moment of the target appearance to the moment of button pressing. Two subjects were excluded from the final MEG/EEG analyses because they could not perform the tasks.

Data acquisition

We recorded 306-channel MEG (Elekta-Neuromag, Helsinki, Finland) and 74-channel EEG data simultaneously in a magnetically shielded room (sampling rate 1 kHz, passband 0.03–330 Hz). The average reference was utilized for all analyses of

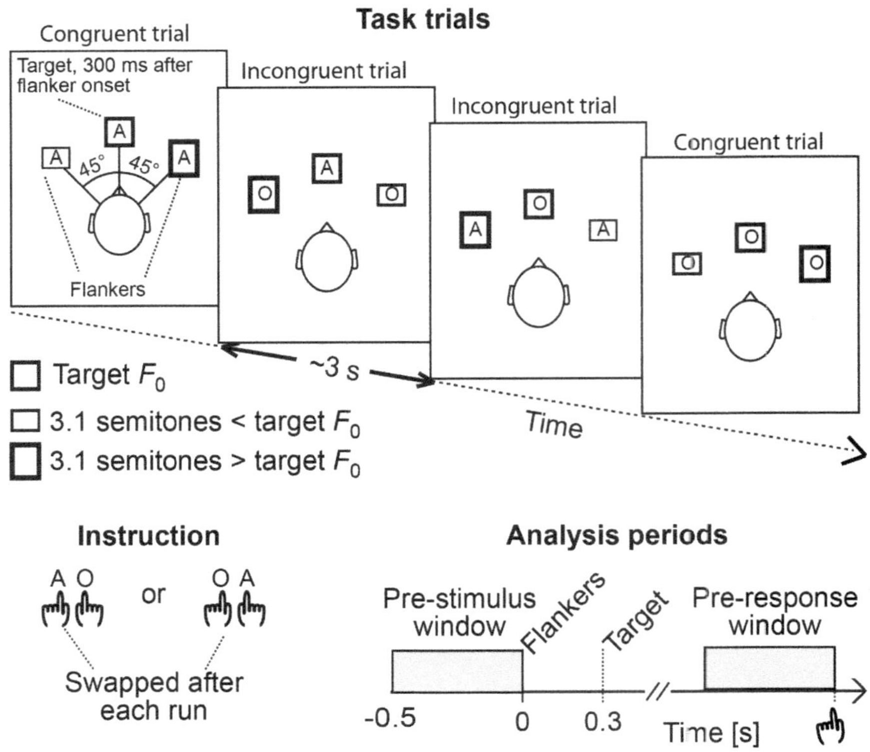

Figure 1. Task design and oscillatory analysis periods. *Task trials*: Subjects were instructed to pay attention to the target sounds and ignore flanking distractor sounds, which were phonetically either congruent (50%) or conflicting (50%) with the target. The flankers arrived 45° to the right and left of the target, at a 3.1 semitones lower or higher pitch than the target. *Instruction*: In a counterbalanced order across runs/subjects, subjects were asked to press a button either with the left index finger to "A" and with the right index finger to "O", or vice versa. *Analysis periods*: To determine oscillatory power and phase locking patterns that predict efficient conflict processing, the analyses were concentrated on the time periods that preceded each stimulus trial ("Pre-stimulus window") and each behavioral response ("Pre-response window").

EEG data. The position of the head relative to the MEG sensor array was monitored continuously using four head position indicator (HPI) coils attached to the scalp. Electrooculogram (EOG) was also recorded to monitor eye artifacts. T1-weighted structural MRIs were obtained for combining anatomical and functional data using a multi-echo MPRAGE pulse sequence (TR = 2510 ms; 4 echoes with TEs = 1.64 ms, 3.5 ms, 5.36 ms, 7.22 ms; 176 sagittal slices with $1\times1\times1$ mm^3 voxels, 256×256 mm^2 matrix; flip angle = 7°). Multi-echo FLASH data were obtained with 5° and 30° flip angles (TR = 20 ms, TE = 1.89+2n ms [n = 0–7], 256×256 mm^2 matrix, 1.33-mm slice thickness) for reconstruction of head boundary-element models (BEM).

Data analysis

Neuronal bases of auditory conflict processing were studied using a cortically constrained MEG/EEG MNE approach [24,38]. The MNE method reconstructs the intracranial sources of activity by identifying the distribution of dipoles with minimum total power that accounts for the magnetic field distribution recorded over the scalp. The cortically constrained approach takes into account the shape of the cortex and thus provides a better spatial resolution than an MNE only confined to the intracranial volume [39,40]. Our overall workflow consists of (i) preprocessing of the MEG/EEG data (removal of artifacts and estimation of noise covariance matrix), (ii) preprocessing of the anatomical MRI data (reconstruction of the cortical surface to set up individual MEG/EEG source space, and the reconstruction of the scalp, outer skull, and inner skull surfaces), (iii) alignment of the MEG and MRI coordinate frames and computing forward solutions, and (iv) computing the MNE inverse operator for source estimates.

External MEG noise was suppressed and subject movements, estimated continuously at 200-ms intervals, were compensated for using the signal-space separation method [49] (Maxfilter, Elekta-Neuromag, Helsinki, Finland). The MEG/EEG data were down-sampled (333 samples/s, passband 0.5–110 Hz). Epochs coinciding with over 150 µV EOG, 100 µV EEG, 2 pT/cm MEG gradiometer, or 4 pT MEG magnetometer peak-to-peak signals were excluded from further analyses.

For building the cortically constrained source space, we used FreeSurfer 5.3 [50] (http://surfer.nmr.mgh.harvard.edu/) to determine the shapes of the surfaces separating the scalp, skull, and brain compartments, and to build the triangular cortical surface mesh from T1-weighted anatomical 3D-volume MRI data by exploiting the gray-white matter boundary generated by the software. The FreeSurfer software was used due to the following advantages [50–52]: first, in addition to folded surfaces, it also computes inflated and flattened representations of the cortex, and can thus expose the parts of the cortex embedded in the sulci. Further, it provides an automated parcellation of the cortex that can be used in inquiring source waveforms in specific ROI. Finally, an additional benefit of the surface-based analysis is that cortical surfaces can be aligned across individuals for the computation of group statistics using a morphing procedure in a spherical coordinate system [50] and several recent studies have shown that the method has the highest stability in gray matter volume estimate compared to two other volume-based methods [53], and better alignments of cortical landmarks than volume-based registrations [54]. To achieve sufficient anatomical detail for the visualization of the folded cortical mantle, the triangular tessellations of each hemisphere contain roughly 100,000 potential vertices, spaced at ~1 mm. For inverse computations, the dense triangulations were decimated to ~1,000 vertices per hemisphere for computational efficiency.

To calculate MRI-guided depth-weighted ℓ_2 MNE [55], the information from structural segmentation of the individual MRIs and the MEG sensor and EEG electrode locations were used to compute the forward solutions for all putative source locations in the cortex using a three-compartment BEM [55].

The covariance matrix and the forward solution computed in the previous procedures were used to obtain a distributed cortically constrained minimum-norm inverse operator that relates the sensor measurements to dipole current estimates in the source space. The individual forward solutions for current dipoles placed at these vertices comprised the columns of the gain matrix (**A**). A noise covariance matrix (**C**) was estimated from the raw MEG/EEG data during a 20–200-ms pre-stimulus baseline. These two matrices, along with the source covariance matrix (**R**), were used to calculate the MNE inverse operator $\mathbf{W} = \mathbf{RA}^T (\mathbf{ARA}^T + \mathbf{C})^{-1}$, which is applied to the sensor-level data to yield the source time courses.

To investigate seed-based cortico-cortical phase locking patterns, the entire MEG/EEG raw data time series at each time point were multiplied by the inverse operator **W** and noise normalized to yield the estimated source activity as a function of time across the entire cortex [40]. In addition, the frontal seed regions, including cACC and DLPFC, were selected from each hemisphere using the Freesurfer anatomical atlas [43]. The DLPFC was, specifically, defined based on the "rostral middle-frontal cortex" label [43], which encompasses the junction of Brodmann's areas 9, 10, and 46 [56]. An average raw data time course was then calculated within these seed regions, with the waveform signs of sources aligned on the basis of surface-normal orientations to avoid phase cancellations.

Accepted MEG/EEG trial epochs were analyzed using the MNE and MNE-Python [57], and FieldTrip tools (http://www.ru.nl/fcdonders/fieldtrip). To investigate the phase locking between the cACC and DLPFC seed regions and all cortical locations, a FFT with Hanning window was applied on (**a**) the raw data epochs in each vertex of the right and left hemisphere and (**b**) on the corresponding trials of the pooled raw time courses of the right and left seed regions, separately for the 500-ms periods preceding each sound triplet and each behavioral response. Our presumption was that long-range inter-regional phase locking patterns would occur in theta and alpha, and lower beta ranges. Therefore, the FFT was applied at 2-Hz intervals at 6–20 Hz at the 500-ms windows and a Hanning taper. The 500-ms window length was selected on the basis of the RT data, such that the analysis window would not overlap with the target sound onset. We then calculated the phase locking between the seeds and each vertex the left and right hemisphere using the debiased wPLI. In addition to controlling for the sample-size bias, the debiased wPLI provides an index of nonzero phase lags across the regions/locations of interest that helps avoid spurious inflation of synchronization indices due to EEG and MEG point spread and crosstalk [58]. The resulting seed-based debiased wPLI estimates, mapped across all cortical locations in each subject, were then normalized to the Freesurfer standard brain representation for surface-based group statistical analyses [59].

In addition to the main analysis concentrating on the seed-based phase locking, we also estimated the power of neuronal oscillations across the available band during 500-ms pre-stimulus and pre-response periods, using a FFT with a Hanning taper at 2-Hz intervals between 4 and 30 Hz and an adaptive time-window of 3 cycles. At 30–110 Hz, 3-Hz frequency smoothing was used, resulting in three orthogonal Slepian tapers being applied to the 500-ms time window [60]. Analogous to [38], the available frequency band was divided to consecutive one-octave wide sub ranges, which corresponded to theta (4–7.5 Hz), alpha (7.5–15 Hz), beta (15–30 Hz), lower gamma (30–60 Hz), and higher gamma (60–110 Hz) bands (*i.e.*, the highest band was less than one octave).

Statistical analysis

RT and hit rate (HR) differences were analyzed using t-tests. The HR distributions were cubically and the RT distributions logarithmically transformed to render them approximately Gaussian [61], as confirmed by using the Jarque-Bera test. To test our specific hypotheses, we examined correlations between behavioral performance (RT to incongruent normalized by the RT to congruent trials) *vs.* cortical phase locking and power changes during periods preceding stimulus presentation and during the 500-ms period preceding the behavioral responses. For the pre-stimulus analyses, we calculated the correlations between the baseline preceding the incongruent trials and the normalized RT conflict effect. For the pre-response analyses, a 2×2 factorial design was utilized to control for the effects of responding hand (right *vs.* left) and task type (incongruent *vs.* congruent). To control for multiple comparisons, the resulting statistical estimates were tested against an empirical null distribution of maximum cluster size across 10,000 iterations with a vertex-wise threshold of $P<0.05$ and cluster-forming threshold of $P<0.05$ (Bonferroni corrected by the number of hemispheres), yielding clusters corrected for multiple comparisons across the surface.

Results

The behavioral analyses showed a significant conflict effect, demonstrating that the task was functioning as anticipated. RTs to the incongruent trials were significantly longer than those to the congruent trials ($t_9 = 7.5$, $p<0.001$; mean ± SD $RT_{Congruent} = 569 \pm 116$ ms; mean ± SD $RT_{Incongruent} = 637 \pm 118$ ms), and HRs were significantly lower to the incongruent than congruent trials ($t_9 = -3.2$, $p = 0.01$; mean ± SD $HR_{Congruent} = 98 \pm 2\%$; mean ± SD $HR_{Incongruent} = 95 \pm 4\%$).

Seed-based phase locking patterns correlating with behavioral conflict processing

Our main purpose was to examine cortico-cortical functional connectivity patterns that predict efficient behavioral performance during the modified auditory flanker task. This analysis concentrated on two distinct time periods, preceding the stimulus trials and preceding each behavioral response that followed the stimuli. **Figure 2** shows estimates of "sustained" baseline connectivity patterns, which predicted fast and efficient conflict processing, i.e., reduced RT lags, in the subsequent stimulus trials. Significant correlations ($p<0.05$, cluster-based Monte Carlo simulation test) between reduced RT lags and increased phase locking patterns (debiased wPLI) were observed at the theta range (6 Hz) between the right cACC and right lateral frontal regions, including FEF. Reduced conflict-induced RT lags also correlated with increased theta/alpha connectivity between cACC and medial frontal cortex regions bilaterally at 6 Hz, and between the right cACC and left medial/superior frontal cortex at 8 Hz. Note that in this case the connectivity patterns are unlikely to be explained by biases caused

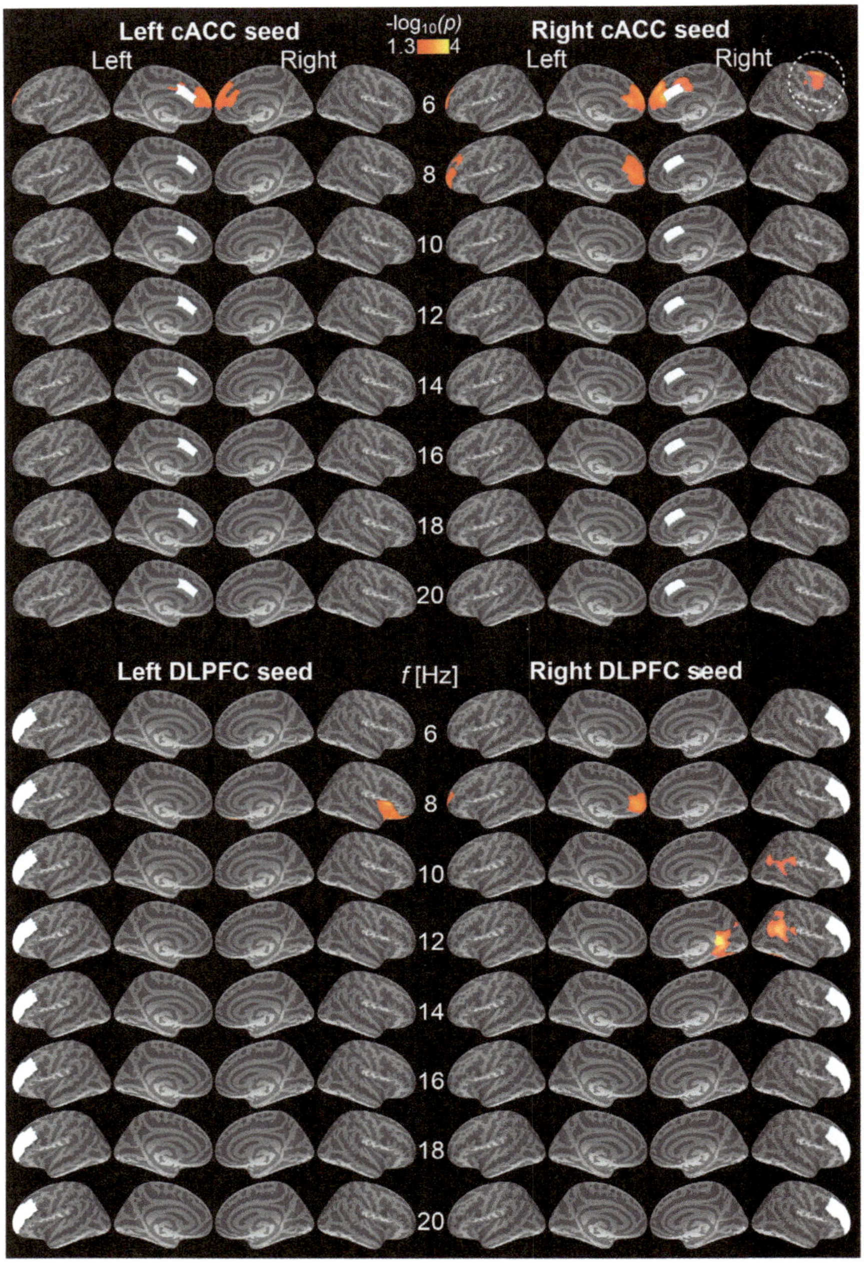

Figure 2. Baseline correlations between conflict-induced RT lags and cortical phase locking to the caudal anterior cingulate (cACC) and dorsolateral prefrontal cortex (DPLPC) seeds during 500-ms periods preceding conflicting trials. All significant findings reflect correlations between reduced RT lags and increased seed-based phase locking patterns ($p<0.05$, cluster-based Monte Carlo simulation test). (Top) Left and right cACC seed data. Interestingly, at 6 Hz (i.e., theta), faster RTs after conflicting sounds correlated with increased connectivity between the right cACC and right lateral prefrontal areas (encircled), and between bihemispheric cACC seeds and adjacent medial frontal cortex locations. (Bottom) Left and right DLPFC seed data. Faster RTs after incongruent trials were strongly correlated with increased alpha phase locking between the right DLPFC and right retrosplenial (12 Hz) and inferior parietal/TPJ regions (10–12 Hz), as well as at 8 Hz, between the left DLPFC and right anterior insula and between right DLPFC and left anteromedial frontal cortex. The results reflect $-\log_{10}(p)$ of the initial t-statistics, masked to the locations where the cluster-based Monte Carlo simulation test was significant ($p<0.05$).

by the anatomical adjacency, i.e., EEG/MEG point spread and cross talk, because the debiased wPLI index emphasizes synchronization patterns with nonzero phase lags [58].

During the pre-stimulus baseline period, the strongest behavioral correlations involving the DLPFC seed connectivity patterns were observed at the alpha range (10–12 Hz): Reduced RT lags associated with incongruent trials correlated with increased phase locking between the right DLPFC and right inferior parietal/temporoparietal junction (TPJ), as well as the right retrosplenial cortices. In addition, analogous behavioral correlations were observed with increased 8-Hz phase locking between the left DLPFC and right anterior insula as well as with phase locking between the right DLPFC and left anterior medial frontal cortex. **Table 1** shows the details of the cluster statistics reflecting correlations between the conflict-induced RT lags and the phase

Table 1. Correlations between RT lags caused by conflict and seed-based phase locking patterns during the pre-stimulus baseline period.

Target hemisphere	Seed	f [Hz]	Max value	Size (mm^2)	x_{MNI}	y_{MNI}	z_{MNI}	Cluster-wise *P*	Anatomical coverage
Left									
	Left cACC								
		6	−2.2	3922	−8	58	17	0.0022	Superior frontal
	Right cACC								
		6	−2.4	4118	−5	38	8	0.0017	Medial frontal
		8	−2.2	6661	−6	35	8	0.0001	Medial frontal
	Right DLPFC								
		8	−2.4	3347	−7	42	2	0.0116	Medial frontal
Right									
	Left cACC								
		6	−2.0	3149	9	41	35	0.0111	Superior frontal
	Right cACC								
		6	−3.0	4605	6	33	18	0.0001	Medial frontal
		6	−2.3	3126	27	8	47	0.0112	Lateral prefrontal
	Left DLPFC								
		8	−2.5	3657	26	12	−17	0.0047	Anterior insula, IFC, orbitofrontal
	Right DLPFC								
		10	−1.9	2930	47	−35	28	0.0155	TPJ/inferior parietal
		12	−3.7	4975	14	−48	3	0.0001	Retrosplenial/precuneus
		12	−2.8	5534	44	−54	23	0.0001	IPS, TPJ/inferior parietal

Monte Carlo simulation results of the data in **Fig. 2** are demonstrated. The maximum values of initial GLM reflect $-\log10(p) \times \mathrm{sign}(t)$.

locking differences after incongruent vs. congruent stimuli, as measured from the 500-ms periods preceding each stimulus.

Figure 3 shows the results reflecting efficient conflict processing, during the post-stimulus/pre-response period, as estimated from a full factorial model estimating the correlations between the RT lags to incongruent vs. congruent trials and phase locking differences after incongruent vs. congruent stimuli. Most importantly, consistent with the hypothesis that efficient conflict processing depends on cingulofrontal connectivity, we found that reduced conflict-induced RT lags correlated with increased 8-Hz alpha phase locking between the bilateral cACC seeds and right lateral prefrontal regions. In the right lateral prefrontal cortex, these behavioral correlation patterns encompassed the likely location of right FEF, associated with the dorsal attention network, and the right DLPFC. In addition, behavioral correlations emerged with increased phase locking between the following regions: the left cACC and right medial parietal cortex at 12 Hz, left DLPFC and left superior/medial pre- and post-central regions at 8 Hz, and right DLPFC seed and right superior frontal gyrus regions at 18 Hz.

Figure 4 highlights the effects, concentrating on the theta/alpha phase locking between the cACC seeds and right lateral frontal cortices before (at 6 Hz) and after the occurrence of the conflicting information (at 8 Hz), which predict efficient/fast conflict processing performance. In addition to the significant behavioral correlations, the data in **Figure 4** also show that when the contribution of behavioral performance has been removed from the model, during the post-stimulus/pre-response period of the main contrast, a significant ($p<0.05$, cluster-based Monte Carlo simulation test) decrease of debiased wPLI between the cACC and right lateral frontal regions is observed after the incongruent vs. congruent trials. This leaves room for an interpretation that the occurrence of a conflicting information has a tendency to disrupt an existing phase locking pattern between the cACC and lateral frontal cortex, rather than eliciting a new functional connectivity pattern, and that the resolution of a conflict depends on the restoration of the sustained functional coupling between the medial and lateral frontal regions. **Table 2** shows the cluster statistics of correlations between conflict-induced RT lags and connectivity patterns emerging during the 500-ms periods preceding each behavioral response.

Cortical power mapping patterns correlating with behavioral conflict resolution

Finally, we also correlated behavioral measures with cortical power mapping results during the same time periods that were examined in the functional connectivity analyses. These analyses revealed a significant correlation between increased left lateral prefrontal cortex high-gamma power (60–110 Hz) during the pre-stimulus baseline period and reduced conflict-induced RT lags (**Figure 5**). No significant correlations emerged in the other frequency bands during the baseline period, or in any frequency band during the period preceding the behavioral responses.

Discussion

We studied seed-based oscillatory phase locking patterns associated with conflict processing during an auditory flanker interference task. Consistent with our hypothesis, the results demonstrate that efficient conflict resolution during sound object selection, as measured with reduced conflict-induced RT lags, is predicted by theta/alpha phase coupling between the cACC and right lateral frontal cortex regions intersecting FEF and DLPFC. Notably, the correlation patterns observed were not fully consistent with a hypothesis that cACC is a region only transiently recruited to detect conflicting coactivations of information processing streams. On the contrary, our statistical model showed that, when the variability of behavioral performance was regressed out, the occurrence of conflict actually disrupts the sustained connectivity between the cACC and lateral frontal regions. Our results, thus, seem to suggest that the cACC is involved in networks that bias processing of task-relevant sound information in situations requiring sustained engagement of control mechanisms.

It is generally agreed that cognitive control utilizes a network of brain regions including DLPFC, ACC, and posterior parietal regions [62]. Further, an emerging view is that discrete areas process information in a coordinated manner rather than as distinct modules [63]. Coordinated activity between neurons in different networks and brain regions may be mediated by spike synchrony with local field potential (LFP) oscillations [64] as well as synchrony of LFP oscillations, which provide windows of time when the effectiveness of a proximal spike on a distal neuron's postsynaptic potential is enhanced [20,63,65]. Our finding of the cACC phase-locked with the FEF and portions of DLPFC in theta/alpha band during conflict resolution is in line with this proposal, and further demonstrates a functional correlation of cognitive control processes and oscillatory theta-band activity between the ACC, the FEF, and the DLPFC.

Our results that the ability to allocate attention to relevant sound objects and disregard those with conflicting information correlates with cACC connectivity with lateral frontal cortices are consistent with previous studies that link cACC with conflict processing [66–68], error-related reinforcement learning [69], selection of goal-directed actions [70], and allocation of attentional resources [71,72]. Although most previous studies consider vision, there is an abundance of evidence that ACC also plays a role in auditory attention and cognitive control [12,31–33]. For example, there is evidence [73] that conflict-related EEG activations, which presumably originate in ACC [74], correlate with the degree of ambiguity of choice-tasks trials that do not involve actual conflicts. This suggests that the underlying circuits might also contribute to disambiguation of complex stimulus scenes. Further, conflict-related mid frontal theta oscillations have been previously identified in a number of EEG studies [27,75]. By exploiting the temporal and spatial resolution of combined MEG/EEG methods and anatomical MRI, our findings provide convincing evidence regarding the source of the mid frontal theta, as well as its involvement in early stage of perceptual processing before the response selection. Importantly, our findings extend previous literature and show that the functional network involving cACC, FEF, and DLPFC, not only monitors instantaneous occurrences of conflicts, but also exerts sustained attentional control needed for the selection of relevant sound objects in complex auditory environments.

During the post-stimulus/pre-response period, most significant correlations with cACC theta/alpha phase locking patterns emerged in the right FEF. Accumulating evidence suggests that the right FEF is a key part of the dorsal attention network (DAN) that governs voluntary deployment of spatial attention to task-relevant locations (for a review, see [76]), and this area could also be associated with auditory spatial attention [77]. Recent neurophysiological studies in non-human primates further suggest that FEF initiates top-down signals that helps bias saliency maps in posterior parietal cortices (e.g., in the monkey homologue of human intraparietal sulcus, IPS) that prioritize stimuli occurring in task relevant locations [78]. One might therefore conclude that cACC provides top-down feedback that, analogously to its proposed role during visual attention [79], helps the network

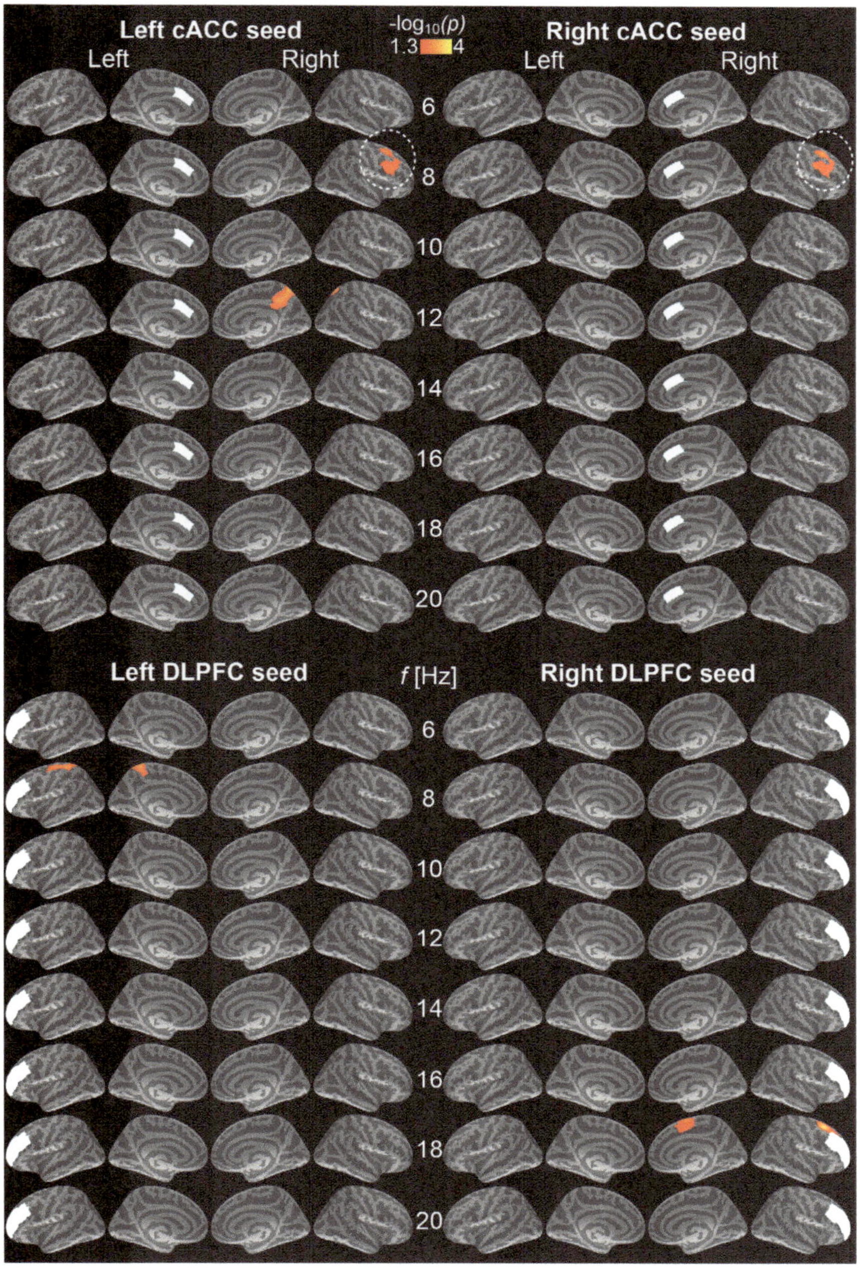

Figure 3. Correlations between conflict-induced RT lags and phase locking to the caudal anterior cingulate (cACC) and dorsolateral prefrontal cortex (DPLPC) seeds during 500-ms periods preceding incongruent trials. All statistically significant findings reflect correlations between reduced RT lags and increased seed-based phase locking after incongruent vs. congruent trials ($p<0.05$, cluster-based Monte Carlo simulation test). (Top) Left and right cACC seed data. Most interestingly, at 8 Hz, reduced conflict-induced RT lags correlated with increased connectivity between the bilateral cACC and right lateral prefrontal areas encompassing FEF and posterior aspects of DLPFC (encircled). At 12 Hz, reduced conflict-induced RT lags also correlate with increased phase locking between the left cACC and right medial parietal cortex. (Bottom) Left and right DLPFC seed data. Reduced conflict-induced RT lags correlated with increased 8-Hz alpha phase locking between the left DLPFC and left postcentral/precentral regions, as well as increased 18-Hz beta phase locking between the right DLPFC and right superior frontal/pre-supplementary motor area (pre-SMA) regions. The results reflect $-\log_{10}(p)$ of the initlal t-statistics, masked to the locations where the cluster-based Monte Carlo simulation test was significant ($p<0.05$).

involving FEF and IPS boost attention toward sound objects originating from the task-relevant spatial direction (here, straight ahead) and suppress those from task-irrelevant directions (here, 45° right/left) during auditory attention. Notably, it has been long speculated that altered connectivity of cingulate regions with FEF and parietal cortices underlies impaired selective attention in schizophrenia, reflected by the patients' inability to distinguish relevant vs. irrelevant objects in their perceptual field [80].

In addition to FEF, we also found the cACC phase-locked with the posterior aspects of right DLPFC at the theta/alpha bands. This finding is consistent with the known bidirectional anatomical connections between ACC and DLPFC [81], and with observations that these two areas work in concert to enhance top-down

Table 2. Correlations between the RT lag caused by conflict and seed-based phase locking differences between periods preceding behavioral responses to incongruent vs. congruent sounds.

Target hemisphere	Seed	f [Hz]	Max value	Size (mm^2)	x_{MNI}	y_{MNI}	z_{MNI}	Cluster-wise *P*	Anatomical coverage
Left									
	Left DLPFC	8	−2.4	3659	−28	−35	58	0.0038	SMA, postcentral
Right									
	Left cACC	8	−1.9	3325	29	13	46	0.0095	Lateral PFC, FEF
		12	−2.6	2983	5	−63	55	0.0130	Precuneus
	Right cACC	8	−2.1	3740	29	13	46	0.0018	Lateral PFC, FEF
	Right DLPFC	18	−2.7	3531	28	14	44	0.0068	Lateral PFC, FEF

Monte Carlo simulation results of the data in **Fig. 3** are demonstrated. The maximum values of initial GLM reflect $-\log10(p) \times \text{sign}(t)$.

control [82]. Our findings are also in line with a proposition that theta oscillations are the electrophysiological mechanism underlying these interactions [83]. For example, a recent animal study reported extensive interactions between ACC and lateral frontal cortices at the theta range [84]. An open question, however, is how the functions of ACC vs. DLPFC are orchestrated during attentional control in the face of interferences and conflicts. The "conflict monitoring" hypothesis [85] suggests a system where ACC monitors and detects conflicts caused by distracting stimuli, and signals them to DLPFC that exerts the ultimate control [86]. The present results are not fully consistent with this notion, as the significant correlation between efficient behavioral conflict resolution and cACC–DLPFC/FEF connectivity was also observable during the pre-stimulus period, that is, before the conflict had even occurred. The presence of effects during the baseline period resembles recent observations in monkey neurophysiological studies [87]. Moreover, when the between-subject behavioral variability was covaried out from our statistical models concerning the post-stimulus/pre-response period, it appeared that the occurrence of a conflict results in a transient decrease in cACC–DLPFC/FEF phase locking. Overall, the results would seem to be most consistent with the notion that cACC and DLPFC work together in a more sustained fashion to suppress distraction and boost attention to relevant stimuli.

However, it is important to note that the present MEG/EEG source estimates are likely less anatomically specific than those achievable with fMRI, not to mention invasive recordings. That is, there is fMRI evidence that the different subregions of ACC may be differentially recruited during conflict processing and distraction suppression. Specifically, a recent study [88] suggested that whereas dorsal aspects of ACC, which overlap with the present cACC seed regions, are associated with biasing attention toward relevant stimuli, the more rostral ACC areas were associated only with conflict detection.

Another interesting finding of the current study is the link between pre-stimulus alpha and performance. Specifically, during the pre-stimulus baseline period, it was found that increased alpha phase locking between the left DLPFC and right AI, as well as between the right DLPFC vs. left anterior MFC and right inferior parietal/TPJ, correlated with fast and efficient behavioral conflict. Although alpha power increases have been often linked to cortical "idling", there is accumulating evidence that inter-regional phase locking at this frequency range mediates top-down effects of attention. Evidence supporting this notion has been shown in animal studies suggesting that interregional alpha and beta synchronization in areas roughly corresponding to primate DLPFC and ACC that generated top-down attentional signals [63], as well as in animal and human studies reporting increases of alpha coherence in visual cortices [29,89] and strengthening of alpha phase synchrony between occipital visual cortex and parietal [90] or PFC [91] regions by attention.

At the beta frequency range, we found that auditory-behavioral conflict resolution correlated with increased phase locking between the right DLPFC and the right pre-SMA. The pre-SMA has anatomical connections with the DLPFC [92,93], and these regions have been implicated in the internally generated aspects of action planning, such as choice and intention. Numerous studies have documented beta oscillations associated with movement behavior and response inhibition, but beta power has also been implicated in broader cognitive processes (for a review, see [94]). In fact, it has been proposed that inter-areal coherence, at the beta frequency range, may have an essential role in cognitive functions including selective attention, working memory, object recognition, perception or sensory-motor integration, due to the prominent

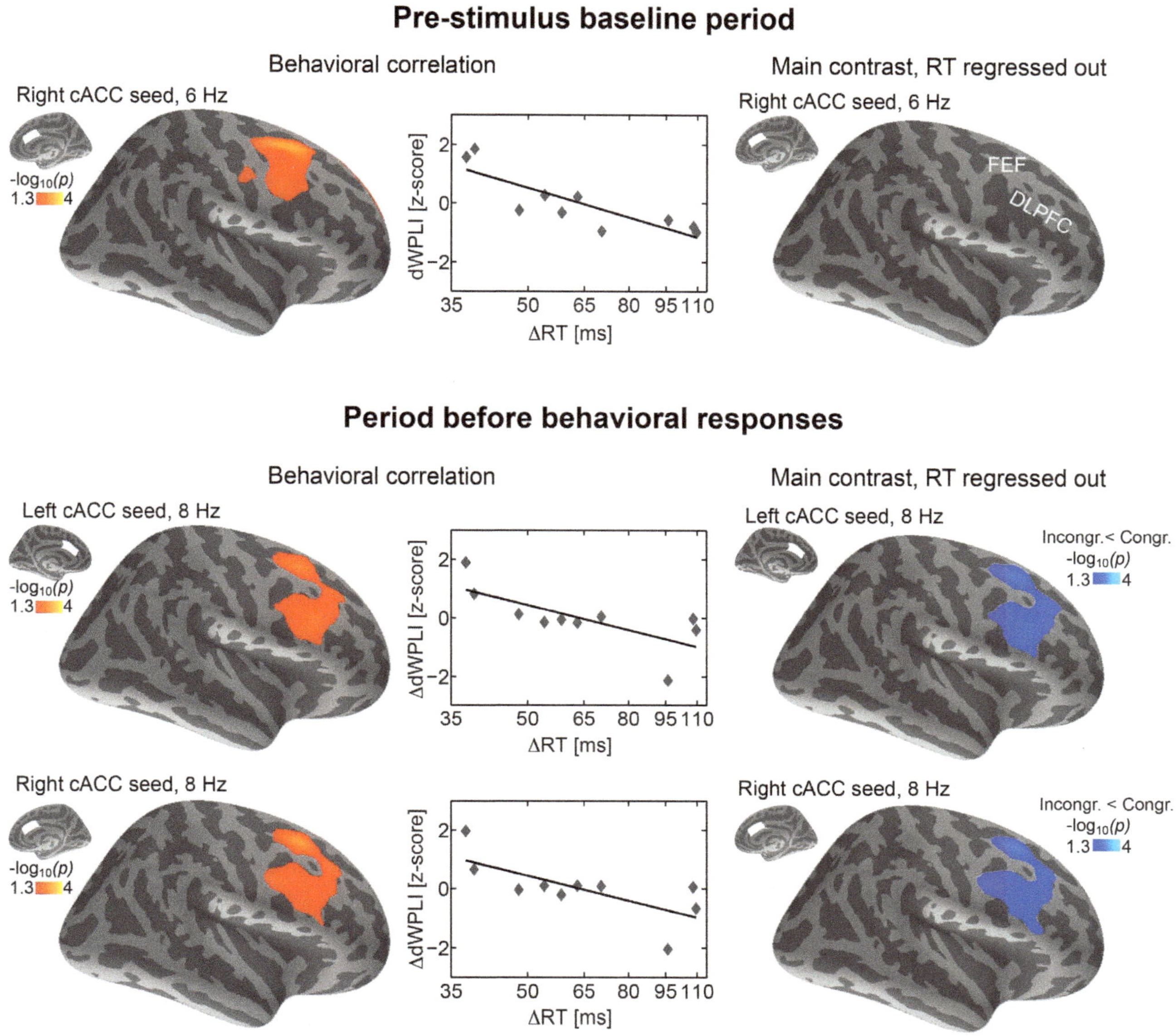

Figure 4. Behavioral conflict resolution and theta/alpha connectivity patters between medial and lateral frontal cortices. (**Top**) The results during the baseline periods. The connectivity between cACC and lateral frontal cortex, specifically FEF, at 6 Hz predicted faster conflict processing, possibly associated with sustained allocation of attention that is necessary for efficient conflict monitoring and resolution during selective listening. The scatter diagram shows the ΔRT (natural logarithmic scale) plotted against lateral frontal cluster average debiased weighted phase lag index (wPLI), with a best-fitting linear trend, depicting the correlation between fast conflict resolution and cACC-lateral frontal theta phase locking. (**Bottom**) Analyses during the 500-ms period preceding each behavioral response are shown. Stronger connectivity between the bilateral cACC and right lateral frontal cortices (FEF, DLPFC) at 8 Hz predicted fast conflict resolution performance, i.e., reduced ΔRT between incongruent and congruent trials. When the effect of behavioral variability was covaried out, the main contrast showed a significant decrease of post-conflict connectivity between the approximately same regions. The scatter diagrams show the ΔRT (natural logarithmic scale) plotted against the lateral frontal debiased wPLI cluster averages for the cACC seed, with the best-fitting linear trend.

role of beta-band oscillations in top-down projections [94]. Interestingly, there is evidence from modeling studies showing that synchronization can tolerate longer synaptic delays for beta than gamma oscillation [23,95], suggesting that long-distance oscillatory synchronization may be more robustly realized at beta frequencies. Our data confirms and extends pervious findings of pre-SMA's involvement in conflict situations [96] and demonstrates that synchronized beta-band oscillations may be the underlying neural mechanism supporting inter-regional communication during conflict processing. Future studies are needed to discern whether its exact role is related to resolving competition between motor plans during response selection, or to conflict-related information processing *per se*.

Our finding that the subjects' ability to resolve conflicts between competing auditory inputs correlated with alpha-band phase locking between the right DLPFC and the retrospenial/precuneus cortex during the baseline period is consistent with recent resting state studies in monkeys and humans demonstrating functional connectivity between the DLPFC and the retrospenial/precuneus regions [97]. It has been proposed that the retrospenial cortex might be the neural substrate between the interaction between the DLPFC and hippocampus [98], and that it plays an essential role

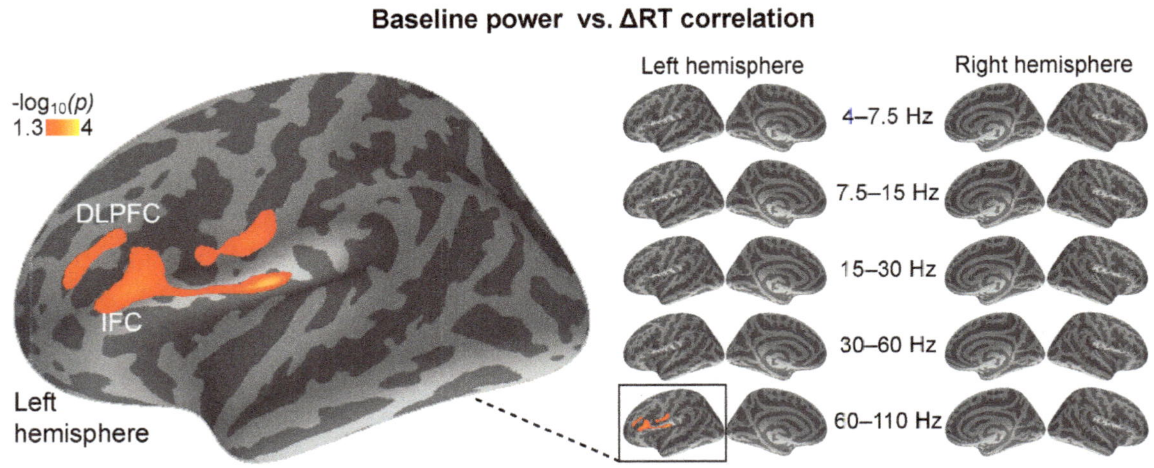

Figure 5. Correlation analyses between the power of pre-stimulus baseline oscillations and behavioral performance. Efficient behavioral conflict processing, as reflected by shorter conflict-induced RT lags, correlated with increased oscillatory power at the higher (60–110 Hz) gamma band during the pre-stimulus period ($p<0.05$, cluster-based Monte Carlo simulation test). The significant correlation were concentrated in the left lateral and inferior frontal cortices, consistent with previous fMRI studies suggesting their role in speech-sound related auditory attention tasks [102]. No significant correlations were observed in the other frequency bands, in the other brain regions, or during the periods immediately before the behavioral responses. The figure shows the significance of initial GLM, masked to the locations that survived the post-hoc correction based on the cluster-based Monte Carlo simulation test.

in cognitive context processing [for a review, see 99]. For example, in an fMRI/MEG study investigating neural synchronization in the contextual processing, activations associated with stronger contextual association were found in retrospenial, parahippocampal and occipital cortices. Importantly, greater phase locking at beta band between these regions were also observed. Taken together, we speculate that the increased phase locking between the right DLPFC and the retrospenial/precuneus cortex observed in the current study might reflect enhanced contextual processing originates in the DLPFC in the face of increasing conflicts/interferences.

Notably, there was a significant correlation between efficient behavioral conflict resolution and increased oscillatory power at the higher (60–110 Hz) gamma band, which concentrated in the left inferior frontal cortex (IFC) during the pre-stimulus period. Previous fMRI studies have shown that IFC are associated with proactive interference [100,101] and may play an important role in speech-related auditory attention tasks [102]. Further, several neurophysiological studies have also observed sustained gamma oscillations in left IFC associated with phonological processing [103] and maintaining auditory patterns in short-term memory [104]. Our results suggest that IFC gamma oscillations may be essential in maintaining relevant auditory objects during selective attention tasks, and support the concept that attention can rely on gamma-band synchronization that helps integrate neural activities related to a specific sensory object into a stable, salient and coherent representation [19]. More generally, this result is consistent with previous findings associating sustained prefrontal gamma-power increases with successful auditory attention performance [38].

Finally, it is noteworthy that the degree of conflict in each individual trial is essentially modulated by what happened during the preceding trials. The conflict monitoring theories [105] suggest that such a "conflict adaptation' occurs because the preceding conflicts trigger stronger top-down control, which improves performance on subsequent trials of similar context. An alternative theory, however, suggested that these effects are related to a priming effect through episodic memory [106]. Although the exact mechanisms may still be debatable, the trial structure is nevertheless a factor that could affect responses and brain activations at the level of individual trials. Relevantly to the current study, previous fMRI studies have shown that the DLPFC activity gets stronger with an increasing predictability and decreasing experience of conflict, that is, when the probability of conflicts increases [9] or an increasing number of incongruent trials occur in a row during visual flanker task studies, respectively [11,107,108]. Future studies with runs having different probabilities of conflict could help elucidate how such a factor may affect cortico-cortical phase locking between cACC and DLPFC.

Conclusions

Our results demonstrate the importance of sustained connectivity, observed as theta/alpha phase locking between ACC and lateral frontal cortices including the right FEF and DLPFC, for efficient auditory conflict processing, and suggest brain regions of control and attention networks may communicate through synchronous oscillations to manage auditory scenes with multiple overlapping signals. The broader functional relevance of this observation is supported by recent results that pre-stimulus preparatory cACC–FEF alpha coherence is reduced in subjects with autism spectrum disorders during antisaccade tasks [109]. In the context of previous theories, the present results are most consistent with a prediction that ACC may play a role in "regulatory" networks that suppress distractions and boost attention to relevant objects in multisource acoustic environments. The cortical power estimates suggest that gamma-band activity in the left IFC plays a role in selective attention to speech-sound objects.

Acknowledgments

We thank Nao Suzuki, and Drs. Wei-Tang Chang and John W. Belliveau for their advice and support.

Author Contributions

Conceived and designed the experiments: JA. Performed the experiments: JA SH SR. Analyzed the data: JA. Contributed reagents/materials/analysis tools: MH. Contributed to the writing of the manuscript: SH JA MH.

References

1. Shinn-Cunningham BG (2008) Object-based auditory and visual attention. Trends Cogn Sci 12: 182–186.
2. Jääskeläinen IP, Ahveninen J (2014) Auditory-cortex short-term plasticity induced by selective attention. Neural Plast 2014: 216731.
3. Larson E, Lee AK (2013) The cortical dynamics underlying effective switching of auditory spatial attention. Neuroimage 64: 365–370.
4. Alain C, Arnott SR (2000) Selectively attending to auditory objects. Front Biosci 5: D202–212.
5. Eriksen B, Eriksen C (1974) Effects of noise letters upon identification of a target letter in a nonsearch task. Percept Psychophys 16: 143–149.
6. Stroop JR (1935) Studies of interference in serial verbal reactions. Journal of Experimental Psychology 12: 643–662.
7. Simon JR, Rudell AP (1967) Auditory S-R compatibility: the effect of an irrelevant cue on information processing. J Appl Psychol 51: 300–304.
8. Luks TL, Simpson GV, Dale CL, Hough MG (2007) Preparatory allocation of attention and adjustments in conflict processing. Neuroimage 35: 949–958.
9. Casey BJ, Thomas KM, Welsh TF, Badgaiyan RD, Eccard CH, et al. (2000) Dissociation of response conflict, attentional selection, and expectancy with functional magnetic resonance imaging. Proc Natl Acad Sci U S A 97: 8728–8733.
10. MacDonald AW 3rd, Cohen JD, Stenger VA, Carter CS (2000) Dissociating the role of the dorsolateral prefrontal and anterior cingulate cortex in cognitive control. Science 288: 1835–1838.
11. Kerns JG, Cohen JD, MacDonald AW 3rd, Cho RY, Stenger VA, et al. (2004) Anterior cingulate conflict monitoring and adjustments in control. Science 303: 1023–1026.
12. Roberts KL, Hall DA (2008) Examining a Supramodal Network for Conflict Processing: A Systematic Review and Novel Functional Magnetic Resonance Imaging Data for Related Visual and Auditory Stroop Tasks. Journal of Cognitive Neuroscience 20: 1063–1078.
13. Liu X, Banich MT, Jacobson BL, Tanabe JL (2004) Common and distinct neural substrates of attentional control in an integrated Simon and spatial Stroop task as assessed by event-related fMRI. Neuroimage 22: 1097–1106.
14. Fan J, Flombaum JI, McCandliss BD, Thomas KM, Posner MI (2003) Cognitive and brain consequences of conflict. Neuroimage 18: 42–57.
15. Folstein JR, Van Petten C (2008) Influence of cognitive control and mismatch on the N2 component of the ERP: a review. Psychophysiology 45: 152–170.
16. Szucs D, Soltesz F (2012) Functional definition of the N450 event-related brain potential marker of conflict processing: a numerical stroop study. BMC Neurosci 13: 35.
17. Larson MJ, Clayson PE, Clawson A (2014) Making sense of all the conflict: A theoretical review and critique of conflict-related ERPs. International Journal of Psychophysiology 93: 283–297.
18. Cohen MX (2014) Advantages and Limitations of Time- and Time-Frequnecy-Domain Analysis. Analyzing Neural Time Series Data: Theory and Practice. Cambridge, MA: MIT. 15–29.
19. Jensen O, Kaiser J, Lachaux JP (2007) Human gamma-frequency oscillations associated with attention and memory. Trends Neurosci 30: 317–324.
20. Womelsdorf T, Fries P (2007) The role of neuronal synchronization in selective attention. Curr Opin Neurobiol 17: 154–160.
21. Engel AK, Fries P, Singer W (2001) Dynamic predictions: oscillations and synchrony in top-down processing. Nat Rev Neurosci 2: 704–716.
22. von Stein A, Sarnthein J (2000) Different frequencies for different scales of cortical integration: from local gamma to long range alpha/theta synchronization. International Journal of Psychophysiology 38: 301–313.
23. Kopell N, Ermentrout GB, Whittington MA, Traub RD (2000) Gamma rhythms and beta rhythms have different synchronization properties. Proc Natl Acad Sci U S A 97: 1867–1872.
24. Huang S, Chang WT, Belliveau JW, Hamalainen M, Ahveninen J (2014) Lateralized parietotemporal oscillatory phase synchronization during auditory selective attention. Neuroimage 86: 461–469.
25. Schack B, Klimesch W, Sauseng P (2005) Phase synchronization between theta and upper alpha oscillations in a working memory task. Int J Psychophysiol 57: 105–114.
26. Moore RA, Gale A, Morris PH, Forrester D (2006) Theta phase locking across the neocortex reflects cortico-hippocampal recursive communication during goal conflict resolution. Int J Psychophysiol 60: 260–273.
27. Nigbur R, Cohen MX, Ridderinkhof KR, Stürmer B (2011) Theta Dynamics Reveal Domain-specific Control over Stimulus and Response Conflict. Journal of Cognitive Neuroscience 24: 1264–1274.
28. Doesburg SM, Green JJ, McDonald JJ, Ward LM (2012) Theta modulation of inter-regional gamma synchronization during auditory attention control. Brain Res 1431: 77–85.
29. von Stein A, Chiang C, König P (2000) Top-down processing mediated by interareal synchronization. Proc Natl Acad Sci U S A 97: 14748–14753.
30. Gross J, Schmitz F, Schnitzler I, Kessler K, Shapiro K, et al. (2004) Modulation of long-range neural synchrony reflects temporal limitations of visual attention in humans. Proc Natl Acad Sci U S A 101: 13050–13055.
31. Benedict RH, Shucard DW, Santa Maria MP, Shucard JL, Abara JP, et al. (2002) Covert auditory attention generates activation in the rostral/dorsal anterior cingulate cortex. J Cogn Neurosci 14: 637–645.
32. Haupt S, Axmacher N, Cohen MX, Elger CE, Fell J (2009) Activation of the caudal anterior cingulate cortex due to task-related interference in an auditory Stroop paradigm. Hum Brain Mapp 30: 3043–3056.
33. Christoffels IK, Formisano E, Schiller NO (2007) Neural correlates of verbal feedback processing: An fMRI study employing overt speech. Hum Brain Mapp 28: 868–879.
34. Westerhausen R, Moosmann M, Alho K, Belsby SO, Hamalainen H, et al. (2010) Identification of attention and cognitive control networks in a parametric auditory fMRI study. Neuropsychologia 48: 2075–2081.
35. Chan JS, Merrifield K, Spence C (2005) Auditory spatial attention assessed in a flanker interference task. Acta Acust United Ac 91: 554–563.
36. Espinoza-Varas B, Jang H (2011) Selective attention to pitch amid conflicting auditory information: context-coding and filtering strategies. Psychol Res 75: 159–178.
37. Ahveninen J, Jääskeläinen IP, Belliveau JW, Hämäläinen M, Lin FH, et al. (2012) Dissociable influences of auditory object vs. spatial attention on visual system oscillatory activity. PLoS ONE 7: e38511.
38. Ahveninen J, Huang S, Belliveau JW, Chang WT, Hamalainen M (2013) Dynamic oscillatory processes governing cued orienting and allocation of auditory attention. J Cogn Neurosci 25: 1926–1943.
39. Dale AM, Sereno MI (1993) Improved Localizadon of Cortical Activity by Combining EEG and MEG with MRI Cortical Surface Reconstruction: A Linear Approach. Journal of Cognitive Neuroscience 5: 162–176.
40. Hämäläinen MS, Lin FS, Mosher JC (2010) Anatomically and Functionally Constrained Minimum-Norm Estimates. In: Hansen O, Kringelbach M., and Salmelin, R., editor. MEG: An Introduction to Methods. New York, NY: Oxford University Press. 186–215.
41. Buzsaki G, Anastassiou CA, Koch C (2012) The origin of extracellular fields and currents–EEG, ECoG, LFP and spikes. Nat Rev Neurosci 13: 407–420.
42. Sharon D, Hämäläinen MS, Tootell RB, Halgren E, Belliveau JW (2007) The advantage of combining MEG and EEG: comparison to fMRI in focally stimulated visual cortex. Neuroimage 36: 1225–1235.
43. Desikan R, Segonne F, Fischl B, Quinn B, Dickerson B, et al. (2006) An automated labeling system for subdividing the human cerebral cortex on MRI scans into gyral based regions of interest. Neuroimage 31: 968–980.
44. Shenhav A, Botvinick MM, Cohen JD (2013) The expected value of control: an integrative theory of anterior cingulate cortex function. Neuron 79: 217–240.
45. Algazi VR, Duda RO, Thompson M, Avendano C (2001) The CIPIC HRTF database; 2001 October 21–24; Mohonk Mountain House, New Paltz, NY. 99–102.
46. Kopp B, Rist F, Mattler U (1996) N200 in the flanker task as a neurobehavioral tool for investigating executive control. Psychophysiology 33: 282–294.
47. Machado L, Guiney H, Struthers P (2013) Identity-based inhibitory processing during focused attention. Q J Exp Psychol (Hove) 66: 138–159.
48. DeWitt I, Rauschecker JP (2012) Phoneme and word recognition in the auditory ventral stream. Proc Natl Acad Sci U S A 109: E505–514.
49. Taulu S, Simola J, Kajola M (2005) Applications of the Signal Space Separation Method. IEEE Trans Signal Proc 53: 3359–3372.
50. Fischl B, Sereno MI, Dale AM (1999) Cortical surface-based analysis. II: Inflation, flattening, and a surface-based coordinate system. Neuroimage 9: 195–207.
51. Fischl B, Liu A, Dale AM (2001) Automated manifold surgery: constructing geometrically accurate and topologically correct models of the human cerebral cortex. IEEE Trans Med Imaging 20: 70–80.
52. Fischl B, Salat DH, van der Kouwe AJ, Makris N, Segonne F, et al. (2004) Sequence-independent segmentation of magnetic resonance images. Neuroimage 23 Suppl 1: S69–84.
53. Klauschen F, Goldman A, Barra V, Meyer-Lindenberg A, Lundervold A (2009) Evaluation of automated brain MR image segmentation and volumetry methods. Hum Brain Mapp 30: 1310–1327.
54. Ghosh SS, Kakunoori S, Augustinack J, Nieto-Castanon A, Kovelman I, et al. (2010) Evaluating the validity of volume-based and surface-based brain image registration for developmental cognitive neuroscience studies in children 4 to 11 years of age. Neuroimage 53: 85–93.
55. Hämäläinen M, Hari R, Ilmoniemi R, Knuutila J, Lounasmaa O (1993) Magnetoencephalography - theory, instrumentation, and applications to noninvasive studies of the working human brain. Rev Mod Phys 65: 413–497.
56. Yendiki A, Greve DN, Wallace S, Vangel M, Bockholt J, et al. (2010) Multi-site characterization of an fMRI working memory paradigm: reliability of activation indices. Neuroimage 53: 119–131.

57. Gramfort A, Luessi M, Larson E, Engemann DA, Strohmeier D, et al. (2013) MNE software for processing MEG and EEG data. Neuroimage.
58. Vinck M, Oostenveld R, van Wingerden M, Battaglia F, Pennartz CM (2011) An improved index of phase-synchronization for electrophysiological data in the presence of volume-conduction, noise and sample-size bias. Neuroimage 55: 1548–1565.
59. Fischl B, Sereno MI, Tootell RB, Dale AM (1999) High-resolution intersubject averaging and a coordinate system for the cortical surface. Hum Brain Mapp 8: 272–284.
60. Percival DB, Walden AT (1993) Spectral analysis for physical applications: multitaper and conventional univariate techniques. Cambridge, UK: Cambridge University Press.
61. Bland JM, Altman DG (1996) Transforming data. BMJ 312: 770.
62. Lesh TA, Westphal AJ, Niendam TA, Yoon JH, Minzenberg MJ, et al. (2013) Proactive and reactive cognitive control and dorsolateral prefrontal cortex dysfunction in first episode schizophrenia. NeuroImage: Clinical 2: 590–599.
63. Totah NKB, Jackson ME, Moghaddam B (2012) Preparatory Attention Relies on Dynamic Interactions between Prelimbic Cortex and Anterior Cingulate Cortex. Cerebral Cortex.
64. Varela F, Lachaux JP, Rodriguez E, Martinerie J (2001) The brainweb: phase synchronization and large-scale integration. Nat Rev Neurosci 2: 229–239.
65. Buzsaki G, Draguhn A (2004) Neuronal oscillations in cortical networks. Science 304: 1926–1929.
66. Braver TS, Barch DM, Gray JR, Molfese DL, Snyder A (2001) Anterior cingulate cortex and response conflict: effects of frequency, inhibition and errors. Cereb Cortex 11: 825–836.
67. Botvinick MM, Cohen JD, Carter CS (2004) Conflict monitoring and anterior cingulate cortex: an update. Trends Cogn Sci 8: 539–546.
68. Carter CS, Braver TS, Barch DM, Botvinick MM, Noll D, et al. (1998) Anterior cingulate cortex, error detection, and the online monitoring of performance. Science 280: 747–749.
69. Holroyd CB, Coles MG (2002) The neural basis of human error processing: reinforcement learning, dopamine, and the error-related negativity. Psychol Rev 109: 679–709.
70. Rushworth MF, Walton ME, Kennerley SW, Bannerman DM (2004) Action sets and decisions in the medial frontal cortex. Trends Cogn Sci 8: 410–417.
71. Fan J, McCandliss BD, Fossella J, Flombaum JI, Posner MI (2005) The activation of attentional networks. Neuroimage 26: 471–479.
72. Sauseng P, Hoppe J, Klimesch W, Gerloff C, Hummel FC (2007) Dissociation of sustained attention from central executive functions: local activity and interregional connectivity in the theta range. Eur J Neurosci 25: 587–593.
73. Szmalec A, Verbruggen F, Vandierendonck A, De Baene W, Verguts T, et al. (2008) Stimulus ambiguity elicits response conflict. Neurosci Lett 435: 158–162.
74. van Veen V, Carter CS (2002) The anterior cingulate as a conflict monitor: fMRI and ERP studies. Physiol Behav 77: 477–482.
75. Cohen MX, Donner TH (2013) Midfrontal conflict-related theta-band power reflects neural oscillations that predict behavior. Journal of Neurophysiology 110: 2752–2763.
76. Corbetta M, Shulman GL (2002) Control of goal-directed and stimulus-driven attention in the brain. Nat Rev Neurosci 3: 201–215.
77. Huang S, Belliveau JW, Tengshe C, Ahveninen J (2012) Brain networks of novelty-driven involuntary and cued voluntary auditory attention shifting. PLoS One 7: e44062.
78. Miller EK, Buschman TJ (2013) Cortical circuits for the control of attention. Curr Opin Neurobiol 23: 216–222.
79. Weissman DH, Gopalakrishnan A, Hazlett CJ, Woldorff MG (2005) Dorsal anterior cingulate cortex resolves conflict from distracting stimuli by boosting attention toward relevant events. Cereb Cortex 15: 229–237.
80. Benes FM, Cunningham GC, Berretta S, Gisabella B (2009) Course and pattern of cingulate pathology in schizophrenia. In: Vogt BA, editor. Cingulate Neurobiology and Disease Oxford University Press. 679–705.
81. Barbas H (2000) Connections underlying the synthesis of cognition, memory, and emotion in primate prefrontal cortices. Brain Research Bulletin 52: 319–330.
82. Badre D, Wagner AD (2004) Selection, Integration, and Conflict Monitoring: Assessing the Nature and Generality of Prefrontal Cognitive Control Mechanisms. Neuron 41: 473–487.
83. van Driel J, Ridderinkhof KR, Cohen MX (2012) Not All Errors Are Alike: Theta and Alpha EEG Dynamics Relate to Differences in Error-Processing Dynamics. The Journal of Neuroscience 32: 16795–16806.
84. Womelsdorf T, Johnston K, Vinck M, Everling S (2010) Theta-activity in anterior cingulate cortex predicts task rules and their adjustments following errors. Proceedings of the National Academy of Sciences 107: 5248–5253.
85. Cohen JD, Botvinick M, Carter CS (2000) Anterior cingulate and prefrontal cortex: who's in control? Nat Neurosci 3: 421–423.
86. Biehl S, Ehlis AC, Muller L, Niklaus A, Pauli P, et al. (2013) The impact of task relevance and degree of distraction on stimulus processing. BMC Neuroscience 14: 107.
87. Johnston K, Levin HM, Koval MJ, Everling S (2007) Top-down control-signal dynamics in anterior cingulate and prefrontal cortex neurons following task switching. Neuron 53: 453–462.
88. Orr JM, Weissman DH (2009) Anterior Cingulate Cortex Makes 2 Contributions to Minimizing Distraction. Cerebral Cortex 19: 703–711.
89. Fries P, Womelsdorf T, Oostenveld R, Desimone R (2008) The Effects of Visual Stimulation and Selective Visual Attention on Rhythmic Neuronal Synchronization in Macaque Area V4. The Journal of Neuroscience 28: 4823–4835.
90. Doesburg SM, Green JJ, McDonald JJ, Ward LM (2009) From local inhibition to long-range integration: a functional dissociation of alpha-band synchronization across cortical scales in visuospatial attention. Brain Res 1303: 97–110.
91. Palva S, Palva JM (2007) New vistas for ± frequency band oscillations. Trends in neurosciences 30: 150–158.
92. Luppino G, Matelli M, Camarda R, Rizzolatti G (1993) Corticocortical connections of area F3 (SMA-proper) and area F6 (pre-SMA) in the macaque monkey. The Journal of Comparative Neurology 338: 114–140.
93. Johansen-Berg H, Behrens TEJ, Robson MD, Drobnjak I, Rushworth MFS, et al. (2004) Changes in connectivity profiles define functionally distinct regions in human medial frontal cortex. Proc Natl Acad Sci U S A 101: 13335–13340.
94. Wang XJ (2010) Neurophysiological and Computational Principles of Cortical Rhythms in Cognition. Physiological Reviews 90: 1195–1268.
95. Bibbig A, Traub RD, Whittington MA (2002) Long-Range Synchronization of γ and β Oscillations and the Plasticity of Excitatory and Inhibitory Synapses: A Network Model. Journal of Neurophysiology 88: 1634–1654.
96. Soutschek A, Taylor PC, Muller HJ, Schubert T (2013) Dissociable networks control conflict during perception and response selection: a transcranial magnetic stimulation Study. J Neurosci 33: 5647–5654.
97. Petrides M, Pandya DN (1984) Projections to the frontal cortex from the posterior parietal region in the rhesus monkey. J Comp Neurol 228: 105–116.
98. Morris R, Pandya DN, Petrides M (1999) Fiber system linking the mid-dorsolateral frontal cortex with the retrosplenial/presubicular region in the rhesus monkey. J Comp Neurol 407: 183–192.
99. Bar M (2004) Visual objects in context. Nat Rev Neurosci 5: 617–629.
100. Jonides J, Smith EE, Marshuetz C, Koeppe RA, Reuter-Lorenz PA (1998) Inhibition in verbal working memory revealed by brain activation. Proc Natl Acad Sci U S A 95: 8410–8413.
101. Badre D, Poldrack RA, Pare-Blagoev EJ, Insler RZ, Wagner AD (2005) Dissociable controlled retrieval and generalized selection mechanisms in ventrolateral prefrontal cortex. Neuron 47: 907–918.
102. Yoncheva YN, Zevin JD, Maurer U, McCandliss BD (2010) Auditory selective attention to speech modulates activity in the visual word form area. Cereb Cortex 20: 622–632.
103. Mainy N, Kahane P, Minotti L, Hoffmann D, Bertrand O, et al. (2007) Neural correlates of consolidation in working memory. Hum Brain Mapp 28: 183–193.
104. Kaiser J, Ripper B, Birbaumer N, Lutzenberger W (2003) Dynamics of gamma-band activity in human magnetoencephalogram during auditory pattern working memory. Neuroimage 20: 816–827.
105. Botvinick MM, Braver TS, Barch DM, Carter CS, Cohen JD (2001) Conflict monitoring and cognitive control. Psychol Rev 108: 624–652.
106. Mayr U, Awh E, Laurey P (2003) Conflict adaptation effects in the absence of executive control. Nat Neurosci 6: 450–452.
107. Botvinick M, Nystrom LE, Fissell K, Carter CS, Cohen JD (1999) Conflict monitoring versus selection-for-action in anterior cingulate cortex. Nature 402: 179–181.
108. Durston S, Davidson MC, Thomas KM, Worden MS, Tottenham N, et al. (2003) Parametric manipulation of conflict and response competition using rapid mixed-trial event-related fMRI. Neuroimage 20: 2135–2141.
109. Kenet T, Orekhova EV, Bharadwaj H, Shetty NR, Israeli E, et al. (2012) Disconnectivity of the cortical ocular motor control network in autism spectrum disorders. Neuroimage 61: 1226–1234.

Adults with Dyslexia Demonstrate Large Effects of Crowding and Detrimental Effects of Distractors in a Visual Tilt Discrimination Task

Rizan Cassim, Joel B. Talcott, Elisabeth Moores*

School of Life and Health Sciences, Aston University, Birmingham, West Midlands, United Kingdom

Abstract

Previous research has shown that adults with dyslexia (AwD) are disproportionately impacted by close spacing of stimuli and increased numbers of distractors in a visual search task compared to controls [1]. Using an orientation discrimination task, the present study extended these findings to show that even in conditions where target search was not required: (i) AwD had detrimental effects of both crowding and increased numbers of distractors; (ii) AwD had more pronounced difficulty with distractor exclusion in the left visual field and (iii) measures of crowding and distractor exclusion correlated significantly with literacy measures. Furthermore, such difficulties were not accounted for by the presence of covarying symptoms of ADHD in the participant groups. These findings provide further evidence to suggest that the ability to exclude distracting stimuli likely contributes to the reported visual attention difficulties in AwD and to the aetiology of literacy difficulties. The pattern of results is consistent with weaker and asymmetric attention in AwD.

Editor: Lawrence M. Ward, University of British Columbia, Canada

Funding: This work constitutes part of RC's PhD thesis for which he received a scholarship from Aston University. The funders had no role in study design, data collection and analysis, decision to publish, or preparation of the manuscript.

Competing Interests: The authors have declared that no competing interests exist.

* Email: e.j.moores@aston.ac.uk

Introduction

Although phonological difficulties are well-established as core features underlying literacy impairments [2–4], focus is being increasingly devoted to the role of visual attention difficulties in reading disorders, including developmental dyslexia. A variety of attention difficulties have been reported in dyslexia, including asymmetric attention distribution [5], reduced visual attention span [6], increased crowding effects [1,7–11], difficulty in using cues [12–14] and less effective mechanisms for noise exclusion [15,16]. Controversially, it has been argued that even core phonological language difficulties shown in dyslexia can be statistically accounted for by an underlying visual deficit [17]. The majority of research implicates a model of dyslexia based on multiple underlying deficits [18], with attention difficulties as an additional contributing factor to the genesis of reading impairments in some individuals. Moreover, the high comorbidity between dyslexia and attention deficit hyperactivity disorder (ADHD) [19] may also account for some of the covariance between deficits in visual attention and core reading skills. Here, we examined three specific aspects of visual attention: (i) visual crowding, (ii) the ability to exclude distractors and (iii) the distribution of attention across the visual field. We also investigated the relationship of these three aspects of attention with four different measures of literacy and with the presence of sub-clinical ADHD symptoms, in our sample.

1.1 Effects of visual crowding

Visual crowding occurs when stimuli become more difficult to either detect or discriminate when surrounded by other stimuli, compared to when they are presented in isolation. Crowding is a phenomenon that occurs in nearly every visual context. It can occur with simple stimuli - such as orientation gratings – and also with complex stimuli such as letters [20]. Efficient allocation and control of visual attention can ameliorate the negative effects of crowding [21,22], although Dakin, Bex, Cass and Watt [23] have argued that crowding does not specifically reflect a limitation in attention. He, Cavanagh and Intriligator have provided alternative evidence from an orientation adaptation and discrimination task that suggests that it is attention – rather than visual acuity – that ultimately limits spatial resolution under normal circumstances [24]. Several studies have suggested that persons with reading impairments such as dyslexia suffer more from crowding than do similarly aged control readers [1,7–11,25]. Research in this area, however, has mainly used letter or letter-like stimuli to investigate this hypothesis. Because dyslexia is also associated with deficits in recognition and processing of linguistic stimuli – including letters – it is difficult to adjudicate between effects linked to visual attention and those associated with processing the symbols of language in such tasks.

1.2 Noise (distractor) exclusion

In addition to evidence for increased crowding effects in dyslexia, other studies also identify difficulties in excluding distracting stimuli. Sperling *et al.* [15,16] showed that performance of adults in a visual motion detection task only correlated with their reading ability in conditions where the signal to noise ratio was low. Using a visual search paradigm, Roach and Hogben [26] measured psychophysical thresholds of adults with dyslexia (AwD) and controls for detection of a tilted target stimulus presented amongst vertical distractors. Although the set size effect of the control group, but not the AwD, was diminished when targets were cued, they provided evidence [13,14] to suggest that the difficulty of the AwD was one of ineffective noise exclusion, rather than problems detecting and localising the cue *per se*. Using a similar paradigm, Moores *et al.* [1] also reported that AwD could use pre-cues to modulate attention, but that they were less successful at using them to counter effects of increasing numbers of distractors on target detectability. A limitation of these studies, however, is that visual search paradigms were used, in which - for uncued conditions - the target location was not known. Therefore, any potential beneficial effects of cueing for either group could reflect reduced spatial uncertainty regarding target location, rather than the effects of enhanced attention or distractor exclusion. As an alternative, the current study presented the target stimulus at one of only two possible fixed locations in the left and right visual fields. This manipulation minimised the potential for eye movements towards a fixed stimulus location. Also, because previous research has shown an asymmetrical distribution of attention in dyslexia, it allowed us to replicate this effect here.

1.3 Distribution of attention

Facoetti, Paganoni and Lorusso [27] have previously reported that a group of children with dyslexia (CwD) showed more distributed or diffuse attentional focus, evidenced by a relatively flat profile of reaction times for stimulus detection with increasing retinal eccentricity. Facoetti and Molteni [28] demonstrated that this profile only occurred for stimuli presented in the right visual field, whereas responses of CwD in the left visual field were slower than those of controls overall, but were faster for stimuli presented at central compared to peripheral locations. They proposed that an attention disorder affecting the left visual field would explain the slower responses overall, with the lack of a performance gradient across eccentricity accounting for the over-distractibility associated with stimulus processing in the right visual field. Hari, Renvall and Tanskanen [29] also reported slower performance in AwD in the left visual field on two psychophysical tasks and from this evidence proposed a left-sided 'minineglect' in dyslexia. Consistent with this hypothesis, Waldie and Hausmann [30] reported a reversal of the normal leftward bias observed in a line bisection task in CwD and in children with ADHD (see also [31]). Further evidence for an asymmetry was provided by Facoetti and Turatto [5], who reported a reduced effect of flankers in the left visual field, and by Facoetti, Turatto, Lorusso and Mascetti [32], who showed slower reaction times to invalidly cued targets in the left compared to the right visual field. A body of psychophysical evidence therefore points toward an asymmetric and more diffuse distribution of attention in dyslexic readers.

1.4 Relationship between literacy and effects of crowding, set-size and visual field asymmetry

It is important to determine whether the differences in attention associated with dyslexia are related to measures of literacy, or more to third variables which also co-occur with dyslexia and other development disorders. Relationships between measures of visual attention and of literacy have previously been demonstrated. Sperling *et al.* [16] reported a moderate [33] correlation between reading ability and ability to detect visual coherent motion amongst noise in adults. Moores *et al.* [1] reported moderate to strong correlations between literacy measures and dependence on attentional cues, effects of crowding and the impact of a greater number of distractors. Facoetti *et al.* [34] reported a strong correlation in dyslexic readers between nonword reading accuracy and the extent of a deficit in attentional inhibition in the right visual field (i.e. the finding that when cued to the left visual field, targets in the right visual field are not inhibited). All these associations between reading and attention variables, however, might plausibly be related to the overlapping dimensions dyslexia shares with ADHD, rather than to literacy skills directly. In the present study, we examined the relationships between four measures of literacy (word reading accuracy, word spelling accuracy, real word reading efficiency and nonword reading efficiency) and our measures of crowding, distractor exclusion and attention asymmetry.

1.5 Associations with ADHD

Previous research has suggested that dyslexic readers suffer more from crowding, are less effective at excluding distractors, and have a different distribution of attention compared to controls. Furthermore, these difficulties correlate with literacy abilities. However, it has been estimated that upwards from 15% of children with dyslexia also have co-occurring attention deficit hyperactivity disorder (ADHD) and around 36% of children with ADHD are estimated to have dyslexia [19]. According to the Diagnostic and Statistical Manual of Mental Disorders 5th Edition [35] the primary symptoms of ADHD are 'inattention' (which includes poor sustained attention, forgetfulness and distractibility) and 'hyperactivity/ impulsivity'. Most contemporary theories of ADHD argue that the core deficits are associated with either poor inhibitory control [36] or aversion to delay [37]. However, an alternative explanation may be that reported 'attention' difficulties in dyslexia may be accounted for by concomitant ADHD symptoms. The dimensions of literacy and attention are continuous variables, with categories derived from rather arbitrary statistical cut-offs. Although many dyslexia studies investigating aspects of visual attention have excluded participants with actual diagnoses of ADHD from their studies, few have specifically investigated the potential role of sub-clinical ADHD symptoms by controlling statistically for their presence. It should be noted, however, that 'inattention' type symptoms as discussed in the context of ADHD may be conceptually different from the type of visual selective attention difficulties investigated in this study and other research in this area. A lack of sustained attention or a general distractibility would be expected to adversely affect performance across *all* conditions of any task, whereas research into visual attention difficulties in dyslexia invariably reports dissociated patterns of deficit which only present in particular conditions; for example only when a display is crowded, or only in the left visual field. Nonetheless, in a different context, it has been shown that ADHD symptoms can mediate the effects of differences in performance variables between groups of persons with dyslexia and controls [38], so in the current study it was important to assess the potential impact of sub-clinical ADHD effects as an alternative hypothesis.

1.6 Limitations, summary and overview

Moores *et al.* [1] showed that a greater dependence on pre-cues, larger effects of crowding and the impact of increased numbers of distractors all correlated strongly with measures of literacy skill. However, as discussed in *section 1.2*, this task was a visual search task in which the target location was not known (unless pre-cued). The advantage of pre-cueing in this task could therefore have been due to a reduced spatial uncertainty over target location as well as – or instead of – enhanced attention and/ or noise exclusion. In addition, crowding could have simply made the target more difficult to locate, rather than more difficult to discriminate *per se* [39]. Furthermore, our previous study did not investigate the potential role of ADHD symptomatology on task performance. With any potential effects of ADHD statistically removed, the present study therefore investigated whether: (i) AwD experienced increased crowding effects and difficulty excluding distractors even when target location was known, (ii) any increased difficulties in excluding distractors or in crowding showed any asymmetry in AwD and (iii) any difficulties with crowding, excluding distractors, or any asymmetry had any relationship with four different measures of literacy.

Materials and Methods

2.1 Participants

Participants provided informed written consent which conformed to the procedures approved by the Aston University's Ethics Committee on use of human participants. The study was approved by Aston University Ethics Committee. Sixteen control adults (7 males) and eighteen AwD (8 males) equated for age and full scale IQ took part in this study (Eleven control adults (7 males) and thireteen AwD (6 males) also took part in our previous study [1]). Participants were also asked to provide ratings of their behaviour across the dimensions of inattention and hyperactivity/ impulsivity on the Barkley Current Symptoms Scales [40]. Scores of greater than 6 on either measure, or exceeding 9 for the sum of inattention and hyperactivity scores, are indicative of dimensions in which further exploration toward a clinical diagnosis of ADHD is usually suggested [40]. The selection criteria required that each participant had a profile of enduring reading and spelling difficulties and/or previous clinical diagnosis, but no prior history of any other developmental disorder. The control group was required to have no previously reported problems in spelling or reading. All participants were required to have a minimum full scale IQ of 90, English as their first language and normal or corrected-to-normal vision. All participants also had completed at least some higher education (on average 12.8 years of schooling, SD = 0.49) and most of them (15 controls and 15 AwD) were either previously or currently enrolled in university degree programmes.

Participants from both groups were initially screened using a battery of assessments for cognitive skills and literacy achievement. All AwD provided a recent report from an educational psychologist at the time of testing, which provided the estimate of full-scale IQ used in the study (using the Wechsler Adult Intelligence Scale (WAIS) [41]). The IQ test for control participants was administered on the day of testing (using the Wechsler Abbreviated Scale of Intelligence (WASI) [42]), unless they had been previously assessed with either the Wechsler Adult Intelligence Scale or the Wechsler Abbreviated Scale of Intelligence. Reading and spelling achievement was measured using the Wechsler Individual Achievement Test (WIAT-II UK) reading and spelling subtests [43] unless these measures had already been administered within the previous 12 months. The Test of Word Reading Efficiency (TOWRE) [44] - a speeded reading test designed to measure word reading accuracy and fluency - was also conducted. The Sight Word Efficiency (SWE) test provided a fluency measure for real words, whilst the Phonemic Decoding Efficiency (PDE) test provided a decoding measure for accuracy and fluency of pronounceable non-words.

A comparison of demographic and psychometric data for both the controls and AwD is summarised in Table 1. Independent sample t-tests (with Levene's correction for unequal variances when appropriate) showed no significant differences between groups for age [t $(28.08) = 0.46$], level of education [t $(22.14) = 1.27$] or IQ [t $(31.98) = 2.51$]. The average performance of the AwD group was significantly lower than the controls for all measures of literacy: WIAT-II word reading [t $(31.53) = 9.54$, $p<.001$], WIAT-II spelling [t $(28.26) = 6.11$, $p<.001$], TOWRE SWE [t $(32.00) = 3.79$, $p<.001$] and TOWRE PDE [t $(28.06) = 19.46$, $p<.001$]. AwD also had higher scores on the ADHD measure [t $(29.62) = -3.87$, $p<.001$].

2.2 Stimuli and apparatus

The tilt discrimination experiment was developed using E-Prime Version 2-Professional [45] and conducted on a P4 Dell Optiplex GX 260 desktop computer displaying the output on a 19-inch CRT Vision Master Pro 510 monitor (1024×768-pixel screen resolution, 60-Hz refresh rate).

The stimuli consisted of five greyscale sine-phase Gabor patches generated using Matlab (MathWorks Ltd) comprising wavelength ($\lambda = 10$ pixels per cycle) and a Gaussian standard deviation ($\sigma = 10$). The target Gabors were tilted (θ) at different angles relative to the vertical distractors in two conditions which varied in difficulty: i) $\theta = \pm 5°$ ('easy' condition) and, ii) $\theta = \pm 2°$ ('difficult' condition).

The participants were asked to support their head within a chin rest while seated at a viewing distance of 57 cm in a dimly lit room. Participant responses were entered using specific key presses on a standard computer keyboard.

2.3 Design

The independent variables of interest were group (AwD or Control), display type (zero distractors, two-spaced distractors, two-crowded distractors, four distractors or eight distractors), task difficulty (easy or difficult tilt) and visual field (VF: left or right). The direction of tilt was also randomised. The dependent variable was percent correct for the detection of the correct orientation of the target stimulus.

Participants performed a two alternative forced choice task (see Figure 1) in which they were required to indicate the orientation (left or right tilt) of a single tilted target stimulus that was always presented in the centre of a variable length string of vertically oriented distractors. On a given trial, there was an equal probability of the target stimulus having a tilt of either $\pm 2°$ (easy) or $\pm 5°$ (difficult). The string was comprised of varying configurations presented with equal probability: zero distractors, two crowded distractors, two spread distractors, four distractors or eight distractors. The stimuli (target and distractors) were positioned either to the left-VF or right-VF (50% probability) of the display on the circumference of an imaginary semi-circle located 5° of visual angle peripheral to the central fixation point. In either VF, the target stimulus always appeared at a fixed central position (indicated by the arrow placeholder as in Figure 1) whilst the distractors were arranged symmetrically above and below it in the same hemifield. To evaluate the effect of distractors alone, crowding effects in the different array conditions were kept constant by separating the distractors closest to the target by an interstimulus distance of 3.5° visual angle from the target while the distance between distractors was constant throughout at 1.6° visual angle. The exception to this was in the two distractor crowded condition in which the effects of crowding were systematically manipulated by positioning the two distractors nearer to the target (target-distractor separation of 1.6° visual angle). Although our spacing manipulation led to unequal spacing of stimuli in four and eight distractor conditions, it enabled us to manipulate the number

Table 1. Demographic and psychometric group data.

	Control (n = 16)		AwD (n = 18)		*p*-value
	Mean	**SD**	**Mean**	**SD**	
Age (years)	26.69	5.65	25.89	4.35	ns
Education[a]	12.94	0.25	12.72	0.67	ns
Full-Scale IQ	124.19	6.53	118.11	7.58	ns
Spelling (WIAT-II UK)[b]	116.50	5.39	100.72	9.25	<.001
Reading (WIAT-II UK)[b]	110.31	3.18	98.44	4.06	<.001
TOWRE (SWE)[b]	107.69	6.09	99.28	6.86	<.001
TOWRE (PDE)[b]	116.63	3.44	95.94	2.65	<.001
ADHD	1.44	1.15	3.39	1.75	<.05

[a]The level of education represents years of schooling from year 1 (infant school) to year 13 (college/sixth form).
[b]The composite standard scores (SS). For the TOWRE these were calculated using the norms 17:0–24:11 (years: months).

of distractors presented in a single hemifield *without* varying the spacing between the central target and its nearest distractors (i.e. without varying the degree of crowding of the target). Stimuli were presented with consistent spacing in the two conditions where we specifically investigated crowding effects (since only two distractors were used in each case).

2.4 Procedure

Initiated by a single key press, each trial sequence commenced with an onset of a blank grey screen with a central fixation point (+) of 40 ms duration. Participants were instructed to visually fixate this position throughout the entire duration of each trial. A second fixation screen followed for 110 ms which had arrows on each side of the display corresponding to the two specific locations at which the target could appear. This was followed by a variable duration display (containing any one of the five display types) and then by a further fixation screen until response (see Figure 1 for a visual schematic of the experimental set-up). If a response was not made a reminder screen followed after 3000 ms.

The display was of a variable duration titrated to achieve individual accuracy levels of between 60% and 90%. The experimental session had a total of 15 blocks with each block having 40 trials (total of 600 trials). In each block, two trials (one target tilting right and one left) of each of 20 conditions were conducted and the detection accuracy calculated for that block. When overall response accuracy either surpassed 90% or fell below 60% a 10 ms reduction or increase (respectively) was made to the stimulus duration. Before commencing the main experiment, the participants performed two blocks of practice and calibration sessions (20 trials each) to ensure that they were sufficiently familiar with the procedure and to establish an accuracy level within the 60%–90% range. The average display durations of the AwD and the control group did differ significantly (119 ms vs. 98 ms, $t(32) = 1.47$, $p < .05$).

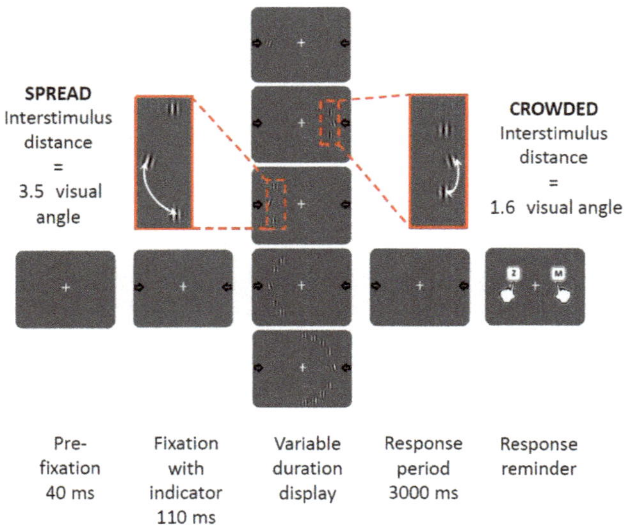

Figure 1. Schematic representation of the stimulus sequence for the tilt discrimination task. The two possible target locations (left and right sides of the screen) were indicated on the display screen with arrows. Targets could be presented either alone, or surrounded by two, four or eight distractors arranged symmetrically above and below the target. In conditions in which two distractors were presented they could be presented with an interstimulus distance of either 3.5 degrees (spread) or 1.6 degrees (crowded). Participants responded whether the target tilted left or right using the z and m keys on the computer keyboard.

Results

The results comprised the proportion of correct discriminations in each of the 20 conditions and are available in the Dataset S1. We first investigated effects of visual crowding using ADHD score as a covariate. Second, we investigated the effects of increasing distractor set size and visual field, again using ADHD as a covariate. Third, we examined the relationship between literacy measures and measures of crowding, distractor set-size and asymmetry of attention with statistical effects of ADHD partialled out from the correlations.

3.1 Effects of Crowding

To assess the potential effects of crowding, a four-way ANCOVA was conducted using the variables: group (controls, AwD); set-size-two display type (spread, crowded); task difficulty (easy, hard) and visual field (left, right). Analyses indicated a significant main effect of group ($F_{(1,31)} = 43.77$, $p < .001$, $\eta^2_p = .59$) with higher performance in controls. There were also significant main effects of display type ($F_{(1,31)} = 6.46$, $p < .05$, $\eta^2_p = .17$) and task difficulty ($F_{(1,31)} = 13.02$, $p < .001$, $\eta^2_p = .30$), showing inferior performance in crowded and difficult conditions. The effect of visual field was not significant ($F_{(1,31)} = 2.46$). ADHD was not a significant covariate ($F_{(1,31)} = 0.69$). Significant interactions between display type and group ($F_{(1,31)} = 8.67$, $p<.01$, $\eta^2_p = .22$) and task difficulty and group ($F_{(1,31)} = 10.66$, $p<.01$, $\eta^2_p = .26$) suggested a different pattern of performance by AwD when the discrimination task was difficult and the display was crowded. No other interactions reached statistical significance.

To investigate the significant interactions, analyses were conducted on each group separately with ADHD as a covariate. The descriptive statistics are summarised graphically in Figure 2. A significant effect of display type emerged for AwD ($F_{(1,16)} = 14.18$, $p<.001$, $\eta^2_p = .47$) but not for controls ($F_{(1,14)} = .108$). Both the control group ($F_{(1,14)} = 9.18$, $p<.05$, $\eta^2_p = .40$) and the AwD ($F_{(1,16)} = 6.97$, $p<.05$, $\eta^2_p = .30$) showed a significant effect of task difficulty. ADHD was not a significant covariate for either the controls ($F_{(1,14)} = .001$) or the AwD ($F_{(1,16)} = 1.05$). The main effect of visual field was not significant for either AwD or controls (Fs<1), although in controls there was a significant interaction between visual field and difficulty ($F_{(1,14)} = 4.97$, $p<.05$, $\eta^2_p = .26$) with similar performance across visual fields in the easy condition, but slightly lower performance in the left visual field in the difficult condition.

3.2 Effects of distractor set size and visual field

The effect of distractor set-size on target discrimination was investigated using a four-factor ANCOVA: group (controls, AwD), distractor set-size (zero, two-spread, four, eight), task difficulty (easy, hard) and visual field (left, right). The descriptive statistics are summarised graphically in Figure 3. Again, a significant main effect of group ($F_{(1,31)} = 39.40$, $p<.001$, $\eta^2_p = .56$) was demonstrated, with higher performance in controls. There were also significant main effects of set-size ($F_{(1,31)} = 15.56$, $p<.001$, $\eta^2_p = .33$), task difficulty ($F_{(1,31)} = 11.31$, $p<.001$, $\eta^2_p = .27$) and visual field ($F_{(1,31)} = 10.98$, $p<.001$, $\eta^2_p = .26$), demonstrating higher performance with fewer distractors, less difficult discriminations, and in the right visual field. ADHD was not a significant covariate (F<1).There were significant two-way group interactions between group and: set-size ($F_{(1,31)} = 13.81$, $p<.001$, $\eta^2_p = .31$), task difficulty ($F_{(1,31)} = 8.72$, $p<.05$, $\eta^2_p = .22$); and visual field ($F_{(1,31)} = 42.49$, $p<.001$, $\eta^2_p = .58$). Also significant were interactions between set-size and task difficulty ($F_{(1,31)} = 4.88$, $p<.05$, $\eta^2_p = .14$), set-size and visual field ($F_{(1,31)} = 10.54$, $p<.001$, $\eta^2_p = .25$), set-size, task difficulty and group ($F_{(1,31)} = 3.84$, $p<.05$, $\eta^2_p = .11$), set-size, visual field and group ($F_{(1,31)} = 30.04$, $p<.001$, $\eta^2_p = .49$)], and set-size, task difficulty, visual field and group ($F_{(3,93)} = 6.71$, $p<.001$, $\eta^2_p = .18$).

To aid interpretation, a three factor ANOVA (visual field×set-size×task difficulty) was conducted for each group separately. The control group showed no main effect of set-size ($F_{(1,42)} = 1.61$) or visual field ($F_{(1,14)} = 0.15$), although there was a significant main effect of task difficulty ($F_{(1,14)} = 8.36$, $p<.05$, $\eta^2_p = .37$) in the expected direction. ADHD did not act as a significant covariate ($F_{(1,14)} = 2.63$). The interactions between set-size and visual field ($F_{(1,14)} = 0.57$); task difficulty and visual field ($F_{(1,14)} = 0.19$); and set-size, task difficulty and visual field ($F_{(1,14)} = 0.16$) were not statistically significant. However, a significant set-size by task difficulty interaction ($F_{(1,14)} = 3.95$, $p<.05$, $\eta^2_p = .22$) suggested that larger set sizes negatively affected control performance when the orientation discrimination judgement was also difficult.

In contrast to controls, the AwD showed significant main effects of set-size ($F_{(1,16)} = 14.47$, $p<.001$, $\eta^2_p = .48$); task difficulty ($F_{(1,16)} = 5.35$, $p<.05$, $\eta^2_p = .25$); and visual field ($F_{(1,16)} = 11.53$, $p<.001$, $\eta^2_p = .42$). ADHD did not act as a significant covariate (F<1). There were significant interactions between set-size and task difficulty ($F_{(1,16)} = 3.57$, $p<.05$, $\eta^2_p = .24$); and set-size and visual field ($F_{(1,16)} = 12.29$, $p<.001$, $\eta^2_p = 0.43$). The interactions between task difficulty and visual field ($F_{(1,12)} = 0.76$), and set-size, task difficulty and visual field ($F_{(1,16)} = 1.36$) were not statistically significant. Unlike the controls, AwD were significantly affected by increasing numbers of distractors regardless of task difficulty and showed lower performance in the left compared to the right visual field. Similar to the controls, AwD were more affected by larger distractor set sizes when the discrimination was also difficult.

3.3 Relationship between literacy measures, crowding, visual field & set-size effects

First, to evaluate the potential predictive relationships for crowding, visual field asymmetry and set size effects on literacy measures three summary variables were created. By using comparisons across conditions for these measures - rather than absolute performance levels in any single condition - these

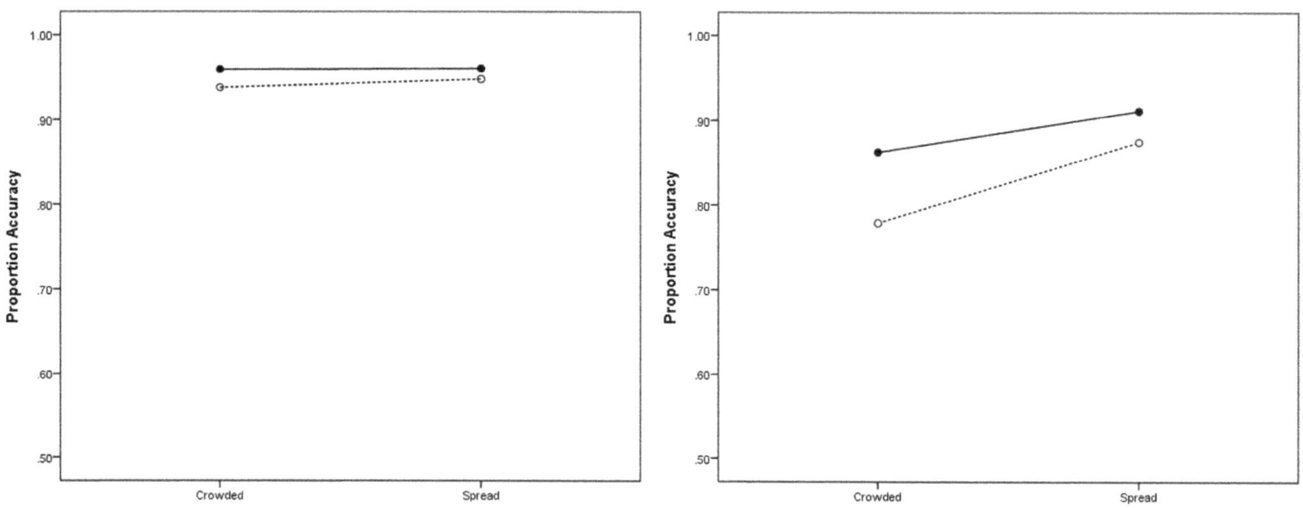

Figure 2. Interaction plots indicating performance accuracy for both controls (left panel) and AwD (right panel) plotted as a function of display type (crowded vs. spread) and task difficulty (solid lines - easy conditions and dotted lines - hard conditions).

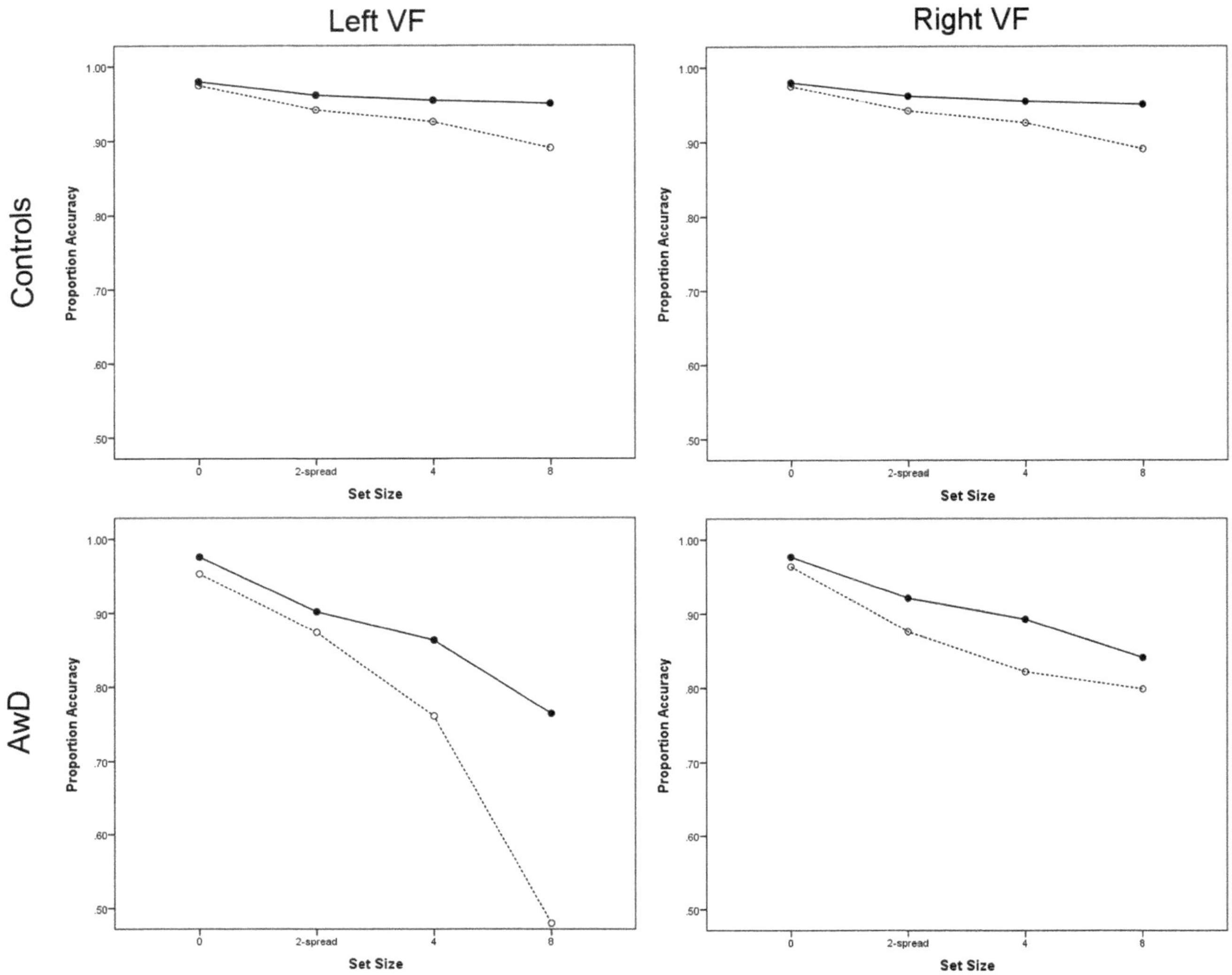

Figure 3. Descriptive statistics showing performance accuracy for both controls (top horizontal panel) and AwD (bottom horizontal panel) for the stimulus display side conditions (left vs. right-VF) plotted as a function of set-size and task difficulty (solid lines representing easy conditions and dotted lines representing hard conditions).

measures tapped crowding, asymmetry and set size effects independent of overall performance.

a) Crowding: The mean difference in accuracy between spread and crowded display types for set size 2

b) Set size: The mean difference in accuracy between set-size eight and set-size zero display types

c) Asymmetry: The mean set size effect (as calculated above in b) for the right visual field minus that for the left visual field

These variables were then entered in to a series of partial correlation analyses (ADHD scores statistically removed) with the literacy variables: WIAT-II spelling, WIAT-II reading, TOWRE-SWE and TOWRE-PDE ($n = 34$ in all cases, approximate critical value of r for a two-tailed 5% confidence level = 0.38). Figure 4 shows scatter plots of these relationships.

The crowding measure correlated significantly with WIAT-II reading ($r = -.54$, $p<.001$) and TOWRE-PDE ($r = -.50$, $p<.01$), suggesting that the larger the impact of crowding the lower the scores on these measures, but not with WIAT-II spelling ($r = -.19$) or TOWRE-SWE ($r = -.17$). The set size measure correlated significantly with WIAT-II spelling ($r = -.50$, $p<.001$), WIAT-II reading ($r = -.77$, $p<.001$) and TOWRE-PDE ($r = -.70$, $p<.001$) but not TOWRE-SWE ($r = -.16$). Again, the significant correlations suggested that the greater the impact of set size on performance, the lower were the scores on the literacy measures. The asymmetry measure correlated significantly with WIAT-II spelling ($r = -.47$, $p<.01$), WIAT-II reading ($r = -.57$, $p<.001$), TOWRE-SWE ($r = -.44$, $p<.01$) and TOWRE-PDE ($r = -.80$, $p<.001$). Here, the more rightward the asymmetry (i.e. better performance on the right vs. the left), the lower the scores on the literacy measures. In order to help clarify the meaning of these correlations, the same partial correlations were repeated, but split by group (AwD/ control). These analyses yielded only one significant correlation for the control group – a negative correlation between WIAT-II reading and set size ($r = -.52$, $p<.05$). For the AwD, there were two significant negative correlations between WIAT-II reading and set size ($r = -.50$, $p<.05$) and WIAT-II reading and crowding ($r = -.67$, $p<.01$).

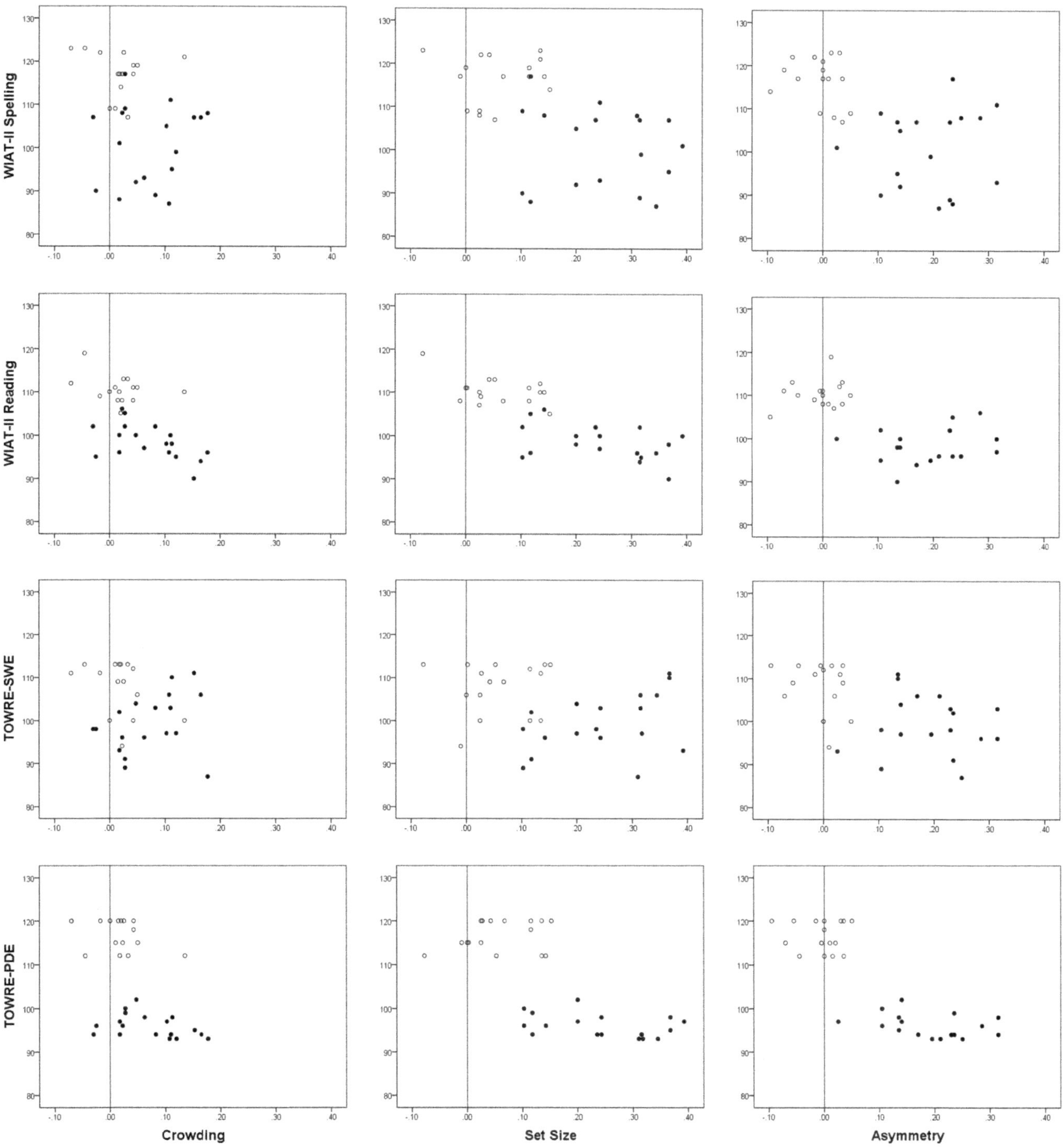

Figure 4. Scatter plots showing the relationships between measures of WIAT-II Spelling, WIAT-II Reading, TOWRE-PDE and TOWRE-SWE with measures of crowding, set size and asymmetry. Controls (empty dots). AwD (filled dots).

Discussion

This study compared adults with dyslexia and controls on a target orientation discrimination task with varying numbers of distractors presented at different spatial proximities to the target. We showed that AwD experienced detrimental effects of crowding and increased numbers of distractors even when the target location was known, and when effects of ADHD were statistically controlled. Difficulty with distractor exclusion in AwD was more pronounced in the left visual field and this asymmetry was also not explained by the magnitude of ADHD symptoms. In AwD, measures of crowding and distractor exclusion correlated significantly with the WIAT-II reading measure, even after removing any effects of co-occurring ADHD symptoms. This suggests that visual attention impacts upon literacy skill directly in dyslexia and not through third variables such as ADHD symptoms.

4.1. Effects of visual crowding

This study confirmed previous findings that AwD are more adversely affected by crowded displays than controls [1,7–11,25], but in a paradigm in which non-complex stimuli were used and in which target location was known. Moores *et al.* [1] demonstrated an effect of crowding in AwD in a visual search task, but performance was equivalent to that of controls when the target stimuli were pre-cued. In that study, the pre-cue may have helped participants to locate the target as well as to enable attentional enhancement of its properties. In the present study, the target was always in one of two possible locations (and was always located on the same side as the distracting stimuli). This result counters any explanation for this pattern of results involving target search, rather than attention enhancement or distractor exclusion. It is not difficult to envisage how crowding effects might impact negatively on reading performance via detrimental effects on letter or word identification [8,9]. Indeed, increased letter spacing has been shown to improve reading in dyslexia [9,46], although it does not provide complete remediation.

4.2. Noise (distractor) exclusion

This study confirmed previous findings that detection performance of AwD suffers more than that for controls from the presence of additional distractors in a display [1,13–16,26]. Moores *et al.* [1] demonstrated an increased impact of number of distractors in AwD whether or not the target was cued. Overall, it was clear that AwD did use information from cues, but employed it less successfully. The present study supports the conclusion that AwD have difficulty excluding distractors, because target discrimination was adversely impacted in displays with increased numbers of distractors even when target location was known. Inter-individual differences on a self-report ADHD measure were unable to account for these effects.

4.3. Distribution of attention

Our results demonstrate that difficulties with distractor exclusion in AwD are asymmetric across the right and left visual fields, with lower performance on the left. As discussed in *section 1.3*, there is increasing evidence for an asymmetric distribution of spatial attention of this type in dyslexia [29]. Whereas Facoetti and Turatto [5] reported a reduced effect of flankers in the left visual field, our data point towards a *difficulty with* distractor exclusion in the left visual field. However, in their paradigm the target was presented centrally with only the flanker presented in the left visual field, whereas in our study both target and distractors were presented in the left visual field. Facoetti and Molteni [28] suggested an inattention disorder in the left visual field (to explain the slower responses in their paradigm overall), but right visual field over-distractibility (to explain the lack of a performance gradient across the eccentricities). The results from all three studies can therefore be explained by weaker attention in the left visual field. Such an asymmetric distribution of attention can explain reduced performance levels overall in the left visual field (the present study and [28]), reduced left flanker effects for a *centrally* presented target [5] and difficulty excluding distractors from a target presented in the left visual field in the present study.

4.4 Relationship between literacy and effects of crowding, set-size and visual field asymmetry

Even when the potential mediating effects of ADHD symptoms were removed statistically, for both AwD and controls the effect of set-size correlated significantly with reading (see Figure 4). For the AwD the effect of crowding additionally correlated with WIAT-II reading. Correlation analyses across both groups suggested that, the effect of asymmetry correlated significantly with all four literacy measures used. However, the removal of this effect in the separate group analyses, suggested that these effects were better explained by asymmetry being an effective discriminator of AwD and control groups rather than there necessarily being any linear relationship between asymmetry and literacy *per se*. The relationships between reading, crowding and set size are consistent with previous research [1,16,34]. In addition, Facoetti *et al.* [34] reported correlations between nonword reading accuracy and the extent of a right attentional inhibition deficit in dyslexic readers. Interestingly, however, they only showed this deficit in dyslexic readers who had impaired non-word reading. On the basis of previous research into neglect dyslexia Facoetti *et al.* [34,47,48], argued that efficient focusing of visuo-spatial attention is crucial for the phonological reading route, but has little effect on lexical-semantic access. It should be noted, of course, that the presence of correlational (or other) effects shown in our study does not necessarily mean that these effects are the *cause* of any reading difficulties exhibited. However, other recent longitudinal research *has* provided evidence to implicate visual attention as a causal factor in dyslexia [49–51], with preschool performance predicting later difficulties.

Summary and Conclusions

These findings provide further evidence to suggest that distractor exclusion difficulties can explain the reported visual attention difficulties in AwD and that such difficulties are associated with literacy. The effects cannot be accounted for by ADHD. Furthermore, they cannot be accounted for by phonological difficulties alone; the task was purely visual and had identical cognitive requirements in all conditions. Weaker and asymmetric attention can explain the crowding and distractor exclusion deficits presented. Visual attention therefore plays an important role in the aetiology of dyslexia.

Supporting Information

Dataset S1 Data collected. This spreadsheet includes psychometric details of participants and their percentage accuracy in the different conditions of the experiment. Information on the different column headings are provided below the dataset.

Author Contributions

Conceived and designed the experiments: EM RC. Performed the experiments: RC. Analyzed the data: RC EM. Wrote the paper: EM JT RC.

References

1. Moores E, Cassim R, Talcott JB (2011) Adults with dyslexia exhibit large effects of crowding, increased dependence on cues, and detrimental effects of distractors in visual search tasks. Neuropsychologia 49: 3881–90.
2. Snowling M (1987) Dyslexia: A Cognitive Developmental Perspective. Blackwell, Oxford.
3. Stanovich KE (1988) Explaining the differences between the dyslexic and the garden variety poor reader: The phonological-core variable-difference model. J Learn Disabil 21: 590–612.
4. Vellutino FR (1979) Dyslexia: Theory and Research. Cambridge, MA: MIT Press.
5. Facoetti A, Turatto M (2000) Asymmetrical visual fields distribution of attention in dyslexic children: a neuropsychological study. Neurosci Lett 290: 216–218.

6. Bosse ML, Tainturier MJ, Valdois S (2007) Developmental dyslexia: the visual attention span hypothesis. Cognition 104: 198–230
7. Bouma H, Legein Ch P (1977) Foveal and parafoveal recognition of letters and words by dyslexics and by average readers. Neuropsychologia 15: 69–80.
8. Spinelli D, DeLuca M, Judica A, Zoccolotti P (2002) Crowding effects on word identification in developmental dyslexia. Cortex 38: 179–200.
9. Martelli M, DiFilippo G, Spinelli D, Zoccolotti P (2009) Crowding, reading, and developmental dyslexia. J Vis 9: 1–18.
10. Pernet C, Valdois S, Celsis P, Démonet JF (2006) Lateral masking, levels of processing and stimulus category: A comparative study between normal and dyslexic readers. Neuropsychologia 44: 2374–2385.
11. Callens M, Whitney C, Tops W, Brysbaert M (2013) No deficiency in left-to-right processing of words in dyslexia but evidence for enhanced visual crowding. Q J Exp Psychol 66: 1803–1817.
12. Facoetti A, Paganoni P, Turatto M, Marzola, Mascetti GG (2000) Visual-spatial attention in developmental dyslexia. Cortex 36: 109–123.
13. Roach NW, Hogben JH (2007) Impaired filtering of behaviourally irrelevant visual information in dyslexia. Brain 130: 771–785.
14. Roach NW, Hogben JH (2008) Spatial cueing deficits in dyslexia reflect generalised difficulties with attentional selection. Vision Res 48: 193–207.
15. Sperling AJ, Lu Z-L, Manis FR, Seidenberg MS (2005) Deficits in perceptual noise exclusion I developmental dyslexia. Nat Neurosci 8: 862–863.
16. Sperling AJ, Lu Z-L, Manis FR, Seidenberg MS (2006) Motion-Perception Deficits and Reading Impairment: It's the noise, not the motion. Psychol Sci 17: 1047–1053.
17. Vidyasagar TR, Pammer K (2010) Dyslexia: a deficit in visuo-spatial attention, not in phonological processing. Trends Cogn Sci 14: 57–63.
18. Pennington BF (2006) From single to multiple-deficit models of developmental disorders. Cognition 10: 385–413.
19. Shaywitz S E, Fletcher JM, Shaywitz BA (1994) Issues in the definition and classification of attention deficit disorder. Top Lang Disord 14: 1–25.
20. Whitney D, Levi DM (2011) Visual crowding: a fundamental limit on conscious perception and object recognition. Trends Cogn Sci 15: 160–168.
21. Yeshurun Y, Rashal E (2010) Precueing attention to the target location diminishes crowding and reduces the critical distance. J Vis 10: 1–12.
22. Freeman J Pelli DG (2007) An escape from crowding. J Vis 7: 1–14.
23. Dakin S, Bex PJ, Cass JR, Watt RJ (2009) Dissociable effects of attention and crowding on orientation averaging. J Vis 9: 1–16.
24. He S, Cavanagh P, Intriligator J (1996) Attentional resolution and the locus of visual awareness. Nature 383: 334–7
25. Pelli DG, Tillman KA, Freeman J, Su M, Berger TD et al. (2007) Crowding and eccentricity determine reading rate. J Vis 7: 1–36.
26. Roach NW, Hogben JH (2004) Attentional modulation of visual processing in adult dyslexia: a spatial cueing deficit. Psychol Sci 15: 650–654.
27. Facoetti A, Paganoni P, Lorusso ML (2000) The spatial distribution of visual attention in developmental dyslexia. Exp Brain Res 132: 531–538.
28. Facoetti A, Molteni M (2001) The gradient of visual attention in developmental dyslexia. Neuropsychologia 39: 352–357.
29. Hari R, Renvall H, Tanskanen T (2001) Left minineglect in dyslexic adults. Brain 124:1373–80.
30. Waldie KE, Hausmann M (2010) Right fronto-parietal dysfunction in children with ADHD and developmental dyslexia as determined by line bisection judgements. Neuropsychologia 48: 3650–3656.
31. Sireteanu R, Goertz R, Bachert I, Wandert T (2005) Children with developmental dyslexia show a left visual "minineglect". Vision Res 45: 3075–3082.
32. Facoetti A, Turatto M, Lorusso ML, Mascetti GG (2001) Orienting of visual attention in dyslexia: evidence for asymmetric hemispheric control of attention. Exp Brain Res 138: 46–53.
33. Cohen J (1998) *Statistical Power Analysis for the Behavioral Sciences* (second ed.) Lawrence Erlbaum Associates.
34. Facoetti A, Zorzi M, Cestnick L, Lorusso ML, Molteni M et al. (2006) The relationship between visuo-spatial attention and nonword reading in developmental dyslexia. Cogn Neuropsychol 23: 841–855.
35. American Psychiatric Association (2013) Diagnostic and Statistical Manual of Mental Disorders (5th Edition).
36. Barkley RA (1997) Behavioral inhibition, sustained attention, and executive functions: constructing a unifying theory of ADHD. Psychol Bull 121: 65–94.
37. Sonuga-Barke EJS (2005) Causal models of attention-deficit/ hyperactivity disorder: from common simple deficits to multiple developmental pathways. Biol Psychiatry 57: 1231–1238.
38. Rochelle KSH, Witton C, Talcott JB (2008) Symptoms of hyperactivity and inattention can mediate deficits of postural stability in developmental dyslexia. Exp Brain Res 192: 627–633.
39. Cohen A, Ivry RB (1990) Density effects in conjunction search: Evidence for a coarse location mechanism of feature integration. J Exp Psychol: Hum Percept Perform 17: 891–901.
40. Barkley RA, Murphy KR (2006) Attention Deficit Hyperactivity Disorder: - A Clinical Workbook. New York: Guilford
41. Wechsler D (1999a) Wechsler Adult Intelligence Scale – Third UK edition. Pearson Assessment.
42. Wechsler D (1999b). Wechsler Abbreviated Scale of Intelligence. Pearson Assessment.
43. Wechsler D (2005) Wechsler Individual Achievement Test – Second UK edition. Pearson Assessment.
44. Torgesen J, Wagner R, Rashotte C (1999) Test of Word Reading Efficiency.
45. Schneider W, Eschmann A, Zuccolotto A (2002) E-Prime user's guide. Pittsburgh, PA: Psychology Software Tools.
46. Zorzi M, Barbiero C, Facoetti A, Lonciari I, Carozzi M et al. (2012) Extra-large letter spacing improves reading in dyslexia. ProcNatl AcadSci U S A 28: 11455–11459
47. Ladavas E, Shallice T, Zanella MT (1997) Preserved semantic access in neglect dyslexia. Neuropsychologia 35: 257–270.
48. Ladavas E, Umiltà C, Mapelli D (1997) Lexical and semantic processing in the absence of word reading: evidence from neglect dyslexia. Neuropsychologia 35: 1075–1085.
49. Plaza M, Cohen H (2007) The contribution of phonological awareness and visual attention in early reading and spelling. Dyslexia 13: 67–76.
50. Kevan A, Pammer K (2009) Predicting early reading skills from pre-reading measures of dorsal stream functioning. Neuropsychologia 47: 3174–3181.
51. Franceschini S, Gori S, Ruffino M, Pedrolli M, Facoetti A (2012) A causal link between visual spatial attention and reading acquisition. Curr Biol 22: 814–819.

Permissions

All chapters in this book were first published in PLOS ONE, by The Public Library of Science; hereby published with permission under the Creative Commons Attribution License or equivalent. Every chapter published in this book has been scrutinized by our experts. Their significance has been extensively debated. The topics covered herein carry significant findings which will fuel the growth of the discipline. They may even be implemented as practical applications or may be referred to as a beginning point for another development.

The contributors of this book come from diverse backgrounds, making this book a truly international effort. This book will bring forth new frontiers with its revolutionizing research information and detailed analysis of the nascent developments around the world.

We would like to thank all the contributing authors for lending their expertise to make the book truly unique. They have played a crucial role in the development of this book. Without their invaluable contributions this book wouldn't have been possible. They have made vital efforts to compile up to date information on the varied aspects of this subject to make this book a valuable addition to the collection of many professionals and students.

This book was conceptualized with the vision of imparting up-to-date information and advanced data in this field. To ensure the same, a matchless editorial board was set up. Every individual on the board went through rigorous rounds of assessment to prove their worth. After which they invested a large part of their time researching and compiling the most relevant data for our readers.

The editorial board has been involved in producing this book since its inception. They have spent rigorous hours researching and exploring the diverse topics which have resulted in the successful publishing of this book. They have passed on their knowledge of decades through this book. To expedite this challenging task, the publisher supported the team at every step. A small team of assistant editors was also appointed to further simplify the editing procedure and attain best results for the readers.

Apart from the editorial board, the designing team has also invested a significant amount of their time in understanding the subject and creating the most relevant covers. They scrutinized every image to scout for the most suitable representation of the subject and create an appropriate cover for the book.

The publishing team has been an ardent support to the editorial, designing and production team. Their endless efforts to recruit the best for this project, has resulted in the accomplishment of this book. They are a veteran in the field of academics and their pool of knowledge is as vast as their experience in printing. Their expertise and guidance has proved useful at every step. Their uncompromising quality standards have made this book an exceptional effort. Their encouragement from time to time has been an inspiration for everyone.

The publisher and the editorial board hope that this book will prove to be a valuable piece of knowledge for researchers, students, practitioners and scholars across the globe.

List of Contributors

Nina Neuhoff, Jennifer Bruder, Jürgen Bartling and Gerd Schulte-Körne
Department of Child and Adolescent Psychiatry, Psychosomatics and Psychotherapy, University of Munich, Munich, Germany

Andreas Warnke
Department of Child and Adolescent Psychiatry and Psychotherapy, University of Würzburg, Würzburg, Germany

Helmut Remschmidt
Department of Child and Adolescent Psychiatry and Psychotherapy, University Hospital Gießen and Marburg, Marburg, Germany

Bertram Müller-Myhsok
Statistical Genetics Max Planck Institute of Psychiatry, Munich, Germany

Wim Tops, Maaike Callens and Marc Brysbaert
Department of Experimental Psychology, Ghent University, Ghent, Belgium

Ellen Verguts
vzw Kinsbergen Oriëntatiecentrum, Antwerp, Belgium

Itamar Sela
The Edmond J. Safra Brain Research Center for the Study of Learning Disabilities, University of Haifa, Haifa, Israel

Avi Karni
The Edmond J. Safra Brain Research Center for the Study of Learning Disabilities, University of Haifa, Haifa, Israel
The Segol Department of Neurobiology & Ethology, and the Department of Human Biology, Faculty of Natural Sciences, University of Haifa, Haifa, Israel

Dianne F. Newbury, Andrew P. Morris and Anthony P. Monaco
Wellcome Trust Centre for Human Genetics, University of Oxford, Oxford, United Kingdom

Thomas S. Scerri
Wellcome Trust Centre for Human Genetics, University of Oxford, Oxford, United Kingdom
The Walter and Eliza Hall Institute for Medical Research, Melbourne, Australia

Fahimeh Darki and Torkel Klingberg
Department of Neuroscience, Karolinska Institutet, Stockholm, Sweden

Andrew J. O. Whitehouse
Telethon Institute for Child Health Research, Centre for Child Health Research, University of Western Australia, West Perth, Australia

Myriam Peyrard-Janvid and Hans Matsson
Department of Biosciences and Nutrition at Novum, Karolinska Institutet, Stockholm, Sweden

Qi W. Ang and Craig E. Pennell
School of Women's and Infants' Health, University of Western Australia, Crawley, Australia

Susan Ring
School of Social and Community Medicine, University of Bristol, Bristol, United Kingdom

John Stein
Department of Physiology, University of Oxford, Oxford, United Kingdom

Juha Kere
Department of Biosciences and Nutrition at Novum, Karolinska Institutet, Stockholm, Sweden
Molecular Medicine Research Programme, University of Helsinki, and Folkhälsan Institute of Genetics, Helsinki, Finland
Science for Life Laboratory, Karolinska Institutet, Stockholm, Sweden

Joel B. Talcott
Aston Brain Centre, School of Life and Health Sciences, Aston University, Birmingham, United Kingdom

Silvia Paracchini
Wellcome Trust Centre for Human Genetics, University of Oxford, Oxford, United Kingdom
School of Medicine, University of St Andrews, St Andrews, United Kingdom

Darina Czamara and Bertram Müller-Myhsok
Max Planck Institute of Psychiatry, Munich, Germany
Munich Cluster for Systems Neurology (SyNergy), Munich, Germany

Gabriele Kohlböck and Joachim Heinrich
Helmholtz Zentrum München, German Research Center for Environmental Health, Institute of Epidemiology I, Neuherberg, Germany

Carla M. T. Tiesler
Helmholtz Zentrum München, German Research Center for Environmental Health, Institute of Epidemiology I, Neuherberg, Germany
Ludwig-Maximilians-University of Munich, Dr. von Hauner Children's Hospital, Division of Metabolic Diseases and Nutritional Medicine, Munich, Germany

Dietrich Berdel and Andrea von Berg
Marien-Hospital Wesel, Department of Pediatrics, Wesel, Germany

Barbara Hoffmann
IUF Leibniz Research Institute for Environmental Medicine and Medical Faculty, Heinrich Heine University of Düsseldorf, Düsseldorf, Germany

Carl-Peter Bauer
Technical University of Munich, Department of Pediatrics, Munich, Germany

Sibylle Koletzko
Ludwig-Maximilians-University of Munich, Dr. von Hauner Children's Hospital, Division of Paediatric Gastroenterology and Hepatology, Munich, Germany

Beate Schaaf
Medical Practice for Pediatrics, Bad Honnef, Germany

Irina Lehmann
Helmholtz Centre for Environmental Research - UFZ, Department for Environmental Immunology, Leipzig, Germany

Olf Herbarth
University of Leipzig, Faculty of Medicine, Environmental Medicine and Hygiene, Leipzig, Germany

Gerd Schulte-Körne
Department of Child and Adolescent Psychiatry, Psychosomatics and Psychotherapy, Ludwig Maximilians-University of Munich, Munich, Germany

Matthew H. Schneps and Gerhard Sonnert
Science Education Department, Harvard-Smithsonian Center for Astrophysics, Cambridge, Massachusetts, United States of America

James R. Brockmole
Department of Psychology, University of Notre Dame, Notre Dame, Indiana, United States of America

Marc Pomplun
Department of Computer Science, University of Massachusetts at Boston, Boston, Massachusetts, United States of America

Susan Whitfield-Gabrieli, Joanna A. Christodoulou and John D. E. Gabrieli
Department of Brain and Cognitive Sciences, McGovern Institute for Brain Research, Massachusetts Institute of Technology, Cambridge, Massachusetts, United States of America

Ying Zhang
Department of Brain and Cognitive Sciences, McGovern Institute for Brain Research, Massachusetts Institute of Technology, Cambridge, Massachusetts, United States of America
State Key Laboratory of Brain and Cognitive Science, Institute of Biophysics, Chinese Academy of Science, Beijing, China

Maki S. Koyama
Rutgers University Center for Molecular and Behavioral Neuroscience, Newark, New Jersey, United States of America
Phyllis Green and Randolph Cowen Institute for Pediatric Neuroscience, New York University Child Study Center, NYU Langone Medical Center, New York, New York, United States of America

Adriana Di Martino, Clare Kelly, Devika R. Jutagir and Jessica Sunshine
Phyllis Green and Randolph Cowen Institute for Pediatric Neuroscience, New York University Child Study Center, NYU Langone Medical Center, New York, New York, United States of America

Francisco X. Castellanos
Phyllis Green and Randolph Cowen Institute for Pediatric Neuroscience, New York University Child Study Center, NYU Langone Medical Center, New York, New York, United States of America
Nathan Kline Institute for Psychiatric Research, Orangeburg, New York, United States of America

Susan J. Schwartz
Center for the Developing Brain, Child Mind Institute, New York, New York, United States of America

Michael P. Milham
Center for the Developing Brain, Child Mind Institute, New York, New York, United States of America
Nathan Kline Institute for Psychiatric Research, Orangeburg, New York, United States of America

Stephanie N. Del Tufo, John Lymberis and Satrajit S. Ghosh
McGovern Institute for Brain Research and Department of Brain and Cognitive Sciences, Massachusetts Institute of Technology, Cambridge, Massachusetts, United States of America

Joanna A. Christodoulou
McGovern Institute for Brain Research and Department of Brain and Cognitive Sciences, Massachusetts Institute of Technology, Cambridge, Massachusetts, United States of America
MGH Institute of Health Professions, Boston, Massachusetts, United States of America
Harvard Graduate School of Education, Cambridge, Massachusetts, United States of America

Patricia K. Saxler
McGovern Institute for Brain Research and Department of Brain and Cognitive Sciences
Harvard Graduate School of Education, Cambridge, Massachusetts, United States of America

John D. E. Gabrieli
McGovern Institute for Brain Research and Department of Brain and Cognitive Sciences
Harvard Graduate School of Education, Cambridge, Massachusetts, United States of America
Athinoula A. Martinos Imaging Center, McGovern Institute for Brain Research, Massachusetts Institute of Technology, Cambridge, Massachusetts, United States of America

Christina Triantafyllou and Susan Whitfield-Gabrieli
McGovern Institute for Brain Research and Department of Brain and Cognitive Sciences, Massachusetts Institute of Technology, Cambridge, Massachusetts, United States of America
Athinoula A. Martinos Imaging Center, McGovern Institute for Brain Research, Massachusetts Institute of Technology, Cambridge, Massachusetts, United States of America

Zoi Kapoula, Chrystal Gaertner and Eric Matheron
IRIS Group, Centre d'Etudes SensoriMotrices UMR8194, CNRS, Université Paris Descartes, Paris, France

Agathe Legrand, Christelle Lemoine and Maria Pia Bucci
Laboratoire de Psychologie et Neuropsychologie Cognitives, IUPDP, Université Paris Descartes, Sorbonne Paris Cité, Institut de Psychologie, Boulogne Billancourt, France

Emmanuel Bui-Quoc
Service d'Ophtalmologie, Hôpital Robert Debré, Paris, France

Karine Doré-Mazars
Laboratoire de Psychologie et Neuropsychologie Cognitives, IUPDP, Université Paris Descartes, Sorbonne Paris Cité, Institut de Psychologie, Boulogne Billancourt, France
Institut Universitaire de France, Paris, France

Christophe-Loïc Gérard
Service de Psychopathologie de l'enfant et de l'adolescent, Hôpital Robert Debré, Paris, France

Maaike Callens, Annemie Desoete, Michaël Stevens and Marc Brysbaert
Ghent University, Ghent, Belgium

Wim Tops
Ghent University, Ghent, Belgium
University of Groningen, Groningen, The Netherlands

Marcella Montico, Lorenzo Monasta, Valentina Ferluga, Anna Bigoni, Alessia Tullio and Luca Ronfani
Epidemiology and Biostatistics Unit, Institute for Maternal and Child Health - IRCCS "Burlo Garofolo", Trieste, Italy

Chiara Barbiero
Epidemiology and Biostatistics Unit, Institute for Maternal and Child Health - IRCCS "Burlo Garofolo", Trieste, Italy
Child Neurology and Psychiatry Ward, Institute for Maternal and Child Health - IRCCS "Burlo Garofolo", Trieste, Italy

Isabella Lonciari and Marco Carrozzi
Child Neurology and Psychiatry Ward, Institute for Maternal and Child Health - IRCCS "Burlo Garofolo", Trieste, Italy

Roberta Penge
Child Neuropsychiatry Department, UOC NPI B La Sapienza University, Rome, Italy

Claudio Vio
Child Neuropsychiatry Unit, Hospital of San Donàdi Piave, San Donàdi Piave, Italy

Patrizio Emanuele Tressoldi
Psychology Department, University of Padua, Padua, Italy

Theodore Chiang, Zeynep Baskurt and Weili Li
Child Health Evaluative Sciences, The Hospital for Sick Children, Toronto, Canada

Lisa J. Strug
Child Health Evaluative Sciences, The Hospital for Sick Children, Toronto, Canada
Dalla Lana School of Public Health, University of Toronto, Toronto, Canada

Laura Addis
Department of Clinical Neurosciences, Institute of Psychiatry, King's College London, London, United Kingdom

Tara Clarke
Department of Epidemiology, Mailman School of Public Health, Columbia University Medical Center, New York, New York, United States of America

Huntley Hardison
St. Christopher's Hospital for Children, Philadelphia, Pennsylvania, United States of America

Steven L. Kugler
Children's Hospital of Philadelphia and University of Pennsylvania School of Medicine, Philadelphia, Pennsylvania, United States of America

David E. Mandelbaum
Hasbro Children's Hospital and The Warren Alpert Medical School of Brown University, Providence, Rhode Island, United States of America

Edward J. Novotny
Yale University Medical Center, New Haven, Connecticut, United States of America

Steven M. Wolf
Beth Israel Medical Center, New York, New York, United States of America

Deb K. Pal
Department of Clinical Neurosciences, Institute of Psychiatry, King's College London, London, United Kingdom
Department of Psychiatry, Columbia University Medical Center, New York, New York, United States of America

Martina Hedenius, Per Alm and Margareta Jennische
Department of Neuroscience, Uppsala University, Uppsala, Sweden

Michael T. Ullman
Brain and Language Lab, Department of Neuroscience, Georgetown University, Washington, D.C., United States of America

Jonas Persson
Aging Research Center, Karolinska Institute and Stockholm University, Stockholm, Sweden

Emma E. Birkett and Joel B. Talcott
Aston Brain Centre, School of Life and Health Sciences, Aston University, Birmingham, United Kingdom

Ou Lin
Department of Psychology, Peking University, Beijing, China

Fang Wang and Yan Song
State Key Laboratory of Cognitive Neuroscience and Learning & IDG/McGovern Institute for Brain Research, Beijing Normal University, Beijing, China
Center for Collaboration and Innovation in Brain and Learning Sciences, Beijing Normal University, Beijing, China

Yuzheng Jiang
School of languages and communication, Beijing Jiaotong University, Beijing, China

Xiangzhi Meng
Department of Psychology, Peking University, Beijing, China
The Joint PekingU-PolyU Center for Child Development and Learning, Peking University, Beijing, China

Yatin Mahajan, Chris Davis and Jeesun Kim
The MARCS Institute, University of Western Sydney, Penrith, New South Wales, Australia

Gojko Žarić, Leo Blomert and Milene Bonte
Department of Cognitive Neuroscience, Faculty of Psychology and Neuroscience, University of Maastricht, Maastricht, Netherlands
Maastricht Brain Imaging Center (M-BIC), Maastricht, Netherlands

Jurgen Tijms
Department of Psychology, University of Amsterdam, Amsterdam, Netherlands
IWAL Institute for Dyslexia, Amsterdam, Netherlands
Rudolf Berlin Center, Amsterdam, Netherlands

Gorka Fraga González
Department of Psychology, University of Amsterdam, Amsterdam, Netherlands
Rudolf Berlin Center, Amsterdam, Netherlands

Maurits W. van der Molen
Department of Psychology, University of Amsterdam, Amsterdam, Netherlands
Rudolf Berlin Center, Amsterdam, Netherlands
Amsterdam Brain and Cognition, University of Amsterdam, Amsterdam, Netherlands

Samantha Huang, Stephanie Rossi and Jyrki Ahveninen
Harvard Medical School, Athinoula A. Martinos Center for Biomedical Imaging, Department of Radiology, Massachusetts General Hospital, Charlestown, Massachusetts, United States of America

Matti Hämäläinen
Harvard Medical School, Athinoula A. Martinos Center for Biomedical Imaging, Department of Radiology, Massachusetts General Hospital, Charlestown, Massachusetts, United States of America
Harvard-MIT Division of Health Sciences and Technology, Cambridge, Massachusetts, United States of America

Rizan Cassim, Joel B. Talcott and Elisabeth Moores
School of Life and Health Sciences, Aston University, Birmingham, West Midlands, United Kingdom

Index